CARDIOVASCULAR GENOMICS

CONTEMPORARY CARDIOLOGY

CHRISTOPHER P. CANNON, MD
SERIES EDITOR

CARDIOVASCULAR GENOMICS

Edited by

MOHAN K. RAIZADA, PhD

Department of Physiology and Functional Genomics,
University of Florida College of Medicine, Gainesville, FL

JULIAN F. R. PATON, PhD
SERGEY KASPAROV, MD, PhD

Department of Physiology, School of Medical Sciences,
University of Bristol, Bristol, UK

MICHAEL J. KATOVICH, PhD

Department of Pharmacodynamics, University of Florida College of Pharmacy,
Gainesville, FL

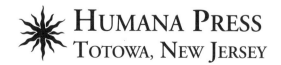
HUMANA PRESS
TOTOWA, NEW JERSEY

© 2005 Humana Press Inc.
999 Riverview Drive, Suite 208
Totowa, New Jersey 07512

www.humanapress.com

Production Editor: Amy Thau
Cover design by Patricia F. Cleary
Cover Illustration: Figure 4A and B from Chapter 13, "Application of Viral Gene Transfer in Studies of Neurogenic Hypertension," by Sergey Kasparov, A. G. Teschemacher, and Julian F. R. Paton.

For additional copies, pricing for bulk purchases, and/or information about other Humana titles, contact Humana at the above address or at any of the following numbers: Tel.: 973-256-1699; Fax: 973-256-8341, E-mail: humana@humanapr.com; or visit our Website: www.humanapress.com

This publication is printed on acid-free paper. ∞
ANSI Z39.48-1984 (American National Standards Institute) Permanence of Paper for Printed Library Materials.

Printed in the United States of America. 10 9 8 7 6 5 4 3 2 1

eISBN: 1-59259-883-8
Library of Congress Cataloging-in-Publication Data

Cardiovascular genomics / edited by Mohan K. Raizada ... [et al.].
    p. ; cm. -- (Contemporary cardiology)
  Includes bibliographical references and index.
  ISBN 1-58829-400-5 (hardcover : alk. paper)
  1. Cardiovascular system--Diseases--Genetic aspects.
 2. Genomics.   I. Raizada, Mohan K. II. Series: Contemporary
cardiology (Totowa, N.J. : Unnumbered)
  [DNLM: 1. Cardiovascular Diseases--genetics. 2. Cell Transplantation. 3. Gene Therapy. 4. Gene Transfer Techniques.
WG 120 C267475 2005]
RC669.9.C354 2005
616.1'042--dc22
                                        2004012489

PREFACE

With the postgenomic transcriptional era currently flourishing, the time seemed right to put together a book entitled *Cardiovascular Genomics*. Cardiovascular genomics is the study of genes relevant to the function and dysfunction of vital organs that both form and control the cardiovascular system. The book is organized into three parts: Part I: Genes and Polymorphisms in Cardiovascular Disease, Part II: Gene Transfer for Combating Cardiovascular Disease, and Part III: Regenerative Tissues for the Diseased Cardiovascular System.

Cardiovascular Genomics provides an up-to-date account of the most recent molecular approaches adopted to understand the cardiovascular system in both health and disease. The book provides an excellent resource for students, researchers, and clinicians on the potential of development of novel strategies for the control of cardiovascular diseases. The contributors are world leaders and the subject matter stretches from basic science to clinical applications, focusing on all components of the cardiovascular system—including vessels, heart, kidney, and the brain—and covers disease states ranging from vascular and cardiac dysfunction to stroke and hypertension.

Primary hypertension, a disease of the cardiovascular system, is a polygenic disease that has reached epidemic proportions worldwide. Most evidence suggests that susceptibility is genetically linked. Despite more than 50 years of using a large arsenal of antihypertensive agents, successful control of blood pressure is difficult to achieve. We believe this indicates that the time is ripe to explore alternate strategies. Cardiovascular genomics is all about doing just that. Discovering the genes that cause susceptibility to cardiovascular diseases will significantly increase the efficacy of treatment for these diseases. Remarkably, little is known about the numbers of genes involved in hypertension, what they do, their interactions with themselves and with others, and how they are modulated by stressors and diet, for example. *Cardiovascular Genomics* attempts to address these issues by focusing on both the villains and the victims.

Methods for identifying the genes that relate to a cardiovascular disease are discussed in relation to the possibility of discovering new drug targets. These approaches include discussions of genetic linkage analysis substitution mapping using congenic strains as well as microarray techniques. All are discussed as plausible strategies for discovery in animal models of hypertension. Not surprisingly, overactivity of the renin–angiotensin system may be one of the most common ailments and polymorphisms of angiotensin type 1 receptors and angiotensin-converting enzyme could well cause an overactivity of the signaling system. The new transgenic mouse models that either over- or underexpress angiotensinogen discussed within may help in addressing the important issue of the function of the tissue renin angiotensin systems. But an understanding of polymorphisms may also be crucial for the effective design of new drugs as well as successful pharmacotherapy for different patients; these important issues are thoroughly discussed, including those relating to statins.

A number of chapters in this book are dedicated to the theme of gene transfer and gene therapy covering a wide range of topics from clinical applications to using viral vectors as tools. For clinical applications, these include novel approaches to stroke, as well as coronary and peripheral vascular diseases. The efficacy of gene therapy for safe gene delivery in cerebrovascular diseases has been used to stimulate angiogenesis, overexpression of vasodilator agents, or breakdown thrombi and stabilize plaques. These forms of somatic gene transfer have also been used to prevent both restenosis and vascular graft failure. Clear evidence has emerged that enhancing nitric oxide production reduces both oxidative stress and inflammatory responses that assist in lowering BP but also, independently, are beneficial in protecting against cardiac remodeling, renal fibrosis, restenosis and cerebral infarction as exemplified by adeno-associated viral-induced expression of kallikrein. In animal models of cardiovascular disease there are a number of chapters detailing a rapid expansion of viral vector technology in basic science. This includes applications to the heart, vasculature, and brain. The new strategies of virally mediated gene transfer include the design and effective use of expressing dominant negative proteins, siRNA, the employment of cell-specific promoters, and the use of vigilant vectors containing a physiologically operated genetic switch.

Cardiovascular Genomics also contains chapters on regenerative medicine that illustrate how molecular biology is enhancing the production of cardiovascular cells and tissues (e.g., cardiomyocytes and endothelial cells) from embryonic stem cells for repairing a diseased system. It is now clear that transplantation of genetically modified noncontractile cells into ischemic or dilated cardiomyopathic hearts can stimulate cardiomyogenesis that increases cardiac function. Moreover, regenerative medicine approaches now using ex vivo-engineered endothelial progenitor cells to treat peripheral and myocardial ischemia and genetically modified vein grafts have also proven successful.

The chapters in this book provide ample evidence for the considerable benefits that come from the application of genomic information and technologies to an understanding of both fundamental physiological processes and design of better therapies for one of the biggest killers worldwide. However, it is clear that many difficult challenges still lie ahead and must be confronted. Many methodologies and concepts are still evolving, common standards have yet to be established, and various problems with experimental design, variability, and statistical analysis still have to be fully understood and overcome. To fully realize the promise of the genomic approach, it is imperative that both scientists and physicians representing different disciplines work together to enhance progress. Only by means of multidisciplinary experimental approaches and the sharing of ideas can we develop novel cardiovascular therapeutics. Collaboration is the key that will unlock the genome.

The editors extend thanks to Ms. Nichole Herring for valuable assistance in putting together this volume.

Mohan K. Raizada, PhD
Julian F. R. Paton, PhD
Sergey Kasparov, MD, PhD
Michael J. Katovich, PhD

CONTENTS

PART III. REGENERATIVE TISSUES
FOR THE DISEASED CARDIOVASCULAR SYSTEM

CONTRIBUTORS

DENIS ANGOULVANT, MD, MSC • *Division of Cardiac Surgery, Toronto General Hospital, University Health Network, University of Toronto, Toronto, Ontario, Canada*

ANDREW H. BAKER, PhD • *British Heart Foundation Glasgow Cardiovascular Research Centre, Division of Cardiovascular and Medical Sciences, Western Infirmary, University of Glasgow, Glasgow, UK*

BRUNO BAUDIN • *Biochemistry Service, Hospital Saint-Antoine, Paris, France*

NISSIM BENVENISTY, MD, PhD • *Department of Genetics, The Life Sciences Institute, The Hebrew University, Jerusalem, Israel*

LARISA H. CAVALLARI, PharmD • *Department of Pharmacy Practice, University of Illinois at Chicago, Chicago, IL*

JULIE CHAO, PhD • *Department of Biochemistry and Molecular Biology, Medical University of South Carolina, Charleston, SC*

LEE CHAO, PhD *Department of Biochemistry and Molecular Biology, Medical University of South Carolina, Charleston, SC*

ANTHONIUS DE BOER, MD, PhD *Department of Pharmacoepidemiology and Pharmacotherapy, Utrecht Institute of Pharmaceutical Sciences, Utrecht University, Utrecht, The Netherlands*

ANNA F. DOMINICZAK, MD • *British Heart Foundation Glasgow Cardiovascular Research Centre, Division of Cardiovascular and Medical Sciences, Western Infirmary, University of Glasgow, Glasgow, UK*

VICTOR J. DZAU, MD • *Department of Medicine, Brigham and Women's Hospital and Harvard Medical School, Boston, MA*

SHAFIE FAZEL, MD, MSC • *Division of Cardiac Surgery, Toronto General Hospital, University Health Network, University of Toronto, Toronto, Ontario, Canada*

PAUL W. M. FEDAK, MD, PhD • *Division of Cardiac Surgery, Toronto General Hospital, University Health Network, University of Toronto, Toronto, Ontario, Canada*

MICHAEL R. GARRETT, MS, MBA • *Departments of Physiology and Cardiovascular Genomics, Medical College of Ohio, Toledo, OH*

JUSTIN L. GROBE • *Department of Pharmacodynamics, University of Florida College of Pharmacy, Gainesville, FL*

DONALD D. HEISTAD, MD • *Cardiovascular Center, Departments of Internal Medicine and Pharmacology, University of Iowa College of Medicine and Veterans Affairs Medical Center, Iowa City, IA*

BINA JOE, PhD • *Department of Physiology and Cardiovascular Genomics, Medical College of Ohio, Toledo, OH*

JULIE A. JOHNSON, PharmD • *Departments of Pharmacy Practice, Pharmaceutics, and Medicine (Cardiology), University of Florida, Gainesville, FL*

HIDEKO KASAHARA, MD, PhD • *Department of Physiology and Functional Genomics, University of Florida College of Medicine, Gainesville, FL*

SERGEY KASPAROV, MD, PhD • *Department of Physiology, School of Medical Sciences, University of Bristol, Bristol, UK*

MICHAEL J. KATOVICH, PhD • *Department of Pharmacodynamics, University of Florida College of Pharmacy, Gainesville, FL*

OLAF H. KLUNGEL, PharmD, PhD • *Department of Pharmacoepidemiology and Pharmacotherapy, Utrecht Institute of Pharmaceutical Sciences, Utrecht University, Utrecht, The Netherlands*

ASHOK KUMAR, PhD • *Pathology Department, New York Medical College, Valhalla, NY*

NETA LAVON • *Department of Genetics, The Life Sciences Institute, The Hebrew University, Jerusalem, Israel*

REN-KE LI, MD, PhD • *Division of Cardiac Surgery, Toronto General Hospital, University Health Network, University of Toronto, Toronto, Ontario, Canada*

PAOLO MADEDDU, MD, FAHA • *Department of Internal Medicine, Sassari University; and Experimental Medicine and Gene Therapy, National Institute of Biostructures and Biosystems (INBB), Osilo, Sassari, Italy*

ANKE-HILSE MAITLAND-VAN DER ZEE, PharmD, PhD • *Human Genetics Center, University of Texas Health Center, Houston, TX, and Department of Pharmacoepidemiology and Pharmacotherapy, Utrecht Institute of Pharmaceutical Sciences, Utrecht University, Utrecht, The Netherlands*

LUIS G. MELO, PhD • *Department of Physiology, Queen's University College of Medicine, Kingston, Ontario, Canada*

WILLIAM H. MILLER, PhD • *British Heart Foundation Glasgow Cardiovascular Research Centre, Division of Cardiovascular and Medical Sciences, Western Infirmary, University of Glasgow, Glasgow, UK*

RYUICHI MORISHITA, MD, PhD • *Division of Clinical Gene Therapy, Graduate School of Medicine, Osaka University, Suita, Osaka, Japan*

STUART A. NICKLIN, PhD • *British Heart Foundation Glasgow Cardiovascular Research Centre, Division of Cardiovascular and Medical Sciences, Western Infirmary, University of Glasgow, Glasgow, UK*

ALOK S. PACHORI, PhD • *Department of Medicine, Brigham and Women's Hospital and Harvard Medical School, Boston, MA*

JULIAN F. R. PATON, PhD • *Department of Physiology, School of Medical Sciences, University of Bristol, Bristol, UK*

M. IAN PHILLIPS, PhD, DSC • *Office of Research, University of South Florida, Tampa, FL*

KAMAL RAHMOUNI • *Cardiovascular Center, Department of Internal Medicine, University of Iowa College of Medicine, Iowa City, IA*

MOHAN K. RAIZADA, PhD • *Department of Physiology and Functional Genomics, University of Florida College of Medicine, Gainesville, FL*

CURT D. SIGMUND, PhD • *Department of Internal Medicine, Cardiovascular Center, University of Iowa College of Medicine, Iowa City, IA*

YI TANG, PhD • *Department of Physiology, College of Medicine, University of South Florida, Tampa, FL*

A. G. TESCHEMACHER, PhD • *Department of Pharmacology, School of Medical Sciences, Univesity of Bristol, Bristol, UK*

YOSHIMASA WATANABE, MD • *Cardiovascular Center, Departments of Internal Medicine and Pharmacology, University of Iowa College of Medicine and Veterans Affairs Medical Center, Iowa City, IA*

RICHARD D. WEISEL, MD • *Division of Cardiac Surgery, Toronto General Hospital,
University Health Network, University of Toronto, Toronto, Ontario, Canada*
TERRENCE M. YAU, MD, MSC • *Division of Cardiac Surgery, Toronto General Hospital,
University Health Network, University of Toronto, Toronto, Ontario, Canada*

Value-Added eBook/PDA on CD-ROM

This book is accompanied by a value-added CD-ROM that contains an eBook version of the volume you have just purchased. This eBook can be viewed on your computer, and you can synchronize it to your PDA for viewing on your handheld device. The eBook enables you to view this volume on only one computer and PDA. Once the eBook is installed on your computer, you cannot download, install, or e-mail it to another computer; it resides solely with the computer to which it is installed. The license provided is for only one computer. The eBook can only be read using Adobe® Reader® 6.0 software, which is available free from Adobe Systems Incorporated at www.Adobe.com. You may also view the eBook on your PDA using the Adobe® PDA Reader® software that is also available free from Adobe.com.

You must follow a simple procedure when you install the eBook/PDA that will require you to connect to the Humana Press website in order to receive your license. Please read and follow the instructions below:

1. Download and install Adobe® Reader® 6.0 software.
You can obtain a free copy of the Adobe® Reader® 6.0 software at www.adobe.com.
*Note: If you already have the Adobe® Reader® 6.0 software installed, you do not need to reinstall it.
2. Launch Adobe® Reader® 6.0 software.
3. Install eBook: Insert your eBook CD into your CD-ROM drive PC: Click on the "Start" button, then click on "Run."
   At the prompt, type "d:\ebookinstall.pdf" and click "OK."
*Note: If your CD-ROM drive letter is something other than d: change the above command accordingly.
MAC: Double click on the "eBook CD" that you will see mounted on your desktop. Double click "ebookinstall.pdf."
   4. Adobe® Reader® 6.0 software will open and you will receive the message "This document is protected by Adobe DRM." Click "OK."
*Note: If you have not already activated the Adobe®Reader® 6.0 software, you will be prompted to do so. Simply follow the directions to activate and continue installation.

Your web browser will open and you will be taken to the Humana Press eBook registration page. Follow the instructions on that page to complete installation. You will need the serial number located on the sticker sealing the envelope containing the CD-ROM.

If you require assistance during the installation, or you would like more information regarding your eBook and PDA installation, please refer to the eBookManual.pdf located on your cd. If you need further assistance, contact Humana Press eBook Support by e-mail at ebooksupport@humanapr.com or by phone at 973-256-1699.

*Adobe and Reader are either registered trademarks or trademarks of Adobe Systems Incorporated in the United States and/or other countries.

I GENES AND POLYMORPHISMS IN CARDIOVASCULAR DISEASE

1 Angiotensin II Receptor Polymorphisms and Hypertension

Bruno Baudin

SUMMARY

Molecular variants of individual components of the renin–angiotensin system have been thought to contribute to inherited predisposition toward essential hypertension. Angiotensin II type 1 receptor (AT-1) mediates the major pressor and trophic actions of angiotensin II (Ang II). Moreover, polymorphisms in genes of angiotensinogen and angiotensin-converting enzyme (ACE) have been associated with arterial hypertension and cardiovascular diseases, and some of them have been related to differential responses to antihypertensive drugs. So far, at least 25 different polymorphisms have been described in *AT-1* gene (*AT_1R* gene), both at the 3' untranslated region and in its promoter region. Best evaluated with respect to the association with cardiovascular phenotypes is the +1166 A/C polymorphism. In particular, the C allele has been associated with the severe form of essential hypertension and in some studies an association was found between C allele in *AT_1R* gene and D allele in ACE gene; but large discrepancies arise from ethnic variability. The role of AT_1R A1166C polymorphism is ambiguous in pathologies related to high Ang II levels, such as deterioration of renal function (for example in diabetes), arterial stiffness, and hypertrophic cardiomyopathy. Recently, polymorphisms have also been described in angiotensin II type 2 receptor (AT-2) gene (*AT_2R* gene), AT-2 being the mediator for vasodilatation, natriuresis, and apoptosis of smooth muscle cells. Associations were found between some of these polymorphisms and left ventricular structure, whereas the response to Ang II infusion did not differ across AT_1R and

From: *Contemporary Cardiology: Cardiovascular Genomics*
Edited by: M. K. Raizada, et al. © Humana Press Inc., Totowa, NJ

AT$_2$R genotypes. On the other hand, a relationship was suggested between AT$_1$R A1166C polymorphism and the humoral and renal hemodynamic responses to losartan, an antihypertensive drug acting as an AT-1 blocker, as well as with enhanced Ang II vascular reactivity or sensitivity even when conflicting results were observed. The variability in the individual response to AT-1 antagonists could also result from variations in the pharmacokinetics of the drugs; in particular, losartan is essentially metabolized to its active form by cytochrome P450 2C9, which biotransforms many cardiovascular drugs but at different rates in function of both ethnic and individual genotypes. The other angiotensin II receptor, AT-2, should also be investigated because the different AT-1 antagonists do not share the same selectivity for both subtypes but all are able to increase Ang II levels, which enhances AT-2 related effects. Arterial hypertension is one of the main risk factors for stroke and coronary artery disease (CAD); however, no clear association was found between AT$_1$R gene polymorphisms and the development of white matter lesions, stroke, CAD, or myocardial infarction, although some studies described relationships between AT$_1$R A1166C polymorphism and hypercholesterolemia, or greater induced arterial vasoconstriction in CAD. Moreover, AT$_1$R C allele, when associated with ACE D allele (of I/D polymorphism), could contribute to susceptibility to CAD and to interindividual differences in severity of cardiovascular disease. Further evaluation in adequately powered studies is necessary for final assessment of allelic markers in RAS component genes, namely *AT$_1$R* and *AT$_2$R* genes, as well as to determine predisposition to hypertension or related diseases, and to choose an antihypertensive drug for an individual and to develop more specifically targeted drugs.

Key Words: Renin–angiotensin system; angiotensin II receptors; single nucleotide polymorphism (SNP); antihypertensive therapy; angiotensin II receptor antagonists; cardiovascular disease.

INTRODUCTION

High blood pressure (BP) is an important risk factor for cardiovascular diseases, kidney failure, and stroke. It is recognized as a multifactorial trait resulting from a combination of environmental and genetic factors. The genetic influences (or heritability) were examined in both cross-sectional samples of data and longitudinal studies. Efforts to date have identified several candidate genes involved in blood pressure or primary hypertension. Special attention has been paid to the study of genes implicated in the renin–angiotensin system (RAS) because its activation and the subsequent generation of angiotensin II (Ang II) both play important roles in normal physiology and in the progression of cardiac and renal diseases. Most of the known actions of Ang II are mediated by the Ang II type 1 receptor (AT-1), including vascular contraction, pressor responses, renal tubular sodium transport and aldosterone secretion. Antagonists of the AT-1 have been developed and are now widely used in the treatment of hypertension *(1)*. Recently, a polymorphism in AT-1 gene (*AT$_1$R* gene) has been related to arterial hypertension and other cardiovascular impairments. Moreover, a relationship was suggested between this polymorphism and the humoral and renal hemodynamic responses to losartan, the first AT-1 blocker. This chapter will present the actual knowledge of the Ang II receptors and the polymorphisms in their genes related to hypertension, and others related to cardiovascular diseases. We will also discuss these data from the area of pharmacogenomics, including variations in the pharmacokinetics of the antihypertensive drugs.

THE ANGIOTENSIN II RECEPTORS

The RAS is a major physiological regulator of body fluid volume, electrolyte balance, and arterial pressure. Originally, the RAS was viewed solely as an endocrine system;

angiotensinogen of hepatic origin is secreted into the systemic circulation and cleaved to Ang I by renin (in its active form as found in blood plasma), and then by both plasma and endothelial membrane-bound ACE to produce the active octapeptide Ang II. Increasing evidence suggests that other complete RAS may reside within individual organs or tissues such as kidney, lung, heart, and vascular smooth muscle cells, where they could act in a functionally independent paracrine/autocrine fashion *(2,3)*.

Ang II is the major effector peptide of this system and the biological actions of Ang II are mediated by at least two different receptor subtypes, AT-1 and AT-2. Because AT-2 has a low degree of expression compared with that of AT-1, virtually all of the biological actions of Ang II, as well as its paracrine and autocrine regulations including cell growth, proliferation, and extracellular matrix formation have been attributed to its binding to AT-1 *(4)*. Both Ang II receptors have been cloned and their signal transduction mechanisms have been clarified. We have now gained a great deal of knowledge concerning the receptor genes, molecular and protein structures, sites, and regulation of expression and mechanisms of action. The gene coding for AT-1 (*AT₁R* gene) is located on human chromosome 3 (q22 band), whereas the gene coding for AT-2 (*AT₂R* gene) is located on chromosome X (q23-24 locus). AT-2 is only 34% identical with its AT-1 counterpart. Both receptors belong to the G protein-coupled receptor superfamily containing seven hydrophobic transmembrane segments forming α helices in the lipid bilayer of the cell membrane. The binding of Ang II to the agonist site of the AT-1 receptor induces a conformational change in the receptor molecule that promotes its interaction with G proteins, which in turn mediate signal transduction via the phospholipases C, D, A_2, and adenylyl cyclase, followed mainly by phosphoinositide hydrolysis and Ca^{2+} signaling *(4–6)*. Based on imidazole derivatives first described by Furukama et al. (*patent*), it became possible to develop specific nonpeptide Ang II receptor antagonists that specifically and selectively block AT-1. The first of this series to reach the clinic, losartan, was followed by a large number of orally active AT-1 antagonists *(1)*. Blockade of AT-1 not only inhibits smooth muscle contraction, but also reduces the production of pressor agents including aldosterone, vasopressin, catecholamines, and endothelin. The AT-1 antagonists are approved for the treatment of hypertension, and in early clinical studies also appear to be of use in the treatment of congestive heart failure, postmyocardial infarction, and renal failure *(7)*. Moreover, treatment with AT-1 antagonists has been found to abolish the growth-promoting actions of Ang II in vitro and in vivo *(1,4)*.

AT-2 is clearly distinct from AT-1 in tissue-specific expression, signaling mechanisms, and diversity in molecular weight. Almost complete divergence between AT-1 and AT-2 is seen in the third intracellular loop, and more extensive differences in the carboxyl terminal tail. The structural diversity of AT-2 is still a complex and unresolved issue, even when oligomerization and differences in the extent of glycosylation are involved. In contrast to the hypertension and impaired vascular responses observed in AT-1-deficient mice (knockout mice for *AT₁R* gene), knockout of the AT-2 leads to elevation of BP and increased vascular sensitivity to Ang II; it stimulates vasodilatation and natriuresis by an autocrine cascade including bradykinin, nitric oxide, and cyclic GMP. This has suggested that AT-2 may exert a protective action in BP regulation by counteracting AT-1. Moreover, whereas the AT-1 stimulates cell proliferation, AT-2 inhibits proliferation and promotes cell differentiation. These differences in growth responses have been ascribed to different cell signalling pathways in which AT-1 stimulates protein phosphorylation and AT-2 stimulates dephosphorylation. In particular, AT-2 could negatively modulate the AT-1-mediated activation of both phospholipase C (for control of vascular tone and natriuresis) and MAPkinase (for control of cell growth). Moreover, AT-2 is able to induce apoptosis and may play a role in cognitive functions and certain types of behavior. By inhibiting the AT-1-mediated negative feedback of Ang II on renin release in the kidney, AT-1 antagonists evoke an overstimulation of the uninhibited AT-2 by enhancing Ang II levels in plasma. However, because the exact physiological roles of AT-2 are not well defined, it is uncertain as to whether this overstimulation of AT-2 would produce beneficial or harmful side effects *(4,8)*.

Recently AT-4, a new angiotensin receptor type, that preferentially binds Ang II (3-8) (a fragment of Ang II, now referred to as Ang IV) has been discovered and characterized. This receptor is prominent among brain structures concerned with cognitive processing and motor and sensory functions. Like AT-2, it may also oppose the effect of AT-1 as it regulates blood flow, inhibits tubular sodium reabsorption, and affects cardiac hypertrophy *(4)*.

In conclusion, most of the known effects of Ang II are mediated through AT-1, including vasoconstriction, aldosterone and vasopressin release, salt and water retention and sympathetic activation, in addition to the important autocrine and paracrine effects of Ang II on cell proliferation and tissue remodeling. Accumulated published data suggest that AT-2 and AT-4 counterbalance the effects of AT-1 in both physiological and pathophysiological situations.

SNP IN AT_1R GENE

Polymorphisms (genetic variations of high frequency) may be the result of variations in the DNA sequence, such as the change of only one nucleotide (single nucleotide polymorphism [SNP]), or an insertion or deletion of one to several hundred bases resulting from the DNA recombination failures, or insertion/deletion of DNA repeating sequences, such as tandem repeat sequences, microsatellites, or AluI sequences. The human AT_1R gene has a length of greater than 55 kb and is composed of five exons and four introns, and has been found highly polymorphic. In particular, an SNP has been described in which there is either an adenine (A) or a cytosine (C) base (A/C transversion) in position 1166 in the 3' untranslated region of the gene *(9)*; until now this +1166 A/C polymorphism was the best evaluated. The A allele that lacks the enzyme-restriction site is designated as the larger fragment, whereas the C allele that has an enzyme-restriction site at nucleotide position 1166 is designated as the smaller fragment. The physiological significance of this polymorphism is uncertain because of its location in an untranslated region. Another SNP at nucleotide position +573 was investigated in hypertension and diabetes *(10,11)*. Erdmann et al. *(12)* characterized nine other SNPs, which may have the potential to influence AT_1R gene expression given their location in the functional promoter region of the gene; these variants were found to be strongly linked, such that the analysis of three SNPs should provide information for all possible haplotypes, i.e., –2228 G/A, –1424 C/G, and –521 C/T. Two other groups found many other SNPs in the 5'-flanking region of the gene: Poirier et al. *(13)* detected seven polymorphisms, i.e., at –1424, –810, –713, –521, –214, –213, and –153 positions, not in linkage equilibrium with A1166C polymorphism, and some of them having also be found by Erdmann et al. *(12)*. Takahashi et al. *(14)* identified seven other polymorphisms, i.e., at –1154, –825, –729, –535, –227, –226, and –166 positions; these polymorphisms also do not occur at random, leading to the classification into three haplotypes. Recently, Zhu et al. *(15)* described five other SNPs at both 5'- and 3'-flanking regions, i.e., –777, –680, –119, +43732, and +44221.

AT_1R GENE POLYMORPHISMS AND HYPERTENSION

Hypertension has a multifactorial etiology with a strong genetic component. Of many human candidate gene loci examined, those encoding components of the RAS are considered to be among the most plausible candidates. The association of *renin* gene polymorphism with essential hypertension has been scarcely reported *(16)*. On the contrary, several studies have demonstrated a link between the *angiotensinogen* (*AG*) gene and hypertension *(17–19)*, particularly the M235T variant which correlates with both plasma angiotensinogen concentration and elevated BP variation; nevertheless, large ethnic discrepancies make this genotyping difficult to use.

The cloning of *ACE* gene enabled the detection of many polymorphisms *(20,21)*, one of which consists of the presence (insertion allele I) or absence (deletion allele D) of a 287-bp DNA fragment in intron 16 of the *ACE* gene. A strong association was detected between the alleles of this polymorphism and the level of serum ACE, individuals homozygous for the D allele (genotype DD) displaying serum ACE levels almost twice as high as those in individuals homozygous for the I allele (genotype II) but without clear correlation to BP *(20,22,23)*. In particular, no association was found between this I/D polymorphism in the *ACE* gene and essential hypertension in young, middle-aged, or elderly populations, even when interindividual variation in BP could be dependent on contexts that are indexed by gender, age, and measures at body size. One possible explanation is that this polymorphism is in linkage disequilibrium with functional variants elsewhere in the *ACE* gene that are responsible for the BP.

For AT_1R gene, the silent A1166C SNP has been associated with the severe form of essential hypertension, and in particular in resistant hypertensive patients taking two or more antihypertensive drugs *(9,24)*. The C allele was particularly overrepresented in Caucasian hypertensive subjects with a strong family history *(25)*, and it was also significantly more frequent in women with pregnancy-induced hypertension, whereas *ACE* I/D and *AG* M235T polymorphisms were not associated with predisposition to development of hypertension in pregnant women *(26)*. However, a significant interaction between the *ACE* I/D and AT_1R A1166C polymorphisms in terms of influence on BP variation has been reported *(27)*, but their linkage mechanism remains unclear. Henskens et al. *(28)* recently confirmed an association of both these polymorphisms with BP in healthy normotensive subjects, although synergistic effects did not seem to be present; in these studies *ACE* D allele and AT_1R C allele were associated with highest pressures, either systolic, diastolic, or both. Berge et al. *(29)* also found an association of AT_1R C allele with systolic BP in normotensive subjects. But large interethnic differences in the frequencies of genotype polymorphisms of the RAS exist; for example, the *ACE* DD and the AT_1R CC genotypes have low prevalence in Chinese subjects compared with whites, whereas the *AG* M235T variant is much higher in Asian populations compared with white populations. Moreover, a higher prevalence of the AT_1R CC genotype was found in Chinese hypertensive patients than in controls *(30)*, whereas the A1166C genotype distribution did not differ between hypertensive and normotensive subjects from Japan *(31)* or Taiwan *(32)*. In a sample of Swedish twins, Iliadou et al. *(33)* did not find any significant linkage and association between *ACE* I/D polymorphism or AT_1R A1166C polymorphism and BP. In Caucasoid subjects from Germany, Schmidt et al. *(34)* did not detect any association of A1166C polymorphism with hypertension, but a trend towards a decreased prevalence of the C allele among hypertensive patients with a late age at diagnosis (>50 yr) was observed. Tiret et al. *(35)* showed a higher prevalence of C allele among female hypertensives than in controls but no such difference was observed for men. Szombathy et al. *(36)* did not find any difference for this polymorphism in AT_1R gene between normotensive controls and subjects with resistant essential hypertension, but high values of systolic BP were associated with the C allele in older and overweight patients. Moreover, Castellano et al. *(37)* found that BP values were lower in CC homozygotes in an Italian population; these homozygotes also presented a lower incidence of family history of hypertension.

The molecular basis of salt sensitivity in human hypertension was explored by De la Sierra's team, and in particular by the evaluation of *RAS* gene polymorphisms; patients with *ACE* II or ID genotype had significantly higher prevalence of salt sensitivity than DD hypertensives, whereas AT_1R A1166C polymorphism had no effect *(38,39)*. Moreover, Tabara et al. *(40)* did not find any significant associations between orthostatic hypotension and gene polymorphisms of *ACE* I/D, *AG* M235T, and AT_1R A1166C, orthostatic hypotension being an important risk factor for future cardiovascular morbidity and mortality. Several studies explored the sensitivity to Ang II in relation to AT_1R A1166C polymorphism; for example, in normotensive subjects, Paillard et al. *(41)* did not find any genotype effect of this polymorphism on the Bmax and K_D values of AT-1 on platelets. Testing for the response to short term infusion of Ang II in normotensive and moderately hypertensive subjects, Hilgers et al. *(42)* also concluded that the A1166C polymorphism does not have a major effect on the action of Ang II, i.e., increases in BP, plasma aldosterone, glomerular filtration rate, and decrease in renal blood flow.

Hypertension is a major risk factor for stroke, renal failure, and cardiovascular diseases. RAS gene polymorphism was studied in patients with cerebral white matter lesions assessed by brain magnetic resonance imaging; these lesions represent a subclinical form of ischemic brain damage and hypertension is one of the most important factors for their development. Sierra et al. *(43)* showed that the presence of the *ACE* D allele may be a predisposing factor for developing white matter lesions in essential hypertensive patients, whereas no significant association for the *AG* M235T and AT_1R A1166C polymorphisms was found. Moreover, no association was shown between AT_1R gene polymorphisms and stroke *(35)*. On the contrary, the presence of the C allele in AT_1R gene might be associated with faster deterioration of renal function, i.e., progression to end-stage renal disease, and whatever the aetiology of the renal failure *(44,45)*. Originally, a synergistic effect was suggested for AT_1R A1166C polymorphism and poor glycemic control on the risk of diabetic nephropathy in insulin-dependent diabetic patients *(11)*. But the subsequent studies performed failed to find any association between this polymorphism in AT_1R gene and diabetic nephropathy *(46–50)*. RAS gene polymorphism was also investigated in obesity, and particularly in obesity-associated hypertension. No association was detected between *AG* M235T or AT_1R A1166C polymorphism and anthropometric indexes or BP, whereas the *ACE* I/D polymorphism was a significant predictor of overweight and abdominal adiposity in man, the DD homozygosity being associated with larger increases in body weight and BP in aging persons, as well as with higher incidence of overweight *(51)*.

Arterial stiffness is associated with excess morbidity and mortality, independently of other cardiovascular risk factors. Age is the main determinant responsible for arterial wall changes leading to arterial stiffening. However, arterial stiffness is also influenced by vasoactive systems, and particularly the RAS. When *AG* M235T, *ACE* I/D, and *aldosterone synthase* gene polymorphisms were not associated with aortic stiffness as assessed by carotid-femoral pulse valve velocity, the 1166C allele in AT_1R gene influenced the relationship between age and arterial pulse valve velocity and in an additive effect with another SNP in AT_1R gene, the –153 A/G *(52)*. The C allele was also associated with aortic stiffness in both normotensive and hypertensive subjects *(53)*, and moreover in correlation with the ratio of total cholesterol on high-density lipoprotein cholesterol *(54)*. Conversely, Girerd et al. *(55)* did not find such a correlation with vascular hypertrophy as assessed by high resolution echography in subjects with no evidence of cardiovascular disease.

Hypertrophic cardiomyopathy occurs as a familial disorder with at least six genes clearly identified; but other factors, genetic as well as environmental, may modify the phenotypic expression of the mutated gene. Ang II is an important modulator of cardiac hypertrophy, and ACE inhibition induces regression of cardiac hypertrophy and prevents dilatation and remodelling of the ventricle after myocardial infarction. Osterop et al. *(56)* investigated whether the *ACE* I/D and AT_1R A1166C polymorphisms influence left ventricular hypertrophy in subjects with hypertrophic cardiomyopathy and concluded that the C allele in AT_1R gene modulates the phenotype of hypertrophy as determined by two-dimensional echocardiography, and independently of *ACE* I/D polymorphism. Takami et al. *(57)* also reported an association between C allele and left ventricular mass index, but in normotensive subjects without hypertrophic cardiomyopathy. These results are not in accordance with the study of Hamon et al. *(58)*, which does not find any association of the AT_1R A1166C polymorphism with left ventricular hypertrophy in subjects with normal coronary arteries; however, a strong association was observed between left ventricular mass and systemic hypertension. Ishanov et al. *(59)* also concluded that this polymorphism does not contribute to the development of cardiac hypertrophy in patients with hypertensive left ventricular hypertrophy or hypertrophic cardiomyopathy. Moreover, no kind of relationship between AT-1 density and/or function and AT_1R gene C allele has yet been observed *(60)*. Investigating patients by echocardiography for idiopathic heart failure diagnosis, Andersson et al. *(61)* found that patients with *ACE* DD and AT_1R CC or AC genotypes tented to have lower ejection fraction and increased left ventricular mass, suggesting an interaction of these two genetic traits on disease severity. Hamon et al. *(58)* also observed that the subjects homozygous for the AT_1R CC genotype had a significantly lower ejection fraction than those with A allele. These studies appear to suggest that in severe forms of hypertension, the AT_1R A1116C SNP is potentially involved in the regulation of BP; even when contrasted with other components of RAS, no direct effect of this polymorphism on the gene product has been demonstrated until now. Moreover, results from one ethnic group cannot be extrapolated to another.

Among the other polymorphisms in AT_1R gene, at 5'-flanking region a higher frequency of the T allele (–535C/T SNP) was observed in hypertensive patients *(14)*, whereas Zhang et al. *(62)*, evaluating nine newly characterized SNPs, did not show any association with arterial hypertension. Poirier et al. *(13)* also noticed that among seven new polymorphisms, all different from those formerly described, none was associated with pressor levels in control subjects, whereas Chaves et al. *(10)* found that the +573C/T polymorphism might be a genetic protective factor for urinary albumin excretion in a population of essential hypertensives. Investigating 25 new polymorphisms in RAS genes, Zhu et al. *(15)* particularly described an association between two AT_1R gene polymorphisms, located at the 3'-flanking region, and hypertension in African Americans but not in European Americans.

Recently, polymorphism in *Ang II type 2 receptor* (AT_2R) gene was also shown and investigated, in particular the A3123C located in the 3' untranslated region of exon 3 in a study showing that this polymorphism may contribute to cardiac hypertrophy in women with hypertrophic cardiomyopathy *(63)*. Conversely, no association was detected between

AT_2R polymorphism and hypertension *(57)*. Delles et al. *(64)* tested another SNP in AT_2R gene, namely +1675 G/A polymorphism, and in parallel of a SNP in AT_1R gene, i.e., -2228 G/A polymorphism; the response to Ang II infusion did not differ across the AT_1R and AT_2R genotypes. Conversely, this latter polymorphism in AT_2R gene was associated with left ventricular structure in young adults with normal or mildly elevated BP; in particular, as stated by echocardiography, hypertensive subjects with the A allele had greater left ventricular thickness and mass index than those with the G allele, suggesting early structural changes of the heart owing to hypertension in association with a genetic trait in RAS *(65)*. Research on AT-2 has unveiled hitherto unknown functions of the RAS extending beyond the classical role of this hormonal system in cardiovascular control, providing a solid basis for further research variation *(66)*, and in particular using AT-1 antagonists.

AT_1R GENE POLYMORPHISM
AND ATHEROSCLEROSIS-RELATED DISEASES

Coronary artery disease (CAD) is a major public health problem in industrialized countries. Dyslipidemia, arterial hypertension, and diabetes mellitus, the main risk factors for CAD apart tobacco consumption, are influenced by both environmental and genetic factors. Several studies have suggested that the activation of the RAS could be an important contributor to CAD. The best-documented of associations between the occurrence of CAD and polymorphisms in genes RAS component is the I/D polymorphism of the *ACE* gene. After the initial work of Cambien et al. *(67)*, who first suggested the potential role of the *ACE* D allele as an independent risk factor for myocardial infarction (MI), other case-control studies either confirmed or were in disagreement with their findings *(68–70)*. The M235T variant of *AG* gene has also been associated with MI but, as in hypertension, with ethnic variability *(19)*. A1166C polymorphism in AT_1R gene does not seem to be a direct risk factor for CAD or MI, but, in many studies, it has been observed to have synergistic effects with *ACE* I/D polymorphism *(53,71–73)*; in particular the highest risks were shown for patients with both *ACE* DD and AT_1R CC genotypes. Conversely to the former studies, other examinations did not find an association between A1116C polymorphism in AT_1R gene and CAD or MI, as well as no interaction between this polymorphism and I/D polymorphism in *ACE* gene *(74–76)* or independently of BP *(77)*. Moreover, Olivieri et al. *(78)* did not find associations between *AG* M235T or AT_1R A1116C polymorphism and atheromatous renal artery stenosis, whereas their results suggested a predisposing role for *ACE* D allele in the development and progression of this atherosclerosis related disease. AT_1R A1116C polymorphism was also not related to hypercholesterolemia, in particular in subjects with essential hypertension *(79)*; but in another study C allele was overrepresented in familial hypercholesterolemia with CAD *(80)*. An association was found between AT_1R C allele and *ACE* D allele in patients with CAD and malignant ventricular arrhythmia treated with an implantable cardioverter defibrillator *(81)*. Recently, Gruchala et al. *(82)*, evaluating left ventricular size and performance of patients with angiographically confirmed CAD by echocardio-graphy, did not find relationships between AT_1R A1116C polymorphism and left ventricular parameters. In two studies, patients carrying the AT_1R CC genotype have greater vasoconstriction in coronary vessels, as well as in response to Ang II infusion (83), than after intravenous injection of methylergonovine maleate, a potent vasoconstrictor whose effects have been explored in CAD *(84)*; but Steeds et al. *(85)* did not find differences in vasomotor function in isolated human mesenteric resistance arterioles, but an increase in sensitivity to prostaglandin F2α in arterioles from patients with C allele in AT_1R gene. Vuagnat et al. *(86)* found the same following Ang II infusion to assess familial resemblance in hypertensive patients. Ortlepp et al. *(87)* concluded that left ventricular hypertrophy in patients with aortic stenosis was not determined by five genetic polymorphisms in RAS, particularly in *ACE, AT_1R,* and *AG* genes. In a large population-based cohort of older adults, Hindorff et al. *(88)* did not observe any association of this AT_1R gene polymorphism with incident cardiovascular events. Thus, taken alone, the A1166C polymorphism in AT_1R gene neither represents a risk factor for adverse events complicating coronary interventions nor seems to have significant impact on further long-term processes such as development and severity of CAD *(89–91)*. Recently, polymorphisms in AT_2R gene were explored as predictors of CAD. Ye et al. *(73)* did not find any association between +1291 G/T or +1297 G/A polymorphism and coronary extent scores defined essentially by the number of coronary segments with significative stenosis. On the other hand, Jones et al. *(77)* demonstrated that hypertensive carriers with AT_2R 1675A/3123A haplotype were at most risk for a cardiovascular event.

In conclusion, among these three well-documented polymorphisms in RAS, i.e., I/D polymorphism in the *ACE* gene, M235T variant of *AG*, and A1166C SNP in AT_1R gene, only two types of relationships seem to be confirmed: (1) D allele of the *ACE* gene as risk factor for CAD and MI; and (2) C allele of A1166C in the AT_1R gene, when associated with *ACE* D allele, as contributor to susceptibility of CAD and to interindividual differences in severity of cardiovascular disease.

PHARMACOGENOMIC CONSIDERATIONS ON ANG II RECEPTORS

The response of patients to antihypertensive therapy is variable; individuals may respond differently to different medications, suggesting that treatment should be matched to individual responsiveness. The two main targets in RAS for an antihypertensive therapy are ACE and AT-1, with ACE inhibitors and AT-1 antagonists (or blockers), respectively. Then, polymorphisms in *ACE* and AT_1R genes may have influence on the antihypertensive response after, of course, ACE inhibitor or AT-1 blocker treatment, but also after other antihypertensive drugs such as diuretics, β-blockers, calcium channel antagonists, or drugs acting on the central nervous system. For *ACE* I/D polymorphism, a recent review has assessed the first conclusions arising from pharmacogenomic studies *(23)*. But few data are available for polymorphisms in AT_1R gene *(92)*. Miller et al. *(93)* hypothesized that renal and systemic Ang II activity would be augmented in subjects with C allele of AT_1R gene A1116C polymorphism, and tested this hypothesis by comparing hemodynamic and humoral responses to AT-1 blockade with losartan (the first AT-1 antagonist) and with low-dose suppressor infusions of Ang II. In this study, glomerular filtration rate, renal plasma flow, and renal blood flow were significantly lower in subjects with C allele and during Ang II infusion; subjects with C allele maintained glomerular filtration rate despite equivalent declines in renal blood flow, suggesting an enhanced efferent arteriolar constrictive response. Losartan increased the glomerular filtration rate and decreased mean arterial pressure in this group of subjects; conversely, aldosterone responses to losartan were blunted in the AA subgroup. This study demonstrates an association between the C allele and the hemodynamic response to losartan treatment. Spiering et al. *(94)* also showed that hypertensive patients had decreased glomerular filtration rate and aldosterone but increased atrial natriuretic peptide. Moreover, Kurland et al. *(95)* showed that C allele is associated with a reduction in both endothelium-dependent and -independent vasodilatations in normotensive individuals, whereas D allele in *ACE* gene was only reduced in endothelium-dependent vasodilatation. Nevertheless, these and the former authors did not discuss the interest in considering A1166C SNP in AT_1R gene an important factor when deciding on antihypertensive therapy for individuals with primary hypertension. Several studies examined relationships between *ACE* and AT_1R genes during antihypertensive therapy, but without AT-1 receptor antagonists. Dieguez-Lucena et al. *(96)* quantitated both the AT-1 and AT-2 messengers in peripheral blood mononuclear cells, and concluded that AT-1, but not AT-2, messenger level varies in relation to *ACE* I/D genotype, because AT-1 messenger and plasma Ang II levels were positively correlated with the D allele in the same individuals, and because AT-1 messenger levels decreased significantly with ACE inhibitor treatment in subjects with DD genotype. These effects were not seen with a β-blocker or a calcium channel antagonist in place of an ACE inhibitor, confirming close relationships between *ACE* and AT_1R genes. Moreover, Benetos et al. *(97)* showed that according to the A1166C genotype in AT_1R gene, an ACE inhibitor and a calcium channel antagonist affect pulse wave velocity (which evaluates aortic stiffness) but in opposite ways—i.e., baseline pulse wave velocity values were higher in subjects with C allele, and perindopril (an ACE inhibitor) decreased much more pulse wave velocity in these subjects, whereas nitrendipine (a calcium channel antagonist) decreased pulse wave velocity only in subjects with AA genotype. In another study, *ACE* and AT_1R genotypes were not related to BP responses after ACE inhibition; only the *AG* M235T variant was an independent predictor of the BP response, with a fall in both systolic and diastolic pressures lowest in homozygotes for the M form compared with hypertensive subjects bearing one or two copies of the variant allele *(98)*. Conversely, Dudley et al. *(99)* did not find any association between response to atenolol (a β-blocker), or lisinopril (an ACE inhibitor), or nifedipine (a calcium channel antagonist) and either the *AG* or *ACE* I/D polymorphisms; and Kurland et al. *(100)* did not show relationships between *AG* M235T or AT_1R A1116C polymorphism and response for 3 mo to treatment with irbesartan (an AT-1 antagonist) or atenolol, whereas *ACE* I/D predicted the blood-lowering response to these antihypertensive therapies.

The variability in the individual response to AT-1 antagonists could also result from variations in the pharmacokinetics of the drugs; in particular, losartan is essentially metabolized to its active form by cytochrome P450 2C (CYP2C9), which biotransforms many cardiovascular drugs *(16,101)*. CYP2C9 activity varies markedly among different ethnic populations, particularly in relation to the frequencies of three alleles in *CYP2C9* gene, thus leading to different interethnic responsiveness to a given drug; this could also be the case for losartan *(16)*. Interestingly, Uchida et al. *(102)* recently described the case of a man with a poor metabolizer genotype of *CYP2C9* who was hospitalized with severe hypotension 2 d after treatment of hypertension with candesartan, another AT-1 blocker. For other AT-1 blockers, such as irbesartan, other allelic variations could be involved for predicting antihypertensive response, but the enzymes responsible for their metabolism in humans have not been reported hitherto.

CONCLUSIONS

Genetic heterogeneity is involved in the metabolism of cardiovascular drugs and the pathogenesis of inherited cardiovascular disorders. Molecular genetic technologies can now provide efficient genetic testing, not only to identify disease-associated genes for diagnosis and risk stratification of many cardiovascular diseases, such as arterial hypertension, coronary artery disease, and diabetic nephropathy, but also to determine the responsiveness to a given drug, particularly in the area of antihypertensive therapy. Identification of the genes responsible for severe inherited forms of hypertension may provide novel diagnostic tools, as well as an opportunity for targeted therapeutic intervention. Candidate genes have been selected from the systems physiologically implicated in BP regulation, namely genes of the renin–angiotensin system as susceptible genes interacting with environmental factors for developing essential hypertension. *Renin, angiotensinogen, angiotensin I-converting enzyme*, and *angiotensin II receptor* genes have been evaluated, and emerging evidence has suggested that polymorphisms in both *AG* and *AT_1R* genes are associated with certain forms of hypertension. Moreover, even when conflicting results were seen, polymorphisms in *AG* and *ACE* genes seem to be useful in the determination of the responsiveness to antihypertensive therapies, at least when using ACE inhibitors for the latter. For the polymorphisms detected in *AT_1R* gene, and moreover in *AT_2R* gene, the pharmacogenomic studies are still scarce, but interestingly, both *ACE* and *AT_1R* genes loci could be associated. Clearly, further evaluation in adequately powered studies is necessary for final assessment. Perhaps when we are able to determine a few genotypes, such as some useful allelic marker SNPs in RAS genes, we might better choose an antihypertensive drug (or an association of drugs), maybe not positively but negatively, eliminating the worst and therefore making the choice easier among the remaining drugs.

REFERENCES

1. Burnier M. Brunner, HR. Angiotensin II receptor antagonists. Lancet 2000;335:637–645.
2. Lindpainter K, Ganten D. The cardiac renin angiotensin system: an appraisal of present experimental and clinical evidence. Cir Res 1991;68:905–921.
3. Dzau VJ. Circulating versus local renin–angiotensin system in cardiovascular homeostasis. Circulation 1988;77(Suppl I):I4–I13.
4. Degasparo M, Catt KJ, Inagami T, Wright JW, Unger T. The angiotensin II receptors. Pharmacol. Rev. 2000;52:415–472.
5. Lucius R, Gallinat S, Busche S, Rosentiel P, Unger T. Beyong blood pressure: new role for angiotensin II. Cell Mol Life Sci 1999;56:1008–1019.
6. Carey RM, Wang ZQ, Siragy HM. Role of the angiotensin type 2 receptor in the regulation of blood pressure and renal function. Hypertension 2000;35(Pt2):155–163.
7. Gradman AH. Long-term benefits of angiotensin II blockade: is the consensus changing? Am J Cardiol 1999;84:16 S–21 S.
8. Gallinat S, Busche S, Raizada MK, Summers C. The angiotensin II type 2 receptor: an enigma with multiple variations. Am J Physiol Endocrinol Metab 2000;278:E357–E374.
9. Bonnardeaux A, Davies E, Jeunemaitre X, et al. Angiotensin II type 1 receptor gene polymorphisms in human essential hypertension. Hypertension 1994;24:63–69.
10. Chaves FJ, Pascual JM, Rovira E, Armengod ME, Redon J. Angiotensin II AT1 receptor gene polymorphism and microalbuminuria in essential hypertension. Am J Hypertens 2001;14(4Pt1):364–370.
11. Doria A, Onuma T, Warram JH, Krolewski AS. Synergistic effect of angiotensin II type 1 receptor genotype poor glycaemic control on risk of nephropathy in IDDM. Diabetologia 1997;40:1293–1299.
12. Erdmann J, Riedel K, Rohde K, et al. Characterization of polymorphisms in the promoter of the human angiotensin II subtype 1 (AT1) receptor gene. Ann Hum Genet 1999;63:369–374.
13. Poirier O, Georges JL, Ricard S, et al. New polymorphisms of the angiotensin II type 1 receptor gene and their associations with myocardial infarction and blood pressure: the ECTIM study. Etude castémoin de l'infarctus du myocarde. J Hypertens 1998;16:1443–1447.
14. Takahashi N, Murakami H, Kodama K, et al. Association of a polymorphism at the 5'-region of the angiotensin II type 1 receptor with hypertension. Ann Hum Genet 2000;64:197–205.

15. Zhu X, Chang YPC, Yan D, et al. Associations between hypertension and genes in the renin–angiotensin system. Hypertension 2003;41:1027–1034.

16. Nakagawa K, Ishizaki T. Therapeutic relevance of pharmacogenetic factors in cardiovascular medicine. Pharmacol Therap 2000;86:1–28.

17. Schmidt S, Sharma AM, Zilch O, et al. Association of M235T variant of the angiotensinogen gene with familial hypertension of early onset. Nephrol Dial Transplant 1995;10:1145–1148.

18. Hata A, Namikawa C, Sasaki M, et al. Angiotensinogen as a risk factor for essential hypertension in Japan. J Clin Invest 1994;93:1285–1287.

19. Tiret L, Ricard S, Poirier O, et al. Genetic variation at the angiotensinogen locus in relation to high blood pressure and myocardial infarction : the ECTIM study. J Hypertens 1995;13:311–317.

20. Rigat B, Hubert C, Alhenc-Gelas F, Cambien F, Corvol P, Soubrier F. An insertion/deletion polymorphism in the angiotensin I-converting enzyme gene accounting for half the variance of serum levels. J Clin Invest 1990;86:1343–1346.

21. Villard E, Tiret L, Visvikis S, Rakotovao R, Cambien F, Soubrier F. Identification of new polymorphisms of the angiotensin I-converting enzyme (ACE) gene and study of their relationship to plasma ACE levels by two-QTL segregation-linkage analysis. Am J Hum Genet 1996;58:1268–1278.

22. Faure-Delanef L, Baudin B, Bénéteau-Burnat B, Beaudoin JC, Giboudeau J, Cohen D. Plasma concentration, kinetic constants and gene polymorphism of angiotensin I-converting enzyme in centenarians. Clin Chem 1998;44:2083–2087.

23. Baudin B. Angiotensin I-converting enzyme gene polymorphism and drug response. Clin Chem Lab Med 2000;38:853–856.

24. Kainulainen K, Perola M, Terwilliger J, et al. Evidence for involvement of the type 1 angiotensin II receptor locus in essential hypertension. Hypertension 1999;33:844–849.

25. Wang WY, Zee RY, Morris BJ. Association of angiotensin II type 1 receptor gene polymorphism with essential hypertension. Clin Genet 1997;51:31–34.

26. Nalogowska-Glosnicka K, Lacka BI, Zychma MJ, et al. Angiotensin II type 1 receptor gene A166C polymorphism associated with the increased risk of pregnancy-induced hypertension. Med Sci Monitor 2000;6:523–529.

27. Wang JG, Staessen JA. Genetic polymorphisms in the renin–angiotensin system: relevance for susceptibility to cardiovascular disease. Eur J Pharmacol 2000;410:289–302.

28. Henskens LH, Spiering W, Stoffers E, et al. Effects of ACE I/D and AT_1R-A[1666]C polymorphisms on blood pressure in a healthy normotensive primary care population: first results of the Hippocrates study. J Hypertens 2003;21:81–86.

29. Berge KE, Berg K. Polymorphisms at the angiotensinogen (AGT) and angiotensin II type 1 (AT1R) loci and normal blood pressure. Clin Genet 1998;53:214–219.

30. Jiang Z, Zhao W, Yu F, Xu G. Association of angiotensin II type 1 receptor gene polymorphism with essential hypertension. Chin Med J 2001;114:1249–1251.

31. Ono K, Mannami T, Baba S, Yasui N, Ogihara T, Iwai N. Lack of association between angiotensin II type 1 receptor gene polymorphism and essential hypertension in Japanese. Hypertens Res 2003;26:131–134.

32. Tsai CT, Fallin D, Chiang FT, et al. Angiotensinogen gene haplotype and hypertension. Interaction with ACE gene I allele. Hypertension 2003;41:9–15.

33. Iliadou A, Lichtenstein P, Morgenstern R, et al. Repeated blood pressure measurements in a sample of Swedish twins: heritabilities and associations with polymorphisms in the renin–angiotensin-aldosterone system. J Hypertens 2002;20:1543–1550.

34. Schmidt S, Beige S, Walla-Friedel M, Michel MC, Sharma AM, Ritz E. A polymorphism in the gene for the angiotensin II type 1 receptor is not associated with hypertension. J Hypertens 1997;5:1385–1388.

35. Tiret L, Blanc H, Ruidavets JB, et al. Gene polymorphisms of the renin–angiotensin system in relation to hypertension and parental history of myocardial infarction and stroke: the PEGASE study. J Hypertens 1998;16:37–44.

36. Szombathy T, Szalai C, Katalin B, Palicz T, Romics L, Csaszar A. Association of angiotensin II type 1 receptor polymorphism in resistant hypertension. Clin Chim Acta 1998;269:91–100.

37. Castellano M, Muiesan ML, Beschi M, et al. Angiotensin II type 1 receptor A/C[1166] polymorphism. Relationships with blood pressure and cardiovascular structure. Hypertension 1996;28:1076–1080.

38. Giner V, Poch E, Bragulat E, et al. Renin–angiotensin system genetic polymorphisms and salt sensitivity in essential hypertension. Hypertension 2000;35(Pt2):512–517.

39. Poch E, Gonzalez D, Giner V, Bragulat E, Coca A, De La Sierra A. molecular basis of salt sensitivity in human hypertension. Evaluation of the renin–angiotensin-aldosterone system gene polymorphisms. Hypertension 2001;38:1204–1209.

40. Tabara Y, Kohara K, Miki T. Polymorphisms of genes encoding components of the sympathetic nervous system but not the renin–angiotensin system as risk factors for orthostatic hypotension. J Hypertens 2002;20:651–656.

41. Paillard F, Chansel D, Brand E, et al. Genotype-phenotype relationships for the renin–angiotensin-aldosterone system in a normal population. Hypertension 1999;34:423–429.

42. Hilgers KF, Langenfeld MRW, Schlaich M, Veelken R, Schmieder R. 1166 A/C polymorphism of the angiotensin II type 1 receptor gene and the response to short-term infusion of angiotensin II. Circulation 1999;100:1394–1399.

43. Sierra C, Coca A, Gomez-Angelats E, Poch E, Sobrino J, De La Sierra A. Renin–angiotensin system genetic polymorphisms and cerebral white matter lesions in essential hypertension. Hypertension 2002;39(Pt2):343–347.

44. Buraczynska M, Ksiazek P, Zaluska W, Spasiewicz D, Nowicka T, Ksiazek A. Angiotensin II type 1 receptor gene polymorphism in end-stage renal disease. Nephron 2002;92:51–55.

45. Coll E, Campos B, Gonzalez-Nunez D, Botey A, Poch E. Association between the A1166C polymorphism of the angiotensin II receptor type 1 and progression of chronic renal insufficiency. J Nephrol 2003;16:357–364.

46. Tarnow L, Cambien F, Rossing P, et al. Angiotensin II type 1 receptor gene polymorphism and diabetic microangiopathy. Nephrol Dial Transplant 1996;11:1019–1023.

47. Chowdhury TA, Dyer PH, Kumar S, et al. Lack of association of angiotensin II type 1 receptor gene polymorphism with diabetic nephropathy in insulin-dependant diabetes mellitus. Diabet Med 1997; 14:837–840.

48. Marre M, Jeunemaitre X, Gallois Y et al. Contribution of genetic polymorphism in the renin–angiotensin system to the development of renal complication in insulin-dependent diabetes. J Clin Invest 1997;99:1585–1595.

49. Savage DA, Feeney SA, Fogarty DG, Maxwell AP. Risk of developing diabetic nephropathy is not associated with synergism between the angiotensin II (type 1) receptor C1166 allele and poor glycaemic control. Nephrol Dial Transplant 1999;14:891–894.

50. Tarnow L, Kjeld T, Knudsen E, Major-Pedersen A, Parving HH. Lack of synergism between long-term poor glycaemic control and three gene polymorphisms of the renin–angiotensin system on risk of developing diabetic nephropathy in type I diabetic patients. Diabetologia 2000;43:794–799.

51. Strazzullo P, Iacone R, Iacoviello L, et al. Genetic variation in the renin–angiotensin system and abdominal adiposity in men: the Olivetti prospective heart study. Ann Intern Med 2003;138:17–23.

52. Lajemi M, Labat C, Gautier S, et al. Angiotensin II type 1 receptor $^{-153}$A/G and ^{1166}A/C gene polymorphisms and increase in aortic stiffness with age in hypertensive subjects. J Hypertens 2001;19:407–413.

53. Benetos A, Gautier S, Ricard S, et al. Influence of angiotensin-converting enzyme and angiotensin II type 1 receptor gene polymorphisms on aortic stiffness in normotensive and hypertensive patients. Circulation 1996;94:698–703.

54. Benetos A, Topouchian J, Ricard S, et al. Influence of angiotensin II type 1 receptor gene polymorphisms on aortic stiffness in never-treated hypertensive patients. Hypertension 1995;26:44–47.

55. Girerd X, Hanon O, Mourad JJ, Boutouyrie P, Laurent S, Jeunemaitre X. Lack of association between renin–angiotensin system, gene polymorphisms, and wall thickness of the radial and carotid arteries. Hypertension 1998;32:579–583.

56. Osterop A, Kofflard M, Sandkuijl L, et al. AT_1 receptor A/C^{1166} polymorphism contributes to cardiac hypertrophic cardiomyopathy. Hypertension 1998;32:825–830.

57. Takami S, Katsuya T, Rakugi H, et al. Angiotensin II type 1 receptor gene polymorphism is associated with increase of left ventricular mass but not with hypertension. Am J Hypertens 1998;11:316–321.

58. Hamon M, Amant C, Bauters C, et al. Association of angiotensin-converting enzyme and angiotensin II type 1 receptor genotypes with left ventricular function and mass in patients with angiographically normal coronary arteries. Heart 1997;77:489–490.

59. Ishanow A, Okamoto H, Watanabe M, et al. Angiotensin II type 1 receptor gene polymorphisms in patients with cardiac hypertrophy. Jap Heart J 1998;39:87–96.

60. Danser AH, Schunkert H. Renin–angiotensin system gene polymorphisms: potential mechanisms for their association with cardiovascular diseases. Eur J Pharmacol 2000;410:303–316.

61. Andersson B, Blange I, Sylven C. Angiotensin-II type 1 receptor gene polymorphism and long-term survival in patients with idiopathic congestive heart failure. Eur J Heart Fail 1999;1:363–369.

62. Zhang X, Erdmann J, Regitz-Zagrosek V, Kurzinger S, Hense HW, Schunkert H. Evaluation of three polymorphisms in the promoter region of the angiotensin II type 1 receptor gene. J Hypertens 2000;18:267–272.

63. Deinum J, Van Gool J, Kofflard M, Ten Kate F, Jan Danser AH. Angiotensin II type 2 receptors and cardiac hypertrophy in women with hypertrophic cardiomyopathy. Hypertension 2001;38:1278–1281.

64. Delles C, Erdmann J, Jacobi J, Fleck E, Regitz-Zagrosek V, Schmieder RE. Lack of association between polymorphisms of angiotensin II receptor genes and response to short-term angiotensin II infusion. J Hypertens 2000;18:1573–1578.

65. Schmieder RE, Erdmann J, Delles C, et al. Effect of the angiotensin II type 2-receptor gene (+1675G/A) on left ventricular structure in humans. J Am Coll Cardiol 2001;37:175–182.

66. Unger T. Björn Fokow Award Lecture: The angiotensin type 2 receptor, variations on an enigmatic theme. J Hypertens 1999;17:1775–1786.

67. Cambien F, Poirier O, Lecerf L, et al. Deletion polymorphism in the gene for angiotensin-converting enzyme is a potent risk factor for myocardial infarction. Nature 1992;359:641–644.

68. Samani NJ, Thompson JR, O'Toole L, Channer K, Woods KL. A meta-analysis of the angiotensin-converting enzyme gene with myocardial infarction. Circulation 1996;94:708–712.

69. Swales JD. ACE gene: the plot thickens. Lancet 1993;342:1065–1066.

70. Lindpainter K, Pfeffer MA, Kreutz R, et al. A prospective evaluation of an angiotensin-converting enzyme gene polymorphism and the risk of ischemic heart disease. N Engl J Med 1995;332:706–711.

71. Tiret L, Bonnardeaux A, Poirier O, et al. Synergistic effects of angiotensin-converting enzyme and angiotensin II type 1 receptor gene polymorphisms on risk of myocardial infarction. Lancet 1994;344:910–913.

72. Nakauchi Y, Suehiro T, Yamamoto M, et al. Significance of angiotensin I-converting enzyme and angiotensin II type 1 receptor gene polymorphisms as risk factors for coronary heart disease. Atherosclerosis 1996;125:161–169.

73. Ye S, Dhillon S, Seear R, et al. Epistatic interaction between variations in the angiotensin I converting enzyme and angiotensin II type 1 receptor genes in relation to extent of coronary atherosclerosis. Heart 2003;89:1195–1199.

74. Gardemann A, Nguyen QD, Humme J, et al. Angiotensin II type 1 receptor A1116C gene polymorphism: absence of an association with the risk of coronary artery disease and myocardial infarction and of synergistic effect with angiotensin-converting enzyme gene polymorphism on the risk of these diseases. Eur Heart J 1998;19:1657–1665.

75. Steeds RP, Wardle A, Smith PD, Martin D, Channer KS, Samani NJ. Analysis of the postulated interaction between the angiotensin II sub-type 1 receptor gene A1166C polymorphism and the insertion/deletion polymorphism of the angiotensin-converting enzyme gene on risk of myocardial infarction. Atherosclerosis 2001;154:123–128.

76. Kee F, Morrison C, Poirier O, et al. Angiotensin II type-1 receptor and ACE polymorphism as risk of myocardial infarction in men and women. Eur J Clin Invest 2000;30:1076–1082.

77. Jones A, Dhamrait S, Hawe E, et al. Genetic variants of angiotensin II receptors and cardiovascular risk in hypertension. Hypertension 2003;42:500–506.

78. Olivieri O, Trabetti E, Grazioli S, et al. Genetic polymorphisms of the renin–angiotensin system and atheromatous renal artery disease. Hypertension 1999;34:1097–1100.

79. Morisawa T, Kishimoto Y, Kitano M, Kawasaki H, Hasegawa J. Influence of angiotensin II type 1 receptor polymorphism on hypertension in patients with hypercholesterolemia. Clin Chim Acta 2001;304:91–97.

80. Wierzbicki AS, Lambert-Hammill M, Lumb PJ, Crook MA. Renin-angiotensin system polymorphisms and coronary events in familial hypercholesterolemia. Hypertension 2000;36:808–812.

81. Anvari A, Turel Z, Schmidt A, et al. Angiotensin-converting enzyme and angiotensin II receptor type 1 polymorphism in coronary disease and malignant ventricular arrhythmias. Cardiovasc Res 1999;43:879–883.

82. Gruchala M, Ciecwierz D, Ochman K, et al. Left ventricular size, mass and function in relation to angiotensin-converting enzyme gene and angiotensin-II type 1 receptor gene polymorphisms in patients with coronary artery disease. Clin Chem Lab Med 2003;41:522–528.

83.   Van Geel PP, Pinto YM, Voors AA, et al. Angiotensin II type 1 receptor A1166C gene polymorphism is associated with an increased response to angiotensin II in human arteries. Hypertension 2000;35:717–721.

84.   Amant C, Hamon M, Bauters C, et al. The angiotensin II type 1 receptor gene polymorphism is associated with coronary artery vasoconstriction. J Am Cell Cardiol 1997 29:486-490.

85.   Steeds RP, Toole LO, Channer KS, Morice AH. Human vascular reactivity and polymorphisms of the angiotensin-converting enzyme and the angiotensin type 1 receptor genes. J Vasc Res 1999;36:445–455.

86.   Vuagnat A, Giacche M, Hopkins PN, et al. Blood pressure response to angiotensin II, low-density lipoprotein cholesterol and polymorphisms of the angiotensin II type 1 receptor gene in hypertensive sibling pairs. J Mol Med 2001;79:175–183.

87.   Ortlepp JR, Breithardt O, Ohme F, Hanrath P, Hoffmann R. Lack of association among five genetic polymorphisms on the renin–angiotensin system and cardiac hypertrophy in patients with aortic stenosis. Am Heart J 2001;141:671–676.

88.   Hindorff LA, Heckbert SR, Tracy R, et al. Angiotensin II type 1 receptor polymorphisms in the cardiovascular health study: relation to blood pressure, ethnicity and cardiovascular events. Am J Hypertens 2002;15:1050–1056.

89.   Stangl K, Cascorbi I, Stangl V, et al. A1166C polymorphism of the angiotensin II type 1 receptor gene and risk of adverse events after coronary catheter interventions. Am Heart J 2000;140:170–175.

90.   Brscic E, Bergerone S, Gagnor A, et al. Acute myocardial infarction in young adults: prognostic value of angiotensin-converting enzyme, angiotensin II type 1 receptor, apolipoprotein E, endothelial constitutive nitric oxide synthase, and glycoprotein IIIa genetic polymorphisms at medium-term follow-up. Am Heart J 2000;139:979–984.

91.   Hamon M, Amant C, Bauters C et al. Dual determination of angiotensin-converting enzyme and angiotensin II type 1 receptor genotypes as predictors of restenosis after coronary angioplasty. Am J Cardiol 1998;81:79–81.

92.   Baudin B. Angiotensin II receptor polymorphisms in hypertension. Pharmacogenomic considerations. Pharmacogenomics 2002;3:1–9.

93.   Miller JA, Thai K, Scholey JW. Angiotensin II type 1 receptor gene polymorphism predicts response to losartan and angiotensin II. Kidney Inter 1999;56:2173–2180.

94.   Spiering W, Kroon AA, Fuss-Lejeune M, Daemen M, De Leeuw P. Angiotensin II sensitivity is associated with the angiotensin II type 1 receptor A1166C polymorphism in essential hypertensives on a high sodium diet. Hypertension 2000;36:411–416.

95.   Kurland L, Melhus H, Sarabi M, Millgard J, Ljunghall S, Lind L. Polymorphisms in the renin–angiotensin system and endothelium-dependent vasodilation in normotensive subjects. Clin Physiol 2001;21:343–349.

96.   Dieguez-Lucena JL, Aranda-Lara P, Ruiz-Galdon M, Garcia-Villanova J, Morell-Ocana M, Reyes-Engel A. Angiotensin I-converting enzyme genotypes and angiotensin II receptors. Response to therapy. Hypertension 1996;28:98–103.

97.   Benetos A, Cambien F, Gautier S, et al. Influence of the angiotensin II type 1 receptor gene polymorphism on the effects of perindopril and nitrendipine on arterial stiffness in hypertensive patients. Hypertension 1996;28:1081–1084.

98.   Hingorani AD, Jia H, Stevens PA, Hopper R, Dickerson JEC, Brown MJ. Renin–angiotensin system gene polymorphisms influence blood pressure and the response to angiotensin-converting enzyme inhibition. J Hypertens 1995;13:1602–1609.

99.   Dudley C, Keavney B, Casadei B, Conway J, Bird R, Ratcliffe P. Prediction of patient responses to antihypertensive drugs using genetic polymorphisms: investigation of renin–angiotensin system genes. J Hypertens 1996;14:259–262.

100. Kurland L, Melhus H, Karlsson J, et al. Angiotensin converting enzyme gene polymorphism predicts blood pressure response to angiotensin II receptor type 1 antagonist treatment in hypertensive patients. J Hypertens 2001;19:1783–1787.

101. Stearns RA, Chakravarty PK, Chen R, Chiu SH. Bio-transformation of losartan to its active carboxylic acid metabolite in human liver microsomes. Role of cytochrome P450 2C and 3A subfamily members. Drug Metab Dispos 1995;23:207–215.

102.   Uchida S, Watanabe H, Nishio S, et al. Altered pharmacokinetics and excessive hypotensive effect of
       candesartan in a patient with the CYP2C91/3 genotype. Clin Pharmacol Ther 2003;74:505–508.

PATENTS

Furukawa Y, Kishimoto S, Nishikawa T. Hypotensive imidazole derivatives. US Patent 4340598 issued to Takada Chemical Industries, Ltd, Osaka, Japan.

2

Angiotensinogen Gene Polymorphisms and Hypertension

Ashok Kumar, PhD

CONTENTS

From: *Contemporary Cardiology: Cardiovascular Genomics*
Edited by: M. K. Raizada, et al. © Humana Press Inc., Totowa, NJ

SUMMARY

Hypertension is a serious risk factor for myocardial infarction, heart failure, vascular disease, stroke, and renal failure. Hypertension affects 50 million Americans with a prevalence rate of 25–30% in the adult Caucasian population. The incidence of hypertension and complications resulting from hypertension are even greater in the African-American population. The renin-angiotensin system plays an important role in the regulation of blood pressure, and previous studies have suggested that the angiotensinogen (*AGT*) gene locus is linked with human essential hypertension. Previous studies have suggested that a single nucleotide polymorphism that converts methionine to threonine at amino acid 235 is associated with hypertension in Caucasian population. This polymorphism is in linkage disequilibrium with A/G polymorphism at –6 position in the promoter of *AGT* gene. Reporter constructs containing variant A at –6 have increased promoter activity on transient transfection in human liver cells, suggesting that this variant may have increased transcriptional activity. However, this polymorphism is not associated with hypertension in the African-American and Chinese populations. We have found an A/G polymorphism at –217 of the human *AGT* gene promoter and have shown that frequency of allele A at –217 is significantly increased in the DNA of African-American hypertensive patients. We have also shown that: (a) reporter constructs containing *AG* gene promoter with nucleoside A at –217 have increased promoter activity on transient transfection; and (b) the C/EBP family of transcription factors and glucocorticoid receptor (GR) bind preferentially to this region of the promoter when nucleoside A is present at –217. In addition, variant –217A is always present with variants –532T, –793A, and –1074T in the human *AGT* gene promoter. We have also shown that liver enriched transcription factor HNF-3β binds more strongly when nucleoside T is present at –1074. Previous studies have shown that HNF-3β interacts with GR and plays an important role in liver-specific gene expression. These data suggest that *AGT* haplotype containing –217A, –532T, –793A, and –1074T may be involved in increased expression of this gene, and may play a role in human hypertension. It will be important to confirm this observation in future human studies and to understand the role of this haplotype in transcriptional regulation using transgenic animals.

Key Words: Human essential hypertension; molecular genetics; angiotensinogen gene; transcription factors; single nucleotide polymorphism (SNP); haplotype; C/EBP; HNF-3.

INTRODUCTION

Hypertension is a serious risk factor for myocardial infarction, heart failure, vascular disease, stroke, and renal failure. It is estimated that hypertension affects 50 million Americans with a prevalence rate of 25–30% in the adult Caucasian population. In the United States, the prevalence of hypertension is 50% greater in blacks than in whites. In blacks, hypertension appears earlier, is generally more severe, and results in high rates of morbidity and mortality from stroke, heart failure, left ventricular hypertrophy, and end-stage renal disease. Both genetic and environmental factors may contribute to the higher prevalence of hypertension in blacks. In addition, a genetic contribution to the increased prevalence of renal disease among hypertensive blacks has been proposed on the basis of family studies and studies of associated histocompatibility antigens. Hypertension is a polygenic disease, and it has been estimated by segregation analysis and twin studies that approx 45% of the interindividual differences in blood pressure (BP) can be accounted by genetic differences *(1)*. In the past two decades, many genes that were implicated in simple (Mendelian) diseases have been identified using genetic linkage and positional cloning methods *(2)*. Although these methods have been remarkably success-ful in identifying high relative risk genes, they have not been successful in identifying genes that are involved in the complex forms of disease such as hypertension and diabetes type II. This failure is the result of three main features of complex diseases. First, such diseases typically vary in severity of symptoms and age of onset, which results in diffi-culty in defining an appropriate phenotype and selecting the best population to study. Second, they can vary in the etiological mechanisms, which might involve various bio-logical pathways. Third, and perhaps most importantly, complex diseases are more likely to be caused by several, and even numerous genes, each with a small overall contribution and relative risk. In addition, hypertension is an arbitrary definition and not a quantitative trait that appears relatively late in life. Nothing is known about the number of genes involved, their mode of transmission, their quantitative effect on BP, their interaction with other genes, or their modulation by environmental factors. Parameters such as ethnicity and body weight increase the genetic heterogeneity and the difficulty of repli-cation from one study to another.

GENOME-WIDE ANALYSIS TO IDENTIFY
HYPERTENSION-RELATED GENES

Krushkal et al. *(3)* performed a genome-wide linkage analysis of systolic BP on 427 sibling pairs and identified four regions of the human genome that show statistical sig-nificant linkage. These regions are on chromosomes 2, 5, 6, and 15. These chromosomal regions include numerous potential candidates, such as phospholamban, estrogen recep-tor (ER), aminopeptidase *N*, α 1B-adrenergic receptor, dopamine receptor type 1A (DR-1A), calmodulin, and sodium-calcium exchanger. However, none of these genes has been confirmed to be associated with human hypertension.

Hunt et al. *(4)* performed a genome-wide analysis using 2959 individuals in 500 white families from the National Heart, Lung and Blood Institute (NHLBI) family heart study and identified five regions of the genome with logarithm of odds (LOD) scores higher than 2.0 for hypertension. These included chromosomes 1, 7, 12, and 15. On the other hand, chromosome 6 showed the best evidence for linkage with systolic BP (SBP). It is important to note that angiotensinogen and renin genes are located on chromosome 1.

Kristjansson et al. *(5)* performed a genome-wide scan with 904 microsatellite markers using 120 extended Icelandic families with 490 hypertensive patients. After adding 5 markers, they found linkage to chromosome 18q with an allele-sharing LOD score of 4.60. These results provide evidence for a novel susceptibility gene for essential hyper-tension on chromosome 18q, and show that it is possible to study the genetics of essential hypertension without stratifying by subphenotypes. Although melanocortin receptor 4 is located in this region of the chromosome, it is not known whether this gene is involved in hypertension.

Rice et al. *(6)* performed a genome-wide scan on 317 black individuals from 114 families and 519 white individuals from 99 families using a multipoint variance-compo-nents linkage model and a panel of 509 markers. Promising results were primarily, but not exclusively, found in the black families. Linkage evidence ($p < 0.0023$) with baseline BP replicated other studies within a 1-LOD interval on 2p, 3p.3 and 12q.33.

Levy et al. *(7)* performed a genome-wide scan in the largest families from two generations of Framingham Heart study participants. Genotyping was performed on 1702 subjects from 332 large families, and BP data were available for 1585 (93%) genotyped
subjects who contributed 12,588 longitudinal BP observations. For diastolic BP, LOD
scores greater than 2.0 were identified on chromosome 17 (74cM, LOD 2.1) and chromosome 18 (7cM, LOD 2.1). Using a genome-wide scan, they found strong evidence for
a BP quantitative trait locus on chromosome 17. The stroke-prone, spontaneously hypertensive rat and the Dahl salt-sensitive, hypertensive rat proved to be useful tools in
identifying quantitative trait loci (QTL) that contribute to BP variations. Evidence of BP
QTL was found on rat chromosomes 2, 10, and X. Human chromosome 17 is syntenic
with rat chromosome 10, and the rat chromosome 10QTL is located near the angiotensin-
converting enzyme (ACE) locus. The ACE locus is an attractive candidate gene because
of its role in the renin-angiotensin system (RAS) and the association between several
polymorphisms in the ACE locus with BP levels in some studies, although other studies
failed to confirm this finding. Other potential candidate genes on this segment of chromosome 17 include the Cl-HCO exchanger, phenylethanolamine *N*-methyltransferase,
nerve growth factor receptor, and pseudohypoaldosteronism type IIB genes.

Caulfield et al. *(8)* recently phenotyped 2010 affected sibling pairs drawn from 1599
severely hypertensive families in a large white European population (BRIGHT study).
Linkage analysis identified a principle locus on chromosome 6q with an LOD score of
3.21, which attained genome-wide significance ($p = 0.042$). The inclusion of three further
loci with LOD scores higher than 1.57 (2q, 5q, and 9q) also show genome-wide significance ($p = 0.017$) when assessed under a locus-counting analysis. There is a region of
overlap with other studies on chromosome 2 (140–170 cM). This region was linked to
hypertension in Chinese sibling pairs and Finnish twins, and linkage is suggested in a
discordant sibling-pair screen. In addition, linkage signals are located proximally to the
BRIGHT locus on chromosome 2p, documented by two genome scans in a genome scan
of families of African ancestry. Furthermore, this region has also been linked to the
hypertension-associated phenotype preeclampsia in some genome-wide screens. Preliminary analysis of each region with an LOD score higher than 1.57 has identified a small
number of good candidates that map to the chromosome 2 and 9 regions of interest. These
candidates include the genes encoding serine-threonine kinases (STK39, STK17B, chromosome 2q), a protein kinase (PKNBETA on 9q), G protein-coupled receptors (GPR21
on 9q33, GPR107 9q, and GPR1 on 2q33) and a potassium channel (KCNJ3 on 2q24.1).
Several BP QTL from hypertensive rat models exhibit homology with the BRIGHT
regions of interest. For instance, rat 3q11–q23 is homologous to the human 9q region, rat
2q14–q16 with the human chromosome 5p region, and rat chromosome 9q22–q34 is
homologous to the human 2q locus. Examination of databases reveals many known genes
and expressed sequence tags in or near the 16cM QTL interval at 17q12–21. Although
no genes that have been strongly implicated in BP variation lie in this interval, potential
candidate genes in the interval include the α-1 thyroid receptors, the neuronal homolog
of the amiloride sensitive epithelial sodium channel, the corticotropin-releasing hormone
receptor 1, insulin-like growth factor-binding protein-4, hepatocyte nuclear factor (HNF)
1-β, and the chloride/bicarbonate exchanger AE1. In addition to the chromosome 17q12–
21 interval, there were two additional regions yielding LOD scores over 2.0 in multipoint
analyses. One of these lies just distal on chromosome 17, and it is possible that this locus
is independent of their largest peak. This second chromosome 17 peak overlaps the locus

encoding the ACE locus, a much-studied candidate gene for hypertension. The final locus that has not been previously implicated in BP variation is on chromosome 18. An interesting candidate gene in the chromosome 18 interval is the melanocortin receptor 2, which is the physiological receptor for corticotropin. Given the known effects of glucocorticoids on BP, it is of interest that receptors involved in the regulation of cortisol secretion lie in both the chromosome 17 and chromosome 18 intervals.

From this brief review it is clear that although different regions of the chromosome have been shown to be involved in the regulation of BP, these studies are often nonreproducible and genes involved in hypertension remain to be identified.

ROLE OF AGT IN HYPERTENSION

The RAS plays an important role in the regulation of BP. The octapeptide, angiotensin II (Ang II), is one of the most active vasopressor agents and is obtained by the proteolytic cleavage of a larger precursor molecule, angiotensinogen (AGT), which is primarily synthesized in the liver and to a lesser extent in the kidney, brain, heart, adrenal, fat, and vascular walls. The human AGT cDNA is 1455 nucleotides long and codes for a 485-amino acid protein (9). AGT is first converted by renin to produce a decapeptide, Ang I, and is then converted to Ang II by the removal of a C-terminal dipeptide by ACE (10). In experimental as well as clinical studies, chronic administration of renin-angiotensin inhibitors has proven effective in lowering BP in hypertension. Genes that encode components of the RAS are therefore potential candidate genes that may play a role in the regulation of BP.

The plasma concentration of AGT is close to the Michaelis constant of the enzymatic reaction between renin and AGT (11). For this reason, a rise in plasma AGT levels can lead to a parallel increase in the formation of Ang II that may ultimately result in hypertension. In fact, recent studies have suggested a direct correlation between AGT and BP. These studies include a highly significant relationship between plasma concentration of AGT and BP in human subjects (4); higher plasma AGT levels in hypertensive subjects and in offspring of hypertensive parents compared with normotensives (12,13); expression of *AGT* gene in multiple tissues—such as brain, kidney, heart, adrenals, placenta, and vascular walls—that are directly involved in BP regulation (14); elevation of BP in transgenic animals that overexpress *AGT* gene (7–9); and reduction of BP in *AGT* gene knockout mice (15). In addition, Kim et al. have introduced up to four copies of the *AGT* gene in mice, with each copy of the gene resulting in a successive increase in BP (16). These results directly demonstrated that small increases in plasma AGT level can quantitatively influence the fine control of renal vascular resistance and increase BP in a gene dose-dependent manner. A similar *ACE* gene duplication in mice led to an increase in plasma ACE level but no increase in BP (17), which supports the importance of the *AGT* gene in human hypertension.

M235T POLYMORPHISM OF *AGT* GENE AND HYPERTENSION

The *AGT* gene contains five exons and four introns, which span 13 kb (18). An extensive study of the potential role of the *AGT* gene in human essential hypertension was performed on two large series of hypertensive siblingships yielding 379 sibling pairs. The highly polymorphic CA dinucleotide repeat marker located in the 3'-region of the *AGT* gene and the powerful affected sibling pair methodology were used to obtain evidence of a genetic linkage between the *AGT* gene and hypertension in this study *(19)*. A 17% excess of AGT allele sharing was found in severely hypertensive sibling pairs. Whereas significant linkage was obtained in male pairs in both the Utah and Paris groups, no excess of shared AGT alleles was observed in female subjects, suggesting the influence of an epistatic hormonal phenomenon. These studies also showed that variants 235T and 174M of the *AGT* gene are associated with hypertension. From these studies, it was estimated that mutations at the AGT locus might be a predisposing factor in at least 3–6% of hypertensive individuals younger than 60 yr of age in the Caucasian population. When the same methodology was used to analyze the same hypertensive sibling pairs from Utah or Paris, it showed no linkage with other genes of the renin system: namely renin *(20)*, ACE *(21)*, or Ang II type I receptor *(22)*.

Two other linkage studies also indicate a relationship between the AGT locus and hypertension. This linkage was observed in the subgroup of patients with diastolic pressure above 100 mmHg, but there was no difference among female–female pairs. However, there was no association between hypertension and the 235T AGT variant in this population *(23)*. The same group also found linkage and association of the AGT locus with high BP in 63 affected sibling pairs of African-Caribbean origin, suggesting some similarity in the genetic basis of essential hypertension in populations of different ethnicity *(24)*. The corroboration of these linkage studies indicate that molecular variants of the *AGT* gene, such as M235T, or those in linkage disequilibrium with this variant are inherited predispositions to essential hypertension in humans.

However, results of these studies must be interpreted with caution for several reasons. First, the frequency of the 235T AGT allele varies in different ethnic groups. The 235T allele is more frequent in the Asian than in the Caucasian population and is by far the predominant allele in the African population. As a consequence, positive results may arise from population admixture, and negative results in populations in which this allele is predominant may result from the constraint of limited statistical power. Second, differences in the design of each study and the choice of the control group make any overall comparison difficult. Finally, most of the results reported to date have been obtained with relatively small numbers of patients, which can also generate false negative or false positive results.

There are divergent results on the association between variants in AGT at position 235 (235T) or 174 (174M) and hypertension in Caucasians. In their original study, Jeunemaitre et al. found that the M235T variant was more frequent in hypertensive probands from Utah and Paris, especially in the more severe index cases *(19)*. A subsequent study by the same group on 136 mild to moderate hypertensive subjects also found that the frequency of the 235T allele was increased, although the increase was significant only for patients with a family history of hypertension. Schmidt also found a higher frequency of the 235T allele in subjects with hypertension, a family history of the disease, and early onset of hypertension *(25)*.

However, other studies have not found any association between the 235T variant and hypertension. Hingorani et al. found no difference in the frequency of M235T in 223 hypertensive subjects and 187 normotensive individuals in Anglia in the United Kingdom *(26)*. A more powerful study performed in Finland by Kiema gave negative results with 508 mild hypertensives and 523 population-based controls *(27)*. On the other hand, four large studies recently showed a positive association between the M235T allele and essential hypertension. An association with severe hypertension with stronger relationship for men than for women was found in a sample from the Framingham Heart study and from the Atherosclerosis Risk in Community (ARIC) study, when the effect of body mass index and triglycerides were taken into account *(28)*. The proportions of cases attributable to the 235 allele were 8% in the ARIC population and 20% in the Framingham population. In a study testing a large number of AGT alleles, the frequency of the 235T allele was 0.47 in the 477 probands of hypertensive families and 0.38 in the 364 Caucasian controls *(29)*. In a cross-section sample of 634 middle-aged subjects from the MONIC Angsburg cohort, Schunkert found that individuals carrying at least one copy of the T235 allele had high SBP and diastolic BP(DBP)s and were more likely to use antihypertensive drugs *(30)*. Finally, another case-control study involving 802 hypertensive subjects and 658 Caucasian controls has shown a significant increase in the frequency of the T235 allele in men and in women whose hypertension was diagnosed before they were 45 yr of age *(31)*. These studies emphasize the importance of sample size testing for susceptibility locus in a complex disease such as hypertension *(32)*.

The frequency of the T235 allele is invariably high in the Japanese population, ranging from 0.65 to 0.75. An association between hypertension and molecular variants of AGT in the Japanese population has been found in several independent studies *(33–35)*. All of the studies reported so far indicate that frequency of the 235T variant is higher in Japanese hypertensive subjects. A more homogeneous genetic and environmental background may explain why the results reported for Japanese populations are more uniform. However, Ishigami et al. *(36)* showed that the –20C variant of the human *AGT* gene plays an important role in hypertension in Japanese population.

Walker et al. showed a remarkably high correlation between plasma AGT concentration and elevated BP ($p < 0.0001$) in a large study involving 574 black subjects *(4)*. Bloem et al. *(37)* showed that (1) plasma AGT level is about 19% higher in black children as compared with white children; and (2) BP is normally higher and increases faster over time in black children as compared with white children. Caulfield et al. *(24)* found an association between the *AGT* gene locus and high BP in 63 affected sibling pairs of African-Carribean origin using CA dinucleotide marker. However, these workers could not find an association between variants M235T and hypertension in the African-American population. Various recent studies have suggested that although the frequency of 235T allele is increased in the African-American population (0.8–0.9), there is no association between 235T allele and hypertension in this population *(38)*.

LINKAGE DISEQUILIBRIUM BETWEEN 235T AND –6A IN *AGT* GENE

Because amino acid 235 is located far away from the renin cleavage site, this polymorphism does not explain the molecular mechanism involved in increased plasma AGT levels by the 235T variant. The human *AGT* gene has an A/G polymorphism at nucleoside –6. It has been shown that nucleoside A is present at –6 in the ancestral *AGT* gene and –6G is a neomorph. Sequence analysis of the human *AGT* gene has shown that molecular variants 235T and –6A are in complete association *(39)*. In addition, Inoue et al. synthesized reporter constructs containing 256 and 70 basepairs (bp) of the 5'-flanking region of the human *AGT* gene containing either nucleoside A or G at –6 position. Transient transfection of these reporter constructs in human liver cells (HepG2) have shown that reporter constructs containing human *AGT* gene promoter with nucleoside A at –6 have increased promoter activity compared to nucleoside G at –6. These experiments suggested that increased plasma AGT levels by the 235T variant in hypertensive patients may actually be a result of increased transcriptional activity of the human *AGT* gene by nucleoside A at –6. However, the molecular mechanism involved in increased transcription of the human *AGT* gene by nucleoside A at –6 as compared with nucleoside G at –6 is not known, and transcription factors that may be involved in this process have not been identified. In addition, as discussed later, experiments using transgenic mice have shown that this polymorphism neither alters the expression of the *hAGT* gene nor increases BP in transgenic mice *(40)*.

ASSOCIATION OF THE –217A VARIANT OF *AGT* GENE WITH HYPERTENSION

Because hypertension is more common in African-American subjects, our laboratory is interested in understanding molecular mechanisms involved in hypertension in the African-American population. We have therefore analyzed 186 African-American and 127 Caucasian subjects with hypertension (mean age: 59 ± 10 yr) and 156 African-American and 135 Caucasian normotensive controls (mean age 58 ± 10 yr). All of these subjects were recruited from the outpatient department of The State University of New York Health Science Center in Brooklyn, New York and Westchester Medical Center, Valhalla, New York. All case and control subjects gave informed consent before participating in the research. All cases were diagnosed as having primary hypertension and patients with secondary hypertension, diabetes mellitus, or ischemic heart disease were excluded. The criteria for hypertension was defined as a SBP greater than 140 mmHg, a DBP greater than 90 mmHg, or under antihypertensive therapy. BP was measured twice with the subject seated and a 5-min interval between measurments. The normotensives (with SBP/DBP <140/90 mmHg) without a history of hypertension and without diabetes mellitus were recruited from the same population and matched for sex and age. All participants completed a standard questionnaire on personal medical history and family history of hypertension. All patients and control subjects were in Hardy–Weinberg equilibrium. The frequency of the –217A allele in hypertensive patients was 0.29 as compared with 0.19 in the normotensive population, which is highly significant ($p = 0.0017$ and OR =1.792) (Table 1). To compare the role of this polymorphic site on hypertension in the African-American and Caucasian populations, we also analyzed genomic DNA from 127 Caucasian hypertensive subjects and 135 normotensive controls. The frequency of –217A allele was 0.15 in Caucasian hypertensive subjects and 0.11 in normotensive controls which is not significant ($p = 0.12$) (Table 1). Statistical analysis based on the –217 A/G genotype (using A allele as a dominant model) also suggested a significant role of the –217A allele in hypertension in African-Americans ($p = 0.0021$ and OR = 2.015) and not in Caucasians (Table 2). Because an A/G polymorphism at –6 has previously been associated with hypertension, we also analyzed genomic DNA from the African-American and Caucasian populations for this polymorphism. The frequency of –6A allele was 0.87 in African-American hypertensive subjects and 0.85 in normotensive controls, which was not significant ($p = 0.58$). However, the frequency of –6A allele was marginally significant in Caucasian subjects ($p = 0.06$). These experiments suggested that –217A allele of the human *AGT* gene plays a significant role in essential hypertension in African-Americans *(41)*. However, if we double the number of total Caucasian subjects, then the role of –217A becomes significant. It is therefore possible that this polymorphism will be significant in Caucasian subjects if we analyze more samples.

Table 1
Statistical Analysis of –217 A/G Polymorphism of Human
Angiotensinogen Based on Allele Frequency

	A allele	G allele	p value
African-American hypertensive (n = 186)	0.29	0.71	p = 0.0017
			OR = 1.792
Normotensive (n = 156)	0.19	0.81	[1.247, 2.575]
Caucasian hypertensive (n = 127)	0.15	0.85	p = 0.1208
			OR =1.507
Normotensive (n = 135)	0.11	0.89	[0.901, 2.522]

Table 2
Statistical Analysis of –217 A/G Polymorphism of Angiotensinogen Gene
Based on the Genotype Distribution Using A Allele Dominant Model

	(AA + AG)		GG	p value
African-American hypertensive (n = 186)	12	84	90	p = 0.0021
				OR = 2.015
Normotensive (n = 156)	4	50	102	[1.301, 3.121]
Caucasian hypertensive (n = 127)	4	31	92	p = 0.1433
				OR =1.595
Normotensive (n = 135)	3	23	109	[0.894, 2.844]

TRANSCRIPTION FACTORS INVOLVED IN THE EXPRESSION OF *AGT* GENE

The activation of eukaryotic genes in vivo often requires the coordinated binding of multiple transcription factors to the promoter–enhancer region. It has been shown that distinct signal transduction pathways regulate activity of many of these transcription factors. In several cases, it has been shown that binding of multiple transcription factors to a specific promoter–enhancer region is cooperative and requires a unique composition and spatial arrangement of transcription factor binding sites. The assembly of these enhancer complexes is facilitated by protein–protein interactions between DNA-bound factors and protein-induced DNA bending. These features are important for transcriptional regulation because combination of multiple transcription factors generates a diverse pattern of regulation, and highly cooperative binding ensures the specificity of transcriptional control *(42–44)*. Most eukaryotic transcription factors contain one or more transactivation domains that are involved in interaction with downstream coactivators (such as CREB binding protein, CBP/p300, and steroid receptor coactivators) and this interaction plays a crucial role in transcriptional activation of a gene *(45,46)*. It is possible that polymorphisms in the promoter of a gene may affect the binding of transcription factors to this region of the promoter and alter the transcriptional regulation of the gene. For example, it has been shown that a single nucleotide polymorphism in the CD14 promoter decreases the affinity of SP1 transcription factor binding and enhances transcriptional activity *(47)*. Similarly two mutations in the promoter of human protein-C gene cause type-1 protein-c deficiency by disruption of two HNF-3 binding sites *(48)*. A polymorphism of the human matrix γ-carboxy glutamic acid protein promoter alters the binding of AP-1 complex and is associated with altered expression and serum levels of this protein *(49)*.

The nucleotide sequence of the human *AGT* gene promoter containing nucleotide sequence from –1223 to +27 and potential *cis*-acting DNA elements that may bind to different transcription factors are shown in Fig. 1. Comparatively little is known about transcriptional regulation of the human *AGT* gene expression. We have shown that the nucleotide sequence located between –99 and –91of the human *AGT* gene binds to the C/EBP family of transcription factors and this region of the promoter plays an important role in DBP and C/EBP-β-induced expression of this gene *(50)*. There is an adjacent SP1 binding site located around –87 and our recent data have suggested that SP1 and C/EBP-β cooperatively regulate the expression of human *AG* gene. It has been previously shown that human *AGT* gene has a C/A polymorphic site at –20 (located between TATA box and transcriptional initiation site). We have shown that USF binds to this sequence when nucleoside C is present at –20 and ER binds to this sequence when nucleoside A is present at –20 *(51)*. We have also shown that cotransfection of ER increases the expression of reporter constructs containing human *AGT* gene promoter with nucleoside A at –20 as compared with the same reporter constructs containing nucleoside G at this position. Orphan receptor Arp-1 also binds to this sequence and reduces ER-induced promoter activity *(52)*. Yanai et al. have also shown that the nucleotide sequence located between the TATA box and transcriptional initiation site of the human *AGT* gene binds to USF and plays a critical role in its expression *(53)*. In addition, we have shown that the liver-enriched transcription factor HNF-3 binds to the nucleotide sequence located between +10 and +20 of the human *AGT* gene promoter *(54)*. It has been shown recently that human *AGT* gene expression is increased by interleukin (IL)-6 treatment and a STAT-3 binding site is located at –274 *(55)*. Our gel shift and transient transfection assays have shown that nucleotide sequence around –240 is an HNF-1 site. HNF-1 plays an important role in liver and kidney specific expression of a gene. Nucleotide sequence of the human *AGT* gene around –217 contains a full palindromic GRE and there are three glucocorticoid receptor-binding site (GRE), half sites in other regions of the promoter (at –673, –130 and +15). We have also shown that the transcription factor CREB binds to the nucleotide sequence located between –840 and –830 of the human *AGT* gene and this sequence is involved in cAMP-induced expression of this gene *(56)*. This is a composite element and has sequence homology with a C/EBP binding site. Nucleotide sequence located between –323 and 490 contains multiple hormone receptor binding sites. There are at least three HNF-4 binding sites (DR-1) between –363 and –423. In addition, this sequence contains DR-4 sites that may be involved in binding with thyroid hormone receptor. Although it has been shown that this region of the promoter is important in the regulation of *AGT* gene expression by HNF-4 *(57)*, it is not known whether it plays any role in TR-induced expression of this gene. It has been shown previously that CREB, HNF-4, ER, USF, C/EBP and GR (which bind to different regions of the human AGT gene) interact with transcriptional coactivator CBP and coordinately regulate the expression of a gene. However, the role of CBP in transcriptional activation of human AGT gene, which is regulated by multiple transcription factors that can individually bind to CBP, is not known.

AGT gene is expressed in multiple tissues such as liver, fat, kidney, brain, and adrenals. However, molecular mechanisms involved in tissue specific expression of this gene are not known. It has been shown that the rat *AGT* gene expression is regulated by glucocorticoids, estrogens, androgens, and thyroid hormones, and by different cytokines during inflammation *(10)*. Glucocorticoids are the most important regulatory agents, and cell culture studies have shown that they increase the expression of *AGT* gene in liver and fat cells. Glucocorticoids can modulate the expression of *AGT* gene by interaction with multiple transcription factors. It has been shown that GR interacts with STAT-3 and C/EBP-β. Because IL-6 increases the expression of a gene through STAT-3 and C/EBP pathways, glucocorticoids may increase the expression of *AGT* gene through the action of IL-6. In addition, GR interacts with cAMP and increases the expression of various liver specific genes. In the case of rat *AGT* gene, a nucleotide sequence called acute phase responsive element (APRE) is located around –545 *(58)*. This nucleotide sequence is flanked by two GREs: a full palindromic sequence located around –580, and a half palindromic sequence located around –470. The nucleotide sequence of APRE has strong homology with NFκB site and partial homology with C/EBP binding site. Gel shift analysis has shown that both of these transcription factors can bind to APRE. Under basal conditions, a constitutively synthesized transcription factor (most probably C/EBP-α) binds to this sequence. However, on lipopolysaccharide (LPS) treatment, an inducible factor (most probably NFκB) binds to this sequence and displaces C/EBP-α. Transient transfection analysis has shown that presence of both of the GREs is required for maximum increase in the expression of rat *AGT* gene by IL-1 and LPS treatment. These experiments suggested that expression of the rat AG gene is increased during acute phase reaction mainly through the NFκB pathway. On the other hand, Brasier's group has shown that expression of the human *AG* gene is increased mainly by the IL-6 pathway *(55)*. However, the molecular mechanism involved in the regulation of human *AGT* gene expression by glucocorticoids is not known, and the role of GREs in this gene has not been analyzed.

The promoters of rat and human *AGT* genes are very different with respect to the location and sequence of GRE. The palindromic GRE of the rat gene has stronger homology with the consensus GRE, but is located far away from the transcriptional initiation site, at –580. On the other hand, although the GRE in the promoter of human *AGT* gene has only partial homology with consensus GRE, it is located much closer to the transcriptional initiation site, at –217. This site in the human gene is located in close proximity with the C/EBP and STAT-3 binding sites.

HUMAN *AGT* GENE PROMOTER WITH –217A VARIANT HAS INCREASED PROMOTER ACTIVITY

To understand the role of A/G polymorphism at –217 on transcription of the human *AGT* gene, we have synthesized reporter constructs where different regions of the human *AGT* gene promoter were attached to the luciferase gene in pGL3 basic vector (Promega Biotec). This vector does not contain any promoter or enhancer sequence. The reporter construct pHAGT1.3*luc* has 1223 bp of the 5'- flanking sequence and 70 bp of exon-I of the human AGT gene, and contains nucleoside A at –6 and G at –217. This construct was then mutated from –217G to –217A using a STRATAGENE site-specific mutagenesis kit. The resulting reporter construct had nucleoside A at –6 and at –217 as determined by nucleotide sequence analysis. These reporter constructs were transiently transfected in

-1223	CCAGACAAGT GATTTTTGAG GAGTCCTAT CTATAGGAAC AAAGTAATTA
-1173	AAAAAATGTA TTTCAGAATT ATACAGGCCA TGTGAGATAT GATTTTTTTA
	HNF-3
-1123	AATGAAGATT TAGATAATG GGTAAAAAAG AGGTATTTGT GTGTTTGTTG
	*
-1073	ATTGTTCAGT CAGTGAATGT ACAGCTTCTG CCTCATATCC AGGCACCATC
-973	TGCCATCGTG GATATGCCGT GGCTCCTTGA ACCTGCTTGT GTTGAAGCAG
-923	GATCTTCTT CCTGTCCCTT CAGTGCCCTA ATACCATGTA TTTAAGGCTG
	AP-1 CREB
-873	GACACATCAC CACTCCCAAC CTGCCTCACC CACTGCGTCA CTTGTGATCA
-823	CTGGCTTCTG GCGACGTCTCA CCAAGGTCTC TGTCATGCCC TGTTATAACG
	* *
-773	ACTACAAAG CAAGTCTTAC CTATAGGAAA ATAAGAATTA TAACCCTTTT
-723	ACTGGTCATG TGAAACTTAC CATTTGCAAT TTGTACAGCA TAAACACAGA
-673	ACAGCACATA TTTCAATGCC TGCATCCTGA AGGCATTTTG TTTGTGTCTT
-623	TCAATCTGGA TGTGCTATTG TTGGTGTTTA ACAGTCTCCC CAGCTACACT
-573	GGAAACTTCC AGAAGGCACT TTTCACTTGC TTGTGTGTTT TCCCCAGTGT
	*
-523	CTATTAGAGG CCTTTGCACA GGGTAGGCTC TTTGGAGCAG CTGAAGGTCA
-473	CACATCCCAT GAGTGGGCAG CAGGGTCAGA AGTGGCCCCC GTGTTGCCTA
	HNF-4/PPAR
-423	AGCAAGACTC TCCCCTGCCC TCTGCCCTCT GCACCTCCGG CCTGCATGTC
	SP1/AP-1
-373	CCTGTGGCCT CTTGGGGGGTA CATCTCCCGG GGCTGGGTCA GAAGGCCTGG
	APRE
-323	GTGGTTGGCC TCAGGCTGTC ACACACCTAG GGAGATGCTC CCGTTTCTGG
	HNF-1
-273	GAACCTTTGGC CCCGACTCCT GCAAACTTCG GTAAATGTGT AACTCGACCC
	CEBP/GRE
-223	TGCACCGGCT CACCTCTGTTC AGCAGTGAAA CTCTGCATCG ATCACTAAGA
	APRE * GRE
-173	CTTCCTGGGAA GAGGTCCCAG CGTGAGTGTC GCTTCTGGCA TCTGTCCTTC
	CEBP
-123	TGGCCAGCCT GTGGT CTGGC CAAGTGATGT AACCCTCCTC TCCAGCCTGT
-73	GCACAGGCAG CCTGGGAACA GCTCCATCCC CACCCCTCAG CTATAAATAG
	ERE/USF +1
-23	GGCATCGTGA CCCGGCCGGG GGAAGAAGCT GCCGTTGTTC TGGGTACTAC
	* *

Fig. 1. Nucleotide sequence of the 1223 bp 5'-flanking region and 27 bp of the first exon of human angiotensinogen gene. Potential *cis*-acting DNA elements that may be involved in transcriptional regulation of this gene are underlined. The transcriptional initiation site is marked as +1.

HepG2 cells. The promoter activity was analyzed after 48 h of transfection, and normalized with the β-gal activity. Results of this experiment showed that reporter construct pHAGT1.3*luc* with nucleoside A at –217 gave a 28% increase in the promoter activity as compared with the reporter construct pHAGT1.3*luc* with nucleoside G at –217 ($p <$ 0.001) (mean value of six experiments) *(41)*. We have recently used these reporter constructs in transient transfection in Hep3B (another human liver-derived cell line) and immortalized human hepatocytes (TPH cells obtained from Dr. Ranjit Ray). TPH cells were obtained by transduction of Hepatitis C virus core protein in primary human hepatocytes, and we have shown that these cells synthesize human AGT mRNA by RT-PCR. Results of these experiments have shown that the reporter construct containing –217A had 20–30% increased basal promoter activity as compared with the reporter construct containing –217G.

NUCLEOTIDE SEQUENCE OF *AGT* GENE AROUND –217 HAS HOMOLOGY WITH GRE AND C/EBP BINDING SITE

The nucleotide sequence of human *AGT* gene promoter from –203 to –226 containing A/G polymorphic site at –217 is shown in the top line of Fig. 2. It has homology with the C/EBP binding site (the consensus C/EBP binding site TT/GNNGCAAT/G is shown in the reverse orientation in line 2). The –217 polymorphic site is the first nucleotide of the consensus C/EBP site. In addition, a consensus GRE (third line) is present in this region of the promoter. The first nucleoside of the palindromic GRE corresponds to the polymorphic site –217 of the *AGT* gene promoter. It has been shown previously that GR cooperatively interacts with other transcription factors and this combinatorial interaction is involved in glucocorticoid induced promoter activity in PEPCK and TAT genes. It has also been shown that C/EBP-β and CREB can interact with GR and cooperatively increase the GR-induced promoter activity by cAMP.

In order to examine whether polymorphism at –217 affects the binding of transcription factors to this region of the promoter, we synthesized two oligonucleotides containing either nucleoside A or G at –217 position and used them in gel shift assays. Our gel shift analysis has suggested that the oligonucleotide containing nucleoside A at –217 binds more strongly to C/EBP family of transcription factors and GR as compared to the same oligonucleotide containing nucleoside G at this position *(41)*.

GLUCOCORTICOIDS AND C/EBP INCREASE THE PROMOTER ACTIVITY OF –217A VARIANT

In order to understand the physiological significance of the GR binding site at –217 region of the *hAGT* gene promoter, we synthesized reporter constructs where six copies each of either oligonucleotide 223A or 223G were attached in front of the pGL2-luc vector (obtained from Promega). These reporter constructs were transiently transfected in HepG2 cells in the presence of an expression vector that contained rat GR coding sequence. After transfection, cells were treated with 100 n*M* dexamethasone, and promoter activity was analyzed after 24 h. Results of this experiment showed that promoter activity of reporter construct containing –217A increased by about 18-fold over the basal value. On the other hand, promoter activity of reporter construct containing –217G increased only two- to threefold. Because PGC-1 acts as a coactivator and increases GR induced promoter activity, we also cotransfected an expression vector containing hPGC-1 in this experiment.

```
-226              -217                                               -195
C C C T G C A C C A/G G C T C A C T C T G T T C A G C A G T G A  A   AGT Gene
                                                                    Cons C/EBP
    C T TG C N  N C  A

        A   G  A A C A N N N T G T T C T                          Cons GRE
```

Nucleotide sequence homology between human AG gene promoter around nucleotide polymorphism A/G at -217 with consensus C/EBP and GR binding sites

Fig. 2. Nucleotide sequence homology between human *AG* gene promoter around nucleotide polymorphism A/G at –217 with consensus C/EBP and GR-binding sites.

Results of this experiment showed that PGC-1 further increased the GR induced promoter activity. The same results were obtained by transient transfection in other cells such as human embryonic kidney cells (HEK 293) and 3T3L1. Taken together, results of these experiments suggested that reporter a construct containing six copies of an oligonucleotide containing –217A has increased GR induced promoter activity as compared with the reporter construct containing six copies of an oligonucleotide containing 217G.

Because C/EBP-β and -δ play an important role in acute phase reaction, and *AGT* gene expression is upregulated during acute phase reaction, we were interested in studying the effect of these transcription factors in the expression of human *AGT* gene containing A/G polymorphic site at –217. Expression vectors containing the coding sequence of either C/EBP-β or C/EBP-δ were cotransfected with reporter constructs containing different regions of the human AGT gene linked to the luciferase gene containing either nucleoside A or G at –217 in HepG2 cells. Transfected cells were then treated with IL-6 and promoter activity was analyzed by luciferase assay. Results of cotransfection experiments with C/EBP-β show that reporter construct pHAGT1.3*luc* containing nucleoside A at –217 had 30% increased promoter activity and reporter construct pHAGT303*luc* containing nucleoside A at –217 had 43% increased promoter activity as compared with corresponding reporter constructs containing nucleoside G at –217. Similarly, results of co-transfection experiments with C/EBP-δ show that reporter construct pHAGT1.3*luc* containing nucleoside A at –217 has 17% increased promoter activity, reporter construct pHAGT303*luc* containing nucleoside A at –217 had 32% increased promoter activity as compared with corresponding reporter constructs containing nucleoside G at –217 *(41)*. It is possible that combinatorial interaction of C/EBP, GRE, and STAT-3 is involved in the induced expression of the human *AG* gene by the IL-6 pathway, and polymorphism at –217 may play an important role in this process.

ASSOCIATION OF VARIANT –217A WITH OTHER POLYMORPHIC SITES OF *AGT* GENE

Previous studies have identified seven polymorphic sites in the 1.2 Kb promoter of human *AGT* gene *(29)*. These polymorphic sites are A/G at –6, A/C at –20, C/T at –532, C/T at –776, G/A at –793, T/A at –830, and G/T at –1074, and are shown in Fig. 3. Jeunemaitra et al. *(29)* have shown that polymorphisms at –532, –793, and –1074 always occur together. Surprisingly, these authors did not find the A/G polymorphism at –217 in the AGT gene promoter. In order to understand the linkage disequilibrium of these polymorphic sites in African-American subjects, we have performed sequence analysis of DNA samples isolated from African-American subjects and have found that variant

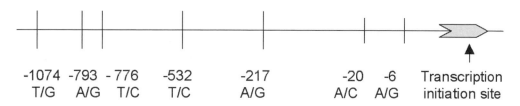

Fig. 3. Position of single nucleotide polymorphisms in the 1.2 kb promoter region of the human angiotensinogen gene.

-217A always occurs with –532T, –793A, and –1074G. The frequency of haplotype AA was 0.237 and that of haplotype AG was 0.086 in African-American subjects, which was statistically significant. This suggests that transcription factors binding to these sites in the AGT gene promoter may interact with each other and regulate the expression of this gene in subjects that contain allele –217A.

NUCLEOTIDE SEQUENCE AROUND –1074T OF *AGT* GENE HAS HOMOLOGY WITH HNF-3 BINDING SITE

The nucleotide sequence of *AGT* gene promoter around –1074 has partial sequence homology with the consensus HNF-3 binding site (Fig. 4). The nucleotide sequence of *AGT* gene with nucleoside G at –1074 has two mismatches with the consensus HNF-3 binding site, whereas the nucleotide sequence of *AGT* gene with nucleoside T at -1074 has one mismatch. Liver-enriched transcription factor HNF-3 belongs to the winged helix/forkhead family of transcription factors, which plays an important role in transcription of liver specific genes. Previous studies have suggested that HNF-3 acts as an accessory factor in GR-induced promoter activity of phosphoenolpyruvate carboxykinase (*PEPCK*) and *TAT* genes in the liver cells. Our unpublished data has shown that an oligonucleotide from this region of the promoter binds more strongly to HNF-3β when nucleoside T is present at –1074. It is tempting to speculate that increased binding of GR and C/EBPβ at -217A and increased binding of HNF-3β at –1074T is involved in increased expression of the *hAGT* gene in this haplotype.

HAPLOTYPE –6A: –217A: –1074 OF *AGT* GENE HAS INCREASED PROMOTER ACTIVITY

Because variant –217A always occurs in association with –532T, –793A, and –1074T, we were interested in examining whether *AGT* gene promoter containing this haplotype AA (containing nucleoside A at –6 and A at –217) has increased promoter activity as compared with the haplotype AG (containing nucleoside A at –6 and nucleoside G at –217). For this purpose, we amplified 1.3 Kb *AGT* gene promoter from a hypertensive and a normotensive subject. These amplified sequences contained –6A, –20A, –217A, –532T, –776T, –793A, and –1074T (haplotype AA) and –6A, –20A, –217G, –532C, –776T, –793G, and –1074G (haplotype AG). These amplified sequences were ligated in pGL3*luc* to produce reporter constructs containing these haplotypes. These reporter constructs were then used in transient transfections in HepG2, Hep3B, TPH, and differentiated and undifferentiated 3T3L1 cells. In all the cells, haplotype AA gave increased basal promoter activity as compared with haplotype AG. Because immortalized human liver cells are the closest representatives of the primary human liver cells, results of this experiment are

**Homology between nucleotide sequence around T/G polymorphic site
at -1074 of human AGT gene promoter with HNF-3 binding site**

T A T T T/G A/G T/C T T/C   CONS. HNF-3 SITE

T G T T T   G   T   T T/G   AGT GENE

Fig. 4. Homology between nucleotide sequence around T/G polymorphic site at –1074 of human AGT gene promoter with HNF-3 binding site

presented here. Reporter constructs (1 µg) and RSV-gal (50 ng) were cotransfected in TPH cells (400,000 cells per well) in triplicates using six-well plates in the presence of lipofectamine reagent (Qiagene). The promoter activity was analyzed after 48 h of transfection and normalized with the β-gal activity. Results of this experiment showed that the promoter activity of haplotype AA was 1.9-fold higher than that of haplotype AG.

TRANSGENIC MICE TO STUDY THE EFFECT OF POLYMORPHISMS OF *AGT* GENE IN VIVO

Transient transfection in cultured cells has provided important information about tissue-, hormonal-, and developmental-specific transcriptional regulation of a number of genes. However, such studies are often hampered by the limited selection and state of differentiation of cell lines used in transient transfection assay. For example, transcription rates of numerous liver-specific genes are greatly reduced in cultured hepatoma cells and primary hepatocytes. In many instances, cultured cells have lost functional hormone receptors (such as glucocorticoid, estrogen, and angiotensin-II receptors in HepG2 cells) and expression vectors containing coding region of these receptors have to be cotransfected to analyze the effect of a particular hormone. These experiments raise another serious problem—the number of transfected receptors may far exceed its physiological level in transfected cells, and may provide false information. Transgenic mice are at present the most rigorous system available for identifying and characterizing *cis*-acting DNA elements. In addition, transgene expression can be assessed in numerous cell types as well as during both embryonic and fetal development.

The transgenic-mice approach has been successfully used to identify *cis*-acting DNA elements involved in liver, kidney, and adipose-specific expression of the rat *PEPCK* gene *(59,60)*. These studies have also provided information about *cis*-acting DNA elements involved in developmental, glucocorticoid, and dietary-regulated expression of this gene. These transgenic experiments have complemented some of the results obtained by transient transfection assay in an in vivo setting. In some cases, mutations were made in selected *cis*-acting DNA elements and the effect of these mutations on tissue-specific expression of the mutated promoter was analyzed by the expression of transgene in mice *(60)*. In recent years, transgenic mice have been generated by the injection of fusion genes containing promoter sequences attached to the β-galactosidase gene. These transgenic mice provide a better colorimeteric assay to analyze the expression of transgene in different tissues. A fusion gene was synthesized by attaching the *lac Z* gene in front of a thymidine kinase promoter sequence attached to a NF-IL6 binding site. Transgenic mice containing this fusion gene were then used to study the effect of hypoxia in an in vivo situation. Results of these experiments indicated that expression of the fusion gene containing the NF-IL6 sequence was increased under hypoxic conditions as measured by the β-gal assay. On the other hand, transgenic mice containing a mutated NF-IL6 site did not show an increase in β-gal activity under hypoxic conditions *(61)*. In a similar way, cell-specific expression of the mouse glycoprotein hormone β-subunit gene was analyzed by *lac Z* gene expression of expression vectors containing a different region of its promoter in transgenic mice *(62)*.

One of the main problems in these transgenic studies is that transgene can integrate at different sites in the chromosome and, depending on the site of integration, promoter activity may vary from experiment to experiment. Another problem is that a different number of transgene copies may integrate in the genome of different mice and promoter activity may vary depending on the number of transgenes in a particular line. However, experiments with *PEPCK* gene have shown that promoter activity did not vary significantly as a result of the number of transgenes in different animals.

In order to overcome these limitations, Sigmund's group has developed another experimental model system to assess the physiological significance of the human *AGT* gene *(63)*. In this model, gene targeting at the HPRT locus was used to selectively target a single copy of the human AGT gene to a known site in the genome. They showed that insertion of the single copy transgene upstream of HPRT does not affect the overall tissue- and cell-specific expression or hormonal regulation of human AGT. This study provides an important proof-of-principle that the functional significance of allelic variation in human AGT can be assessed by examining mice carrying transgenes targeted in a single copy to an identical insertion site. They targeted the human *AGT* gene to the mouse HPRT locus by employing embryonic stem (ES) cells harboring a deletion in the endogenous *HPRT* gene, and a special targeting vector capable of restoring its full functionality upon homologous recombination. The use of gene targeting is essential in developing a model for studying effects of allelic gene variants in vivo because it nullifies the copy number and positional effects associated with transgene expression in transgenic mouse models generated by pronuclear injection. It allows reproducible insertion of the single copy of a transgene in a predetermined locus, permitting direct comparison with individually generated transgenic lines. Furthermore, independently derived transgenic mice generated by gene targeting are genetically identical, abolishing the need for multiple transgenic mouse lines harboring the same construct. An important practical benefit of their strategy is the highly reproducible efficiency in selecting single homologous recombination events. This is because, unlike the common approach to homologous recombination in which the targeting construct carries a positive selectable marker, the HPRT system carries sequences that can repair the deletion of HPRT found in the specific ES clone that is suitable for these studies. The selection for growth in HAT medium allows only targeted clones to survive, so all clones that survive selection have been targeted. This should allow for relatively easy development of a number of transgenic ES cell clones that harbor specific variants of a gene of interest, and the subsequent generation of transgenic mice.

However, there are certain potential drawbacks of using a nonnative locus, such as HPRT, for gene targeting. Exogenous genes may not harbor all of the sequences necessary and sufficient for proper regulation of expression and may therefore be influenced by *cis*-acting regulatory elements in the vicinity of the *HPRT* gene. However, previous studies by Sigmund's group have shown that the 13.8-kb genomic human AGT transgene is expressed in a tissue- and cell-specific and copy-number proportional fashion in transgenic mice, suggesting that all essential regulatory elements are present in the transgene. Another potential drawback of targeting the HPRT locus is that it is located on the X chromosome and the transgene expression is affected by random X inactivation. This means that one can effectively achieve an equivalent of 1°copy (in the case of male and homozygous transgenic female mice) or 0.5°copy (in the case of heterozygous transgenic female mice) transgene expression. Taken together, their data indicated that the human *AGT* gene was apparently unaffected by the HPRT locus. It exhibited correct tissue and cell specificity and was properly regulated by the changes in testosterone levels. Furthermore, the human AGT protein was normally processed, and its plasma concentration was proportional to the level of human AGT mRNA, indicating proper regulation. The protein in plasma is readily cleaved by human renin, resulting in the acute pressor response, which could be easily detected by changes in BP.

In a recent paper, this group has used this model to specifically test the physiological effects of variants at nucleoside –6 and amino acid 235 in the *AGT* gene in vivo *(40)*. For this purpose, they generated two different hAGT transgenes, representative of the two haplotypes observed in humans, by site-directed mutagenesis, and inserted both transgenes in a single copy at HPRT in the mouse genome. The identical genetic environment in both genetic background and transgene location allowed them to directly compare the transcriptional and functional activity of each haplotype and to link any significant difference in phenotype(s) to the sequence differences of the hAGT transgenes. The molecular analysis of the two hAGT haplotypes showed that variation at nucleotide –6 and amino acid 235 positions have no effect on the tissue- and cell-specific expression pattern in either males or females, and that both variants are transcribed with equal efficiency in liver, kidney, brain, and aorta. This result was unexpected, because previous reports indicated that the –6 variant affects baseline transcriptional efficiency both in vitro (in the context of a reporter construct), and in vitro, in that it may influence the steady-state level of AGT mRNA in the decidual spiral arteries of first trimester pregnant women. They have argued that there are several possibilities for this disparity. As was previously shown by the work in their laboratory, the *hAGT* gene can behave differently when studied in vitro and in vivo *(46)*. Whereas deletion mutations in the promoter and 3' enhancer of the *hAGT* gene were shown to have an obvious effect on the transcription of the gene in HepG2 cells, no effect on gene regulation was detected in vivo when these mutations were studied in transgenic mice. The reason for this remains elusive, although it is conceivable that the HepG2 cell culture model is lacking all of the factors involved in the normal regulation of the hAGT expression, because it is an immortalized cell line. It is also possible that the environment of a mouse cell does not allow for the effect of the hAGT variants to be revealed. This could result either from the absence of cellular factors that can recognize specific elements of the hAGT promoter, or the fact that those factors are significantly different from their human counterparts so that they cannot serve the same function.

It is important to recognize that Sigmund's group has specifically analyzed the effect of only one polymorphism, namely at –6 position, in the *hAGT* gene on its transcriptional regulation *(40)*. However, studies by Inoue et al. have shown the effect of only 256 bp of the 5'-flanking region of the human *AGT* gene on transient transfection in HepG2 cells. It is important to note that the effect of –6A variant was very small (only 14–19%) on transient transfection. It is possible that experiments using transgenic animals containing different haplotypes of the human *AGT* gene may provide meaningful results. It is also important to mention that in order to examine the effect of promoter variants of the *AGT* gene on the BP in transgenic animals, one has to use double transgenic mice containing human AGT, as well as human renin genes. Very little is known about the tissue-specific regulation of human renin gene expression and therefore, although these experiments are very interesting, there are many unsolved problems. In addition, mouse physiology may be different from the human physiology and this haplotype, though important in the regulation of BP in human subjects, may not show its effect in mice.

CONCLUSIONS AND PERSPECTIVES

Hypertension is a polygenic disease, and most probably multiple genes are involved in the etiology of this disease in different ethnic groups. Although initial studies, based on microsatellite markers, had shown that renin, ACE, and angiotensin receptor type 1 genes are not involved in hypertension, recent studies have suggested that certain polymorphic variants of renin and angiotensin receptor may be involved in human essential hypertension *(64)*. It is also important to mention that other genes such as adducin *(65)*, β2-adrenergic receptor *(66)*, and G protein β3 subunit *(67)* have also been suggested to be involved in human hypertension. It will be important to examine whether interaction of these genes leads to hypertension.

ACKNOWLEDGMENTS

Work in the author's laboratory was supported by NIH grants HL49884, HL59547, HL66296, and a grant from Philip Morris Inc.

REFERENCES

1. Luft FC. Hypertension as a complex genetic trait. Semin Nephrol 2002;22:115–126.
2. Lifton RP, Gharavi AG, Geller DS. Molecular mechanisms of human hypertension. Cell 2001;104:545–556.
3. Krushkal J, Ferrell R, Mockrin SC, Turner ST, Sing CF, Boerwinkle E. Genome-wide linkage analyses of systolic blood pressure using highly discordant siblings. Circulation1999;99:1407–1410.
4. Hunt SC, Ellison RC, Atwood LD, Pankow JS, Province MA, Leppert MF. Genome scans for blood pressure and hypertension: the National Heart, Lung, and Blood Institute Family Heart Study. Hypertension 2002;40:1–6.
5. Kristjansson K, Manolescu A, Kristinsson A, et al. Linkage of essential hypertension to chromosome 18q. Hypertension 2002;39:1044–1049.
6. Rice T, Rankinen T, Chagnon YC, et al. Genomewide linkage scan of resting blood pressure: HERITAGE Family Study. Health, Risk Factors, Exercise Training, and Genetics. Hypertension 2002;39:1037–1043.
7. Levy D, DeStefano AL, Larson MG, et al. Evidence for a gene influencing blood pressure on chromosome 17. Genome scan linkage results for longitudinal blood pressure phenotypes in subjects from the framingham heart study. Hypertension 2000;36:477–483.
8. Caulfield M, Munroe P, Pembroke J, et al. Genome-wide mapping of human loci for essential hypertension. Lancet 2003;361:2118–2123.
9. Kageyama R, Ohkubo H, Nakanishi S. Primary structure of human preangiotensinogen deduced from the cloned cDNA sequence. Biochemistry 1984;23:3603–3609.
10. Corvol P, Jeunemaitre X. Molecular genetics of human hypertension: role of angiotensinogen. Endocr Rev 1997;18:662–677.
11. Gould AB, Green D. Kinetics of the human renin and human substrate reaction. Cardiovasc Res 1971;5:86–89.
12. Fasola AF, Martz BL, Helmer OM. Renin activity during supine exercise in normotensives and hypertensives. J Appl Physiol 1966;21:1709–1712.

13. Watt GC, Harrap SB, Foy CJ, et al. Abnormalities of glucocorticoid metabolism and the renin- angiotensin system: a four-corners approach to the identification of genetic determinants of blood pressure. J Hypertens 1992;10:473–482.

14. Campbell DJ, Habener JF. Angiotensinogen gene is expressed and differentially regulated in multiple tissues of the rat. J Clin Invest 1986;78:31–39.

15. Tanimoto K, Sugiyama F, Goto Y, et al. Angiotensinogen-deficient mice with hypotension. J Biol Chem 1994;269:31334–31337.

16. Kim HS, Krege JH, Kluckman KD, et al. Genetic control of blood pressure and the angiotensinogen locus. Proc Natl Acad Sci USA 1995;92:2735–2739.

17. Krege JH, Kim HS, Moyer JS, et al. Angiotensin-converting enzyme gene mutations, blood pressures, and cardiovascular homeostasis. Hypertension 1997;29:150–157.

18. Gaillard I, Clauser E, Corvol P. Structure of human angiotensinogen gene. DNA 1989;8:87–99.

19. Jeunemaitre X, Soubrier F, Kotelevtsev YV, et al. Molecular basis of human hypertension: role of angiotensinogen. Cell 1992;71:169–180.

20. Jeunemaitre X, Rigat B, Charru A, Houot AM, Soubrier F, Corvol P. Sib pair linkage analysis of renin gene haplotypes in human essential hypertension. Hum Genet 1992;88:301–306.

21. Jeunemaitre X, Lifton RP, Hunt SC, Williams RR, Lalouel JM. Absence of linkage between the angiotensin converting enzyme locus and human essential hypertension. Nat Genet 1992;1:72–75.

22. Bonnardeaux A, Davies E, Jeunemaitre X, et al. Angiotensin II type 1 receptor gene polymorphisms in human essential hypertension. Hypertension 1994;24:63–69.

23. Caulfield M, Lavender P, Newell Price J, Kamdar S, Farrall M, Clark AJ. Angiotensinogen in human essential hypertension. Hypertension 1996;28:1123–1125.

24. Caulfield M, Lavender P, Newell Price J, et al. Linkage of the angiotensinogen gene locus to human essential hypertension in African Caribbeans. J Clin Invest 1995;96:687–692.

25. Schmidt S, Sharma AM, Zilch O, et al. Association of M235T variant of the angiotensinogen gene with familial hypertension of early onset. Nephrol Dial Transplant 1995;10:1145–1148.

26. Hingorani AD, Sharma P, Jia H, Hopper R, Brown MJ. Blood pressure and the M235T polymorphism of the angiotensinogen gene. Hypertension 1996;28:907–911.

27. Kiema TR, Kauma H, Rantala AO, et al. Variation at the angiotensin-converting enzyme gene and angiotensinogen gene loci in relation to blood pressure. Hypertension 1996;28:1070–1075.

28. Borecki IB, Province MA, Ludwig EH, et al. Associations of candidate loci angiotensinogen and angiotensin-converting enzyme with severe hypertension: The NHLBI Family Heart Study. Ann Epidemiol 1997;7:13–21.

29. Jeunemaitre X, Inoue I, Williams C, et al. Haplotypes of angiotensinogen in essential hypertension. Am J Hum Genet 1997;60:1448–1460.

30. Schunkert H, Hense HW, Gimenez-Roqueplo AP, et al. The angiotensinogen T235 variant and the use of antihypertensive drugs in a population-based cohort. Hypertension 1997;29:628–633.

31. Tiret L, Blanc H, Ruidavets JB, et al. Gene polymorphisms of the renin-angiotensin system in relation to hypertension and parental history of myocardial infarction and stroke: the PEGASE study. Projet d'Etude des Genes de l'Hypertension Arterielle Severe a moderee Essentielle. J Hypertens 1998;16:37–44.

32. Kunz R, Kreutz R, Beige J, Distler A, Sharma AM. Association between the angiotensinogen 235T-variant and essential hypertension in whites: a systematic review and methodological appraisal. Hypertension 1997;30:1331–1337.

33. Hata A, Namikawa C, Sasaki M, et al. Angiotensinogen as a risk factor for essential hypertension in Japan. J Clin Invest 1994;93:1285–1287.

34. Kamitani A, Rakugi H, Higaki J, et al. Association analysis of a polymorphism of the angiotensinogen gene with essential hypertension in Japanese. J Hum Hypertens 1994;8:521–524.

35. Iwai N, Shimoike H, Ohmichi N, Kinoshita M. Angiotensinogen gene and blood pressure in the Japanese population. Hypertension 1995;25:688–693.

36. Ishigami T, Umemura S, Tamura K, et al. Essential hypertension and 5' upstream core promoter region of human angiotensinogen gene. Hypertension 1997;30:1325–1330.

37. Bloem LJ, Foroud TM, Ambrosius WT, Hanna MP, Tewksbury DA, Pratt JH. Association of the angiotensinogen gene to serum angiotensinogen in blacks and whites. Hypertension 1997;29:1078–1082.

38. Larson N, Hutchinson R, Boerwinkle E. Lack of association of 3 functional gene variants with hypertension in African Americans. Hypertension 2000;35:1297–1300.

39. Inoue I, Nakajima T, Williams CS, et al. A nucleotide substitution in the promoter of human angiotensinogen is associated with essential hypertension and affects basal transcription in vitro. J Clin Invest 1997;99:1786–1797.

40. Cvetkovic B, Keen HL, Zhang X, Davis D, Yang B, Sigmund CD. Physiological significance of two common haplotypes of human angiotensinogen using gene targeting in the mouse. Physiol Genomics 2002;11:253–262.

41. Jain S, Tang X, Narayanan CS, et al. Angiotensinogen gene polymorphism at –217 affects basal promoter activity and is associated with hypertension in African-Americans. J Biol Chem 2002;277:36889–36896.

42. Choy B, Roberts SG, Griffin LA, Green MR. How eukaryotic transcription activators increase assembly of preinitiation complexes. Cold Spring Harb Symp Quant Biol 1993;58:199–203.

43. Choy B, Green MR. Eukaryotic activators function during multiple steps of preinitiation complex assembly. Nature 1993;366:531–536.

44. Ptashne M. 1997 Albert Lasker Award for Basic Medical Research. Control of gene transcription: an outline. Nat Med 1997;3:1069–1072.

45. Rosenfeld MG, Glass CK. Coregulator codes of transcriptional regulation by nuclear receptors. J Biol Chem 2001;276:36,865–36,868.

46. Glass CK, Rosenfeld MG. The coregulator exchange in transcriptional functions of nuclear receptors. Genes Dev 2000;14:121–141.

47. LeVan TD, Bloom JW, Bailey TJ, et al. A common single nucleotide polymorphism in the CD14 promoter decreases the affinity of Sp protein binding and enhances transcriptional activity. J Immunol 2001;167:5838–5844.

48. Spek CA, Greengard JS, Griffin JH, Bertina RM, Reitsma PH. Two mutations in the promoter region of the human protein C gene both cause type I protein C deficiency by disruption of two HNF-3 binding sites. J Biol Chem 1995;270:24,216–24,221.

49. Farzaneh-Far A, Davies JD, Braam LA, et al. A polymorphism of the human matrix gamma-carboxyglutamic acid protein promoter alters binding of an activating protein-1 complex and is associated with altered transcription and serum levels. J Biol Chem 2001;276:32466–32473.

50. Narayanan CS, Cui Y, Kumar A. DBP binds to the proximal promoter and regulates liver-specific expression of the human angiotensinogen gene. Biochem Biophys Res Commun 1998;251:388–393.

51. Zhao YY, Zhou J, Narayanan CS, Cui Y, Kumar A. Role of C/A polymorphism at –20 on the expression of human angiotensinogen gene. Hypertension 1999;33:108–115.

52. Narayanan CS, Cui Y, Zhao YY, Zhou J, Kumar A. Orphan receptor Arp-1 binds to the nucleotide sequence located between TATA box and transcriptional initiation site of the human angiotensinogen gene and reduces estrogen induced promoter activity. Mol Cell Endocrinol 1999;148:79–86.

53. Yanai K, Nibu Y, Murakami K, Fukamizu A. A cis-acting DNA element located between TATA box and transcription initiation site is critical in response to regulatory sequences in human angiotensinogen gene. J Biol Chem 1996;271:15981–15986.

54. Cui Y, Narayanan CS, Zhou J, Kumar A. Exon-I is involved in positive as well as negative regulation of human angiotensinogen gene expression. Gene 1998;224:97–107.

55. Sherman CT, Brasier AR. Role of Signal Transducers and Activators of Transcription 1 and -3 in Inducible Regulation of the Human Angiotensinogen Gene by Interleukin-6. Mol Endocrinol 2001;15:441–457.

56. Narayanan CS, Cui Y, Kumar S, Kumar A. cAMP increases the expression of human angiotensinogen gene through a combination of cyclic AMP responsive element binding protein and a liver specific transcription factor. Mol Cell Biochem 2000;212:81–90.

57. Yanai K, Hirota K, Taniguchi-Yanai K, et al. Regulated expression of human angiotensinogen gene by hepatocyte nuclear factor 4 and chicken ovalbumin upstream promoter-transcription factor [In Process Citation]. J Biol Chem 1999;274:34,605–34,612.

58. Brasier AR, Han Y, Sherman CT. Transcriptional regulation of angiotensinogen gene expression. Vitam Horm 1999;57:217–247.

59. Short MK, Clouthier DE, Schaefer IM, Hammer RE, Magnuson MA, Beale EG. Tissue-specific, developmental, hormonal, and dietary regulation of rat phosphoenolpyruvate carboxykinase-human growth hormone fusion genes in transgenic mice. Mol Cell Biol 1992;12:1007–1020.

60. Patel YM, Yun JS, Liu J, McGrane MM, Hanson RW. An analysis of regulatory elements in the phosphoenolpyruvate carboxykinase (GTP) gene which are responsible for its tissue-specific expression and metabolic control in transgenic mice. J Biol Chem 1994;269:5619–5628.

61. Yan SF, Zou YS, Mendelsohn M, et al. Nuclear factor interleukin 6 motifs mediate tissue-specific gene transcription in hypoxia. J Biol Chem 1997;272:4287–4294.
62. Brinkmeier ML, Gordon DF, Dowding JM, et al. Cell-specific expression of the mouse glycoprotein hormone alpha-subunit gene requires multiple interacting DNA elements in transgenic mice and cultured cells. Mol Endocrinol 1998;12:622–633.
63. Cvetkovic B, Yang B, Williamson RA, Sigmund CD. Appropriate tissue- and cell-specific expression of a single copy human angiotensinogen transgene specifically targeted upstream of the HPRT locus by homologous recombination. J Biol Chem 2000;275:1073–1078.
64. Zhu X, Chang YP, Yan D, et al. Associations between hypertension and genes in the renin-angiotensin system. Hypertension 2003;41:1027–1034.
65. Casari G, Barlassina C, Cusi D, et al. Association of the alpha-adducin locus with essential hypertension. Hypertension 1995;25:320–326.
66. Bray MS, Krushkal J, Li L, et al. Positional genomic analysis identifies the beta(2)-adrenergic receptor gene as a susceptibility locus for human hypertension. Circulation 2000;101:2877–2882.
67. Dong Y, Zhu H, Sagnella GA, et al. Association between the C825T polymorphism of the G protein beta3-subunit gene and hypertension in blacks. Hypertension 1999;34:1193–1196.

3

Substitution Mapping

Using Congenic Strains to Detect Genes Controlling Blood Pressure

Bina Joe, PhD
and Michael R. Garrett, MS, MBA

CONTENTS

SUMMARY

Changes in blood pressure (BP) from low to high, are genetically controlled by many genes. Identifying genes that regulate BP is important for two major reasons: (1) for delineating the biochemical/physiological mechanisms for BP control; and (2) for utilizing this knowledge to improve clinical management strategies for maintenance of normal physiological BP, which is an important factor in reducing the risk for susceptibility to cardiovascular diseases.

Genetic approaches to identify BP regulatory genes involve the use of rat models with elevated BP (hypertension). Typically, genetic linkage analyses and substitution mapping using congenic strains are performed. These studies are designed to enable the identification of BP regulatory genes primarily by virtue of their location on the rat genome. This chapter captures the current status of studies aimed at identifying BP causative genes using various congenic rat strains.

Key Words: Hypertension; genetic; rat; animal model; QTL; cardiovascular; renal; disease causative genes.

INTRODUCTION

Monogenic vs Polygenic Diseases

Depending on the number of genes that are responsible for causing disturbances in normal physiology, diseases can be classified as being (1) monogenic, i.e., caused by a

From: *Contemporary Cardiology: Cardiovascular Genomics*
Edited by: M. K. Raizada, et al. © Humana Press Inc., Totowa, NJ

single gene; or (2) polygenic, i.e., caused by many genes. An important aspect of molecular genetics involves the identification of genes causing disease irrespective of whether they are monogenic or polygenic. The first step in discovering disease causative genes involves mapping the gene precisely to a small chromosomal interval. Mapping genes causing monogenic diseases is easier than mapping genes causing polygenic diseases because of the strong correlation between phenotype and genotype. Single recombinants are sufficient to define minimal chromosomal intervals (where the causative gene resides) to less than 1 centimorgan (cM). As a result, discovery of DNA sequence variants that are found only in one of a small number of candidate genes in affected subjects usually provides adequate evidence to establish identity of the disease-causing gene. This technique has been successfully used for gene identification of many monogenic diseases in humans. These are compiled at the following website: http://www.ncbi.nlm.nih.gov/books/bv.fcgi?call=bv.View..ShowSection&rid=gnd; additional information is also available at http://www.ncbi.nlm.nih.gov/entrez/query.fcgi?db=OMIM.

Discovering genes that cause polygenic diseases involves basically the same strategy as for monogenic disorders, but it is not as straightforward (1). When many genes control a single trait, the phenotype–genotype correlations at a gene locus are not nearly as strong as they are for monogenic diseases. This is because a single locus does not define the polygenic trait, but rather it is the net effect over multiple loci, which defines the trait. Moreover, finding genes causing polygenic diseases in humans is further confounded by a variety of factors such as gene–gene interactions, gene–environment interactions, genetic heterogeneity among populations, and incomplete disease penetrance. Considering these complexities combined with the difficulty associated with finding causative genes for polygenic traits, it is a generally well-accepted norm to add the word "complex" as a prefix when referring to polygenic traits/diseases. To date, only a handful of causative genes for complex polygenic diseases have been identified (2,3).

Using Rat Models for Understanding the Genetic Basis of Blood Pressure Regulation

Blood pressure (BP) in humans and rodents is well-recognized as a "quantitative trait" (i.e., variable from low to high) under polygenic control (i.e., controlled by many genes) (4). High BP (hypertension) is an undesirable trait because it is a major risk factor for cardiovascular and renal diseases. The expected result from finding and characterizing the genes that control BP is the gaining of insights into the etiology of hypertension. Several of the complications (such as those listed in the previous paragraph) that are associated with genetic studies of BP in humans are reduced to a large extent in well-defined experimental animal models of hypertension, which therefore serve as useful alternates for the genetic analysis of BP in humans.

Inbred strains of hypertensive rats are used as genetic models to identify genes that control BP. These include the Dahl salt-sensitive (S) rat, the spontaneously hypertensive rat (SHR), stroke-prone SHR (SHRSP), Milan hypertensive strain (MHS), genetically hypertensive (GH) rat, Sabra DOCA salt-sensitive (SBH) rat, Lyon hypertensive (LH) rat, Fawn-hooded hypertensive (FHH) rat, inherited stress-induced arterial hypertension (ISIAH) rat, albino surgery (AS) rat, and the Prague hypertensive rat (PHR) (5). Each of these rat strains represents an individual genetic pool of naturally occurring alleles that account for an overall phenotype of high BP. Determining the identity of each of these BP-increasing alleles is important in order to understand the molecular underpinnings of

BP regulation. Genetic experiments to do so involve mapping the location of the BP causative genes on the rat genome with progressively improving resolution. These experiments are detailed in the following stages.

Stage 1: Genetic Linkage Analysis

The first stage is to establish statistically significant genome-wide evidence for linkage of large regions of the genome to BP. Genomic regions identified to contain genes that regulate a quantitative trait such as BP are called quantitative trait loci (QTL). BP QTL can be identified by whole-genome genetic linkage analysis in segregated populations of hypertensive and relatively normotensive rats. Using this approach, information on chromosomal location, the magnitude of the BP effect, and the mode of inheritance of each causative locus can be obtained. It was, however, not until 1991 that the first full genome scans for BP QTL were done by Hilbert et al. *(6)* and Jacob et al. *(7)* using microsatellite markers on the same F2 population derived from hypertensive SHRSP rats and Wistar Kyoto (WKY) rats. Subsequently, multiple genetic linkage analyses have been performed using various hypertensive-inbred strains. Results from these studies indicate that there are BP QTL widely distributed throughout the rat genome, as is summarized at the following website: http://rgd.mcw.edu/qtls/. Figure 1 summarizes the numbers of articles on QTL that control BP and related phenotypes, sorted by their location on the rat genome by chromosome. The largest number of genetic linkage analyses performed on any single cardiovascular trait in rats is systolic BP. Note in Fig. 1 that every rat chromosome has been reported to contain a BP QTL.

Stage 2: Substitution Mapping

Linkage analysis results in the identification of genomic regions in the range of 10–30 cM. A genetic interval of this size typically corresponds in humans and rodents to 10–30 Mb of DNA, or approx 100 to 300 genes *(1)*, which is far too many candidates to begin functional evaluation of each gene individually. Thus, initial low-resolution linkage studies typically establish the map location to a resolution that is sufficiently precise to justify studies to confirm and define the genomic interval. In rodent model systems, this can be done with the use of consomic strains *(8,9)* and/or congenic strains *(10)*. The use of consomic or congenic strains to confirm and define a QTL is known as substitution mapping. Congenic strains were first utilized by Snell *(11)*. Developing congenic strains involves substituting a segment of chromosome, or in the case of a consomic, the entire chromosome, from one inbred strain (the donor strain) into another inbred strain (the recipient strain). This is done by crossing the donor and recipient strains to produce F1 animals, and then crossing F1 to recipient (first backcross). The offspring of this first backcross are genotyped using tail biopsy DNA for markers across a putative QTL containing region of a chromosome. Because chromosomal crossovers will occur between the donor and recipient chromosomes in the meioses of the F1 animal, recombinant chromosomes will be found in some of the offspring. This means that an animal with a specified donor chromosomal segment can easily be found. Such (heterozygous) offspring are backcrossed again to the recipient strain, and the offspring carrying the specific donor chromosomal segment are again selected. According to the classical approach, this procedure is repeated at least eight times. At each backcross, half of the unlinked heterozygous loci outside the selected (congenic) region become homozygous for the recipient allele; that is, the genetic background progressively becomes that of the recipient strain. After eight backcrosses, rats are selectively bred to fix the donor chromosomal

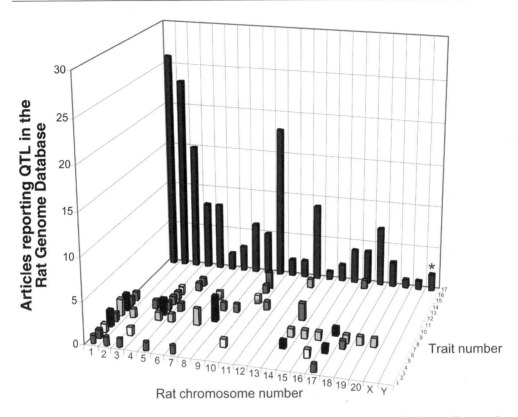

Fig. 1. Quantitative trait loci (QTL) for cardiovascular and related traits. QTL for cardiovascular and related traits that are cataloged by the rat genome database (RGD)(http://rgd.mcw.edu/) were searched in November 2003 and are plotted here against the rat chromosome number on which they are located. Bars represent the number of articles reporting QTL listed for each individual trait. * Refers to refs. *(83,84)* that identified blood pressure (BP) QTL on the Y chromosome, which are not curated in the RGD. The 17 traits listed from the front row (foreground) to the back row are as follows: (1) left-ventricular mass; (2) mean arterial pressure; (3) renal damage; (4) renal disease; (5) aldosterone levels; (6) serum cholesterol levels; (7) serum triglyceride levels; (8) sensitivity to stroke; (9) obesity; (10) serum phospholipid levels; (11) hypercalcinurea; (12) atrial natriuretic peptide concentration; (13) vascular elastic tissue fragility; (14) cardiac mass; (15) proteinuria; (16) hypoxia-induced right ventricular hypertrophy; and (17) systolic BP (the tallest bars are on the back row).

segment in the homozygous state on the background of the recipient strain, producing a congenic strain. Congenic strains are indicated by the following notation: "Recipient strain. Donor strain," wherein, "recipient strain" is the strain to whose genome a known genomic region from the "donor strain" is introgressed. For example, S.LEW refers to the introgression of a segment of LEW rats into the S-rat genetic background.

Recently, a technique called marker-assisted selection, or "speed congenics," has enabled the development of a congenic strain using only 4–5 backcrosses *(12–14)*. This technique involves selecting for the genome of the "donor" strain at the targeted chromosomal region, while simultaneously selecting against retention of the "donor" genome outside of the targeted chromosomal region using microsatellite markers throughout the genome.

There have been extensive linkage analyses performed in order to understand the genetic components of BP regulation, and for many of these studies congenic strains have also been developed to confirm and define the QTL *(2,12,15–40)*. The origins and progress of most, if not all, of these studies were extensively reviewed by Rapp in 2000 *(5)*. The present report focuses on progress during the last 3 yr that has been accomplished using substitution mapping as an approach to finding BP-altering genes.

RESULTS

Note: Data for all the studies reviewed in this article are compiled in Table 1. For clarity of presentation, these results are categorized based on rat chromosome number. Data on congenic strains are emphasized.

Chromosome 1

Initial observations with multiple genetic linkage analyses and subsequent substitution mapping approaches indicated the presence of at least one chromosomal region on rat chromosome (RNO)1 that influenced BP *(5)*. Further substitution mapping from several groups over the past 3 yr revealed that RNO1 contains multiple BP QTL. Congenic substrains with relatively small regions of RNO1 have been developed and tested. These congenic strains include the transfer of Sabra hypertension-prone rat (SBH/y) into Sabra hypertension-resistant rat (SBN/y) and vice versa *(32)*, Brown Norway (BN) into SHR *(22)*, LEW into S *(17,21,27,41)*, SHRSP into WKY *(33)*, SHR into WKY *(35)*, WKY/Izm into SHRSP/Izm *(36)*, and SHRSP/Izm to WKY/Izm *(37)* (Table 1). The locations of all the BP QTL that are confirmed by these substitution mapping studies are presented in Fig. 2A. It is evident from Figure 2A that these studies vary widely in terms of the resolution to which the locations of BP QTL have been determined. For example, Fig. 2A studies 1–4 have reported the localization of BP QTL to be within small regions from 2 to 20 Mb, whereas the majority of the other BP QTL represented in Fig. 2A are within large genomic regions of greater than 125 Mb. Of notable interest is also the fact that several of the BP QTL localized by these studies, with the exception of studies 1 and 6 (Fig. 2A), are clustered around the region of approx 100–225 Mb on RNO1. The present localization of BP QTL on RNO1 from multiple animal models is not sufficient to determine if allelic forms of the same gene(s) underlie the BP QTL found in each of the models.

Chromosome 2

Following several linkage analyses using multiple F2 populations (reviewed in ref. *5*), congenic strains introgressing the low BP QTL alleles from WKY or MNS into the S rat proved the existence of a substantial BP effector QTL on RNO2 *(40)*. The congenic strain with the WKY donor was further genetically dissected by substitution mapping and reported to be clearly comprised of two BP QTL, QTL1 and QTL2 *(29)*. These QTL are represented in Fig. 2B, studies 1 and 2. A third BP QTL called QTL3 was also suggested to be in the region represented in Fig. 2B, study 3 *(29)*. However, experimental evidence for this QTL was weak *(29)*. A congenic strain with the MNS donor on the S background localized a BP QTL to a 15-cM region *(25)*. This BP QTL region is shown in Fig. 2B, study 4. In a second article published by the same group *(42)*, the BP QTL was further localized to a 5.7-cM region on RNO2.

Table 1

Status of Substitution Mapping for Blood Pressure Loci Using Congenic Strains

RNO no.	QTL study number	"From" marker	"To" Marker	Cytogenetic location of QTL	Name of the BP QTL	Congenic strain (Recipient.donor)	Reference
1	1	D1Rat211	D1Rat12	1p11	QTL2 region	S.LEW	41
1	2	D1Mgh7	D1Mco36	1q22	QTL1a region	S.LEW	27
1	3	D1Rat35	D1Rat131	1q22–32	QTL1b region	S.LEW	27
1	4	D1Wox34	D1Rat55	1q32–36	QTL1	SISA1	34
1	5	D1Rat56	D1Rat111	1q36–41	QTL2	WISA1	34
1	6	D1Rat10	D1Rat24	1p11–q12	SS1a	SBH.SBN	32
1	7	D1Rat27	D1Rat74	1q22–43	SS1b	SBH.SBN	32
1	8	D1Rat29	D1Rat57	1q22–q36	No name	WKY-1.SHRSP	33
1	9	D1Rat38	Mtpa	1q32–41	No name	WKY.SHR	35
1	10	D1Rat68	D1Rat71	1q41–43	No name	SHR.BN	22
1	11	D1Wox18	D1Wox10	1q22–43	No name	SHRSP/Izm.WKY/Izm	36
1	12	D1Wox18	D1Smu11	1q22–34	No name	WKY/Izm.SHRSP/Izm	37
1	13	D1Rat29	D1Rat57	1q22–43	No name	WKY.SHRSP	74
2	1	D2Rat35	D2Wox18	2q32	qtl1	S.WKY	29
2	2	D2Wox18	D2Wox25	2q34	qtl2	S.WKY	29
2	3	D2Wox25	D2Rat259	2q34	qtl3?	S.WKY	29
2	4	D2Rat166	D2Mgh10	2q32–34	no name	S.MNS	25
2	5	D2Rat21	D2Rat27	2q22	pBP1 QTL	WKY/lj.SHR/lj	43
2	6	D2Mgh10	D2Rat62	2q34–q43	pBP2 QTL	WKY/lj.SHR/lj	43
2	7	D2Rat40	D2Rat50	2q26	pBP3 QTL	SHR/lj.WKY/lj	43
2	8	D2Rat161	D2Mgh10	2q26–q34	dBPQTL	SHR/lj.WKY/lj	43
2	9	D2Rat171	D2Arb24	2q24–42	no name	SHR.BN	38
2	10	D2Rat43	D2Mgh12	2q32–34	no name	SHRSP.WKY	44
3	1	D3Mco19	D3Mco24	3q42	minus BP QTL	S.R	19
3	2	D3Rat52	D3Rat130	3q12	minus BP QTL	S.LEW	56

(continued)

Chromosome	Study number	From	To	Cytogenetic location	BP QTL	Strain	Reference
3	3	D3Chm63	D3Rat26	3q24	plus BP QTL	S.LEW	56
5	1	D5Uwm31	D5Rjr1	5q34	qtl1	S.LEW	30
5	2	D5Rat154	D5Wox39	5q32	qtl2	S.LEW	30
5	3	D5Wox20	D5Rat63	5q32–36	no name	SHR.BN	28
7	1	D7Mco19	D7Mco7	7q34	no name	S.R	31
8	1	Rbp2	D8Mit6	8q11–24	no name	SHR.BN-Lx	39
9	1	D9Mco14	D9Uia6	9q32–34	no name	S.R	68
10	1	D10Mco1	D10Wox23	10q26	qtl1	S.MNS and S.LEW	26
10	2	D10Mit1	D10Mco6	10q32.1	qtl2	S.MNS	26
10	3	D10Mit11Mit119	D10Rat27	10q26	qtl1	S.LEW	69
10	4	D10Rat204	D10Rat9	10q32.1	qtl2	S.LEW	69
10	5	D10Rat27	D10Rat93	10q26	qtl3	S.LEW	69
10	6	Myhse	D10Mit11	10q24–q32.1	BP/SP-1b	WKY.SHRSP	73
10	7	Myh3	Aldoc	10q24	BP/SP-1a	WKY.SHRSP	74
13	1	Consomic	Consomic	Not applicable	No name	S.BN	75
16	1	D16Rat21	D16Rat88	16p16	No name	S.LEW	76
19	1	D19Rat57	D19Mit7	19q12	SHR.BN-Agt	SHR.BN	78
20	1	D20Cebr215s7	D20Rat23	20p12	No name	SHR.1N	79
X	1	Ar-Mycs/Pfkb1	DXMgh3	Xp14–22	No name	BB/OK.SHR	80
Y	1	Consomic	Consomic	Not applicable	No name	SHR.BN	83
2	2	Consomic	Consomic	Not applicable	No name	SHRSP.WKY and WKY.SHRSP	84

BP quantitative trait loci (QTL) that are reported in the literature are organized in this table by their location on the rat genome by chromosome. For clarity of presentation, a study number identifies each BP QTL. "From" marker indicates the marker that defines the p terminal end of the BP QTL region. "To" marker indicates the marker that defines the q terminal end of the BP QTL region. The cytogenetic location of each BP QTL was obtained by BLAST searching the rat genome using the "From" marker and the "To" marker at the website: http://www.ensembl.org/Rattus_norvegicus/. Whenever the markers were not listed at this website, alternate markers at the closest position on the radiation hybrid map were obtained from http://rgd.mcw.edu/ and used instead for the BLAST search. The name of the BP QTL is entered as reported from the corresponding articles listed in the last column. A congenic strain is represented by names of two strains separated by a period. The recipient strain is the one to the left of the period, and the donor strain from which alleles are introgressed into the recipient genome background is shown to the right of the period.

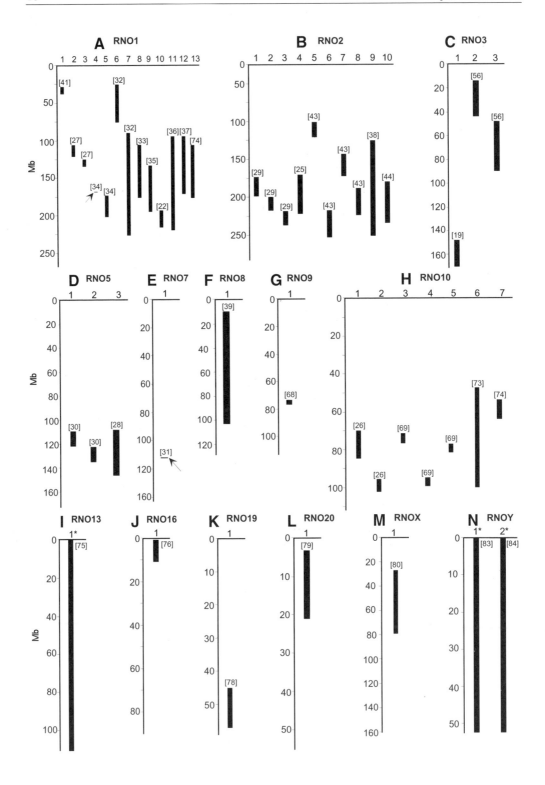

Fig. 2

BP QTL have also been localized on RNO2 using SHR as one of the parental strains. These earlier reports are reviewed elsewhere *(5)*. More recently, Alemayehu and coworkers constructed and studied reciprocal congenic strains using SHR and WKY rats *(43)*. This study resulted in the identification of at least four independent BP QTL *(43)*. The locations of these BP QTL are shown on the physical map of RNO2 (Fig. 2B, studies 5–8). SHR alleles at three of the BP QTL shown in Fig. 2B, studies 5, 6, and 7, increase BP, whereas SHR alleles at the BP QTL shown in Fig. 2B, study 8, decrease BP. Alleles of BN rats from RNO2 introgressed into SHR to derive SHR.BN congenics are also reported to lower BP *(38)*. As seen in Fig. 2B, study 9, the BP QTL detected in this study using SHR.BN congenic strain is large, and overlaps with most of the BP QTL localized by other substitution mapping studies. Taken together, all these results indicate that, like on RNO1, RNO2 is also rich in BP regulatory genes.

In addition to substitution mapping, McBride et al. have reported a study wherein they used microarray gene expression analysis as a complementary technique to detect superior candidate genes from among all the candidate genes within the BP QTL region *(44)* (Fig. 2B, study 10). Their study was aimed at identifying the gene(s) underlying the BP QTL on RNO2 that was previously defined by substitution mapping using SHRSP.WKY congenic strains *(12,45)*. Genome-wide microarray expression profiling was undertaken to identify differentially expressed genes among the parental SHRSP, WKY, and SHRSP.WKY congenic rats. A significant reduction in expression of glutathione S-transferase type 1 (*Gstm1*), a gene involved in the defense against oxidative stress, was observed *(44)*. More importantly, however, Gstm1 mapped within the BP QTL region on RNO2. In the SHRSP rat, endothelial dysfunction has been attributed to increased generation of superoxide anions, which in turn leads to vascular oxidative stress *(46–48)*. Induction of chronic oxidative stress by glutathione depletion can cause severe hypertension in normotensive rats *(49)*. Based on these data the authors have concluded that *Gstm1* is a positional and physiological candidate gene for the BP QTL on RNO2 *(44)*.

Fig. 2. *(continued from facing page)* Schematic representation of locations of blood pressure (BP) QTL on the rat genome that are defined using congenic strains. Data presented in this figure are organized by rat chromosome numbers, i.e., each panel represents the BP QTL defined on one rat chromosome. The *y*-axis for each panel represents the length of the corresponding rat chromosome in megabases (Mb). The length of the rat Y chromosome was not available. Therefore, it was calculated based on the relative length of the human Y chromosome to the human X chromosome. Numbers denoted on the top of the figure represent study numbers assigned to each BP QTL in Table 1. Bars represent the locations of BP QTL that are defined by the "From" marker and "To" marker represented in Table 1. The locations of each of these markers on the physical map of the rat genome (v. 18.3.1; 4 November 2003) were determined by BLAST searching the Ensembl website (http://www.ensembl.org/Rattus_norvegicus/) in November 2003. Whenever the markers were not listed at this website, alternate markers at the closest position on the radiation hybrid map were obtained from http://rgd.mcw.edu/ and used instead for the BLAST search. Number in paranthesis on the top (or, in some cases, alongside) of each bar represents the number of the cited reference. Arrows in panels **(A)** and **(E)** represent BP QTL that have been localized to relatively small genomic intervals of less than 2Mb and 177kb, respectively. * Indicates the study wherein a consomic strain is reported; microsatellite markers used to derive this consomic strain are not mentioned.

Chromosome 3

BP QTL on RNO3 are reported by multiple genetic linkage analyses *(17,19,50–55)*. In 1999, Cicila et al. reported an S.R congenic strain that successfully "trapped" a BP QTL *(19)*. As shown in Fig. 2C, study 1, this QTL on RNO3 is located toward the distal end of RNO3. However, it is only recently that Palijan et al. *(56)* constructed and studied multiple S.LEW congenic strains spanning the proximal region of RNO3, and reported that the proximal region of RNO3 contains a BP QTL (Fig. 2C, study 2) wherein alleles from the LEW rat lowered BP *(56)*. In addition to these two BP QTL, a third BP QTL located towards the middle region of RNO3 (Fig. 2C, study 3) was also identified *(56)*. The BP-enhancing effect of LEW alleles at this QTL was identified in S.LEW congenic rats, thereby demonstrating the utility of congenic strains for dissection and detection of closely linked alleles with opposing effects on BP.

Chromosome 4

Linkage analyses for BP identified QTL on RNO4 *(57–60)*. A congenic strain containing a 12-cM region from the SHR rat introgressed into the BB/OK rat is also reported on chromosome 4 *(61)*. Although these congenics provided strong evidence for the presence of genes on RNO4 involved in obesity and related phenotypes, the mean and diastolic BP of this congenic strain were not different from those in the parental BB/OK rat. Therefore, the existence of a BP QTL on RNO4 could not be confirmed using the BB.SHR congenic strain.

Chromosome 5

Garrett and Rapp *(30)* have developed and tested multiple S.LEW congenic strains on RNO5 and concluded that there are two closely linked interactive BP QTL on RNO5 (Fig. 2D, studies 1 and 2). The QTL was found to be interactive because strains with congenic segments that contained only QTL1 or QTL2 did not show a BP effect, but strains with congenic segments that contained both QTL did show a significant BP effect. BP QTL on RNO5 has also been localized using a SHR.BN congenic strain (Fig. 2D, study 3) *(28)*. As seen in Fig. 2D, this BP QTL spans a large genomic interval that overlaps with both the QTL identified by Garrett and Rapp *(30)* using S.LEW congenic strains. It remains to be seen, however, whether the BP QTL colocalized to this region using SHR.BN congenic strain (Fig. 2D, study 3) is similarly comprised of multiple BP QTL that may interact.

Chromosome 6

No congenic strains for BP are reported on chromosome 6.

Chromosome 7

Substitution mapping for BP QTL on RNO7 *(23,31)* has historical significance for two reasons. First, unlike the other BP QTL that remain unidentified to date, the BP causative gene on RNO7 was suggested as early as the 1970s to be the steroid biosynthetic enzyme 11-β hydroxylase *(62)*. Substitution mapping pursued for the BP QTL on RNO7 can therefore be viewed as "a proof-of-principle" of the approach *per se*, as well as the actual identification of the BP causative gene. Secondly, the introgressed region (177kb) of the S.R causative gene constructed to define the BP QTL on RNO7 represents one of the best "minimal" congenic strains ever constructed to date using rats (Fig. 2E) *(31)*. This study therefore demonstrates that substitution mapping can indeed achieve the limit of resolution required to identify a candidate BP causative gene as one among five or six genes. As a result of compelling evidence supported by coding sequence mutations *(23,63)*, and by functional studies on 11-β hydroxylase *(62,64,65)*, it was concluded that the gene responsible for the observed BP QTL on RNO7 in S rats is indeed 11-β hydroxylase.

Chromosome 8

Several independent genetic linkage studies provide suggestive evidence for BP QTL on RNO8. These have been reviewed previously *(5)*. Two recent genetic linkage analyses using F2 (S × SHR) and F2 (S × AS) populations also indicate BP QTL on RNO8 *(52,60)*. To date, very little progress has been made toward confirming and dissecting these BP QTL using substitution mapping. There has been one report of an SHR.Lx (Lx = BN.Lx/Cub) congenic strain that has successfully "trapped" a BP QTL in the region indicated in Fig. 2F *(39)*.

Chromosome 9

Genetic linkage analyses using F2 populations derived from (SHR × WKY), (S × R), and (S × SHR) rats independently detected BP QTL on RNO9 *(52,55,66,67)*. However, only the study involving the S and R has reported the confirmation of the BP QTL using S.R congenic strains *(67)*. A recent study *(68)* has further localized this BP QTL to be within a relatively smaller genomic region of approx 2.4 cM on rat RNO9 (Fig. 2G). Localization of this BP QTL to this small interval has eliminated, among others, two solute carrier (Na^+/H^+ exchanger) genes, *Nhe2* and *Nhe4*, as positional BP candidate genes. Yet another solute carrier (Cl^-/HCO_3^- exchanger) gene, *Ae3*, which could not be eliminated based on its location (*Ae3* is contained within the 2.4-cM BP QTL region), was however reasonably well-excluded as a BP causative gene based on the absence of sequence variants within the coding regions, and as a result of the lack of differential renal gene expression of *Ae3* between S and R rats *(68)*.

Chromosome 10

The search for BP causative genes on RNO10 began with several genetic linkage analyses detecting the presence of BP QTL on RNO10 (reviewed in ref. *5*). Further linkage analysis indicated the presence of BP QTL on RNO10 in an F2 (S × MNS) and F2 (S × LEW) population, and initial congenic strains confirmed the presence of QTL with either MNS *(16)* or LEW *(17)* as the donor of large regions of RNO10. During the last 3 yr, multiple congenic substrains have been constructed and characterized for fine-mapping these BP QTL *(26,69)*. These studies resulted in the localization of two RNO10 BP QTL, QTL1 and QTL2 (Table 1) to intervals of less than 2.6 cM and less than 3.2 cM, respectively *(26)*. QTL 1 region (Fig. 2H, study 1) from the MNS congenic series also represents the QTL defined with the LEW congenic series. This implies that both LEW and MNS carry alleles that are functionally the same, but are in contrast with those in the S rat for BP QTL1. In contrast with QTL1, the QTL2 region (Fig. 2H, study 2) was identified in the congenic substrains derived from MNS, but not from LEW. Additional studies using S.LEW congenic substrains to localize BP QTL on RNO10 are recently reported *(69,70)*. The method of measuring BP in these studies was by telemetry as opposed to the tail-cuff method used by Garrett et al. *(26)*. Telemetry studies have corroborated the findings of Garrett et al. *(26)*, and additionally resulted in further fine-mapping the QTL1 and QTL2 regions to approx 5.79 Mb and approx 4.75 Mb on RNO10 (Fig. 2H, studies 3 and 4) . Also, this study *(69)* provided evidence for the existence of another BP QTL called as QTL3 (Fig. 2H, study 5), which is localized within the QTL1 region reported by Garrett et al. *(26)*.

Linkage analyses in experimental crosses of SHRSP and WKY rats have suggested the presence of BP QTL on RNO10 in the region around the *Wnk4* (a serine/threonine kinase) locus. *Wnk4* has been implicated in human pseudohypoaldosteronism type II, which is a rare Mendelian form of arterial hypertension *(71,72)*. WKY.SHRSP congenic strains constructed around the *Wnk4* locus were used to analyze the candidacy of Wnk4 for BP control in rats *(73)*. Whereas this congenic strain was proven to encompass a BP QTL represented in Fig. 2H, study 6, *Wnk4* was reasonably ruled out as a candidate gene for this QTL based on lack of mutations in the coding sequences and lack of differential renal gene expression of *Wnk4* between SHRSP and WKY rats *(73)*. In another study by the same group using WKY.SHRSP congenic strains, a genetic interaction for the regulation of systolic BP has also been reported between the BP QTL on RNO10 shown in Fig. 2H, study 7 *(74)* and the BP QTL on RNO1 shown in Fig. 2A, study 13 *(74)*. The congenic strain containing the BP QTL on RNO1 is reported in this study *(74)* to have no significant changes in systolic BP after salt loading compared with that in the parental WKY rats, but was reported to exert its effect only through interaction with RNO10. This is, however, the same congenic strain named WKY-1.SHRSP-Mt1pa/D1Rat200 *(33)*, which was previously reported to have a significant systolic BP effect after salt loading *(33)* independent of RNO10. This inconsistency in the BP effect of the QTL on RNO1 renders the reported genetic interaction between the QTLs on RNO1 and RNO10 inconclusive.

Chromosomes 11 and 12

No studies using substitution mapping for identification of BP QTL have been reported on these chromosomes.

Chromosome 13

Since the review written by Rapp in 2000 *(5)*, no additional congenic strains have been reported on this chromosome. Of related interest, recently a consomic strain constructed through the replacement of the entire RNO13 of the S rat with that of the BN rat was found to have markedly low BP compared with the S rat (Fig. 2I, study 1) *(75)*.

Chromosomes 14 and 15

No congenic strains for BP have been reported on RNO14 or RNO15.

Chromosome 16

Suggestive evidence for linkage of BP to RNO16 on F2 (SHR × BN) *(58)* and F2 (S × LEW) *(17)* populations are reported. A recent report has confirmed the BP QTL on RNO16 using S.LEW congenic strains *(76)*. This BP QTL is located towards the proximal region of RNO16, and is localized to approx 10 Mb region. Figure 2J represents the location of this BP QTL on the physical map of RNO16.

Chromosome 17

Two independent genetic linkage analyses using F2 (S × LEW) *(17)* and F2 (SBH × SBN) *(77)* rats detected BP QTL on RNO17. However, an S.LEW congenic strain did not corroborate the identification of the BP QTL found using the F2 (S × LEW) population. The reason for this remains unknown, although it was suggested that the BP QTL detected by linkage, could have been missed by the introgressed region on the congenic strain *(5)*. Since then, there have been no additional studies for detecting or confirming BP QTL on RNO17 by substitution mapping. Therefore, conclusive experimental evidence for or against the existence of BP QTL on RNO17 is lacking.

Chromosome 18

There are no reports using substitution mapping for BP QTL on RNO18.

Chromosome 19

Linkage studies using the SHR have suggested BP QTL on RNO19 in the vicinity of the angiotensinogen gene *(78)*. An SHR.BN congenic strain was constructed *(78)*. This congenic strain significantly lowered BP compared with SHR parental. The introgressed region in this congenic strain (Fig. 2K) contains BN alleles at the angiotensinogen locus. Despite the BP-lowering effect observed, there were no major changes in plasma angiotensinogen or renin activities between this congenic strain and the parental SHR strain. The BP QTL "trapped" in this congenic strain is not explained by differences in plasma angiotensinogen levels or angiotensinogen expression.

Chromosome 20

Most of the substitution mapping studies for localizing BP QTL on RNO20 have focused on the major histocompatibility complex RT1 (reviewed in ref. *5*). A recent study *(79)* reported the effect of high-fat diet on BP using SHR and SHR.1N (1N = BN.*Lx/Cub*) congenic rats. In these congenic rats, approx 30 cM region including the tumor necrosis factor (TNF)-α locus on RNO20 in the SHR rat was replaced by alleles from the BN.*Lx/Cub* rat (Fig. 2L). BN alleles in the introgressed region resulted in elevated BP compared with SHR rats. In this study, the authors were interested in examining the role of the TNF-α locus. Although they identified a number of sequence differences between SHR and SHR.1N rats in the regulatory regions of the TNF-α gene, no significant gene–diet interactions in mRNA expression were observed *(79)*. TNF-α was therefore excluded as a candidate gene for the QTL on RNO20 that controls high-fat-diet-induced changes in BP.

Chromosome X

Evidence from a genetic linkage analysis using an F2 (SHRSP × WKY) population indicated the presence of a BP QTL on RNO X *(6)*. In another F2 population derived from SBH and SBN rats *(77)*, BP was linked to a broad region of RNO X overlapping with the region indicated by Hilbert et al. *(6)*. Kloting et al. *(80)* constructed a congenic strain introgressing SHR alleles on the normotensive BB/OK background consisting of the genomic region indicated by Hilbert et al. *(6)* (Fig. 2M). This congenic strain had higher

BP compared with BB/OK. Since this study, there are no additional reports of substitution mapping for BP on RNO X.

Chromosome Y

Previous studies indicated that hypertension in the SHR is linked to the Y chromosome *(81,82)*. Replacing the SHR RNOY with the BN (= BN.*Lx/Cub*) RNOY resulted in significant decreases in systolic and diastolic BPs in the SHR.BN-Y consomic strain *(83)* (Fig. 2N, study 1). The effect of the SHRSP and WKY RNOY on BP was also studied using reciprocal consomic strains *(84)*. Transfer of the Y chromosome from WKY onto SHRSP background significantly reduced systolic BP compared with BP of parental SHRSP *(84)* (Fig. 2N, study 2). In the reciprocal WKY.SHRSP consomic strain, systolic BP was increased compared with WKY parental strain *(84)*. Based on these results, it was concluded that the Y chromosome of SHR and SHRSP models of hypertension harbors a locus contributing to systolic BP. In contrast, neither the origin of the Y chromosome nor the sex of the parental strain had any significant impact on the magnitude of the BP response to salt loading in the SBH model of hypertension *(32)*.

PERSPECTIVES

Finding BP Causative Genes by Substitution Mapping: Are We There Yet?

Experiments conducted so far using substitution mapping to localize BP-controlling genes can be viewed as belonging to three categories: (1) construction and characterization of congenic strains with large introgressed segments (>20–30 cM)—such experiments are primarily focused on corroborating the initial BP QTL localization by genetic linkage analysis; (2) construction and characterization of congenic substrains to further localize a BP QTL within a smaller genomic region (<5–20 cM); and (3) construction and characterization of congenic substrains to fine-localize a BP QTL to a region less than 1 cM. Most of the studies conducted in the past 3 yr have advanced from category 1 to category 2. Very few, however, have progressed into category 3. So far, there is only one report that provides a reasonable "proof-of-principle" for substitution mapping using congenic strains as a correct approach for advancing from QTL localization to BP causative gene identification *(31)*. Considering that evidence from genetic linkage analyses and substitution mapping indicate the presence of a large number of BP QTL (compiled at http://rgd.mcw.edu/) coupled with the fact that the identity of only one of them is known, an obvious question faced by investigators is whether to proceed with substitution mapping as a valid approach for finding the remaining BP causative genes. Two factors are in favor of searching for BP causative genes using substitution mapping.

1. *Sequencing of the rat and mouse genomes.* The major limitation in the construction of congenic substrains was that the development of microsatellite markers in a given target region was difficult. The availability of mouse and, subsequently, rat genome sequences has facilitated the identification of microsatellite markers in any targeted region of the rat genome, which can then be easily tested for polymorphisms and used to construct congenic strains. Additionally, now that the genome sequence is available and annotated for human, mouse, and rat genes, candidate genes in a QTL region can sometimes be found by searching a database.

2. *Microarray gene expression analysis.* Aitman et al. *(85)* successfully identified CD36 as a molecule responsible for insulin resistance in the SHR. The technique used by Aitman et al. *(85)* was to perform a comparative global gene expression analysis between a congenic strain with a relatively large introgressed region and one of the parental strains. The success of this study encourages the use of global gene expression analysis as a complementary technique to expedite BP causative gene identification using congenic strains. A recent study by McBride et al. has used gene expression analysis in combination with substitution mapping and identified glutathione *S*-transferase (*Gstm1*) as a BP causative candidate gene *(44)*. Such reports do require additional compelling evidence to progress from the identification of a "BP causative candidate gene" to validation of it being "the BP causative gene." For example, transgenic rescue experiments were used by Pravenec et al. *(86)* to establish unequivocally that CD36 is an insulin resistance QTL in the SHR.

To summarize, the recent reports discussed in this article indicate that it is possible to utilize substitution mapping as an efficient (albeit lengthy) strategy in not only confirming that genomic regions harbor BP QTL, but also defining with improved resolution the physical limits of the genomic regions surrounding each of these BP QTL. Further improving the resolution of localization by additional substitution mapping is, however, essential for advancing from BP QTL detection and confirmation to BP QTL identification. "Is it possible" to identify BP genes *(10)*? Yes. "Are we there yet?" No.

ACKNOWLEDGMENTS

Sincere thanks to Prof. John P. Rapp and Dr. George T. Cicila for their critical reading and valuable suggestions.

REFERENCES

1. Glazier AM, Nadeau JH, Aitman TJ. Finding genes that underlie complex traits. Science 2002;298:2345–2349.
2. Glazier AM, Scott J, Aitman TJ. Molecular basis of the Cd36 chromosomal deletion underlying SHR defects in insulin action and fatty acid metabolism. Mamm Genome 2002;13:108–113.
3. Zhang Y, Leaves NI, Anderson GG, et al. Positional cloning of a quantitative trait locus on chromosome 13q14 that influences immunoglobulin E levels and asthma. Nat Genet 2003;18:18.
4. Luft FC. Hypertension as a complex genetic trait. Semin Nephrol 2002;22:115–126.
5. Rapp JP. Genetic analysis of inherited hypertension in the rat. Physiol Rev 2000;80:135–172.
6. Hilbert P, Lindpaintner K, Beckmann JS, et al. Chromosomal mapping of two genetic loci associated with blood-pressure regulation in hereditary hypertensive rats. Nature 1991;353:521–529.
7. Jacob HJ, Lindpaintner K, Lincoln SE, et al. Genetic mapping of a gene causing hypertension in the stroke-prone spontaneously hypertensive rat. Cell 1991;67:213–224.
8. Cowley AW, Jr, Roman RJ, Jacob HJ. Application of genome substitution techniques in gene-function discovery. J Physiol 2004;554:46–55.
9. Drenjancevic-Peric I, Frisbee JC, Lombard JH. Skeletal Muscle Arteriolar Reactivity in SS.BN13 Consomic Rats and Dahl Salt-Sensitive Rats. Hypertension 2003;41:1012–1015.
10. Rapp JP, Deng AY. Detection and positional cloning of blood pressure quantitative trait loci: Is it possible? Identifying the genes for genetic hypertension. Hypertension 1995;25:1121–1128.
11. Snell GD. Methods for the study of histocompatibility genes. J Genet 1948;49:87–108.
12. Jeffs B, Negrin CD, Graham D, et al. Applicability of a "speed" congenic strategy to dissect blood pressure quantitative trait loci on rat chromosome 2. Hypertension 2000;35:179–187.
13. Wakeland E, Morel L, Achey K, Yui M, Longmate J. Speed congenics: a classic technique in the fast lane (relatively speaking). Immunol Today 1997;18:472–477.

14. Markel P, Shu P, Ebeling C, et al. Theoretical and empirical issues for marker-assisted breeding of congenic mouse strains. Nat Genet 1997;17:280–284.
15. Deng AY, Dene H, Rapp JP. Mapping of a quantitative trait locus for blood pressure on rat chromosome 2. J Clin Invest 1994;94:431–436.
16. Dukhanina OI, Dene H, Deng AY, Choi CR, Hoebee B, Rapp JP. Linkage map and congenic strains to localize blood pressure QTL on rat chromosome 10. Mamm Genome 1997;8:229–235.
17. Garrett MR, Dene H, Walder R, et al. Genome scan and congenic strains for blood pressure QTL using Dahl salt-sensitive rats. Genome Res 1998;8:711–723.
18. Rapp JP, Garrett MR, Deng AY. Construction of a double congenic strain to prove an epistatic interaction on blood pressure between rat chromosomes 2 and 10. J Clin Invest 1998;101:1591–1595.
19. Cicila GT, Choi CR, Dene H, Lee SJ, Rapp JP. Two blood pressure/cardiac mass quantitative trait loci on chromosome 3 in Dahl rats. Mamm Genome 1999;10:112–116.
20. Pravenec M, Krenova D, Kren V, et al. Congenic strains for genetic analysis of hypertension and dyslipidemia in the spontaneously hypertensive rat. Transplant Proc 1999;31:1555–1556.
21. Saad Y, Garrett MR, Lee SJ, Dene H, Rapp JP. Localization of a blood pressure QTL on rat chromosome 1 using Dahl rat congenic strains. Physiol Genom 1999;1:119–125.
22. St Lezin E, Liu W, Wang JM, et al. Genetic analysis of rat chromosome 1 and the Sa gene in spontaneous hypertension. Hypertension 2000;35:225–230.
23. Cicila GT, Garrett MR, Lee SJ, Liu J, Dene H, Rapp JP. High-resolution mapping of the blood pressure QTL on chromosome 7 using Dahl rat congenic strains. Genomics 2001;72:51–60.
24. Deng AY, Dutil J, Sivo Z. Utilization of marker-assisted congenics to map two blood pressure quantitative trait loci in Dahl rats. Mamm Genome 2001;12:612–616.
25. Dutil J, Deng AY. Further chromosomal mapping of a blood pressure QTL in Dahl rats on chromosome 2 using congenic strains. Physiol Genomics 2001;6:3–9.
26. Garrett MR, Zhang X, Dukhanina OI, Deng AY, Rapp JP. Two linked blood pressure quantitative trait loci on chromosome 10 defined by Dahl rat congenic strains. Hypertension 2001;38:779–785.
27. Saad Y, Garrett MR, Rapp JP. Multiple blood pressure QTL on rat chromosome 1 defined by Dahl rat congenic strains. Physiol Genomics 2001;4:201–214.
28. Pravenec M, Kren V, Krenova D, et al. Genetic isolation of quantitative trait loci for blood pressure development and renal mass on chromosome 5 in the spontaneously hypertensive rat. Physiol Res 2003;52:285–289.
29. Garrett MR, Rapp JP. Multiple blood pressure QTL on rat chromosome 2 defined by congenic Dahl rats. Mamm Genome 2002;13:41–44.
30. Garrett MR, Rapp JP. Two closely linked interactive blood pressure QTL on rat chromosome 5 defined using congenic Dahl rats. Physiol Genomics 2002;8:81–86.
31. Garrett MR, Rapp JP. Defining the Blood Pressure QTL on Chromosome 7 in Dahl Rats by a 177kb Congenic Segment Containing Cyp11b1. Mamm Genome 2003;14:268–273.
32. Yagil C, Hubner N, Kreutz R, Ganten D, Yagil Y. Congenic strains confirm the presence of salt-sensitivity QTLs on chromosome 1 in the Sabra rat model of hypertension. Physiol Genomics 2003;12:85–95.
33. Hubner N, Lee YA, Lindpaintner K, Ganten D, Kreutz R. Congenic substitution mapping excludes Sa as a candidate gene locus for a blood pressure quantitative trait locus on rat chromosome 1. Hypertension 1999;34:643–648.
34. Frantz S, Clemitson JR, Bihoreau MT, Gauguier D, Samani NJ. Genetic dissection of region around the Sa gene on rat chromosome 1: evidence for multiple loci affecting blood pressure. Hypertension 2001;38:216–221.
35. Iwai N, Tsujita Y, Kinoshita M. Isolation of a chromosome 1 region that contributes to high blood pressure and salt sensitivity. Hypertension 1998;32:636–638.
36. Kato N, Nabika T, Liang Y-Q, et al. Isolation of a chromosome region affecting blood pressure and vascular disease traits in the stroke-prone rat mode. Hypertension 2003;42:1191–1197.
37. Cui ZH, Ikeda K, Kawakami K, Gonda T, Nabika T, Masuda J. Exaggerated response to restraint stress in rats congenic for the chromosome 1 blood pressure quantitative trait locus. Clin Exper Pharmacol Physiol 2003;30:464–469.
38. Pravenec M, Zidek V, Musilova A, et al. Genetic isolation of a blood pressure quantitative trait locus on chromosome 2 in the spontaneously hypertensive rat. J Hypertens 2001;19:1061–1064.
39. Kren V, Pravenec M, Lu S, et al. Genetic isolation of a region of chromosome 8 that exerts major effects on blood pressure and cardiac mass in the spontaneously hypertensive rat. J Clin Invest 1997;99:577–581.

40. Deng AY, Dene H, Rapp JP. Congenic strains for the blood pressure quantitative trait locus on rat chromosome 2. Hypertension 1997;30[part 1]:199–202.

41. Joe B, Garrett MR, Dene H, Rapp JP. Substitution mapping of a blood pressure quantitative trait locus to a 2.73 Mb region on rat chromosome 1. J Hypertens 2003;21:2077–2084.

42. Dutil J, Deng AY. Mapping a blood pressure quantitative trait locus to a 5.7-cM region in Dahl salt-sensitive rats. Mamm Genome 2001;12:362–365.

43. Alemayehu A, Breen L, Krenova D, Printz MP. Reciprocal rat chromosome 2 congenic strains reveal contrasting blood pressure and heart rate QTL. Physiol Genomics 2002;10:199–210.

44. McBride MW, Carr FJ, Graham D, et al. Microarray analysis of rat chromosome 2 congenic strains. Hypertension 2003;41:847–853.

45. Carr FJ, Negrin CD, Clark JS, et al. Chromosome 2 reciprocal congenic strains to evaluate the effect of the genetic background on blood pressure. Scott Med J 2002;47:7–9.

46. Grunfeld S, Hamilton CA, Mesaros S, et al. Role of superoxide in the depressed nitric oxide production by the endothelium of genetically hypertensive rats. Hypertension 1995;26:854–857.

47. Kerr S, Brosnan MJ, McIntyre M, Reid JL, Dominiczak AF, Hamilton CA. Superoxide anion production is increased in a model of genetic hypertension: role of the endothelium. Hypertension 1999;33:1353–1358.

48. Hamilton CA, Brosnan MJ, McIntyre M, Graham D, Dominiczak AF. Superoxide excess in hypertension and aging: a common cause of endothelial dysfunction. Hypertension 2001;37:529–534.

49. Vaziri ND, Wang XQ, Oveisi F, Rad B. Induction of oxidative stress by glutathione depletion causes severe hypertension in normal rats. Hypertension 2000;36:142–146.

50. Cicila GT, Rapp JP, Bloch KD, et al. Cosegregation of the endothelin-3 locus with blood pressure and relative heart weight in inbred Dahl rats. J Hypertens 1994;12:643–650.

51. Kato N, Hyne G, Bihoreau M-T, Gauguier D, Lathrop GM, Rapp JP. Complete genome searches for quantitative trait loci controlling blood pressure and related traits in four segregating populations derived from Dahl hypertensive rats. Mamm Genome 1999;10:259–265.

52. Garrett MR, Saad Y, Dene H, Rapp JP. Blood pressure QTL that differentiate Dahl salt-sensitive and spontaneously hypertensive rats. Physiol Genomics 2000;3:33–38.

53. Ueno T, Tremblay J, Kunes J, et al. Resolving the composite trait of hypertension into its pharmacogenetic determinants by acute pharmacological modulation of blood pressure regulatory systems. J Mol Med 2003;81:51–60.

54. Stoll M, Kwitek-Black AE, Cowley AW, Jr, et al. New target regions for human hypertension via comparative genomics. Genome Res 2000;10:473–482.

55. Siegel AK, Planert M, Rademacher S, et al. Genetic Loci contribute to the progression of vascular and cardiac hypertrophy in salt-sensitive spontaneous hypertension. Arterioscler Thromb Vasc Biol 2003;23:1211–1217.

56. Palijan A, Dutil J, Deng AY. Quantitative trait loci with opposing blood pressure effects demonstrating epistasis on Dahl rat chromosome 3. Physiol Genomics 2003;15:1–8.

57. Katsuya T, Higaki J, Zhao Y, et al. A neuropeptide Y locus on chromosome 4 cosegregates with blood pressure in the spontaneously hypertensive rat. Biochem Biophys Res Commun 1993;192:261–267.

58. Schork NJ, Krieger JE, Trolliet MR, et al. A biometrical genome search in rats reveals the multigenic basis of blood pressure variation. Genome Res 1995;5:164–172.

59. Kovacs P, Voigt B, Kloting I. Alleles of the spontaneously hypertensive rat decrease blood pressure at loci on chromosomes 4 and 13. Biochem Biophys Res Commun 1997;238:586–589.

60. Garrett MR, Joe B, Dene H, Rapp JP. Identification of blood pressure quantitative trait loci that differentiate two hypertensive strains. J Hypertens 2002;20:2399–406.

61. Kloting I, Kovacs P, van den Brandt J. Congenic BB.SHR (D4Mit6-Npy-Spr) rats: a new aid to dissect the genetics of obesity. Obes Res 2002;10:1074–1077.

62. Rapp JP, Dahl LK. Mendelian inheritance of 18- and 11beta-steroid hydroxylase activities in the adrenals of rats genetically susceptible or resistant to hypertension. Endocrinology 1972; 90:1435-1446.

63. Cicila GT, Rapp JP, Wang J-M, St. Lezin E, Ng SC, Kurtz TW. Linkage of 11β-hydroxylase mutations with altered steroid biosynthesis and blood pressure in the Dahl rat. Nat Genet 1993;3:346–353.

64. Rapp JP, Dahl LK. Mutant forms of cytochrome P-450 controlling both 18- and 11β-steroid hydroxylation in the rat. Biochemistry 1976;15:1235–1242.

65. Nonaka Y, Fujii T, Kagawa N, Waterman MR, Takemori H, Okamoto M. Structure/function relationship of CYP11B1 associated with Dahl's salt-resistant rats. Expression of rat CYP11B1 and CYP11B2 in *Escherichia coli*. Eur J Biochem 1998;258:869–878.

66. Takami S, Higaki J, Miki T, et al. Analysis and comparison of new candidate loci for hypertension between genetic hypertensive rat strains. Hypertens Res 1996;19:51–56.

67. Rapp JP, Garrett MR, Dene H, Meng H, Hoebee B, Lathrop GM. Linkage analysis and construction of a congenic strain for a blood pressure QTL on rat chromosome 9. Genomics 1998;51:191–196.

68. Meng H, Garrett MR, Dene H, Rapp JP. Localization of a blood pressure QTL to a 2.4-cM interval on rat chromosome 9 using congenic strains. Genomics 2003;81:210–220.

69. Palijan A, Lambert R, Dutil J, Sivo Z, Deng AY. Comprehensive congenic coverage revealing multiple blood pressure quantitative trait loci on Dahl rat chromosome 10. Hypertension 2003;42:515–522.

70. Sivo Z, Malo B, Dutil J, Deng AY. Accelerated congenics for mapping two blood pressure quantitative trait loci on chromosome 10 of Dahl rats. J Hypertens 2002;20:45–53.

71. Wilson FH, Disse-Nicodeme S, Choate KA, et al. Human hypertension caused by mutations in WNK kinases. Science 2001;293:1107–1112.

72. Kahle KT, Wilson FH, Leng Q, et al. WNK4 regulates the balance between renal NaCl reabsorption and K+ secretion. Nat Genet 2003;35:372–376.

73. Monti J, Zimdahl H, Schulz H, Plehm R, Ganten D, Hubner N. The role of Wnk4 in polygenic hypertension: a candidate gene analysis on rat chromosome 10. Hypertension 2003;41:938–942.

74. Monti J, Plehm R, Schulz H, Ganten D, Kreutz R, Hubner N. Interaction between blood pressure quantitative trait loci in rats in which trait variation at chromosome 1 is conditional upon a specific allele at chromosome 10. Hum Mol Genet 2003;12:435–439.

75. Cowley AW, Jr, Roman RJ, Kaldunski ML, et al. Brown Norway chromosome 13 confers protection from high salt to consomic Dahl S rat. Hypertension 2001;37:456–461.

76. Moujahidine M, Dutil J, Hamet P, Deng AY. Congenic mapping of a blood pressure QTL on chromosome 16 of Dahl rats. Mamm Genome 2002;13:153–156.

77. Yagil C, Sapojnikov M, Kreutz R, Zurcher H, Ganten D, Yagil Y. Role of chromosome X in the Sabra rat model of salt-sensitive hypertension. Hypertension 1999;33:261–265.

78. St Lezin E, Zhang L, Yang Y, et al. Effect of chromosome 19 transfer on blood pressure in the spontaneously hypertensive rat. Hypertension 1999;33:256–260.

79. Pausova Z, Sedova L, Berube J, et al. Segment of rat chromosome 20 regulates diet-induced augmentations in adiposity, glucose intolerance, and blood pressure. Hypertension 2003;41:1047–1055.

80. Kloting I, Voigt B, Kovacs P. Metabolic features of newly established congenic diabetes-prone BB.SHR rat strains. Life Sci 1998;62:973–979.

81. Ely DL, Turner ME. Hypertension in the spontaneously hypertensive rat is linked to the Y chromosome. Hypertension 1990;16:277–281.

82. Ely D, Turner M, Milsted A. Review of the Y chromosome and hypertension. Braz J Med Biol Res 2000;33:679–691.

83. Kren V, Qi N, Krenova D, et al. Y-chromosome transfer induces changes in blood pressure and blood lipids in SHR. Hypertension 2001;37:1147–1152.

84. Negrin CD, McBride MW, Carswell HV, et al. Reciprocal consomic strains to evaluate y chromosome effects. Hypertension 2001;37:391–397.

85. Aitman TJ, Glazier AM, Wallace CA, et al. Identification of Cd36 (Fat) as an insulin-resistance gene causing defective fatty acid and glucose metabolism in hypertensive rats. Nat Genet 1999;21:76–83.

86. Pravenec M, Landa V, Zidek V, et al. Transgenic rescue of defective CD36 ameliorates insulin resistance in spontaneously hypertensive rats. Nat Genet 2001;27:156–158.

4 Local Production of Angiotensinogen

Insights From Genetic Manipulation of Mice

Kamal Rahmouni and Curt D. Sigmund, PhD

CONTENTS

SUMMARY

Genetic approaches such as gene targeting have been extensively used to gain a better understanding of the role of hormones and pathways involved in cardiovascular physiology. Given its pivotal role in cardiovascular homeostasis the renin–angiotensin system has been one of the most frequently targeted systems. Angiotensinogen (AGT), the only known precursor of the renin–angiotensin system, has received particular attention because genetic and molecular studies have shown that genetic variation at this locus impacts individual differences in blood pressure and the likelihood of developing essential hypertension. Knockout and overexpression of the *AGT* gene lead to adverse cardiovascular phenotypes. In this chapter we will review these data and detail a strategy using well-characterized cell-specific promoters to specifically target the *AGT* gene to defined cells and tissues. The development and characterization of these models has helped uncover the role and significance of local production of AGT in several tissues.

Key Words: Renin–angiotensin system; tissue angiotensinogen; blood pressure; transgenic mice; cell-specific targeting.

INTRODUCTION

The renin–angiotensin system (RAS) is a major regulator of vascular hemodynamics and a determinant of cardiovascular homeostasis. It also contributes to the development and maintenance of various forms of hypertension and other cardiovascular diseases such

From: *Contemporary Cardiology: Cardiovascular Genomics*
Edited by: M. K. Raizada, et al. © Humana Press Inc., Totowa, NJ

as heart failure, cardiac hypertrophy, and atherosclerosis. Angiotensin II (ANG II), the primary effector of the RAS, is produced by the serial cleavage of angiotensinogen (AGT) by renin and angiotensin-converting enzyme (ACE). The actions of ANG II on distinct receptors (AT1a, AT1b, and AT2) located in vascular smooth muscle, kidney, adrenal gland, and brain lead to an elevation of arterial blood pressure through increased vascular resistance, cardiac output, sodium reabsorption and blood volume, and the production of other vasoactive hormones such as aldosterone (1,2). In addition, the RAS has been shown to play a role in regulating cell growth, in vascular smooth muscle proliferation, and during development (3,4). Based on the presence of different components of the RAS at both the protein and mRNA level in a variety of tissues, including adrenal gland, kidney, brain, heart, adipose tissue, and blood vessels, local-tissue RAS has been proposed (2,5,6).

We will describe here some of the genetic manipulations used to study the role of AGT in the control of blood pressure and cardiovascular-related functions. AGT has received particular attention for many reasons. First, AGT is the only known precursor of ANG II. Second, the strongest evidence implicating a gene as a cause of human essential hypertension is for the *AGT* gene, and association of AGT levels and hypertension has been reported in families (7,8). Third, transgenic animals expressing high levels of AGT have elevated blood pressure (9), whereas knockout mice lacking AGT have low blood pressure (10,11).

ANGIOTENSINOGEN (*AGT*) GENE

The human AGT mRNA is encoded from a gene located on chromosome 1, and contains five exons and four introns. The mRNA is 1455 nucleotides long and codes for a globular glycoprotein of 485 amino acids. The coding potential of AGT is located in exons 2 to 5, whereas the first exon encodes only a portion of the 5' untranslated region. Because the K_m of renin is close to the plasma concentration of AGT in humans, a modest change in its plasma concentration can affect the rate of ANG II formation. Mouse and rat renin hydrolyze a Leu–Leu bond in mouse and rat AGT, in contrast to the Leu–Val bond in human AGT. Because of this, and perhaps other differences in the AGT protein, the cleavage of AGT by renin is species-specific (12). Mice or rats producing human renin or human AGT, but not both, do not develop hypertension or any other phenotype (13,14).

Experimental evidence suggests that the liver represents the primary source of plasma AGT. AGT is probably not stored in hepatocytes, but is constitutively secreted into the systemic circulation (15). Production of AGT by the liver is regulated by several hormonal factors including estrogen, glucocorticoids, thyroid hormone, insulin, and ANG II (15,16). In accordance with the local-tissue RAS concept, AGT is synthesized in many tissues other than the liver, for example the brain, kidney, heart, adrenal gland, vasculature, and adipose tissue. The AGT produced by these tissues may be converted locally or released into the bloodstream to contribute to the circulating pool of AGT. The production of AGT in these tissues may also be regulated locally, independently of the circulating system. The presence of other components of the RAS, such as renin and ACE necessary for the biosynthesis of active angiotensin peptides in most of the tissues that produce AGT, provides further evidence for the de novo synthesis of ANG II in these tissues (Fig. 1). However, the existence of alternative pathways for the production of ANG II in tissues where some components of RAS were not found cannot be excluded (6).

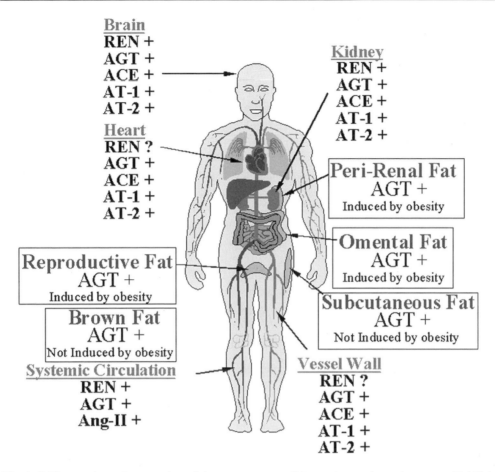

Fig. 1. Different sites of expression of the components of the renin–angiotensin system (RAS) in the body. The classical systemic RAS in which angiotensinogen (AGT) is derived from the liver, renin from the kidney, and angiotensin-converting enzyme from lung is shown. Presence of different components of the RAS in a variety of tissues has led to the concept of local RAS. AGT expression is also detected in adipose tissue and is induced by obesity in some depots. Adipose tissue is becoming recognized as another potential tissue RAS.

TARGETING SYSTEMIC AGT

In order to evaluate the effect of *AGT* gene disruption on blood pressure regulation, conventional gene targeting in embryonic stem cells was used to delete the *AGT* gene *(10,11)*. As expected, homozygous AGT knockout mice had no detectable plasma AGT whereas there was a 58% decrease in heterozygous mutant mice. Survival studies have shown that absence of a functional *AGT* gene is compatible with survival to birth, but postnatal survival is severely compromised, perhaps because of the altered renovascular development in these mice *(17)*. Furthermore, compared to wild-type mice, knockout of the *AGT* gene resulted in a marked decrease in blood pressure.

Further evidence for the crucial role of AGT in blood pressure regulation is derived from studies of mice with different copies of the *AGT* gene *(11)*. Plasma AGT levels increase with the *AGT* gene copy number (by 35% in 1 copy, 124% in 3 copies, and 145% in 4 copies). Interestingly, blood pressure increased in proportion to the increase in *AGT* gene copy number, averaging 8 mmHg per copy. This experiment demonstrates clearly that variation in circulating AGT can affect blood pressure. It also establishes the potential for an effect on blood pressure by genetic influences arising from differences in circulating AGT.

We generated transgenic mice containing the entire *hAGT* gene in order to study its tissue- and cell-specific expression and its role in the pathogenesis of hypertension *(14)*. The transgene employed contains all five exons and intervening intron sequences, and extends approx 1.2 kb upstream and 1.4 kb downstream of the gene. The expression pattern of *hAGT* gene was found to be very consistent with the tissue-specific expression of the mouse and rat *AGT* genes and with the expected pattern of AGT expression in humans. Consistent with previous reports, analysis of the cellular origin of kidney hAGT in these transgenic mice revealed that it was exclusively localized to the epithelial cells of the proximal convoluted tubules *(18)*. All together, these data demonstrated that the *hAGT* transgene was appropriately regulated. It also suggests that these transgenic mice represent a valid model for examining the regulation of *hAGT* gene.

The hAGT released into the plasma of the transgenic mice was determined to be functional because infusion of a single bolus dose of purified human renin resulted in transient increase in blood pressure of approx 30 mmHg within 2 min. Furthermore, crossbreeding of these mice expressing hAGT with transgenic mice containing a genomic clone encoding the human renin resulted in chronic elevation of blood pressure *(19)*. These double-transgenic mice also had an altered baroreflex response (i.e., resetting of the arterial baroreflex of heart rate to a higher pressure without significantly changing the gain or sensitivity of the reflex).

We also evaluated whether elements of the human RAS could functionally overcome the hypotension, renal pathology, and reduced survival observed in the AGT knockout mice. This was achieved by breeding the double-transgenic (hAGT/human renin) mice with the AGT knockout mice *(20)*. We found that the presence of both human transgenes rescued the postnatal lethality in AGT knockout mice. The lower blood pressure and renal lesions observed in AGT knockout mice were also corrected by the presence of the human transgenes. These findings indicate that it is the absence of ANG II, and not AGT *per se*, that is responsible for the abnormalities observed in the AGT mutant mice. These data demonstrate also the ability of human renin and *AGT* genes to replace the mouse *AGT* gene.

TARGETING THE TISSUE AGT

In recent years there has been a refocusing of effort on understanding the role of tissue RAS in the regulation of blood pressure and fluid and electrolyte homeostasis, as well as their involvement in cardiovascular and renal diseases. The advances in genetic manipulation, which allow gene ablation and tissue-specific gene targeting, have provided a new set of tools to experimentally dissect the role of the AGT produced in different tissues. We will illustrate the important role of local AGT synthesis by describing the development and characterization of mouse models in which AGT has been targeted to specific cell types.

Liver AGT

As mentioned previously, the liver is considered the primary site of AGT synthesis and the main source of plasma AGT. We therefore examined the effects of hepatic AGT elimination on the circulating pool of AGT. To knock out AGT specifically in the liver,

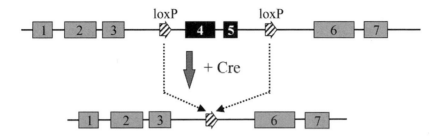

Fig. 2. Schematic of Cre-loxP System. The targeted gene is designed with loxP sites flanking one or more important coding exons (filled boxes). The addition of Cre-recombinase will result in the deletion of the flanked exon, disabling the gene. (For more details, *see* ref. *56).*

we used the Cre–loxP system *(21)* (Fig. 2). We designed a transgene in which exon 2 of the hAGT gene is flanked by loxP sites *(22)*. Efficient recombination was observed in transgenic mouse liver upon intravenous administration of adenovirus that expressed Cre recombinase (Adcre). Systemic administration of Adcre caused hepatic-specific deletion of hAGT, as no hAGT mRNA or protein was detected in the liver, whereas in the kidney its expression was unaltered. This is consistent with the results demonstrating that intravenous administration of adenoviruses affects primarily the liver, but not other tissues *(23)*. Further analyses have shown that the deletion of the *hAGT* transgene in the liver was associated with a significant decrease in the plasma level of hAGT (over 90% of control levels) and a markedly attenuated or absent pressor response to infusion of purified recombinant human renin protein. These results strongly suggest that the liver is by far the main source of AGT. A potential limitation of this Cre–loxP system is its effectiveness for acute, but not chronic, elimination of hepatic hAGT. Indeed, transgenic mice containing the floxed hAGT construct exhibited transient lowered blood pressure in response to Adcre, likely a result of repopulation of the liver with AGT-positive cells *(24)*. Chronic elimination of hepatic hAGT will likely require the use of transgenic mice endogenously expressing Cre recombinase in the liver *(25)*.

Renal AGT

In the kidney, the proximal tubule is the major site of angiotensin production *(18)*. The AGT mRNA is localized predominantly in the proximal renal tubule, with considerably lesser amounts in distal tubular segments and glomerular tufts. AGT and ANG II have been detected in proximal tubule fluid *(26,27)*, and are secreted through the apical membrane in proximal tubule cells in culture *(28)*. The presence of AGT in the urine is an indication of its secretion in the tubular fluid and its transition through the entire nephron. However, it was not clear whether the AGT produced locally in the kidney contributed to the circulating pool of this protein. A role for intrarenal AGT in the regulation of blood pressure and renal function was also hypothesized. This is based on the finding that the kidney contains not only the AT1 and AT2 receptors, but also all of the enzymes required to convert AGT to the active hormone ANG II.

To address the potential role of AGT synthesized within the kidney, we produced transgenic mice with a kidney-specific expression of AGT. This was achieved by designing a transgene that contained the *hAGT* gene driven by the kidney androgen-regulated protein promoter *(29–31)*. This promoter was chosen because, like AGT, it is expressed in the renal proximal tubule cells and is responsive to androgens *(32)*. No hAGT was detected in the plasma of the transgenic mice, which suggests that the kidney does not contribute to the circulating pool of AGT. However, elevated concentrations of hAGT were clearly observed in the urine of the transgenic animals, confirming its release in the tubular lumen. To test the impact of the intrarenal production of AGT on blood pressure, we bred these transgenic mice with the mice that express systemic human renin. Double-transgenic male mice had increased blood pressure but normal circulating ANG II levels *(30)*. The minimal blood pressure response to the acute intravenous infusion of the selective AT1 receptor antagonist losartan in these double-transgenic animals as compared with the systemic model confirms that the elevation in blood pressure is a result of the activation of a selective intrarenal mechanism. Our data support the conclusion that kidney AGT participates in the control of blood pressure and renal homeostasis, suggesting that a dysfunction in the intrarenal production of AGT could likely contribute to hypertension. Furthermore, the usefulness of the kidney androgen-regulated protein promoter to study the kidney AGT illustrates the possibility of specifically targeting the intrarenal systems using gene overexpression.

Brain AGT

The brain RAS has received much attention recently because accumulated experimental evidence has shown its involvement in the development of different forms of hypertension *(33)*. The central action of ANG II is known to regulate several activities that can affect blood pressure, including sympathetic nervous function, vasopressin release, drinking behavior, and the appetite for salt. The expression of AGT is widely distributed throughout the brain, with high expression in those areas involved in cardiovascular regulation, such as the hypothalamus and preoptic areas *(34)*. Renin is also thought to be expressed in the brain and appears localized primarily in neurons but also in some glia *(35,36)*, although this is controversial. To experimentally dissect the role of AGT produced in the brain we developed transgenic mice models that express hAGT in the brain, driven by different promoters. Given that astrocytes are considered as the major source of brain AGT *(37)*, we first generated transgenic mice that express hAGT under the control of the glial-specific, glial fibrillary acidic protein (GFAP) promoter *(38)*. In these mice, hAGT protein was mainly localized in astrocytes, but was also present in neurons in the subfornical organ. Measurement of circulating hAGT has shown that plasma levels of hAGT protein were not elevated over baseline. Direct administration of human renin in the cerebral ventricles of these transgenic mice caused a dose-dependent increase in blood pressure, which was prevented by pretreatment with an AT1 receptor blocker. Furthermore, crossing the GFAP-hAGT mice with mice that express human renin systemically led to the development of mice that exhibited moderate, but chronic elevation in blood pressure (about 15 mmHg). In further studies we found that when these double-transgenic mice were provided a choice between tap water and saline, they exhibited a significantly greater preference for saline, because they drink nearly 40% of their total volume as saline as compared with 26% in control mice. To ascertain that the phenotype observed in these double-transgenic mice is a result of the ANG II produced locally in the brain, we crossed the GFAP-hAGT mice with transgenic mice that express human renin under the control of this GFAP promoter *(39)*. The double-transgenic animals had an increase in blood pressure, drinking volume, and salt intake, which indicates that these alterations are caused by the local production and action of ANG II in the central nervous system. All together, these data demonstrate that the AGT produced by astrocytes plays a major role in blood pressure regulation and fluid homeostasis. Other models using antisense techniques to reduce glial AGT similarly support its importance in blood pressure regulation *(40)*, although this is beyond the scope of this chapter. Interestingly, and perhaps surprisingly, glial-specific expression of ANG II was reported to correct the renal defects observed in AGT knockout mice *(41)*.

Because both in vitro and in vivo studies have shown that neurons also produce AGT, which is in accordance with the status of ANG II as a neurotransmitter, we developed mice that express AGT driven by synapsin I (SYN I), a neuron-specific promoter *(42)*. In these transgenic mice, the hAGT protein was detected exclusively in neurons. However, the widespread expression of hAGT throughout the central nervous system that was observed in these animals does not follow the pattern normally exhibited by AGT. This is an experimental limitation resulting from the absence of an appropriate promoter that would allow us to specifically target only those neurons normally expressing AGT, such as the subfornical organ. The hAGT produced in the brain is active as demonstrated by the dose-dependent response of blood pressure to central injection of purified human renin in these transgenic mice. A moderate chronic hypertension and increased drinking intake and salt preference were obtained when these SYN I-hAGT mice were bred with mice that express the human renin driven by the same promoter *(39)*. These findings indicate that neural-derived AGT can be converted locally to ANG II, acting as an autocrine and/or paracrine effector to alter blood pressure and the equilibrium of fluid and electrolytes. Although similar phenotypes regarding cardiovascular function and fluid–electrolyte homeostasis were obtained in both of our transgenic models (whether the expression of hAGT is driven by GFAP or SYN), further studies are required to examine the consequences of differential expression of hAGT on several other functions in which brain RAS is involved, such as cognition, memory, pain perception, sexual behavior, and stress. Models expressing AT-1 receptors in the brain driven by the rat neuron-specific enolase promoter have also been recently reported *(43)*.

Cardiac AGT

The identification of a local RAS in the heart has led some to speculate that its activation could lead to ventricular hypertrophy and myocardial fibrosis independently of blood pressure. Although the source of cardiac renin (de novo local synthesis vs uptake from the circulation) is still debated, strong evidence supports an intracardiac production of ANG II *(44)*. AGT mRNA and protein has been detected in all parts of the hearts of different species, as well as in cultured cardiac myocytes and fibroblasts *(44,45)*. The cardiac production of AGT seems to be regulated by different stimuli, such as glucocorticoids, β-adrenergic receptor agonists, and stretch *(45)*. Furthermore, the levels of cardiac AGT mRNA were significantly increased in hypertensive rats *(46)*, but also in patients with ventricular hypertrophy and heart failure *(47)*.

In order to examine the consequence of increased local production of AGT on cardiac function, Mazzolai et al. *(48)* produced mice overexpressing the rat *AGT* gene specifically in the heart. The cardiac-specific α-myosin heavy-chain promoter was used to direct AGT synthesis in cardiomyocytes. Cardiac specificity of the transgene was demonstrated by its expression in the heart, but not in the other tissues tested. The increase in AGT production in the heart of transgenic animals resulted in increased cardiac ANG II. Cardiac hypertrophy, characterized by the presence of enlarged cardiomyocytes, was observed in all transgenic mice independently of hypertension. However, no significant development of fibrosis was observed in these transgenic animals. These data underline the pathophysiological role of increased AGT synthesis in the heart, which appears to promote cardiac hypertrophy. The direct targeting of angiotensin peptides to the heart using a novel fusion protein has also been shown to induce the expression of atrial natriuretic peptide mRNA, a marker of cardiac hypertrophy *(49)*.

To further examine the role of heart AGT in cardiac hypertrophy, Kang et al. *(50)* used an approach involving the re-expression of AGT in liver and brain, but not heart, in AGT knockout mice. This was achieved by breeding AGT-deficient mice with transgenic mice expressing rat AGT only in the liver and brain. The resulting animals have increased blood pressure, and rescued the developmental defects in the kidney of AGT knockout animals. Interestingly, the mice with AGT only in the brain and liver developed less cardiac hypertrophy than mice capable of making AGT in the heart. The perivascular and interstitial fibrosis was also less pronounced in the mice lacking AGT only in the heart. These data demonstrate that locally synthesized AGT is important for cardiac damage. However, the fact that mice with blunted cardiac AGT synthesis still develop cardiac hypertrophy and fibrosis suggests that uptake of the AGT or other angiotensin peptides from the circulation may also be very important.

Adipose Tissue AGT

Until recently, adipose tissue was considered exclusively as a body energy store without other function. However, the realization that adipocytes can produce many peptides and hormones including leptin, atrial natriuretic peptide, and AGT has led us to view this tissue as an endocrine secretory organ with consequences on the cardiovascular system *(51)*. For instance, AGT produced by the adipose tissue may act locally to affect adipocyte growth and differentiation, or may be secreted into the bloodstream, thereby contributing to the circulating pool of AGT. Synthesis of AGT in adipose tissue associated with the presence in this tissue of the enzymatic cascade and ANG II receptors makes possible the local production and action of ANG II *(52,53)*. To study the specific role of the adipose AGT on fat mass and blood pressure, Massiera et al. *(54)* have generated transgenic mice in which AGT is restricted to adipose tissue. This was achieved by developing mice that express a transgene containing the full-length rat AGT cDNA driven by the adipocyte-specific aP2 promoter. These transgenic mice were then back-crossed with AGT knockout mice to generate animals whose AGT expression is restricted to adipose tissue. Compared with AGT knockout mice, which have no detectable AGT in the plasma, the circulating levels of AGT in the transgenic mice expressing AGT only in the adipose tissue was about 20–30% of the wild-type mice. It is noteworthy to mention that the analysis of AGT secretion from adipose tissue explants has shown an approximately ten-times higher production of AGT in the transgenic mice than wild-type animals, partially explaining the relatively high plasma AGT levels detected in the mice. Nonetheless, expresson of AGT only in the adipose tissue rescued the hypotensive phenotype as well as the renal dysfunction observed in the AGT knockout mice.

This demonstration that AGT produced by the adipose tissue may be released in the bloodstream suggests that the high circulating levels of AGT associated with obesity may be a result of the increased fat mass. We have recently tested the hypothesis that obesity may be associated with an adipose tissue-specific increase in the *AGT* gene transcription (summarized in Fig. 1) *(55)*. We found that mice with obesity induced by high-fat diet exhibited a greater *AGT* gene expression in visceral fat (omental fat, perirenal fat, repro-

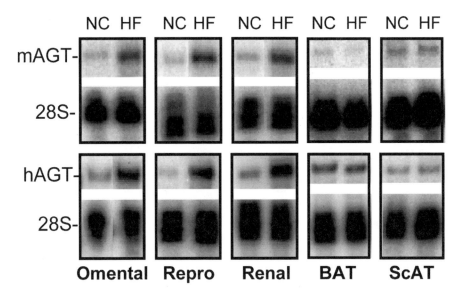

Fig. 3. Effect of the obesity induced by 20 wk of high-fat diet on the expression of mouse angiotensinogen (*AGT*) gene (mAGT) in wild-type mice (top) and hAGT in the transgenic mice (bottom) in the intraabdominal fat depots. The effect of high-fat diet (HF) was compared to normal chow (NC) as a control. mAGT and hAGT mRNA expression was quantified using RNAse protection assay and the 28S rRNA was used as an internal control. Repro, reproductive fat; Renal, peri-renal fat; BAT, brown adipose tissue; ScAT, subcutaneous adipose tissue. (Reprinted from ref. *55*, with permission from the American Physiological Society.)

ductive fat: epididymal fat in males and parametrial fat in females, Fig. 3). However, the expression of the *AGT* gene was not affected by high-fat diet in nonadipose tissues (liver, kidney, and heart), in brown adipose tissue, or in subcutaneous fat. To study the effect of diet-induced obesity on *hAGT* gene expression, we took advantage of the transgenic mice that express the *hAGT* gene. A similar pattern of response was observed for the *hAGT* gene when obesity is induced in these transgenic animals by high-fat diet (Fig. 3), suggesting that the endogenous mouse AGT and transgenic hAGT are regulated in the same fashion. Our findings demonstrate that 1.2 kb of regulatory sequences present in the *hAGT* transgene is sufficient to transcriptionally respond to a high-fat diet, and in an adipose-specific manner. All together, these data indicate that hAGT transgenic mice provide a unique model for studying the regulation of *hAGT* gene in obesity.

CONCLUSION

Gene targeting in the mouse has yielded remarkable advances in our understanding of the role played by specific genes in the regulation of the cardiovascular system. The greatest limitation of this strategy is the lethal phenotype that results from the lack of proteins, such as AGT, serving essential functions. Furthermore, such strategy does not distinguish between the role of an endocrine system and tissue-restricted biological systems. Differentiating between these systems can be technically challenging because of the specificity of pharmacological inhibitors or difficulties in their delivery to appropriate cell types. The strategy of cell-specific targeting coupled with new advances in genetic methodology allowing an investigator to regulate transgene expression or generate cell-specific knockouts is a valid alternative through which to distinguish and elucidate the physiological role of different gene products. We have illustrated that it is feasible to target different locations of AGT to evaluate the contribution of each site of production of this hormone precursor in vivo.

REFERENCES

1. Reid IA, Morris BJ, Ganong WF. The renin–angiotensin system. Annu Rev Physiol 1978;40:377–410.
2. Campbell DJ. Circulating and tissue angiotensin systems. J Clin Invest 1987;79:1–6.
3. Schmidt-Ott KM, Kagiyama S, Phillips MI. The multiple actions of angiotensin II in atherosclerosis. Regul Pept 2000;93:65–77.
4. Gomez RA, Norwood VF. Developmental consequences of the renin–angiotensin system. Am J Kidney Dis 1995;26:409–431.
5. Bader M, Peters J, Baltatu O, Muller DN, Luft FC, Ganten D. Tissue renin–angiotensin systems: new insights from experimental animal models in hypertension research. J Mol Med 2001;79:76–102.
6. Lavoie JL, Sigmund CD. Minireview: overview of the renin–angiotensin system—an endocrine and paracrine system. Endocrinology 2003;144:2179–2183.
7. Jeunemaitre X, Soubrier F, Kotelevtsev YV, et al. Molecular Basis of Human Hypertension: Role of Angiotensinogen. Cell 1992;71:169–180.
8. Watt GC, Harrap SB, Foy CJ, et al. Abnormalities of glucocorticoid metabolism and the renin–angiotensin system: a four-corners approach to the identification of genetic determinants of blood pressure. J Hypertens 1992;10:473–482.
9. Ohkubo H, Kawakami H, Kakehi Y, et al. Generation of transgenic mice with elevated blood pressure by introduction of the rat renin and angiotensinogen genes. Proc Natl Acad Sci USA 1990;87:5153–5157.
10. Tanimoto K, Sugiyama F, Goto Y, et al. Angiotensinogen-deficient mice with hypotension. J Biol Chem 1994;269:31,334–31,337.
11. Kim HS, Krege JH, Kluckman KD, et al. Genetic control of blood pressure and the angiotensinogen locus. Proc Natl Acad Sci USA 1995;92:2735–2739.
12. Hatae T, Takimoto E, Murakami K, Fukamizu A. Comparative studies on species-specific reactivity between renin and angiotensinogen. Mol Cell Biochem 1994;131:43–47.
13. Ganten D, Wagner J, Zeh K, et al. Species-specificity of renin kinetics in transgenic rats harboring the human renin and angiotensinogen genes. Proc Natl Acad Sci USA 1992;89:7806–7810.
14. Yang G, Merrill DC, Thompson MW, Robillard JE, Sigmund CD. Functional expression of the human angiotensinogen gene in transgenic mice. J Biol Chem 1994;269:32497–32502.
15. Brasier AR, Li JY. Mechanisms for inducible control of angiotensinogen gene transcription. Hypertension 1996;27:465–475.
16. Deschepper CF. Angiotensinogen: Hormonal regulation and relative importance in the generation of angiotensin II. Kidney Int 1994;46:1561–1563.
17. Nagata M, Tanimoto K, Fukamizu A, et al. Nephrogenesis and renovascular development in angiotensinogen- deficient mice. Lab Invest 1996;75:745–753.
18. Ingelfinger JR, Zuo WM, Fon EA, Ellison KE, Dzau VJ. In situ hybridization evidence for angiotensinogen messenger RNA in the rat proximal tubule. An hypothesis for the intrarenal renin angiotensin system. J Clin Invest 1990;85:417–423.
19. Merrill DC, Thompson MW, Carney C, Schlager G, Robillard JE, Sigmund CD. Chronic hypertension and altered baroreflex responses in transgenic mice containing the human renin and human angiotensinogen genes. J Clin Invest 1996;97:1047–1055.
20. Davisson RL, Kim HS, Krege JH, Lager DJ, Smithies O, Sigmund CD. Complementation of reduced survival, hypotension and renal abnormalities in angiotensinogen deficient mice by the human renin and human angiotensinogen genes. J Clin Invest 1997;99:1258–1264.
21. Kilby NJ, Snaith MR, Murray JAH. Site-specific recombinases: tools for genome engineering. Trends Genet 1994;9:413–421.
22. Stec DE, Davisson RL, Haskell RE, Davidson BL, Sigmund CD. Efficient liver-specific deletion of a floxed human angiotensinogen transgene by adenoviral delivery of cre-recombinase in vivo. J Biol Chem 1999;274:21,285–21,290.
23. Bosch A, McCray PBJ, Chang SM, et al. Proliferation induced by keratinocyte growth factor enhances in vivo retroviral-mediated gene transfer to mouse hepatocytes. J Clin Invest 1996;98:2683–2687.

24. Stec DE, Keen HL, Sigmund CD. Lower blood pressure in floxed angiotensinogen mice after adenoviral delivery of cre-recombinase. Hypertension 2002;39:629–633.

25. Matsusue K, Haluzik M, Lambert G, et al. Liver-specific disruption of PPARgamma in leptin-deficient mice improves fatty liver but aggravates diabetic phenotypes. J Clin Invest 2003;111:737–747.

26. Wang CT, Navar LG, Mitchell KD. Proximal tubular fluid angiotensin II levels in angiotensin II-induced hypertensive rats. J Hypertens 2003;21:353–360.

27. Kobori H, Harrison-Bernard LM, Navar LG. Urinary excretion of angiotensinogen reflects intrarenal angiotensinogen production. Kidney Int 2002;61:579–585.

28. Loghman-Adham M, Rohrwasser A, Helin C, et al. A conditionally immortalized cell line from murine proximal tubule. Kidney Int 1997;52:229–239.

29. Ding Y, Sigmund CD. Androgen-Dependent Regulation of Human Angiotensinogen Expression in KAP-hAGT Transgenic Mice. Am J Physiol: Renal Physiol 2001;280:F54–F60.

30. Davisson RL, Ding Y, Stec DE, Catterall JF, Sigmund CD. Novel mechanism of hypertension revealed by cell-specific targeting of human angiotensinogen in transgenic mice. Physiol Genomics 1999;1:3–9.

31. Ding Y, Davisson RL, Hardy DO, Zhu L-J, Merrill DC, Catterall JF, Sigmund CD. The kidney androgen-regulated protein (KAP) promoter confers renal proximal tubule cell-specific and highly androgen-responsive expression on the human angiotensinogen gene in transgenic mice. J Biol Chem 1997;272:28,142–28,148.

32. Meseguer A, Catterall JF. Androgen regulated expression of kidney androgen-regulated protein mRNA is localized in the epithelial cells of the murine renal proximal convoluted tubules. Mol Endocrinol 1987;1:535–541.

33. Paul M, Bader M, Steckelings UM, Voigtlander T, Ganten D. The renin–angiotensin system in the brain. Localization and functional significance. [Review]. Arzneimittel-Forschung 1993;43:207–213.

34. Sernia C. Location and secretion of brain angiotensinogen. [Review]. Regulatory Peptides 1995;57:1–18.

35. Morimoto S, Cassell MD, Sigmund CD. The Brain Renin–angiotensin System in Transgenic Mice Carrying a Highly Regulated Human Renin Transgene. Circ Res 2002;90:80–86.

36. Lavoie JL, Cassell MD, Gross KW, Sigmund CD. Localization of Renin Expressing Cells in the Brain Using a REN-eGFP Transgenic Model. Physiol Genomics 2004;16:240–246.

37. Stornetta RL, Hawelu Johnson CL, Guyenet PG, Lynch KR. Astrocytes synthesize angiotensinogen in brain. Science 1988;242:1444–1446.

38. Morimoto S, Cassell MD, Beltz TG, Johnson AK, Davisson RL, Sigmund CD. Elevated blood pressure in transgenic mice with brain-specific expression of human angiotensinogen driven by the glial fibrillary acidic protein promoter. Circ Res 2001;89:365–372.

39. Morimoto S, Cassell MD, Sigmund CD. Glial- and neuronal-specific expression of the renin–angiotensin system in brain alters blood pressure, water intake, and salt preference. J Biol Chem 2002;277:33,235–33,241.

40. Schinke M, Baltatu O, Bohm M, et al. Blood pressure reduction and diabetes insipidus in transgenic rats deficient in brain angiotensinogen. Proc Natl Acad Sci USA 1999;96:3975–3980.

41. Lochard N, Silversides DW, Van Kats JP, Mercure C, Reudelhuber TL. Brain-specific restoration of angiotensin II corrects renal defects seen in angiotensinogen-deficient mice. J Biol Chem 2002;278:2184–2189.

42. Morimoto S, Cassell MD, Sigmund CD. Neuron-specific expression of human angiotensinogen in brain causes increased salt appetite. Physiol Genomics 2002;9:113–120.

43. Lazartigues E, Dunlay SM, Loihl AK, et al. Brain-selective overexpression of angiotensin (AT1) receptors causes enhanced cardiovascular sensitivity in transgenic mice. Circ Res 2002;90:617–624.

44. Bader M. Role of the local renin–angiotensin system in cardiac damage: a minireview focussing on transgenic animal models. J Mol Cell Cardiol 2002;34:1455–1462.

45. Carey RM, Siragy HM. Newly recognized components of the renin–angiotensin system: potential roles in cardiovascular and renal regulation. Endocr Rev 2003;24:261–271.

46. Tamura K, Umemura S, Nyui N, et al. Tissue-specific regulation of angiotensinogen gene expression in spontaneously hypertensive rats. Hypertension 1996;27:1216–1223.

47. Serneri GG, Boddi M, Cecioni I, et al. Cardiac angiotensin II formation in the clinical course of heart failure and its relationship with left ventricular function. Circ Res 2001;88:961–968.

48. Mazzolai L, Nussberger J, Aubert JF, et al. Blood pressure-independent cardiac hypertrophy induced by locally activated renin–angiotensin system. Hypertension 1998;31:1324–1330.

49. Methot D, LaPointe MC, Touyz RM, et al. Tissue targeting of angiotensin peptides. J Biol Chem 1997;272:12,994–12,999.

50. Kang N, Walther T, Tian XL, et al. Reduced hypertension-induced end-organ damage in mice lacking cardiac and renal angiotensinogen synthesis. J Mol Med 2002;80:359–366.

51. Bradley RL, Cleveland KA, Cheatham B. The adipocyte as a secretory organ: mechanisms of vesicle transport and secretory pathways. Recent Prog Horm Res 2001;56:329–358.

52. Engeli S, Negrel R, Sharma AM. Physiology and pathophysiology of the adipose tissue renin–angiotensin system. Hypertension 2000;35:1270–1277.

53. Goossens GH, Blaak EE, van Baak MA. Possible involvement of the adipose tissue renin–angiotensin system in the pathophysiology of obesity and obesity-related disorders. Obes Rev 2003;4:43–55.

54. Massiera F, Bloch-Faure M, Ceiler D, et al. Adipose angiotensinogen is involved in adipose tissue growth and blood pressure regulation. FASEB J 2001;15:2727–2729.

55. Rahmouni K, Mark AL, Haynes WG, Sigmund CD. Adipose depot-specific modulation of angiotensinogen gene expression in diet-induced obesity. Am J Physiol: Endocrinol Metabol 2004;286:E891–E895.

56. Stec DE, Sigmund CD. Modifiable gene expression in kidney: kidney-specific deletion of a target gene via the cre-loxP system. Exp Nephrol 1998;6:568–575.

5 Cardiovascular Pharmacogenomics

Julie A. Johnson, PharmD and
Larisa H. Cavallari, PharmD

SUMMARY

Pharmacogenomics is a field aimed at understanding the genetic contribution to inter-patient variability in drug efficacy and toxicity. The promise of pharmacogenomics is that it will allow for individualized therapy based on a person's genetic makeup, allowing for the selection of the drug that is likely to be the most effective with minimal risk of toxicity. Pharmacogenomics can also be used to help guide the drug discovery process, although this is not discussed in this chapter. This chapter describes the various manners in which pharmacogenomics might be used in the treatment of cardiovascular disease, including those whose treatment is by trial-and-error (like hypertension), and those whose treatment is protocol-driven (like heart failure or myocardial infarction). The current literature on genetic associations with efficacy and toxicity of cardiovascular drug response is reviewed. The approaches to pharmacogenomics research are also reviewed, including a candidate gene-driven approach and genomic approaches. There is discussion of how the approaches to date, usually single-candidate gene, must become more sophisticated in order to better understand the genetic basis for variable drug response. There is also extensive discussion of the various laboratory approaches that are essential to pharmacogenomics, including a number of different polymorphism genotyping methods. Pharmacogenomics holds great promise for enhancing our understanding of cardiovascular drug response and allowing for individualized therapy. There will be substantial work in this field in the coming years, which will hopefully lead to the point of individualization of cardiovascular drug therapy in patients.

Key Words: Pharmacogenetics; pharmacogenomics; drug metabolism; pharmacology; single nucleotide polymorphisms; genotyping methods.

From: *Contemporary Cardiology: Cardiovascular Genomics*
Edited by: M. K. Raizada, et al. © Humana Press Inc., Totowa, NJ

INTRODUCTION

It is well-recognized that there is great interpatient variability in response to drugs, including drugs used in the treatment of cardiovascular disease. Whereas some patients may attain the desired therapeutic response from a given drug, others may show no therapeutic benefit, and others may experience toxicities. Currently, there are limited, if any, tools available to the clinician to help him or her predict into which of these categories a patient might fall if that patient is prescribed a specific drug therapy. There are numerous factors that influence the variability in response to a drug, including the patient's age, race, concomitant diseases, interacting drugs, and renal and hepatic function. However, there is increasing evidence that for a number of drugs, genetic variability plays an important (and sometimes central) role in variable response to drugs. Thus, the field of pharmacogenomics is focused on providing an understanding of the genetic contribution to variable drug response. There is some debate about the differences in definitions of the terms "pharmacogenetics" and "pharmacogenomics," but such discussions seem to have little value. If one chooses to give them different definitions, pharmacogenomics is the broader term, which encompasses pharmacogenetics. As such, we will only use the term pharmacogenomics herein.

There are two broad manners in which pharmacogenomics can be approached from a research perspective. The first is to use genomic information to help identify potential new drug targets. The concept is that if the genetic or genomic basis of a disease is understood, then it might be possible to develop highly targeted therapies. Currently, all drugs used today represent only about 500 different drug targets, although it is estimated that there are probably 5000 to 10,000 potential drug targets in the body. Thus, such an approach clearly has the potential to increase the number of novel drug targets. Although there are certain examples in the area of cancer of marketed drugs that have been developed through such an approach, it would be hard to argue that any marketed cardiovascular drugs have been discovered by this strategy. Because many of the other chapters in this text will deal with ways in which genomics technologies can be useful in understanding cardiovascular disease and therefore in identifying potential new drug targets, we will not focus on these issues in this chapter.

The other manner in which pharmacogenomics can be approached is through attempts to elucidate the genetic (or genomic) contribution to variable drug response of existing drugs, either those on the market or currently under development. The bulk of this chapter will focus on this type of research effort. We will summarize the current literature in the area of cardiovascular pharmacogenomics, discuss the various methodological approaches that can be taken, and review relevant laboratory techniques.

How Pharmacogenomics Might Be Used Clinically

Pharmacological management of cardiovascular diseases is largely based on evidence from clinical trials and guidelines from expert consensus panels. For example, current consensus guidelines recommend the institution of angiotensin-converting enzyme (ACE) inhibitors and β-blockers and consideration of spironolactone in all patients with severe heart failure, based on evidence that these drugs reduced morbidity and mortality in several large clinical trials *(1)*. However, not all participants enrolled in heart failure studies with ACE inhibitors, β-blockers, and spironolactone derived clinical benefits from these drugs, and some study participants experienced serious adverse drug reactions requiring study discontinuation. For instance, in the Studies of Left Ventricular Dysfunc-

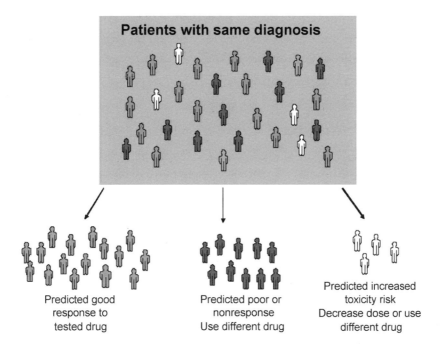

Fig. 1. Clinical potential of pharmacogenetics. Patients with the same empirical diagnosis (e.g., hypertension, leukemia, etc.) are typically treated in the same manner, although their responses to drug therapy will not be the same. Pharmacogenetics has the potential to provide a tool for predicting those patients who are likely to have the desired response to the drug, those who are likely to have little or no benefit, and those at risk for toxicity. This would allow tailored therapy that should reduce adverse reactions to drugs, and increase efficacy rates. (Reproduced with permission from ref. *64.*)

tion (SOLVD), one of the first trials to demonstrate the benefits of ACE inhibitor therapy in heart failure, approx 5% of participants discontinued ACE inhibitor treatment because of worsening disease *(2).* An additional 8% of participants discontinued treatment because of adverse drug effects. Thus, one cannot assume that a given patient will have a favorable response to a particular drug, despite benefits observed in the overall population of a clinical trial.

Pharmacogenomics might enable clinicians to individualize cardiovascular drug therapy based on a person's genotype, as shown in Fig. 1. This approach to cardiovascular disease management has the potential to streamline the management of diseases such as heart failure. Rather than starting all heart failure patients on the same therapy, drug regimens might be tailored according to each individual's genetic predisposition for obtaining benefit or experiencing harm from a particular drug. For instance, patients with heart failure would be genotyped for drug response at the time of heart failure diagnosis. Then, the drug or drugs expected to produce the greatest clinical response for a particular patient with regard to reductions in morbidity and mortality would be started and titrated to maximally tolerated doses. This approach would be particularly beneficial for patients with inadequate blood pressure to safely take recommended doses of both ACE inhibitors and β-blockers. Patients with a genetic predisposition to serious adverse drug effects, such as angioedema from ACE inhibitors, could be started on alternative therapy. Not only would this approach to heart failure management potentially improve clinical outcomes in the heart failure population as a whole, but it might also reduce healthcare costs associated with the management of adverse drug reactions and with unnecessary polypharmacy.

Pharmacogenomics also has the potential to eliminate the trial-and-error approach to the management of diseases such as hypertension. Patients with hypertension are currently started on one or two drugs to lower their blood pressure. Therapy is then continued as initially prescribed if an adequate response is obtained, or, more commonly, therapy is adjusted until there is sufficient blood pressure reduction. Often, initial drug therapy is abandoned because of a lack of response or intolerable adverse effects, and alternative agents are instituted. For example, in the Antihypertensive and Lipid-Lowering Treatment to Prevent Heart Attack Trial (ALLHAT), 15–20% of participants discontinued initial antihypertensive therapy, usually as a result of adverse drug events or therapeutic failure (3). With pharmacogenomics, clinicians might be able to predict a patient's response to various antihypertensive medications prior to drug initiation and then prescribe the drug expected to produce the greatest blood pressure response with the least potential for harm. Such an approach to hypertension management may shorten the duration until blood pressure control is achieved and thus the length of time the patient is at risk for hypertension-related end-organ damage. Additionally, this approach would reduce the number of office visits required to find the best therapy, minimize exposure to agents that will not provide benefit but could still cause adverse effects, and avoid costs for ineffective agents and the adverse events they might cause.

CARDIOVASCULAR PHARMACOGENOMICS: CURRENT EVIDENCE

There are a number of studies in the published literature that provide proof-of-concept that genetic variation contributes to the variable response that is observed upon administration of cardiovascular drugs.

In general, knowledge about drugs is separated into two broad categories: pharmacokinetics and pharmacodynamics. Pharmacokinetics describes the disposition of the drug in the body, including absorption from the gut, distribution to tissues, metabolism (usually in the liver), and elimination from the body (usually by the kidneys). Pharmacodynamics involves the pharmacological action of the drug. Similarly, pharmacogenomics studies are also often separated in this way, as highlighted in Fig. 2. Genetic variability in drug-metabolizing enzymes and drug transporters are the most common causes of variable drug pharmacokinetics, and drug targets (defined as any proteins involved directly or indirectly in the pharmacological action of the drug) are the most common source of variable pharmacodynamics.

Genetic Influences on Pharmacokinetics

DRUG METABOLISM

Drug-metabolism pharmacogenomics has a long history, with work in this field dating to the 1950s. In many cases, patients with extreme response (often toxicity) were found to have excessively high plasma drug concentrations, which were subsequently found to result from variations in the gene for the enzyme important to that drug's metabolism (4). A number of drug-metabolizing enzymes have inactivating mutations, which lead to absent or nonfunctional protein, and for drugs with a high dependence on that particular enzyme, plasma drug concentrations can be 5–10 times that of normal. For drugs with a

Pharmacogenetics

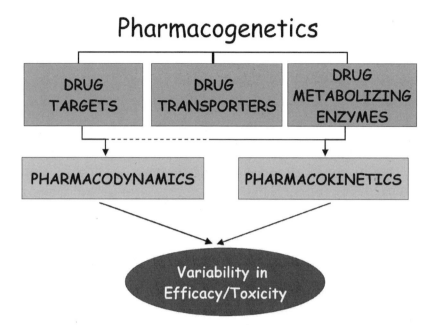

Fig. 2. Key components in pharmacogenetics. Figure highlights the two broad areas for research in pharmacogenetics; specifically, pharmacokinetics and pharmacodynamics. Drug-metabolizing enzymes and drug transporters most often contribute to variable pharmacokinetics. Proteins involved in mediating drug effect are broadly defined as drug targets, and include not just the direct protein targets of the drug but any proteins involved in the drug action (e.g., signal transduction proteins, proteins mediating adverse effects). Any of these types of proteins could contribute to interpatient variability in drug efficacy or toxicity, and thus could be candidate genes in pharmacogenetic studies. (Reproduced with permission from ref. *64*).

narrow therapeutic index (a small range in which the drug is efficacious, without causing toxicity) these polymorphisms can have profound clinical consequences. One of the best examples of clinical application of pharmacogenomics is with the drug-metabolizing enzyme thiopurine *S*-methyltransferase (TPMT), which metabolizes thiopurines commonly used in cancer chemotherapy and for immune suppression *(5)*. This enzyme has several inactivating mutations, and genetic testing for TPMT prior to administration of thiopurines is becoming the standard of practice *(4,5)*.

In the case of cardiovascular drugs, there are some that are substrates for the enzymes that exhibit genetic variability, but in a number of cases, these do not have important clinical consequences. For example, approx 70–80% of the metabolism of the β-blocker metoprolol is controlled by the polymorphic cytochrome P450 2D6 (CYP2D6) enzyme, and those who have inactivating mutations on both alleles have no functional protein present. In these patients, called poor metabolizers, their metoprolol plasma concentrations can be more than five times that of normal *(6–8)*. And although such patients may require lower doses of metoprolol, when it is dose-titrated to response, poor metabolizers do not appear to experience significantly greater rates of toxicity from metoprolol, in large part because its concentration–response curve plateaus. As such, the marked increases in metoprolol plasma concentration seen in CYP2D6 poor metabolizers do not lead to a greater maximal therapeutic effect, but rather just a prolongation of effect *(8)*.

A number of other β-blockers and antiarrhythmic drugs are metabolized by CYP2D6, including timolol, propranolol, carvedilol, propafenone, flecainide, and mexilitene, although none of these are metabolized by CYP2D6 to as great an extent as metoprolol *(9,10)*. CYP2D6 poor metabolizers will have higher concentrations of these drugs as compared to population averages at any given dose, as is seen with metoprolol. However, it is only on occasion that this translates into important problems clinically.

The examples described above are somewhat typical for the cardiovascular drugs in relation to the clinical impact of genetic polymorphisms in the drug-metabolizing enzymes. In general, cardiovascular drugs have very wide therapeutic indexes, so marked increases in plasma drug concentration are typically well tolerated. Thus, drug metabolism pharmacogenomics is less relevant clinically than in areas where the drugs have a much more narrow therapeutic range, such as is the case with cancer chemotherapy, psychiatric medications, and anticonvulsants.

However, there are some interesting exceptions to this rule. Perhaps the one gathering the greatest attention at present is warfarin, an anticoagulant drug with a very narrow therapeutic range, whose metabolism is governed largely by the polymorphic CYP2C9 enzyme. Unlike CYP2D6, CYP2C9 does not have inactivating mutations, but contains several SNPs that change the encoded amino acid, leading to different functional capacities for metabolism. The most common of these polymorphisms are called CYP2C9*2 and CYP2C9*3. Up to 40% of Caucasians (fewer for Asians and those of African descent) carry at least one variant allele, and both variant alleles have significantly reduced catalytic activity *(11)*. Importantly, the presence of one or more variant alleles has been associated in numerous studies with substantially lower warfarin dose requirements, prolongation of the time to stable dosing, and increased risk of bleeding, including serious bleeding episodes *(11–14)*. Given that warfarin requires intensive monitoring and follow-up, the potential benefits of using genetic information to help determine the most appropriate dose for a specific patient are clear. However, studies documenting the benefit of a *priori* genetic information to guide dosing have not yet been done, and until they are, it is unlikely that CYP2C9 genotyping will be used widely in the clinical setting.

Another example in which drug-metabolism genotype is important is with the enzyme *N*-acetyl transferase and the drugs procainamide and hydralazine. The relationship between the genetics and pharmacokinetics of these drugs was among the earliest pharmacogenomic examples. Both of these drugs cause a lupus-like syndrome, and it was recognized decades ago that those who developed this lupus-like syndrome were much more likely to have decreased acetylation as compared with those who did not experience this toxicity *(4,15,16)*. Thus, "slow acetylators," a genetically-determined phenotype, are at increased risk of drug-induced lupus. In the case of procainamide, fast acetylators may also experience genotype-related adverse events. Specifically, procainamide is metabolized to *N*-acetylprocainamide (NAPA), an active metabolite that also possesses antiarrhythmic activity. Fast acetylators accumulate much higher concentrations of NAPA, and as a result are at somewhat increased risk of NAPA-induced QT prolongation and Torsades de Pointes (TdP).

DRUG TRANSPORTERS

Another interesting example that relates to pharmacokinetic differences is digoxin and P-glycoprotein. P-glycoprotein is a membrane-bound adenosine triphosphate (ATP)-dependent efflux pump that is important to the distribution and elimination of a number of drugs, and thus falls into the Fig. 2 "transporter" category *(17,18)*. P-glycoprotein vs gene, *ABCBl* has numerous genetic polymorphisms, some of which have been associated with differences in digoxin plasma concentrations, potentially a result of genotype-dependent bioavail-ability and renal clearance *(19–22)*. Whereas much of the P-glycoprotein literature for other drugs is inconsistent, the findings with respect to digoxin pharmacokinetics and P-glycoprotein are fairly consistent, a finding that may be attributed to the fact that most other P-glycoprotein substrates are confounded by significant metabolism by CYP3A4, while digoxin is not. Other cardiovascular drugs that are substrates for P-glycoprotein include amiodarone, atorvastatin, diltiazem, losartan, quinidine, and verapamil *(17)*. The impact of P-glycoprotein genetic polymorphisms on their pharmacokinetics remains to be elucidated.

Genetic Influences on Pharmacodynamics

As highlighted above, there are some interesting examples of cardiovascular drugs whose pharmacokinetics are affected by genetic variation, leading to differences in efficacy or toxicity. However, it seems that genetic variability in the proteins involved in drug pharmacodynamics will ultimately be more informative to understanding response variability for cardiovascular drugs. Unlike drug metabolism pharmacogenomics, for which there are nearly five decades of research, drug target pharmacogenomics (i.e., that focus on drug pharmacodynamics) is in its infancy, with the first cardiovascular pharmacogenomics papers being published in the mid- to late 1990s. Nonetheless, the literature is expanding rapidly, and a comprehensive review is beyond the scope and goals of this chapter. Table 1 provides some examples from the literature, and the reader is referred to several review articles for more detailed information on the cardiovascular pharmacogenomics literature *(15,16,23)*. Herein, we provide selected examples from the cardiovascular pharmacogenomics literature. The information will be divided into studies showing associations between drug efficacy and genotype and those showing associations between drug toxicity and genotype.

VARIABLE DRUG EFFICACY AND PHARMACOGENOMICS

The two therapeutics areas for which there is the most literature on cardiovascular drug targets and pharmacogenomics are hypertension and lipid disorders. In the area of hypertension, there are data in the literature showing genetic associations between drug targets and antihypertensive response for diuretics, β-blockers, ACE inhibitors, and angiotensin$_1$-receptor blockers. The only first-line drug class with no data is the calcium channel blockers, and this is because there are limited data available on sequence variability in genes relevant to the calcium channel blocker response.

In the case of β-blockers, several different studies have shown an association between polymorphisms in the β$_1$-adrenergic receptor gene and blood pressure lowering *(24–26)*. We and others have found that the strongest predictors of blood pressure lowering are the Arg→Gly polymorphism at codon 389 and the Ser→Gly polymorphism at codon 49. Specifically, those who are Arg389Arg and Ser49Ser had the greatest blood pressure lowering with metoprolol *(25)*. These findings are consistent with in vitro mutagenesis functional studies, which showed that the Arg389 form of the β$_1$-adrenergic receptor had greater basal and agonist-stimulated adenylyl cyclase activity *(27)*. Similarly, the Ser49 form of the β$_1$-adrenergic receptor has been shown to be resistant to agonist-stimulated downregulation *(28,29)*. Thus, in vitro data suggested that the Arg389 and Ser49 forms of the receptor would be associated with the greatest sympathetic nervous system activation, and the β-blocker response data support this. One group has also found an asso-

Table 1
Examples of Cardiovascular Drugs With Evidence
of Association Between Genetics and Efficacy or Toxicity

Drug/Drug class	Gene(s) associated with efficacy or toxicity[a]
β-agonists	β$_2$-adrenergic receptors
β-blockers	β$_1$-adrenergic receptor
	ACE
	Gs protein α subunit
	CYP2D6
ACE inhibitors	ACE
	Angiotensinogen
	AT$_1$ receptor
	Bradykinin B$_2$ receptor
Antiarrhythmics	Various congenital long QT syndrome genes
	N-acetyltransferase (procainamide)
	CYP2D6
Antithrombotics	
Abciximab	Platelet glycoprotein IIIa
Aspirin	Platelet glycoprotein IIIa
Heparin	Platelet Fc γ-receptor
Warfarin	CYP2C9
AT$_1$-receptor blockers	AT$_1$ receptor
Digoxin	P-glycoprotein
Diuretics	G protein β$_3$ subunit
	α-adducin
Hydralazine	N-acetyltransferase
Lipid-lowering drugs	
Statins	Apolipoprotein E
	Cholesteryl ester transfer protein
	Stromelysin-1
	β-fibrogen
	LDL receptor
	Lipoprotein lipase
	ACE
Gemfibrozil	Apolipoprotein E
	Stromelysin-1

[a]The reader is referred to focused reviews for detailed information (15,16,23).
    ACE, angiotensin-converting enzyme; CYP, cytochrome P450; AT$_1$, angiotensin type 1; LDL, low-density lipoprotein.

ciation between a G protein α$_s$ subunit polymorphism and β-blocker response (30). This association is also consistent with pharmacology of the β-blockers, because the β-receptors couple to Gα$_s$.

For the diuretics, a number of different studies have shown genetic associations between blood pressure response and polymorphisms in the G protein β3 gene and the α-adducin gene (31–35). In the case of the α-adducin polymorphism, a nonsynonymous

Arg460Trp cSNP has been associated with increased renal tubular sodium reabsorption, and differential diuretic response *(34–36)*. Perhaps of greatest interest is a study showing that the association between diuretic therapy and reduction in risk of myocardial infarction and stroke differed significantly with α-adducin genotype *(33)*. This case-control study found that the carriers of the wild-type Gly460Gly genotype had no significant benefit from diuretics, whereas those who carried a variant Trp460 allele had a significant 51% reduction in the risk of nonfatal myocardial infarction and stroke. Although these data need to be confirmed in an independent population, they suggest that genotype information might allow us to target therapies to the patient's underlying hypertension pathophysiology.

Genetic association with responses to cholesterol-lowering therapies, particularly statins have also been extensively investigated *(37–47)* and summarized *(37,47)* Genes for which positive associations have been shown include those for apolipoprotein E (Apoε4), stromelysin-1, cholesteryl ester transfer protein (CETP), β-fibrinogen, low-density lipoprotein receptor, lipoprotein lipase, toll-like receptor 4, and CYP3A4, among others. These studies have evaluated a number of different drug-response phenotypes, including lipid lowering, atherosclerosis regression, and cardiovascular outcomes. In the latter category is a study from one of the first statin survival trials, the Scandivavian Simvistatin Surivival Study (4S), which showed that carriers of the Apoε4 allele derived the greatest risk reduction from simvastatin therapy *(41)*.

Cardiovascular Drug Toxicity and Pharmacogenomics

Although cardiovascular drugs tend to be safer than drugs used in other clinical situations (e.g., cancer), there are still some important toxicities for which the ability to predict them based on genetic information would be useful. Perhaps highest on the list for potential benefit is the propensity of certain drugs (both cardiovascular and noncardiovascular) to produce prolongation of the QT interval on the electrocardiogram, and increase the risk of the polymorphic ventricular arrhythmia, TdP. QT prolongation and TdP have been the most common reasons for withdrawal of drugs from the US market over the past 10–15 yr, and all new drugs under investigation must undergo extensive testing to determine their ability to produce QT prolongation. As such, there are extensive efforts underway that seek to identify whether there are genetic factors that predispose a patient to developing QT prolongation and TdP. Numerous studies have found mutations (most have allele frequencies <0.01, thus do not meet the definition of polymorphism) in ion channel genes, particularly the sodium and potassium channels, in patients who have experienced drug-induced QT prolongation or TdP *(23,48–52)*. Although these studies provide clear clues to the genetic basis for risk for drug-induced QT prolongation, there are many challenges. First, QT prolongation and TdP is relatively uncommon, so identifying enough patients who experience this adverse drug effect in order to determine genetic association is a challenge. Additionally, many of the mutations found to date do not occur across a large portion of patients who experience drug-induced QT prolongation. Instead, the data suggest that there are a large number of rare mutations that appear to be associated with QT prolongation risk. Thus, whereas the ultimate goal might be that genetic screening would allow clinicians to select out those patients at risk of QT prolongation from a drug with that propensity, the data are far from that reality. As such, understanding the genetic basis for risk of drug-induced QT prolongation and TdP remains an important research question for basic and clinical scientists.

Another cardiovascular adverse effect that has been extensively studied for its association with genetic polymorphisms is estrogen-induced venous thromboembolism. It is well recognized that estrogen, whether taken as an oral contraceptive or as postmenopausal estrogen replacement therapy, increases a woman's risk of venous thromboembolism. A number of studies have evaluated the role of genetic polymorphisms in proteins in the clotting cascade, particularly prothrombin (Factor II) and Factor V in this adverse event *(53)*. These studies have consistently shown that the G21210A polymorphism in the prothrombin gene and the Leiden mutation (G1691A) in the Factor V gene increase the patient's risk of developing venous thromboembolism. In the case of heterozygotes, the risk is increased approximately three- to eightfold, and in homozygotes about 80-fold *(54)*. The prothrombin and factor polymorphisms occur with allele frequencies in Caucasians of 1–3% and 2–15%, respectively, and thus are common enough in the population to be of interest. Of note is that these mutations are associated with increased risk of venous thromboembolism in the absence of drug therapy, but that risk increases dramatically in the presence of estrogen therapy, particularly through oral contraceptives *(53–59)*. For example, a meta-analysis suggests that the risk of venous thromboembolism is increased 2.3-fold in oral contraceptive users, 5.9-fold in carriers of the Factor V Leiden mutation, and 10.3-fold in carriers of Factor V Leiden who also take oral contraceptives *(54)*. Similar trends have been observed with the prothrombin mutation. As a result of these findings, there has been debate about whether women wishing to use oral contraceptives should first be screened for these mutations *(60,61)*. At present, it is concluded that although the relative risk is markedly increased in individuals with these mutations who also use oral contraceptives, the absolute risk of thromboembolism remains low. Thus, genetic screening at present is not justified, and would likely result in many women being denied oral contraceptives who could take them safely. However, it seems likely that as more factors, both genetic and nongenetic, associated with risk of thromboembolism are identified, such screening might occur in the future.

DISCOVERY OF GENETIC ASSOCIATIONS WITH DRUG RESPONSE

Cardiovascular Pharmacogenomics to Date: A Candidate Gene-Driven Approach

All of the studies highlighted above can be described as following a candidate gene approach. This means that genes and polymorphisms were selected for study based on suspicion that they might be associated with the disease or drug response of interest. In the case of drug response, this tends to work somewhat better than for diseases because intelligent selection of candidate genes is probably easier. This is because we have prior knowledge of the proteins that are important to either the pharmacokinetics or pharmacological action of the drug. Thus, if we know that a drug is metabolized extensively by CYP2D6, then this becomes a good candidate gene for pharmacogenomic study. Likewise, we can use the information we have about a drug's mechanism of action to help select candidate drug target genes. For example, β-blockers work by inhibiting the actions of norepinephrine at the β_1-adrenergic receptor, thus the β_1-adrenergic receptor gene is a good candidate. Similarly, genetic variability in proteins involved in the signal transduction cascade of the drug response may also contribute much to drug response variability. Candidate genes might also be genes for proteins involved in the system that is interfered with the drug; such is the case for the lipid-lowering drugs. In this case, many of the candidate genes are ones that are involved in lipid transport and metabolism, not just genes for those proteins directly involved in the drug response. Thus, candidate gene selection in pharmacogenomic research relies on our current knowledge of the drug's pharmacokinetics, mechanism of action, and the physiologic system in which the drug is acting.

PHARMACOGENOMICS KNOWLEDGE PYRAMID USING THE CANDIDATE GENE APPROACH

Many working in the field of pharmacogenomics view the candidate gene approach as building on a knowledge pyramid, as highlighted in Fig. 3. This is also highlighted in the NIH's Pharmacogenetics and Pharmacogenomics Knowledge Base website (http://www.pharmgkb.org/).

SNP DISCOVERY

Once a candidate gene is selected, based on the above principles, knowledge of the sequence variability in the gene of interest is at the base of the knowledge pyramid. Although information of polymorphisms is increasingly available in public databases, e.g., http://www.ncbi.nlm.nih.gov/SNP/, this information is still often of limited quality, specifically because much of the data currently in the databases has not been validated, or because there is limited information on population allele frequencies. Thus, many pharmacogenomics investigators must first undertake SNP discovery efforts in order identify the relevant sequence variability. This is often done by resequencing the gene of interest in a sufficient number of individuals (e.g., 40 to 100) of diverse ancestral background (e.g., those of African, European, and Asian descent) to capture the population diversity in the gene.

Most current SNP discovery efforts focus on the coding region of the gene, intron/exon junctions, the 5' untranslated region (which is presumed to contain the promoter), and the 3' untranslated region (where sequence variability may influence mRNA stability). Fewer investigators sequence the entire gene, including the full intronic sequence, because the purpose or function of intronic sequence is not yet clear.

IN VITRO FUNCTIONAL STUDIES

Once a genetic polymorphism is identified, there is interest in knowing whether it has functional consequences. Some investigators argue that functional studies should be done prior to any clinical association studies, whereas others suggest that functional studies might be reserved until there is evidence of association with a clinical phenotype. For polymorphisms that occur in the coding region and result in a change in amino acid (nonsynonymous cSNPs), there are also approaches that can be taken to predict the likelihood of functional effect. For example, the Grantham score assesses how radical a change the amino acid substitution is, with the assumption that the more radical the change, the more likely it is to have functional consequence (62). Comparisons of sequence homology across species can also provide insight, as amino acid changes that occur in highly conserved regions are more likely to be of functional consequence. Assessment of the location in the protein can also provide insight, because portions of the protein are known to have specific and more important functions than others. For example, in the case of the β_1-adrenergic receptor codon 389 Arg→Gly polymorphism, functional effect was anticipated prior to any studies, for several reasons. First, the nucleotide change resulted in a moderately radical amino acid change, from a charged to uncharged amino acid. Secondly, codon 389 is in a highly conserved region of the β_1-adrenergic

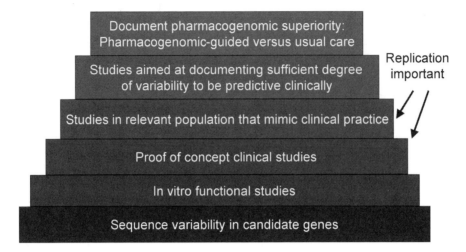

Fig. 3. Moving pharmacogenomics to clinical practice. Pyramid of the steps required to move knowledge from point of sequence variability to clinical utility of pharmacogenetic information in practice. (Reproduced with permission from ref. *64*).

receptor protein, and is located in a region that is critical to G protein coupling. As described previously, functional studies did suggest that this polymorphism is functional *(27)*, which was further supported by clinical studies, including pharmacogenetic studies *(24–26)*. Finally, if the crystallized protein structure is known, it is possible to make predictions *in silico* of the potential effects of the nonsynonymous SNP.

Actual functional studies can be conducted in a number of ways, although in vitro mutagenesis of cell culture systems, with evaluation of the functions of the different forms of the protein, is most common. Transgenic animal models can also be undertaken, but are technically more difficult than the cell culture-based approaches.

Having an understanding of the functional basis for clinical associations with genetic polymorphisms is important, and although some could argue about the point in the process at which these should be conducted, there is little debate about their importance.

CLINICAL STUDIES

With respect to pharmacogenomics research, clinical studies are sometimes first done in normal volunteers (as compared to the relevant patient population). In certain situations this is reasonable, whereas in others it might be misleading and could lead investigators to believe that there are no genetic associations with drug response, when it is just that the magnitude and variability in drug response in normals may simply not be large enough to document the association.

At some point, particularly for drug target-focused pharmacogenomics studies, it is important that these are conducted in a relevant patient population, in a manner that reflects usual treatment practices. Without this, it will not be possible to move the information to the point of clinical utility.

Future Approaches

CANDIDATE GENE APPROACH DRIVEN BY POLYGENIC NATURE OF DRUG RESPONSE

The current literature provides clear proof-of-concept that genetic variability contributes to the interpatient variability in drug response. However, as discussed previously,

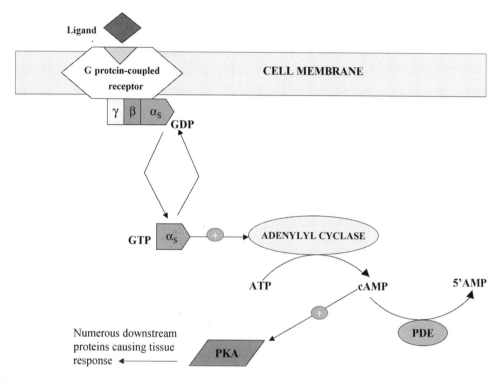

Fig. 4. Representative signal transduction cascade for drug effect. Simplified schematic of signal transduction cascade for receptors coupling to G protein α_s subunit. Abbreviations: ATP, adenosine triphosphate; cAMP, cyclic adenosine monophosphate; PDE, phosphodiesterase; PKA, protein kinase A; GDP, guanosine diphosphate; GTP, guanosine triphosphate. (Reproduced with permission from ref. *64*).

most of the studies have focused on a single gene (and often on a single polymorphism within the gene), and although this might provide evidence of a genetic association with response, it usually does not explain enough of the variability to be utilized clinically. This concept is discussed in detail elsewhere *(63,64)*. In order to move the field to the point where a sufficient amount of the response variability is accounted for, it seems likely that there has to be a move toward a more inclusive candidate gene approach or a genomic approach.

A broader candidate gene approach will probably necessitate consideration of genes that contribute to both the drug's pharmacokinetics and pharmacodynamics, and within the pharmacodynamics, consideration of the complexity of the drug response. By example, Fig. 4 shows a simplified schematic of the signal transduction cascade for the β-adrenergic receptors and other Gα$_s$ protein-coupled receptors. This highlights that there are numerous proteins involved in the signal transduction cascade, and thus many genes whose variability might contribute to variable drug response. This signal transduction cascade is not atypical for those involved in drug action, and is less complicated than many of the other signal transduction cascades relevant to drug action. Additionally, there are often other systems that may be involved, and thus their genes may also contribute to variable drug response. For example, the β-adrenergic receptor system is closely tied to the renin–angiotensin system, and thus data suggesting that an *ACE* gene polymorphism is associated with β-blocker response are not surprising *(65)*.

There are several studies that have begun to follow this multicandidate gene approach, and it seems likely that this approach will be increasingly common. For example, Sciarrone et al. *(32)* examined the *ACE* and *α-adducin* genes as candidates for response to diuretic therapy in hypertension. These genes were chosen based on evidence for their role in blood pressure response to sodium. Greatest blood pressure response to diuretic therapy was observed in patients with at least one insertion allele of the *ACE* gene and one 460Trp allele of the *α-adducin* gene, supporting polygenic determinants of diuretic response.

Studies of warfarin pharmacogenetics have also begun to move to this approach. In a study in our laboratory, we are testing the contribution of seven polymorphisms in three coagulation factor genes and the *CYP2C9* gene for their correlation with warfarin dose requirements. Other groups have taken similar approaches. One group focused on genetic variation in three genes that contribute to warfarin pharmacokinetics, including *CYP2C9*, *CYP3A5*, and *ABCB1 (66)*. Although *ABCB1* variants were overrepresented in the low-dose patients, these polymorphisms were not significant predictors of warfarin dose in multiple regression analysis, whereas *CYP2C9* genotype was. Shikata et al. tested eight different genes, including those for Factors II, VII, IX, and X, protein S, protein C, γ-glutamyl carboxylase and *CYP2C9* relative to warfarin pharmacokinetics and pharmacodynamics *(67)*. They found that they could account for 50% of the variance in warfarin sensitivity based on polymorphisms in *CYP2C9*, Factor II, Factor VII, and γ-glutamyl carboxylase. This level of prediction of variance is higher than nearly all other pharmacogenetic studies to date. These findings illustrate how genetic variation in the proteins involved in both the disposition of a drug and the effects of the drug can contribute to the observed interpatient variability in drug response.

GENOMIC APPROACHES

Although much has been learned through candidate gene-driven pharmacogenomic studies, there are certain limitations to this approach. One important limitation is that the approach is based on our current understanding of the pharmacokinetics, the mechanism of action of the drug, and the disease state. When comparing pharmacogenomic studies to disease-gene studies, pharmacogenomics clearly has the advantage with regard to the candidate gene approach. This is because we do have a fairly good knowledge of the proteins (and thus genes) involved in the pharmacokinetics and action of the drug, therefore there is greater likelihood of the selected candidate genes being associated with variable drug response. Nonetheless, this approach is still limited by our current understanding, and thus prevents us from identifying genes that might contribute to variable drug response because we do not know of their role in the drug's pharmacokinetics or action.

Another limitation inherent in candidate gene studies is that the genetic variation under study may not actually have any functional activity, despite significant associations between the variant and the outcome of interest. Rather, the variant may be a marker for a functionally active variant or variants located elsewhere in the genome. An alternative to the candidate gene approach is a genomically based approach. One advantage of genome-wide approach is that it requires no previous knowledge of gene function or even of proteins involved in disease biology or drug effects. Genome-wide approaches also have the potential to identify unsuspected genetic associations with drug response, and thus may provide insight into previously undescribed disease mechanisms and targets for disease intervention.

A genomic approach commonly used in animal models and certain human diseases is gene expression microarray studies. This requires collection of a tissue of interest and testing for differential expression levels of mRNA. This approach can be very informative and provide new insights into disease or drug response. However, in the setting of human studies of cardiovascular disease, this approach has clear limitations. First, access to tissues of interest in cardiovascular disease represents a significant barrier to these approaches in human studies. But perhaps more importantly, many of the cardiovascular diseases are essentially systemic diseases, e.g., hypertension, heart failure, or lipid disorders. In these diseases, the most appropriate tissue for study would not be clear. For example, in hypertension, the response to antihypertensive drugs may be based on a combination of their effects on the brain, heart, vasculature and kidney. Thus, gene expression microarray studies have limited utility in cardiovascular pharmacogenomics.

Another approach that is common in the search to understand the genetic basis for disease is the genome scanning approach. This approach tests for association with a phenotype with microsattelite markers spread throughout the genome. This allows for localization on the chromosome where causative genes for the disease of interest may lie. Such approaches are common in cardiovascular disease, and there have been numerous recent publications using such an approach to decipher the genetic contribution to hypertension (68,69). However, this approach is also not feasible within the context of pharmacogenomics studies. This is because these are family-based studies that use large pedigrees or discordant siblings to test for the association. Although family studies are common in genetics research, they are not usually feasible within pharmacogenomics because it is rare that multiple family members, particularly across generations, have exposure to the same drug and have had their response to that drug carefully characterized.

For the reasons previously described, several of the common genomic approaches used to aid in understanding of disease are not particularly amenable to cardiovascular pharmacogenomics research. Genomic approaches that focus on genomic DNA and variability within the genome are therefore the approaches that have the greatest potential application in cardiovascular pharmacogenomics (70,71). To date, published data using such approaches for cardiovascular drugs are limited, although such studies are clearly underway.

Approaches utilizing single nucleotide polymorphism (SNP) maps across the genome are likely to be the most commonly used genomic approaches within cardiovascular pharmacogenomics. The objective under this approach is to use SNPs from across the genome to identify those chromosomal locations associated with drug response variability. SNP maps available commercially at present can test for approx 10,000 SNPs using chip technology (e.g., the Gene Chip® 10K Array from Affymetrix; http://www.affymetrix.com/products/arrays/specific/10k.affx) (70). Given that there are an estimated 10 million SNPs, this approach captures only a small portion of the genetic variability, although it is perhaps the best available at this time. A substantial improvement to a genomic SNP map approach occurred in 2004, when Affymetrix marketed a 100,000 SNP chip, based on a similar technology to that of their 10K SNP chip. Eventually, this approach will be perfected further through data generated through the International HapMap Project (http://www.genome.gov/10001688). The HapMap project focuses on the fact that the genetic variability occurs in blocks (called haplotypes) within a chromosome (e.g., certain polymorphisms are inherited together at a frequency higher than expected by chance). The goal of the HapMap project is to determine the SNPs in the haplotype that uniquely define that haplotype, such that only a small portion of the genetic variability in that block would actually have to be tested. It is anticipated that the HapMap project might identify about 500,000 tag SNPs that could be genotyped to represent the genetic diversity across the entire human genome.

The genomic approaches currently available (e.g., the 10K or 100K SNP chips) are expensive, but not prohibitively so. Over the next 5–10 yr, as the costs of genotyping fall further, and the technologies for genome-wide SNP genotyping are enhanced, it is anticipated that costs or feasibility for such approaches will not limit the use of this approach. The greater challenges are likely to lie in the interpretation of the genomic variability data, and the statistical genetics approaches that are needed to analyze these type data.

LABORATORY METHODS IN PHARMACOGENOMICS RESEARCH: SNP GENOTYPING

The pharmacogenomics researcher will use a variety of laboratory methods, depending on his or her work. Those involved in SNP discovery will utilize direct sequencing, perhaps along with other screening methods for variation such as denaturing high-performance liquid chromatography (HPLC) or single-stranded conformation polymorphism (SSCP) analysis. Those conducting functional studies might use a wide array of cell culture, animal, or molecular techniques in order to test for functional effects of polymorphisms. However, the necessity of being able to genotype samples of genomic DNA from patients is essentially universal among pharmacogenomics researchers.

There are a variety of techniques available for screening variations in an amplified segment of genomic DNA. Direct sequencing of products from a polymerase chain reaction (PCR) is considered the "gold standard" of genotyping techniques to which other techniques are compared. Automated, fluorescence-based DNA sequencing was used to draft the sequence of the human genome and largely enabled the early completion of the human genome project (72). The SNP consortium, a collaborative effort of pharmaceutical companies, a large research charity, and academic centers, used a reduced representation shotgun sequencing approach to create a high-density, high-quality SNP map of the human genome (73). Basically, genomic DNA from a group of unrelated individuals was digested by restriction enzymes, and fragments of certain sizes were then directly sequenced. However, for SNP genotyping (as opposed to SNP discovery), sequencing has several limitations. First, it requires equipment that is typically owned by core laboratories, but much less frequently by individual investigators. This limits the ability of an investigator to do his or her own genotyping if sequencing was the approach. Additionally, sequencing is somewhat more cumbersome from a laboratory and analysis approach than other methods, and in most cases is more expensive than other methods. Thus, it is rarely used as a primary genotyping method.

An alternative to sequencing is PCR coupled with restriction fragment length polymorphism (RFLP) analysis (74). This genotyping approach has been widely used for many years to examine a limited number of polymorphisms in a relatively small number of samples. The PCR-RFLP method involves digestion of PCR products containing the polymorphism of interest with an enzyme that recognizes one polymorphic allele but not the other. Resulting DNA fragments are then separated on a gel by electrophoresis and visualized with ethidium bromide staining to determine genotype. Samples for which the genotype has been determined by direct sequencing may be included in PCR-RFLP experiments with DNA samples of unknown genotype to ensure the accuracy of genotyping results.

One limitation with RFLP is that restriction enzymes that discriminate between the polymorphic alleles of interest are not always commercially available. However, this limitation may be overcome by creating a restriction site in the PCR product that will then be recognizable by an available restriction enzyme and will enable enzymatic discrimination between polymorphic alleles. Such restriction sites are created through alteration of one or more bases in the oligonucleotide PCR primer. Another limitation of RFLP analysis is that it is not automated, and thus is relatively time-consuming and labor-intensive (and thus expensive), and not practical or feasible for large-scale pharmacogenomic studies.

High throughput genotyping technologies enable efficient genotyping for large-scale pharmacogenomic studies that involve multiple genetic variations and/or genotyping on large sample sets. The available technologies and their advantages, disadvantages, and costs have been reviewed and we will summarize them here *(75)*. Single nucleotide primer extension (SNPE) followed by fluorescence detection is one method to rapidly determine SNPs in a large number of samples *(76)*. The SNPE method is also referred to as minisequencing because a limited number of bases are sequenced with each reaction. Several SNPE assays have been described *(77)*. These include the PinPoint *(78)* and GOOD *(79)* assays in which an oligonucleotide primer anneals to a template PCR product immediately adjacent to the polymorphic base pair (bp). In the presence of a fluorescently-labeled dideoxynucleotide triphosphate (ddNTP) chain terminator, DNA polymerase extends the primer by a single base that is complementary to the base on the PCR template. Fluorescence detection with an automated gel-based sequencer reveals the identity of the appended DNA base(s).

In contrast to the PinPoint and Good assays, the PROBE assay *(80)* and MassExtend™ *(81)* assay utilize a mixture of deoxynucleotide triphosphates (dNTPs) and a single ddNTP. Deoxynucleotides are incorporated into the primer extension product until the ddNTP is incorporated and the reaction terminates. The resultant primer extension products will differ among heterozygous alleles. Thus the mass of the extension product will differ among alleles. These mass differences can be used to help identify the polymorphism.

Multiplexing, or simultaneous detection of multiple SNPs in a single PCR amplicon, may be done with SNPE and differently-sized primers. Each is designed to end one nucleotide from the polymorphism of interest *(82)*. Separation of differently sized primers on DNA sequencing gels allows for the detection of fluorescently labeled nucleotides appended to each primer. Applied Biosystems (Foster, CA) produces a SnaPshot® Multiplex Kit for commercial use, which allows multiplexing of up to 10 SNPE reactions in a single tube (www.appliedbiosystems.com).

Mass spectrometry through matrix-assisted laser desorption ionization (MALDI) and time-of-flight detectors is an alternative to fluorescent-labeling as a method to detect appended bases from SNPE assays (83). Genotyping by mass spectrometry is based on the molecular weight differences of nucleotide bases, where the identity of the polymorphic nucleotide is determined by its mass. The combination of SNPE and MALDI-mass spectrometry may be fully automated and is adaptable to high throughput SNP analysis. In addition, multiplexing is possible because of the ability of MALDI-mass spectrometry to accurately resolve primers of various masses *(84)*. Kim et al. *(85)* recently reported successful genotyping of three different SNPs in the same PCR amplicon of the β_2-adrenergic receptor gene using SNPE and MALDI-mass spectrometry technology. Several kits are commercially available for SNPE with the MALDI-mass spectrometry genotyping detection platform. These include the Sequazyme™ Pinpoint SNP Assay Kit (Applied Biosystems), and the MassARRAY™ System (Sequenom, San Diego, CA, Caltonics Inc. Billerica, MA, www.bdal.com).

One major limitation with SNPE and MALDI is that they are very sensitive to impurities. Impurities can affect the specificity of nucleotide incorporation by DNA polymerase during the SNPE reaction, in addition to interfering with the mass spectrometry assay (76,77). Thus, purification of the PCR amplicon is necessary prior to the single primer extension, resulting in additional technical time and effort.

Other, non-SNPE methods to produce allele-specific products for mass spectrometry detection include hybridization, oligonucleotide ligation, and cleavage. A detailed review of these technologies in addition to other types of mass spectrometry is provided by Tost and Gut (77). The cost of a mass spectrometer currently limits widespread use of mass spectrometry-based genotyping; however, once the instrumentation is purchased, the cost per sample is comparable with that of other technologies (86).

Pyrosequencing technology is useful for medium- to high-throughput analysis of SNPs and other types of polymorphisms such as insertion/deletions. The methodology of Pyrosequencing is reviewed in detail by Fakhrai-Rad et al. (87). The basic premise of pyrosequencing is that when DNA polymerase incorporates a nucleotide into a DNA strand, pyrophosphate is released. Pyrophosphate is converted to ATP, which provides the necessary energy to generate a detectable light signal that is indicative of the number of incorporated nucleotides. Each of the four dNTPs is added to the pyrosequencing reaction individually. If the base is complementary to the base on a template strand included in the reaction, then the base is incorporated. Unincorporated dNTPs are degraded prior to the addition of the next base. Results from pyrosequencing provide a limited sequence of bases surrounding the polymorphism of interest (usually 20–30 bp). Advantages to pyrosequencing include its accuracy, speed, and automated and multiplexing capabilities. Commercially available models can analyze approx 30,000 polymorphisms in 24 h (www.biotage.com). The sequence surrounding the assayed polymorphism may be used as a control to verify the accuracy of the reaction. The use of pyrosequencing is most limited by the cost of the instrument. However, with the exclusion of instrument cost, the cost of genotyping per sample does not differ significantly from other assay methods. Another limitation is that primers and unincorporated nucleotides from the PCR reaction must be removed prior to pyrosequencing because they may interfere with the pyrosequencing reaction. However, purification strategies amendable to automation are available (87).

Denaturing HPLC is also useful for identifying SNPs, insertions, and deletions (88). Under partial denaturing conditions, PCR products are denatured and reannealed to form homo- and heteroduplexes. Homoduplexes are formed when both DNA strands have the same sequence, whereas heteroduplexes result from the annealing of two strands with differing sequence. Homo- and heteroduplexes are distinguished from one another based on differing retention times. Under complete denaturing conditions, HPLC resolves single-stranded nucleic acids in PCR amplicons based on differences in base composition. Differences in base composition result in differences in hydrophobicity and HPLC retention times. For example, cytosine is the least hydrophobic base and thus has the shortest retention time, whereas the most hydrophobic base, thymidine, is retained the longest *(88)*. A denaturing HPLC system and software for detecting both known and unknown genetic variations in PCR products, marketed as the Wave® System, is commercially available from Transgenomic Inc. (San Jose, CA; www.transgenomic.com).

CONCLUSIONS

The field of pharmacogenomics is a rapidly evolving one, and cardiovascular drugs are among the most extensively studied in the field. There is currently clear evidence that genetic variability influences both the likelihood for efficacy and risk of toxicity of a drug in a given patient. The ultimate goal, from a clinical perspective, is that pharmacogenomics will allow for therapy to be individualized to a specific patient based on his or her genetic profile. This goal is still a long way from reality for cardiovascular drugs; such an approach might be used in limited ways within the 5- to 10-yr time frame, but probably not before that.

The approaches used to address cardiovascular pharmacogenomics questions to date have focused largely on candidate genes. Although a candidate gene approach seems to work better in pharmacogenomics than in studies aimed at uncovering the genetic basis of complex disease, it seems clear that more sophisticated approaches must be taken. These more sophisticated approaches might include either focusing on numerous candidate genes that might influence a drug's action and disposition, or genomic approaches that are not influenced by our current knowledge of the drug.

Technologies to enable pharmacogenomics research are rapidly expanding and the costs for genotyping are dropping quickly. It is anticipated that technologies for genome-wide SNP genotyping will become increasingly affordable, and that the major challenges ahead will center around analysis of the large quantities of data generated by such an approach.

Pharmacogenomics is a field that appears to offer great promise for improving the management of cardiovascular diseases with drug therapy. Research in this field represents a translational approach, with the data collected largely from human subjects, but requiring basic genetic and molecular biology knowledge and techniques in order to conduct the research.

ACKNOWLEDGMENTS

This work was supported in part by NIH grants R01 HL64691, R01 HL74730, K24 HL68834, and R01 HL64924, and a grant from Abbott Laboratories, Inc. to JAJ and AHA Midwest Affiliate Grant #0335361Z to LHC.

REFERENCES

1. Hunt SA, et al. ACC/AHA Guidelines for the Evaluation and Management of Chronic Heart Failure in the Adult: Executive Summary A Report of the American College of Cardiology/American Heart Association Task Force on Practice Guidelines (Committee to Revise the 1995 Guidelines for the Evaluation and Management of Heart Failure): Developed in Collaboration With the International Society for Heart and Lung Transplantation; Endorsed by the Heart Failure Society of America. Circulation 2001;104:2996–3007.
2. Effect of enalapril on survival in patients with reduced left ventricular ejection fractions and congestive heart failure. The SOLVD Investigators. N Engl J Med 1991;325:293–302.
3. Major outcomes in high-risk hypertensive patients randomized to angiotensin-converting enzyme inhibitor or calcium channel blocker vs diuretic: the Antihypertensive and Lipid-Lowering Treatment to Prevent Heart Attack Trial (ALLHAT). JAMA 2002;288:2981–2997.

4. Weinshilboum R. Inheritance and Drug Response. N Engl J Med 2003;348:529–537.

5. Krynetski EY and Evans WE. Genetic Polymorphism of Thiopurine S-Methyltransferase: Molecular Mechanisms and Clinical Importance. Pharmacology 2000;61:136–146.

6. McGourty JC, et al. Metoprolol metabolism and debrisoquine oxidation polymorphism—population and family studies. Br J Clin Pharmacol 1985;20:555–566.

7. Lennard MS, et al. Differential stereoselective metabolism of metoprolol in extensive and poor debrisoquin metabolizers. Clin Pharmacol Ther 1983;34:732–737.

8. Lennard MS, et al. Oxidation phenotype—a major determinant of metoprolol metabolism and response. N Engl J Med 1982;307:1558–1560.

9. Lennard MS, Tucker GT, Woods HF. The polymorphic oxidation of beta-adrenoceptor antagonists. Clinical pharmacokinetic considerations. Clin Pharmacokinet 1986;11:1–17.

10. Buchert E, Woosley RL. Clinical implications of variable antiarrhythmic drug metabolism. Pharmacogenetics 1992;2:2–11.

11. Daly AK, King BP. Pharmacogenetics of oral anticoagulants. Pharmacogenetics 2003;13:247–252.

12. Freeman BD, et al. Cytochrome P450 polymorphisms are associated with reduced warfarin dose. Surgery 2000;128:281–285.

13. Aithal GP, et al. Association of polymorphisms in the cytochrome P450 CYP2C9 with warfarin dose requirement and risk of bleeding complications. Lancet 1999;353:717–719.

14. Higashi MK, et al. Association between CYP2C9 genetic variants and anticoagulation-related outcomes during warfarin therapy. JAMA 2002;287:1690–1698.

15. Johnson JA, Humma LM. Pharmacogenetics of cardiovascular drugs. Brief Functional Genom Proteom 2002;1:66–79.

16. Terra SG, Johnson JA. Pharmacogenetics, pharmacogenomics, and cardiovascular therapeutics: the way forward. Am J Cardiovasc Drugs 2002;2:287–296.

17. Schwab M, Eichelbaum M, Fromm MF. Genetic polymorphisms of the human MDR1 drug transporter. Annu Rev Pharmacol Toxicol 2003;43:285–307.

18. Sakaeda T, Nakamura T, Okumura K. Pharmacogenetics of MDR1 and its impact on the pharmacokinetics and pharmacodynamics of drugs. Pharmacogenomics 2003;4:397–410.

19. Hoffmeyer S, et al. Functional polymorphisms of the human multidrug-resistance gene: multiple sequence variations and correlation of one allele with P-glycoprotein expression and activity in vivo. Proc Natl Acad Sci USA 2000;97:3473–3478.

20. Verstuyft C, et al. Digoxin pharmacokinetics and MDR1 genetic polymorphisms. Eur J Clin Pharmacol 2003;58:809–812.

21. Johne A, et al. Modulation of steady-state kinetics of digoxin by haplotypes of the P-glycoprotein MDR1 gene. Clin Pharmacol Ther 2002;72:584–594.

22. Kurata Y, et al. Role of human MDR1 gene polymorphism in bioavailability and interaction of digoxin, a substrate of P-glycoprotein. Clin Pharmacol Ther 2002;72:209–219.

23. Roden DM. Cardiovascular pharmacogenomics. Circulation 2003;108:3071–3074.

24. Sofowora GG, et al. A common beta1-adrenergic receptor polymorphism (Arg389Gly) affects blood pressure response to beta-blockade. Clin Pharmacol Ther 2003;73:366–371.

25. Johnson JA, Zineh I, Puckett BJ, et al. Beta1-adrenergic receptor polymorphisms and antihypertensive response to metoprolol. Clin Pharmacol Ther 2003;74:44–52.

26. Liu J, et al. Gly389Arg polymorphism of beta1-adrenergic receptor is associated with the cardiovascular response to metoprolol. Clin Pharmacol Ther 2003;74:372–379.

27. Mason DA, et al. A gain-of-function polymorphism in a G-protein coupling domain of the human beta1-adrenergic receptor. J Biol Chem 1999;274:12,670–12,674.

28. Rathz DA, et al., Amino acid 49 polymorphisms of the human beta1-adrenergic receptor affect agonist-promoted trafficking. J Cardiovasc Pharmacol 2002;39:155–160.

29. Levin MC, et al., The myocardium-protective gly-49 variant of the beta 1-adrenergic receptor exhibits constitutive activity and increased desensitization and down-regulation. J Biol Chem 2002;277:30,429–30,435.

30. Jia H, et al. Association of the G(s)alpha gene with essential hypertension and response to beta-blockade. Hypertension 1999;34:8–14.

31. Turner ST, et al. C825T polymorphism of the G protein beta(3)-subunit and antihypertensive response to a thiazide diuretic. Hypertension 2001;37:739–743.

32. Sciarrone MT, et al. ACE and alpha-adducin polymorphism as markers of individual response to diuretic therapy. Hypertension 2003;41:398–403.

33. Psaty BM, et al. Diuretic Therapy, the alpha-adducin gene variant, and the risk of myocardial infarction or stroke in persons with treated hypertension. JAMA 2002;287:1680–1689.

34. Glorioso N, et al. The role of alpha-adducin polymorphism in blood pressure and sodium handling regulation may not be excluded by a negative association study. Hypertension 1999;34:649–654.

35. Cusi D, et al. Polymorphisms of alpha-adducin and salt sensitivity in patients with essential hypertension. Lancet 1997;349:1353–1357.

36. Manunta P, Barlassina C, Bianchi G. Adducin in essential hypertension. FEBS Lett 1998;430:41–44.

37. Dornbrook-Lavender KA, Pieper JA. Genetic polymorphisms in emerging cardiovascular risk factors and response to statin therapy. Cardiovasc Drugs Ther 2003;17:75–82.

38. Boekholdt SM, et al. Variants of toll-like receptor 4 modify the efficacy of statin therapy and the risk of cardiovascular events. Circulation 2003;107:2416–2421.

39. de Maat MP, et al. –455G/A polymorphism of the beta-fibrinogen gene is associated with the progression of coronary atherosclerosis in symptomatic men: proposed role for an acute-phase reaction pattern of fibrinogen. REGRESS group. Arterioscler Thromb Vasc Biol 1998;18:265–271.

40. de Maat MP, et al. Effect of the stromelysin-1 promoter on efficacy of pravastatin in coronary atherosclerosis and restenosis. Am J Cardiol 1999;83:852–856.

41. Gerdes LU, et al. The apolipoprotein epsilon4 allele determines prognosis and the effect on prognosis of simvastatin in survivors of myocardial infarction: a substudy of the Scandinavian simvastatin survival study. Circulation 2000;101:1366–1371.

42. Heath KE, et al. The type of mutation in the low density lipoprotein receptor gene influences the cholesterol-lowering response of the HMG-CoA reductase inhibitor simvastatin in patients with heterozygous familial hypercholesterolaemia. Atherosclerosis 1999;143:41–54.

43. Jukema JW, et al. The Asp9 Asn mutation in the lipoprotein lipase gene is associated with increased progression of coronary atherosclerosis. REGRESS Study Group, Interuniversity Cardiology Institute, Utrecht, The Netherlands. Regression Growth Evaluation Statin Study. Circulation 1996;94:1913–1918.

44. Kajinami K, et al. CYP3A4 genotypes and plasma lipoprotein levels before and after treatment with atorvastatin in primary hypercholesterolemia*1. Am J Cardiol 2004;93:104–107.

45. Kuivenhoven JA, et al. The role of a common variant of the cholesteryl ester transfer protein gene in the progression of coronary atherosclerosis. The Regression Growth Evaluation Statin Study Group. N Engl J Med 1998;338:86–93.

46. Ordovas JM, et al. Effect of apolipoprotein E and A-IV phenotypes on the low density lipoprotein response to HMG CoA reductase inhibitor therapy. Atherosclerosis 1995;113:157–166.

47. Schmitz G, and Drobnik W. Pharmacogenomics and pharmacogenetics of cholesterol-lowering therapy. Clin Chem Lab Med 2003;41:581–589.

48. Yang P, et al. Allelic variants in long-QT disease genes in patients with drug- associated torsades de pointes. Circulation 2002;105:1943–1948.

49. Napolitano C, et al. Evidence for a cardiac ion channel mutation underlying drug-induced QT prolongation and life-threatening arrhythmias. J Cardiovasc Electrophysiol 2000;11:691–696.

50. Drici MD, Barhanin J. Cardiac K+ channels and drug-acquired long QT syndrome. Therapie 2000;55:185–193.

51. Sesti F, et al. A common polymorphism associated with antibiotic-induced cardiac arrhythmia. Proc Natl Acad Sci USA 2000;97:10,613–10,618.

52. Splawski I, et al. Variant of SCN5A sodium channel implicated in risk of cardiac arrhythmia. Science 2002;297:1333–1336.

53. Martinelli I, Battaglioli T, Mannucci PM. Pharmacogenetic aspects of the use of oral contraceptives and the risk of thrombosis. Pharmacogenetics 2003;13:589–594.

54. Emmerich J, et al. Combined effect of factor V Leiden and prothrombin 20210A on the risk of venous thromboembolism—pooled analysis of 8 case-control studies including 2310 cases and 3204 controls. Study Group for Pooled-Analysis in Venous Thromboembolism. Thromb Haemost 2001;86:809–816.

55. Martinelli I, et al. High risk of cerebral-vein thrombosis in carriers of a prothrombin-gene mutation and in users of oral contraceptives. N Engl J Med 1998;338:1793–1797.

56. Martinelli I, et al. Interaction between the G20210A mutation of the prothrombin gene and oral contraceptive use in deep vein thrombosis. Arterioscler Thromb Vasc Biol 1999;19:700–703.

57. Herrington DM, et al. Estrogen-receptor polymorphisms and effects of estrogen replacement on high-density lipoprotein cholesterol in women with coronary disease. N Engl J Med 2002;346:967–974.

58. Martinelli I, Battaglioli T, Mannucci PM. Combined estrogen-progestin oral contraceptives. N Engl J Med 2004;350:307–308; author reply 307–308.

59. Martinelli I, et al. Genetic risk factors for superficial vein thrombosis. Thromb Haemost 1999;82:1215–1217.

60. Creinin MD, Lisman R, Strickler RC. Screening for factor V Leiden mutation before prescribing combination oral contraceptives. Fertil Steril 1999;72:646–651.

61. Walker ID. Factor V Leiden: should all women be screened prior to commencing the contraceptive pill? Blood Rev 1999;13:8–13.

62. Grantham R. Amino acid difference formula to help explain protein evolution. Science 1974;185:862–864.

63. Johnson JA, Lima JJ. Drug receptor/effector polymorphisms and pharmacogenetics: current status and challenges. Pharmacogenetics 2003;13:525–534.

64. Johnson JA. Pharmacogenetics: potential for individualized drug therapy through genetics. Trends Genet 2003;19:660–666.

65. McNamara DM, et al. Pharmacogenetic interactions between beta-blocker therapy and the angiotensin-converting enzyme deletion polymorphism in patients with congestive heart failure. Circulation 2001;103:1644–1648.

66. Wadelius M, et al. Warfarin sensitivity related to CYP2C9, CYP3A5, ABCB1 (MDR1) and other factors. Pharmacogenomics J 2004;4:40–48.

67. Shikata E, et al. Association of pharmacokinetic (CYP2C9) and pharmacodynamic (vitamin K-dependent protein-Factors II, VII, IX, and X, proteins S and C, and γ-glutamyl carboxylase) gene variants with warfarin sensitivity. Blood 2004;103:2630–2635.

68. Caulfield M, et al. Genome-wide mapping of human loci for essential hypertension. Lancet 2003;361:2118–2123.

69. Samani NJ. Genome scans for hypertension and blood pressure regulation. Am J Hypertens 2003;16:167–171.

70. Kennedy GC, et al. Large-scale genotyping of complex DNA. Nat Biotechnol 2003;21:1233–1237.

71. Zhong XB, et al. Single-nucleotide polymorphism genotyping on optical thin-film biosensor chips. Proc Natl Acad Sci USA 2003;100:11559–11564.

72. Hood L, Galas D. The digital code of DNA. Nature 2003;421:444–448.

73. Altshuler D, et al. An SNP map of the human genome generated by reduced representation shotgun sequencing. Nature 2000;407:513–516.

74. Shi MM, Bleavins MR, de la Iglesia FA. Technologies for detecting genetic polymorphisms in pharmacogenomics. Mol Diagn 1999;4:343–351.

75. Chen X, and Sullivan PF. Single nucleotide polymorphism genotyping: biochemistry, protocol, cost and throughput. Pharmacogenomics J 2003;3:77–96.

76. Syvanen AC. From gels to chips: "minisequencing" primer extension for analysis of point mutations and single nucleotide polymorphisms. Hum Mutat 1999;13:1–10.

77. Tost J, Gut IG. Genotyping single nucleotide polymorphisms by mass spectrometry. Mass Spectrom Rev 2002;21:388–418.

78. Haff LA, Smirnov IP. Single-nucleotide polymorphism identification assays using a thermostable DNA polymerase and delayed extraction MALDI-TOF mass spectrometry. Genome Res 1997;7:378–388.

79. Sauer S, et al. Full flexibility genotyping of single nucleotide polymorphisms by the GOOD assay. Nucleic Acids Res 2000;28:E100.

80. Braun A, Little DP, Koster H. Detecting CFTR gene mutations by using primer oligo base extension and mass spectrometry. Clin Chem 1997;43:1151–1158.

81. Buetow KH, et al. High-throughput development and characterization of a genomewide collection of gene-based single nucleotide polymorphism markers by chip-based matrix-assisted laser desorption/ionization time-of-flight mass spectrometry. Proc Natl Acad Sci USA 2001;98:581–584.

82. Kobayashi M, et al. Fluorescence-based DNA minisequence analysis for detection of known single-base changes in genomic DNA. Mol Cell Probes 1995;9:175–182.

83. Griffin TJ, Smith LM. Single-nucleotide polymorphism analysis by MALDI-TOF mass spectrometry. Trends Biotechnol 2000;18:77–84.

84. Yang H, et al. Multiplex single-nucleotide polymorphism genotyping by matrix-assisted laser desorption/ionization time-of-flight mass spectrometry. Anal Biochem 2003;314:54–62.

85. Kim S, et al. Multiplex genotyping of the human beta2-adrenergic receptor gene using solid-phase capturable dideoxynucleotides and mass spectrometry. Anal Biochem 2003;316:251–258.

86. Jackson PE, Scholl PF, Groopman JD. Mass spectrometry for genotyping: an emerging tool for molecular medicine. Mol Med Today 2000;6:271–276.

87. Fakhrai-Rad H, Pourmand N, Ronaghi M. Pyrosequencing: an accurate detection platform for single nucleotide polymorphisms. Hum Mutat 2002;19:479–485.

88. Xiao W, Oefner PJ. Denaturing high-performance liquid chromatography: a review. Hum Mutat 2001;17:439–474.

6

Genetic Polymorphisms and Response to HMG-CoA Reductase Inhibitors

Anke-Hilse Maitland-van der Zee, PharmD, PhD,
Olaf H. Klungel, PharmD, PhD,
and Anthonius de Boer, MD, PhD

CONTENTS

INTRODUCTION
PHARMACOGENETICS
PHARMACOKINETIC INTERACTIONS
GENES IN CAUSAL PATHWAY OF DISEASE
CONCLUSIONS
REFERENCES

SUMMARY

Coronary artery disease is among the leading causes of death worldwide. Clinical trials show a protective effect of statins against coronary artery disease. The mean risk reductions for subjects using statins compared with placebo found in these trials is about 30%. These are average reductions for all patients included in the trials. Important factors in interpreting the variability in outcome of drug therapy include the patient's health profile, prognosis, disease severity, quality of drug prescribing, compliance with prescribed pharmacotherapy, and the genetic profile of the patient. This chapter aims to give an overview of the known polymorphisms that have an influence on the effects of statins in the general population. The expectation is that in the future, a subject's genotype may determine whether he/she will be treated with statins or not. Determining the genotype will not deny therapy to a subject, but will help in the decision as to which therapy suits the patient best.

Key Words: Pharmacogenetics; HMG-CoA reductase inhibitor; Apolipoprotein ε; ACE insertion deletion; CETP; Stromelysin-1; β fibrinogen gene; lipoprotein lipase; hepatic lipase; platelet glycoprotein; toll-like receptor 4; interleukin-1B.

From: *Contemporary Cardiology: Cardiovascular Genomics*
Edited by: M. K. Raizada, et al. © Humana Press Inc., Totowa, NJ

INTRODUCTION

Cardiovascular disease is one of the leading causes of death, especially in developed countries. Several risk factors for cardiovascular disease have now been well established, especially cigarette smoking, hypertension, lipid disorders, and diabetes mellitus. Pharmacotherapeutic interventions such as the use of aspirin and other antithrombotic drugs, antihypertensive drugs, and cholesterol-lowering therapy probably have contributed to the gradual decline in cardiovascular disease over the last decades *(1,2)*. Statins are inhibitors of hydroxy-methylglutaryl coenzyme A (HMG-CoA) reductase, which inhibits cholesterol production in the hepatocyte. This increases the synthesis of low-density lipoprotein (LDL) receptors and thereby lowers cholesterol. In recent years, several landmark trials have been published that establish the efficacy of statin therapy in primary and secondary prevention *(3–7)*. Treatment with statins over a 5-yr period was associated with a statistically significant reduction in mortality and in the number of patients experiencing a heart attack or a stroke, or undergoing a revascularization procedure. The risk reduction for coronary artery disease for subjects using statins was approx 30%. These reductions, however, are average effects for all patients included in the trials; in subpopulations these effects may differ.

Important factors in interpreting variability in the outcome of drug therapy include the patient's overall health, prognosis, disease severity, quality of drug prescribing, compliance with prescribed pharmacotherapy, and the genetic profile of the patient *(8,9)*. In the large trials, several subgroups have been analyzed. In the Cholesterol and Recurrent Events (CARE) trial, the effect of pravastatin on the rates of major coronary events was greater among women (–46% [95% CI –22 to –62%]) than among men (–20% [95% CI –8 to –30%]) *(3)*. In the other trials there were no significant differences between men and women. Other subgroup analyses included age groups; comorbidity such as hypertension, diabetes mellitus, previous myocardial infarction, and smoking; and pretreatment plasma lipid levels, but these yielded no statistically significant differences *(3–7,10,11)*. In the Scandinavian Simivastatin Survival study (4S), measurements of the serum cholestanol concentration revealed a subgroup of patients in whom coronary events were not reduced by simvastatin treatment. The reduction in relative risk increased gradually from 0.62 to 1.17 in the quarters of distribution of cholestanol at baseline. Thus, patients with high baseline synthesis of cholesterol seem to be responders whereas those with low synthesis of cholesterol are nonresponders *(12)*.

PHARMACOGENETICS

Pharmacogenetics and pharmacogenomics are emerging disciplines that focus on genetic determinants of drug response at the levels of single genes or the entire human genome, respectively *(13)*. Polymorphisms may influence drug response in three ways *(14)*. The first way is through pharmacokinetic interactions, caused by genetically based differences in drug absorption, disposition, metabolism and excretion. An important role is played by polymorphisms in the cytochrome P450 (CYP) enzymes. In addition, there are pharmacodynamic gene–drug interactions that involve gene products expressed as receptors or signal transduction molecules, which are relevant to the pharmacodynamics of drugs. After entering the circulation each drug interacts with numerous proteins and multiple types of receptors. These proteins determine the site of action and the pharmacological response. The third possibility of influencing drug response is through genes that are in the causal pathway of disease and are able to modify the effects of drugs. For example, differences in the effects of statins may be measured on cholesterol levels. However, because statins have certain effects that are independent of cholesterol lowering, such as effects on blood pressure, coagulation, cell proliferation, immune function, and macrophage metabolism (15,16), the effects on cholesterol levels alone may not accurately predict the effects on cardiovascular morbidity and mortality (17). Another way to measure the effects of statins is the rate of progression of coronary atherosclerosis measured by coronary angiography. When a difference in response is measured on these endpoints it is not known whether this drug resistance also translates into a lack of effect on important clinical outcomes (fatal and nonfatal coronary disease).

This chapter aims to give an overview of the currently known polymorphisms that influence the effects of statins. This chapter is an update of a previous publication on this subject (18).

PHARMACOKINETIC INTERACTIONS

Although several studies have been published recently on possible pharmacokinetic interactions with statins, currently no useful polymorphisms for the prediction of the pharmacokinetics (and thereby predictions of efficacy and adverse effects) are available. Statins are highly extracted by the liver. The CYP enzyme system plays an important part in the metabolism of statins. Most statins (lovastatin, simvastatin, and atorvastatin) are predominantly metabolized by CYP3A4 (19,20). For this enzyme, no functional polymorphisms have been described so far (21).

Simvastatin is given orally as a prodrug and is converted to the active form simvastatin hydroxy acid. Simvastatin is not only metabolized by CYP3A4, but also by CYP2D6 and CYP2C9 (22). Several studies have been published on the role of the CYP2D6 polymorphism in the efficacy of simvastatin. The in vivo activity of the CYP2D6 enzyme is characterized by extreme individual variability. The variability in the rate of metabolism by CYP2D6 is more than 100-fold, which is genetically determined (23). To date, 30 polymorphisms in the CYP2D6 gene have been described, resulting in classification of the phenotype into three categories (24): subjects with normal activity (extensive metabolizers), subjects with low or absent activity (slow metabolizers), and subjects with high activity (ultraprapid metabolizers). It appears that genotyping for the most common defective alleles will predict the CYP2D6 phenotype with a high amount of certainty (24). In 1997, Nordin et al. found in a study of 10 healthy volunteers that subjects who were ultrarapid metabolizers might need higher dosages of simvastatin to be effective (25). Mulder et al. studied 88 patients, with primary and secondary hypercholesterolemia, to investigate the link between polymorphism of CYP2D6 and the efficacy and tolerability of simvastatin treatment. Mulder et al. found results in line with the results of Nordin et al. Adverse effects were more common in slow metabolizers and the efficacy in lowering cholesterol levels was also higher in this group (26). Geisel et al. did not find such an association in a study of 41 patients with primary hypercholesterolemia (27). Several reasons for the different results were discussed. Mulder et al. included patients with secondary hypercholesterolemia and neglected to analyze several nonfunctional alleles and therefore, may have misclassified subjects. On the other hand, the study of Mulder et al. included more patients and therefore, might have had a better chance of finding significant differences (27,28). Because only a few small studies have been performed, larger studies are necessary to assess whether this interaction is relevant.

Polymorphisms in CYP2C9 have been shown to influence response to warfarin *(29)*. Because fluvastatin is also metabolized via this isoform, studies assessing a possible interaction between fluvastatin and CYP2C9 polymorphisms might be of interest *(21)*. Kirchheiner et al. investigated the pharmacokinetics and the cholesterol-lowering activity of fluvastatin in 24 healthy subjects who took 40 mg fluvastatin for 2 wk *(30)*. The pharmacokinetics depended on the CYP2C9 genotype, but differences in plasma concentrations were not reflected in cholesterol *(30)*. Larger studies in hypercholesterolemic patients are needed to confirm these results.

Another pharmacokinetic interaction was published with pravastatin. Pravastatin is not significantly metabolized by the CYPP450 system *(31)*. Pravastatin is rapidly absorbed from the upper region of the small intestine, and then taken up efficiently from the circulation by the liver through organic anion transporting polypeptide C (OATP-C), a sodium independent bile transporter *(32)*. A number of single nucleotide polymorphisms have been identified that changed the in vitro transport capability *(33)*. Nishizato et al. investigated the significance of polymorphisms in the *OATP-C* and *OAT3* genes in a Japanese population (*n* = 120) with regard to the disposition kinetics of pravastatin. They provide evidence that the *OATP-C* gene polymorphism contributes to in vivo activity of OATP-C and thereby to differences in the pharmacokinetics of pravastatin. This might lead to differences in the efficacy and safety of pravastatin. Because of the small number of subjects in this study, these results should be confirmed in larger studies *(32)*.

All results in the pharmacokinetic studies discussed in this section are still debated and must be further investigated. Alternative candidate genes for pharmacokinetic interactions include the *CYP3A4* gene, the ABC transporter-like *MDR1* gene, or the glucuronyl transferase gene, because these genes are also involved in the excretion an biotransformation of HMG-CoA reductase inhibitors *(21,34)*.

GENES IN CAUSAL PATHWAY OF DISEASE
Cholesteryl Ester Transfer Protein Polymorphism

REVERSE CHOLESTEROL TRANSPORT

The presence of a polymorphism in the cholesteryl ester transfer protein *(CETP)* gene (which is also called *Taq1B*) is associated with alterations in lipoprotein levels and high-density lipoprotein (HDL) concentrations. The CETP enzyme has a central role in reverse cholesterol transport (RCT), whereby cholesterol from peripheral tissues is transported back to the liver, where it is preferentially excreted into bile. There are several proteins crucial for RCT. These proteins include the ATP-binding cassette transporter 1 gene (ABC_I transporter), lecithin cholesterol acyl transferase (LCAT), CETP, hepatic lipase (HL), and scavenger receptor type BI (SR-BI) *(35)*.

The ABC_I gene product has been provisionally termed cholesterol-efflux regulatory protein (CERP). CERP is involved in the transfer of free cholesterol and phospholipids (PLs) form macrophages to apoA-I. Mutations in the ABC_I gene cause plasma HDL deficiency and premature atherosclerosis *(36,37)*.

Nascent HDL particles, mainly consisting of apo-A1 and PLs, are acceptors for free cholesterol. As soon as these HDL discs have absorbed free cholesterol, the LCAT enzyme converts this cholesterol to cholesterol esters, which increase HDL size from disc to spherical. CETP is then capable of transporting these cholesterol esters to very low-density lipoprotein (VLDL) or LDL. In exchange, CETP converts triglycerides (TGs) back to HDL.VLDL and, consequently, LDL transport these cholesterol esters back to the liver, where they are taken up through the LDL receptor system. Conversely, in the other pathway, HL hydrolyzes the TGs in HDL *(35)*, which renders HDL a prime candidate for direct uptake into the liver by the SR-BI receptor

CETP POLYMORPHISM

The presence of the polymorphism in the first intron of the *CETP* gene is referred to as TaqIB. People with the B1 allele have higher CETP concentrations and, because cholesterol esters are extracted from HDL, lower HDL-cholesterol concentrations. CETP levels are highest in subjects with two copies of the B1 allele (B1B1) and lowest in persons with the B2B2 genotype. The mechanism by which the CETP polymorphism may affect CETP activity is not known. It is unlikely that this polymorphism, which is located in an intron, represents a functional mutation. The most plausible explanation is that this polymorphism is in almost complete linkage disequilibrium with a functional polymorphism in the promotor region of the *CETP* gene, the CETP/–629 polymorphism *(38,39)*. This –629 polymorphism, corresponding to a C/A substitution at position –629, exerts a significant effect on transcriptional activity.

Kuivenhoven et al. observed a significant genotype-dependent association of the CETP TaqIB polymorphism with the progression of coronary atherosclerosis in the placebo group; carriers of the B1B1 genotype had the highest CETP concentrations, the lowest HDL-cholesterol (C) concentrations and the fastest progression of coronary atherosclerosis *(40)*. Ordovas et al. found that CETP activity was decreased in men and women with the B2 allele. The HDL concentration for both men and women was lowest in the B1B1 group. For men carrying the B2 allele, the odds ratio for prevalent coronary heart disease was 0.70 (95% CI 0.50–0.98), but after adjustment for HDL-C levels and other known risk factors, the odds ratio was no longer significantly different (0.74 [95% CI 0.46-1.16]). No significant protective effects of this genotype were observed in women *(41)*. There is some controversy in the literature as to whether CETP inhibition is beneficial in preventing ischemic heart disease. Several studies in Japanese populations support the results from Kuivenhoven et al., which showed that CETP deficiency is potentially antiatherogenic and may be associated with an increased life span *(42,43)*. Other studies find an increased risk of ischemic heart disease in subjects with low CETP concentrations even though they have higher HDL-C concentrations *(44–48)*. Van Venrooij et al. found in a 30-wk randomized trial in 217 unrelated diabetic subjects that subjects with the B1B1 genotype or the CC carriers (which were tightly concordant in their study [$p < 0.001$]) had a more atherogenic lipid profile (lower HDL, higher TGs). They also showed that these subjects responded better to atorvastatin with respect to reduction of CETP mass and elevation of HDL-C concentrations *(49)*.

In addition, Kuivenhoven et al. found no difference in plasma lipoprotein response to pravastatin between the different genotypes, but the B2B2 genotype (about 16% of all Caucasian men) with low CETP and high HDL concentrations did not respond to pravastatin in terms of decreased disease progression 40. Furthermore, in a case-control study, Fumeron et al. showed that HDL-C levels were only increased in subjects with the B2B2 genotype after ingesting at least 25 g of alcohol per day *(50)*. In the cohort of Kuivenhoven et al., alcohol consumption did not affect the association between the CETP genotype and the angiographic outcome in the control group, nor in the group treated with pravastatin *(51)*. In the WOSCOPS trial (one of the primary prevention trials) the same association between the B2B2 genotype and cardiovascular events was found. Homozygotes for the B2B2 allele had a higher HDL-C and a 30% reduction of suffering a cardiovascular event compared to B1B1 homozygotes. This association was primarily found in nonsmokers, not in smokers. However, no interaction was observed between the *CETP* genotype and pravastatin treatment *(52)*. They also typed the –631 C/A, –629 C/A, I405V, and D442G CETP polymorphisms but they did not find significant association with risk. Haplotype analysis did not add to the information given by the individual polymorphisms *(52)*. Blankenberg et al. found in the Atherogene study, a cohort study including 1303 patients who had at least one stenosis greater than 30% in a major coronary artery diagnosed with coronary angiography, that in patients with coronary artery disease, the CETP –629 A allele (which is almost completely concordant with the B2 allele of the Taq IB polymorphism) had a strong protective effect on future mortality from cardiovascular causes. Furthermore, a statistically significant interaction between the CETP –629 C/A polymorphism and statin treatment on cardiovascular mortality was found. The benefit of statin treatment was restricted to subjects with the –629 C allele. In these patients, cardiovasular mortality was reduced by about 50% in those taking statin medication, whereas no effect was observed in patients carrying the –629 A allele *(53)*.

Stromelysin-1 Polymorphism

Matrix metalloproteinases (such as stromelysin) have important roles in connective tissue remodeling during tissue repair, cell migration, angiogenesis, tissue morphogenesis, and growth *(54–57)*. These physiological processes require a tightly controlled balance between matrix metalloproteinases and their specific tissue inhibitors. Disruption of this balance may lead to various pathological states. Low tissue levels of these metalloproteinases are associated with atheroscerosis *(54)*. A common polymorphism in the promotor sequence of the stromelysin-1 gene exists, with one allele having a run of six adenosines (6A) and the other of five adenosines (5A). The prevalence of the two alleles 5A and 6A was found to be 51% and 49% in a sample of 354 healthy individuals in the United Kingdom *(54)*. This promotor variant affects transcription. In vitro studies have shown that genotypes with a 5A allele expressed higher activity of stromelysin-1 than the 6A allele in both cultured fibroblasts and vascular smooth muscle cells *(54)*. Compared with other genotypes, individuals homozygous for the 6A allele would have lower stromelysin-1 levels in their arterial walls because of lower transcription level, and this might therefore favor deposition of extracellular matrix in the atherosclerotic lesions. This may lead to the development of an atherosclerotic plaque with a thick cap, and result in a more rapid progression of angiographically defined stenosis *(58)*.

In the REGRESS trial of pravastatin vs placebo, de Maat et al. compared male patients with coronary artery disease with 5A5A, 5A6A, and 6A6A genotypes of the stromelysin polymorphism, with respect to relevant clinical events such as myocardial infarction (fatal or nonfatal), mortality of coronary heart disease, percutaneous transluminal coronary angioplasty or coronary artery bypass graft surgery, stroke and transient ischemic attack, and overall mortality *(59)*. Patients in the placebo group with the 5A6A or 6A6A genotypes had a higher 2-yr cumulative incidence of one of these clinical events than patients with the 5A5A genotype (26% and 12%, respectively; $p = 0.03$). In the pravastatin group, the risk of clinical events in patients with 5A6A or 6A6A genotypes was lower (14%) than in patients on placebo, whereas it was unchanged in those with a 5A5A genotype (17%) (*see* Table 1). These effects were independent of the effects of pravastatin on lipid levels *(59)*.

Table 1
Polymorphisms That Might Influence the Efficacy of Statin Therapy

Polymorphism	Effect	References
Cytochrome P450 2D6	Slow metabolizers may have higher efficacy and more side effects of simvastatin	25–28
Cytochrome P450 2C9	No effect found with fluvastatin	30
OATP-C	Disposition kinetics of pravastatin were different.	32
CETP Taq IB and –629 C/A	Subjects with the B2B2 or with –629 AA allele had no effect from statin therapy on reduction of angiographically defined CHD and on reduction of cardiovascular events.	40,51–53
Stromelysin-1	Subjects with the 5A5A genotype had no effects of pravastatin on incidence of clinical events.	59
β-fibrinogene –455 G/A and TaqI	Subjects with the –455 AA genotype had a greater efficacy of statins.	67
Apolipoprotein E	Subjects with the ε4 allele have the least cholesterol lowering effect with statins, but they have the same or even a better effect of statins (compared with the ε2 and ε3 allele) in reducing CHD.	72,74–85
Lipoprotein lipase gene	Subjects with the Asp9Asn mutation had a greater efficacy of statins on angiographic parameters.	91
ACE insertion deletion	Results for this polymorphism are conflicting.	78,100–103
Hepatic lipase –514 C/T	Subjects with the TT genotype did not have a regression of angiographically determined atherosclerosis after 2.5 y of intensive lipid-lowering therapy.	108
Platelet Glycoprotein	Statin therapy reduced the increased rate of restenosis associated with the P1[A2] allele.	100,110
Toll-like receptor 4	Carriers of the 229 Gly had a much stronger cardiovascular risk reduction, but the interaction was not found in reduction of lipid parameters.	117
Interleukin-1B	Coronary function improves after 6 mo of statin therapy in subjects with the A2- allele but not in subjects with the A2+ allele.	118

OATP, organic anion transporting polypeptide; CETP, cholesteryl ester transfer protein; ACE, angiotensin-coverting enzyme; CHD, coronary heart disease.

–455G/A AND TAQ I POLYMORPHISMS OF THE β-FIBRINOGEN GENE

Several epidemiological studies have reported a strong associaton between elevated plasma levels of fibrinogen and an increased risk of myocardial infarction (60–65) and stroke (66). Because fibrinogen is an acute phase protein, an increased plasma fibrinogen level may reflect the inflammatory state of the vascular wall and may thus be related to cardiovascular risk (64). The three chains of fibrinogen are encoded by three different genes (68). Polymorphisms of the α gene (Taq I) and of the β gene (–455G/A) are associated with differences in plasma levels of fibrinogen.

De Maat et al. found in The REGRESS trial significantly higher fibrinogen levels (3.9 g/L [95% CI 3.2–4.8]) in subjects who where homozygous for the rare –455A allele (the frequency was 0.21%), whereas the homozygotes for the common -455G allele and the heterozygotes had comparable fibrinogen levels (3.2 g/L [95% CI 3.0–3.3], and 3.1 g/L [95% CI 2.9–3.3], respectively) *(67)*. In the placebo group, subjects with the –455AA had a significantly greater progression of coronary artery disease, as reflected by angiographic variables (mean segment diameter decrease 0.24 ± 0.45), than patients with the –455GG and the –455GA genotypes (mean segment diameter decrease 0.09 ± 0.39 and 0.10 ± 0.39, respectively). In patients receiving pravastatin, this difference was not observed. These results suggest that pravastatin is capable of offsetting the deleterious effects of the –455AA genotype of the β-fibrinogen gene *(67)*.

APOLIPOPROTEIN-ε4

Several studies have investigated the relation between apolipoprotein-ε (apoε) genotypes and the LDL cholesterol response to HMG-CoA reductase inhibitors in hypercholesterolemic patients. Human apoε is a genetically polymorphic protein defined by three alleles—ε2, ε3, and ε4—at a single gene locus on chromosome 19; these code for three isoforms (ε2, ε3, and ε4) that differ by an amino acid substitution at residues 112 and 158, and thus determine the six genotypes resulting from the combination of any two of them *(69)*. Apoε allele frequencies in the normal population were assessed in 2457 subjects in the Framingham Offspring study and were 8%, 78%, and 14% *(70)*, respectively, for ε2, ε3, and ε4; Corbo et al. investigated the worldwide distribution of the apoε polymorphism and discovered that the ε3 allele is the most frequent in all human populations and that its frequency is always negatively correlated with that of ε4 *(71)*. The ε4 allele occurs relatively frequently in human populations where foraging still exists or food supplies are scarce or qualitatively poor. Carrying this allele would be favorable, because this allele promotes intestinal cholesterol uptake and increases plasma cholesterol levels which otherwise would be too low *(71)*.

The polymorphism of the apoε genotype influences hepatic cholesterol content because lipoproteins with the ε4 isoform are taken up with greater affinity than those with the common ε3 isoform, which in turn are cleared more efficiently than those with the ε2 isoform. Accelerated lipoprotein clearance by the liver leads to a downregulation of hepatocyte LDL receptors. This, in addition to increased intestinal uptake, underlies the well-known hypercholesterolemic effect of the ε4 allele, with its attendant high risk of atherosclerosis and cardiovascular mortality *(72)*. On the other hand, lipoproteins containing apoε2 have a reduced binding affinity for the LDL receptor; thus their plasma clearance rate is reduced. This lowers intracellular cholesterol levels and upregulates HMG-CoA reductase synthesis. HMG-CoA reductase inhibitors (statins) may be less effective in reducing cholesterol levels in apoε4 individuals, as they may already have low HMG-CoA reductase activities *(44,73)*. Several studies found a significant interaction between an individuals's apoε genotype and plasma lipoprotein–lipid changes with statin therapy *(74–78)*. In these studies, subjects with the ε2 allele, and sometimes subjects with the ε3 allele, were more likely to respond favorably to statin therapy than subjects with at least one ε4 allele. The decrease in both total cholesterol and LDL cholesterol was larger in subjects with the ε2 allele than in subjects with an ε3 or an ε4 allele. In subjects with the ε3 allele, total cholesterol and LDL cholesterol were reduced more than in subjects with at least one ε4 allele. Five other studies did not find significant differences in the cholesterol lowering effects of statins in the different apoε genotypes *(72,79–82)*. However, in two of these studies there was a trend for greater LDL cholesterol reductions in subjects with the ε2 and ε3 allele *(80,82)*. Two studies reported that, whereas men displayed a significant gene–drug response interaction, in women the apoE polymorphism did not account for any significant gene–drug interaction *(76,83)*. It was also found in the REGRESS study that ε2 carriers exhibited the largest improvement in lipoprotein levels upon pravastatin treatment, compared with those having ε3 or ε4 alleles, but the efficacy of pravastatin toward angiographic parameters was less pronounced in carriers of the ε2 allele, although this was not statistically significant *(84)*. Importantly, in a substudy from the 4S study myocardial infarction survivors with the ε4 allele proved to have a nearly twofold increased risk of dying in a follow-up period of about 5.5 yr, compared with other patients. Compared with placebo, the relative risk of mortality in subjects treated with simvastatin was 0.33 (95% CI 0.16–0.69) in ε4 carriers and 0.66 (95% CI 0.35–1.24) in other patients (*see* Table 1). The increased risk of death was not accompanied by an increased risk of a major coronary event, and there was also no difference in the efficacy of statin treatment on reducing coronary events *(81)*.

In a hypercholesterolemic subcohort ($n = 3626$) of the Rotterdam study, a large cohort study that included 7983 subjects of 55 yr and older in a suburb of Rotterdam, no differences in effect were found between subjects with and without the ε4 allele in reducing the risk of coronary artery disease and total mortality. The mortality risk in subjects with the ε4 allele was reduced to 0.71 *(85)* after 2 yr of statin treatment, whereas the mortality risk in subjects without the ε4 allele was reduced to 0.91 *(85)*. The difference with the 4S study might be explained by the difference in mean age of both populations. Subjects in the Rotterdam study had a higher mean age and, unlike the subjects in the 4S study, in the untreated subjects there was no increased risk of dying in subjects with the ε4 allele. Perhaps risk factors other than carrying the ε4 allele became more important at a higher age in predicting the risk of dying *(85)* Furthermore, among subjects in the Rotterdam study that started statin therapy, the risk of discontinuing medication within 3 yr was 3.18 times higher in men with the ε4ε4 genotype compared to men with the ε2ε3 genotype *(86)*. This suggests that subjects who are genetically prone to develop hypercholesterolemia showed the highest risk of discontinuation of statin treatment. A possible explanation for this observation is that these men have the least effect on their cholesterol levels. This may lead to the conclusion that measuring cholesterol levels might not be a good way to evaluate the efficacy of statin therapy *(86)*.

MUTATIONS IN THE LIPOPROTEIN LIPASE GENE

Lipoprotein lipase is a multifunctional protein and pivotal enzyme in lipoprotein metabolism. It is anchored to the vascular endothelium where it constitutes the rate-limiting step in the catabolism of TGs in circulating TG-rich lipoproteins *(87,88)*. The contribution of lipoprotein lipase to atherogenesis is significantly influenced by the balance between vessel wall protein (proatherogenic) and plasma activity (antiatherogenic) *(89)*.

Mailly et al. found in their study that the frequency of healthy Dutch, Swedish, English, and Scottish carriers of the Asp_9Asn mutation (Asp substituted by Asn at position 9 in exon 2) was 1.6 to 4.4% *(90)*. The frequency of the carriers was roughly twice as high (range, 4.0–9.8%) in selected subjects with combined hyperlipidemia (elevated plasma levels of cholesterol and TGs) and in patients with angiographically assessed atherosclerosis (REGRESS) *(91)*. Carriers of the mutation more often had a family history of cardiovascular disease and higher TG and lower HDL-C levels than noncarriers.

The reduction of total and LDL cholesterol appeared to be less in patients with the mutation compared to patients without the mutation. However, the differences between patients with and without the mutation did not differ significantly between the placebo and the pravastatin groups *(91)*. Angiographic results (progression of focal atherosclerosis and percentage diameter stenosis) showed a deleterious effect of the mutation which could be reversed by pravastatin therapy *(91)*. The relative risk of the presence of the Asp9Asn mutation for any clinical event within 2 yr was estimated to be 1.85 (95% CI 0.94–3.66). The effect of pravastatin on the clinical event-free period was not significantly different for patients with and without the mutation *(91)*.

Although the lipid-lowering effect was attenuated in patients carrying the Asp_9Asn mutation, the deleterious effect of this mutant on the progression of atherosclerosis could be reversed by pravastatin.

Two other common polymorphisms in the lipoprotein lipase gene are associated with coronary heart disease. The Ser447X polymorphism is seen in 17–22% of the population. This polymorphism was found to be protective against high TG levels, low HDL-C cholesterol levels, and premature coronary heart disease *(92–94)*. The N291S is seen in 1–7% of the population. This polymorphism is associated with elevated TGs, decreased HDL cholesterol, and, most likely, increased heart disease risk *(93,94)*. It is not yet established if the effects of statins differ in subjects with these polymorphisms.

ACE Deletion-Type Gene

The angiotensin-converting enzyme (ACE) is thought to play an important role in the development of coronary artery disease. In humans, plasma levels of ACE are partly under genetic control. Plasma and cellular levels of ACE are associated with the insertion/deletion (I/D) polymorphism located in intron 16 of the *ACE* gene. DD carriers have about twice the plasma levels of ACE compared with II carriers, whereas heterozygotes have intermediate levels *(95)*. The frequencies of the ACE genotypes differ in various populations. In the control group of the male Caucasian study population of Gardemann et al., the frequencies of II, ID, and DD were 23, 50, and 27%, respectively *(96)*. The angiotensin converting enzyme converts angiotensin I into the bioactive angiotensin II, and is also responsible for the breakdown of bradykinin to kinin degradation products. These processes result in an increased vascular tone, neointimal proliferation, and LDL oxidation, all predisposing to atherosclerosis *(97)*. Many studies have examined the correlation of the different genotypes with various cardiovascular diseases. Cambien et al. were the first to report an association of this deletion polymorphism with an increased risk of coronary artery disease *(98)*. The meta-analysis of Staessen et al. included 145 reports with an overall sample size of 49,959 subjects *(99)*. In comparison with the II reference group, the excess risk in DD homozygotes was 32% for coronary heart disease (CHD; 30 studies) and 45% for myocardial infarction (20 studies). The D allele behaves as a marker of atherosclerotic cardiovascular complications *(99)*. Concerning the influence of the ACE genotype on the effectiveness of statins, however, contradictory results have been published.

Marquez-Vidal et al. found no interaction of the ACE polymorphism and statins on reduction of lipids and lipoproteins in their case-control study *(78)*. In the CARE trial, subjects with the Platelet Pla2 allele ACE D allele carriers had a larger risk reduction than ACE II subjects *(100)*. In the Lipoprotein and Coronary Atherosclerosis study (LCAS) study, subjects with the ACE DD genotype had the strongest reduction of coronary atherosclerosis with pravastatin. The distribution of clinical events among the genotypes was not clinically significantly different *(101)*. In The REGRESS trial comparing pravastatin with placebo, van Geel et al. found that the DD genotype was associated with a significantly higher incidence of ischemic events. Although pravastatin decreased serum lipids to a similar extent in the *DD* as in the ID and II groups, the beneficial effects of pravastatin on angiographically defined coronary atherosclerosis were apparently blunted by the ACE deletion type *DD* gene *(102)*. Treating patients with the DD genotype with pravastatin seems less effective than treating patients with the other genotypes with pravastatin.

In a hypercholesterolemic cohort in the Rotterdam study (*n* = 3624), an association between the ACE genotype and the effectiveness of statins in reducing coronary events was found. The relative risk reduction in DD subjects was 1.29 (95% CI 0.62–2.60), in ID subjects, 0.87 (95% CI 0.52–1.45), and in II subjects, 0.40 (95% CI 0.15–1.10). In men, this interaction was much stronger than in women *(103)*. In men the relative risk reduction in DD subjects was 1.34 (0.44–4.09), and in II subjects 0.23 (0.04–1.28); in women, the relative risk reduction in DD subjects was 1.27 (0.43–3.81), and in II subjects, 0.72 (0.20–2.56). The gender difference in risk reduction is not easily explained. Other studies showed that genetic variance in the region of the *ACE* gene significantly influenced interindividual blood pressure in males, but not in females *(104,105)*. This suggests that there are gender differences in genetic regulation of the ACE system. There might be an interaction between the ACE genotype and statin therapy in men, but these data need to be confirmed in a larger study.

–514 CT POLYMORPHISM IN *HL* GENE

HL is a plasma lipolytic enzyme that plays a major role in the metabolism of LDL cholesterol and HDL cholesterol. HL promotes the conversion of large TG-rich HDL2 to small, dense HDL3 particles. High HL levels are associated with low HDL2 levels. In addition, HL catalyzes the hydrolysis of TGs and PLs of the intermediate density lipoproteins (IDL) and large buoyant LDL to form the more atherogenic small, dense LDL particles *(106)*. Patients with small, dense LDL have an increased risk of coronary artery disease *(107)*. The presence of a C instead of a T at position –514 with respect to the transcription start site of the *HL* gene accounts for 20–30% of the variance in HL activity in men and women *(108)*. The presence of the C allele contributes to increased HL activity, which leads to more atherogenic LDL particles and lower levels of anti-atherogenic HDL cholesterol.

Zambon et al. conducted a study within a small but intense clinical trial *(108)*. They studied 49 dyslipidemic men who were treated for 2.5 yr with intensive lipid-lowering therapy with either lovastatin and colestipol, or niacin and colestipol. The type of lipid-lowering therapy did not affect the association between polymorphism and changes in coronary stenosis. The results from the two different treatment groups were therefore pooled and analyzed together. Homozygous CC patients showed a greater decrease in HL activity and a greater increase in LDL buoyancy with lipid-lowering therapy than subjects with at least one T allele.

Lipid-lowering therapy resulted in a significant improvement of coronary stenosis in CC patients ($\Delta\%_{Sprox}$ –2.1) and to a lesser extent in the TC group ($\Delta\%_{Sprox}$ –1.1), whereas progression of stenosis ($\Delta\%_{Sprox}$ 4.0) was observed in the TT group. Because no distinction was made between the two lipid-lowering therapies, it is not clear if the differences in treatment effect were attributable to statin therapy.

Platelet Glycoprotein

Platelets play a central role in the restenosis process by inducing neointimal proliferation after coronary interventions *(109)*. The glycoprotein IIb/IIIa Pl^{A2} polymorphism has been associated with the occurrence of acute coronary syndromes and increased restenosis rates. Statins have been shown to exert potent antiproliferative, anti-inflammatory, and antithrombotic properties, thereby potentially interfering with the major processes of in-stent restenosis. To investigate if statin therapy affects restenosis rates Walter et al. followed 650 patients for 6 mo after coronary stent insertion. Carriers of the Pl^{A2} allele (22% of the patients) demonstrated a significantly increased restenosis rate, which was diminished by statin therapy (50.9% vs 28.6%, $p = 0.01$). Patients homozygous for the Pl^{A1} allele only had a slight recuction in stenosis rate (27% vs 34%, $p = 0.13$). Moreover, statin therapy was associated with a significant reduction (28.2% vs 49.3%) of myocardial infarction, cardiac death, and target vessel revascularization in the 6 mo after the intervention in patients with the Pl^{A2} allele, and only with a minimal reduction in subjects with the Pl^{A1} allele (32.1% in statin treated patients and 37.5% in patients without treatment). Statin therapy reduces increased stent restenosis rates and improves clinical outcome following coronary stent implantation in patients bearing the Pl^{A2} allele, suggesting that statins interfere with the functional consequence of a genetically determined platelet-mediated risk factor associated with Pl^{A2} polymorphism *(110)*.

The clinical effect of the PI^A genotype has also been investigated in a substudy of the CARE trial *(100)*. The prevalence of the $PI^{A1.A2}$ genotype was 28.8% in the cases and 23.8% in controls; this was not significantly different. The relative risk of CHD death or nonfatal myocardial infarction in the $PI^{A1.A2}$ genotype group was 1.32 (95% CI 0.99–1.76). This suggests that there is a trend towards a higher relative risk, but it is not statistically significant. In patients with the $PI^{A1.A2}$ genotype, treatment with pravastatin reduced the risk of fatal CHD or nonfatal myocardial infarction by 31%, whereas in patients with the $PI^{A1.A1}$ genotype, treatment with pravastatin only reduced these events with 7%. Of the seven patients with the $PI^{A2.A2}$ genotype in the control group only one experienced a fatal CHD or a myocardial infarction, whereas in the pravastatin group six of the nine $PI^{A2.A2}$ patients experienced such an event. These data suggest that the $PI^{A2.A2}$ genotype is not associated with an increased risk of death resulting from CHD or nonfatal myocardial infarction, and that pravastatin might have a detrimental effect on coronary events in patients with this genotype *(100,111)*. Because of the low sample size in this study, these results should be cautiously interpreted.

Toll-Like Receptor 4

Atherosclerosis is increasingly considered to be a chronic inflammatory disease *(112)*. Lipopolysaccharide (LPS) is a product of Gram-negative microorganisms that activates the immune system. LPS in combination with CD14 serves as a ligand to toll-like receptor 4 (TLR4). The presence of LPS in the circulation is not confined to sepsis, but also occurs in healthy subjects *(113,114)* and is associated with early atherosclerosis *(113)*. Two functional SNPs have been discovered in the *TLR4* gene. These variants, Asp299Gly and Thr399Ile, lead to a blunted immunological response to inhaled LPS *(115)* and to lower levels of proinflammatory cytokines, acute-phase reactants, and soluble adhesion molecules *(116)*. Most importantly, they were associated with reduced extent and progression of angiographically-determined carotid atherosclerosis *(116)*. Boekholdt et al. investigated in the REGRESS study whether the Asp299Gly and the Thr399Ile polymorphisms influenced the progression of coronary atherosclerosis and the risk of cardiovascular events (117). There were no significantly differences between genetically defined subgroups with respect to baseline factors, treatment, or in-trial changes of lipid, lipoprotein, or angiographic measurements. Carriership of the 299Gly allele did not significantly affect the risk of cardiovascular events in the entire cohort when compared with noncarriers (11.5% vs 14.9%, $p = 0.58$). However, in the pravastatin group, carriers of the 299Gly allele had a significantly lower risk of cardiovascular events than noncarriers. Among noncarriers, the risk of cardiovascular events was reduced from 18.1% to 11.5%, whereas among carriers of the 229Gly the risk was reduced from 29.6% to 2%. Testing for the interaction between the 299Gly genotype and pravastatin was statistically significant ($p = 0.025$) (117). Analyses were performed to investigate whether the Thr399Ile polymorphism influenced the interaction between 299Gly and pravastatin, but the results did not allow any conclusions because of the low frequency of this genotype (117). This is another observation of an interaction between a genotype and statin treatment in reducing clinical events without an interaction reducing lipid parameters.

INTERLEUKIN-1B GENOTYPE

A polymorphism at position –511 of interleukin (IL)-1B gene promotor regulates IL-1B levels, immune and inflammatory responses, and possible atherogenesis. Lehtimäki et al. found in a small trial ($n = 34$) that at baseline, there was no difference in basal or adenosine-stimulated myocardial flow between subjects with the A2+ and subjects with the A2– genotype. After 6 mo of treatment with pravastatin, the adenosine-stimulated myocardial flow increased by 18.0% in subjects with the A2– genotype ($n = 7$), and decreased by 2% in subjects with the A2+ genotype ($n = 7$). In the placebo recipients there were no significant changes compared with the baseline values. Both genotype groups showed a similar decrease in total LDL cholesterol levels. Coronary function improves after 6 mo of statin therapy in subjects with the IL-1B A2– allele but not in those with the A2+ allele (118).

CONCLUSIONS

In this review, we have discussed a number of polymorphisms which might interfere with the effectiveness of statin therapy. Most polymorphisms described in this chapter have an indirect effect on statin response. Only a few of them are in genes encoding for proteins that are involved in the disposition of statins, or in genes-encoding proteins that are direct targets of statin therapy. More proteins are involved in efficacy and metabolism of statins; therefore, more genes are involved, and probably more polymorphisms will influence the efficacy of statin therapy. The use of other techniques in pharmacogenetic and pharmacogenomic research will enable us to compare gene profiles of patients with differences in reactions to drugs. Instead of looking at one single SNP in a gene, haplotypes might better explain the differences in response to drugs. Furthermore, models need to be developed that enable us to look at combinations of polymorphisms at the same time. Because so many genes are involved, probably more polymorphisms have to be determined to predict a patients response to statins.

What is the clinical relevance of the polymorphisms described in this chapter? Some of them might be useful to select patients with a high risk for coronary artery disease (for example, ACE and ApoE). Subjects with that particular genotype might be treated rigorously, especially in the case of Apoε4 carriers, who are genetically prone to develop coronary artery disease and who are at higher risk to discontinue their therapy (86). Other polymorphisms could predict the effectiveness of statins. For example, carriers of the CETP B2B2 polymorphism or the stromelysin-1 A5A5 polymorphism seem to have no benefit from treatment with statins. Nevertheless, in the study of Kuivenhoven et al., it was only the effect on angiographic progression of coronary disease that was measured, whereas statins do have effects that are independent of cholesterol lowering. Therefore, we do agree with Goldstein *(119)* that at this moment, there is certainly not enough evidence to exclude patients with a certain genotype from statin treatment. However, in the near future, it is likely that genetic information may be used to modify dose and suggest supplemental treatment regimens. Further research in large general population samples and large clinical trials is necessary to assess the importance of these polymorphisms on the effectiveness of statins in the reduction of cardiovascular diseases.

The ethical, legal, and social implications of population-based genotyping are still unresolved and much debated. It is important that distinctions are made between disease susceptibility gene polymorphisms, which provide information about risks of diseases, and pharmacogenetic profiles *(120)*, even though it is not always possible to make this distinction. An example is the Apoε polymorphism. This polymorphism might predict a patient's response to statins *(76)* or the risk for discontinuation of statins *(86)*, but it also predicts a patients risk on developing Alzheimer's disease *(121)*. For such polymorphisms, it might lead to difficult decisions for health care professionals. Is it the task of health care professionals to tell the patient about this risk? The patient has of course the right (not) to know. This information might not only influence the patient, but also members of his family who might carry the same polymorphism. Furthermore, it might not only influence the patient's perception of his health and life, but also his eligibility for healthcare and life insurance. The debate is ongoing in various countries with, so far, an uncertain outcome.

If polymorphisms exist that influence the response to statins, it is also important to evaluate the cost-effectiveness of screening for such genotypes. In a recent study, the cost-effectiveness of screening for the ACE genotype before starting statin therapy was evaluated *(122)*. If the interaction between the ACE genotype and the effectiveness of statin therapy is confirmed in more studies, then screening could save money. The model used in this study can also be used to determine the cost-effectiveness for screening for other polymorphisms.

At present, no single polymorphism has been identified that renders statin treatment ineffective based on clinical outcomes. Therefore, results from large-scale population studies are needed, to complement results from clinical trials and small-scale studies in selected populations.

Possibly, one day a person's genotype might determine if he or she should get a statin or not. Then, determining the genotype will not deny therapy to a subject, but will help in the decision as to which therapy suits the patient best, and potentially increase cost-effectiveness of the treatment

ACKNOWLEDGMENT

The author was financially supported by the Netherlands Heart Foundation, grant number NHF-2000.170.

REFERENCES

1. McGovern PG, Pankow JS, Shahar E, et al. Recent trends in acute coronary heart disease—mortality, morbidity, medical care, and risk factors. The Minnesota Heart Survey Investigators. N Engl J Med 1996;334:884–890.
2. Dobson AJ, McElduff P, Heller R, Alexander H, Colley P, D'Este K. Changing patterns of coronary heart disease in the hunter region of New South Wales, Australia. J Clin Epidemiol 1999;52:761–771.
3. Sacks F, Pfeffer MA, Moye LA, et al. The effect of pravastatine on coronary events after myocardial infarction in patients with average cholesterol levels. N Eng J Med 1996;335:1001–1009.
4. Shepherd J, Cobbe SM, Ford I, et al. Prevention of coronary heart disease with pravastatine in men with hypercholesterolemia. New Eng J Med 1995;333:1301–1307.
5. Downs JR, Clearfield M, Weis S, et al. Primary prevention of acute coronary events with lovastatine in men and women with average cholesterol levels. Results of AFCAPS/TexCAPS. JAMA 1998;279:1615–1622.
6. Heart Protection Study Collaborative Group. MRC/BHF Heart protection study of cholesterol lowering with simvastatin in 20,536 high risk individuals; a randomized placebo controlled trial. Lancet 2002;360:7–22.
7. Sever PS, Dahlof B, Poulter NR. Prevention of coronary and stroke events with atorvastatin in hypertensive patients who have average or lower-than-average cholesterol concentrations; in the Anglo-Scandinavian Cardiac Outcomes Trial-Lipid Lowering Arm (ASCOT-LLA), a multicentre randomised controlled trial. Lancet 2003;361:1149–1158.
8. Sander C. Genomic medicine and the future of health care. Science 2000;287:1977–1978.
9. Vesell ES. Therapeutic lessons from pharmacogenetics. Ann Intern Med 1997;126:653–655.
10. (No authors listed). Randomised trial of cholesterol lowering in 4444 patients with coronary heart disease: the Scandinavian Simvastatine Survival Study. Lancet 1994;344:1383–1389.
11. (No authors listed). Prevention of cardiovascular events and death with pravastatin in patients with coronary heart disease and a broad range of initial cholesterol levels. The Long-Term Intervention with Pravastatin in Ischemic Disease (LIPID) Study Group. N Eng J Med 1998;339:1349–1357.
12. Miettinen TA, Gylling H, Strandberg T, Sarna S. Baseline serum cholestanol as predictor of recurrent coronary events in subgroup of Scandinavian simvastatin survival study. Finnish 4S Investigators. BMJ 1998;316:1127–1130.
13. Sadee W. Pharmacogenomics [interview by Clare Thompson]. BMJ 1999;319:1286.
14. Maitland-van der Zee AH, de Boer A, Leufkens HGM. The interface between pharmaoepidemiology and pharmacogenetics. Eur J Pharmacol 2000;410:13–22.
15. Lefer AM, Scalia R, Lefer DJ. Vascular effects of HMG Co-A reductase inhibitors (statins) unrelated to cholesterol lowering: new concepts for cardiovascular disease. Cardiovasc Res 2001;49:281–287.
16. Vaughan CJ, Murphy MB, Buckley BM. Statins do more than just lower cholesterol. Lancet 1996;348:1079–1082.
17. Psaty BM, Weiss NS, Furberg CD, et al. Surrogate end points, health outcomes, and the drug-approval process for the treatment of risk factors for cardiovascular disease. JAMA 1999;282:786–790.
18. Maitland-van der Zee AH, Klungel OH, Stricker BH, et al. Genetic polymorphisms: importance for response to HMG-CoA reductase inhibitors. Atherosclerosis 2002;163:213–222.
19. Cheng H, Rogers JD, Sweany AE, et al. Influence of age and gender on the plasma profiles of 3-hydroxy-3-methylglutaryl-coenzyme A (HMG-CoA) reductase inhibitory activity following multiple doses of lovastatin and simvastatin. Pharm Res 1992;9:1629–1633.
20. Stern RH, Gibson DM, Whitfield LR. Cimetidine does not alter atorvastatin pharmacokinetics or LDL-cholesterol reduction. Eur J Clin Pharmacol 1998;53:475–478.
21. Schmitz G, Drobnik W. Pharmacogenomics and pharmacogenetics of cholesterol-lowering therapy. Clin Chem Lab Med 2003;41:581–589.
22. Mauro VF. Clinical pharmacokinetics and practical applications of simvastatin. Clin Pharmacokinet 1993;24:195–202.
23. Wolf CR, Smith G. Pharmacogenetics. Br Med Bull 1999;55:366–386.
24. Sachse C, Brockmoller J, Bauer S, Roots I. Cytochrome P450 2D6 variants in a Caucasian population: allele frequencies and phenotypic consequences. Am J Hum Genet 1997;60:284–295.
25. Nordin C, Dahl ML, Eriksson M, Sjoberg S. Is the cholesterol-lowering effect of simvastatin influenced by CYP2D6 polymorphism? Lancet 1997;350:29–30.

26. Mulder AB, van Lijf HJ, Bon MA, et al. Association of polymorphism in the cytochrome CYP2D6 and the efficacy and tolerability of simvastatin. Clin Pharmacol Ther 2001;70:546–551.

27. Geisel J, Kivisto KT, Griese EU, Eichelbaum M. The efficacy of simvastatin is not influenced by CYP2D6 polymorphism. Clin Pharmacol Ther 2002;72:595–596.

28. Mulder AB, van den Bergh FA, Vermes I. Response to "The efficacy of simvastatin is not influenced by CYP2D6 polymorphism" by Geisel et al. Clin Pharmacol Ther 2003;73:475.

29. Aithal GP, Day CP, Kesteven PJ, Daly AK. Association of polymorphisms in the cytochrome P450 CYP2C9 with warfarin dose requirement and risk of bleeding complications. Lancet 1999;353:717–719.

30. Kirchheiner J, Kudlicz D, Meisel C, et al. Influence of CYP2C9 polymorphisms on the pharmacokinetics and cholesterol-lowering activity of (–)-3S,5R-fluvastatin and (+)-3R,5S-fluvastatin in healthy volunteers. Clin Pharmacol Ther 2003;74:186–194.

31. Williams D, Feely J. Pharmacokinetic-pharmacodynamic drug interactions with HMG-CoA reductase inhibitors. Clin Pharmacokinet 2002;41:343–370.

32. Nishizato Y, Ieiri I, Suzuki H, et al. Polymorphisms of OATP-C (SLC21A6) and OAT3 (SLC22A8) genes: consequences for pravastatin pharmacokinetics. Clin Pharmacol Ther 2003;73:554–565.

33. Tirona RG, Leake BF, Merino G, Kim RB. Polymorphisms in OATP-C: identification of multiple allelic variants associated with altered transport activity among European- and African-Americans. J Biol Chem 2001;276:35669–35675.

34. Kusuhara H, Suzuki H, Sugiyama Y. The role of P-glycoprotein and canalicular multispecific organic anion transporter in the hepatobiliary excretion of drugs. J Pharm Sci 1998;87:1025–1040.

35. Hill SA, McQueen MJ. Reverse cholesterol transport—a review of the process and its clinical implications. Clin Biochem 1997;30:517–525.

36. Owen JS. Role of ABC1 gene in cholesterol efflux and atheroprotection. Lancet 1999;354:1402–1403.

37. Tall AR, Wang N. Tangier disease as a test of the reverse cholesterol transport hypothesis. J Clin Invest 2000;106:1205–1207.

38. Dachet C, Poirier O, Cambien F, Chapman J, Rouis M. New functional promoter polymorphism, CETP/-629, in cholesteryl ester transfer protein (CETP) gene related to CETP mass and high density lipoprotein cholesterol levels: role of Sp1/Sp3 in transcriptional regulation. Arterioscler Thromb Vasc Biol 2000;20:507–515.

39. Klerkx AHEM, Tanck MWT, Kastelein JJP, et al. Haplotype analysis of the CETP gene: not TaqIB, but the closely linked –629 C/A polymorphism and a novel promotor variant are independently associated with CETP concentration. Hum Mol Gen 2003;12:111–123.

40. Kuivenhoven J, Jukema JW, Zwinderman AH, et al. The role of a common variant of the cholesteryl ester transfer protein gene in the progression of coronary atherosclerosis. N Eng J Med 1998;338:86–93.

41. Ordovas JM, Cupples LA, Corella D, et al. Association of cholesteryl ester transfer protein-TaqIB polymorphism with variations in lipoprotein subclasses and coronary heart disease risk: the Framingham study. Arterioscler Thromb Vasc Biol 2000;20:1323–1329.

42. Inazu A, Brown ML, Hesler CB, et al. Increased high-density lipoprotein levels caused by a common cholesteryl-ester transfer protein gene mutation. N Engl J Med 1990;323:1234–1238.

43. Inazu A, Jiang XC, Haraki T, et al. Genetic cholesteryl ester transfer protein deficiency caused by two prevalent mutations as a major determinant of increased levels of high density lipoprotein cholesterol. J Clin Invest 1994;94:1872–1882.

44. Hagberg JM, Wilund KR, Ferrell RE. APO E gene and gene-environment effects on plasma lipoprotein-lipid levels. Physiol Genomics 2000;4:101–108.

45. Bruce C, Sharp DS, Tall AR. Relationship of HDL and coronary heart disease to a common amino acid polymorphism in the cholesteryl ester transfer protein in men with and without hypertriglyceridemia. J Lipid Res 1998;39:1071–1078.

46. Zhong S, Sharp DS, Grove JS, et al. Increased coronary heart disease in Japanese-American men with mutation in the cholesteryl ester transfer protein gene despite increased HDL levels. J Clin Invest 1996;97:2917–2923.

47. Agerholm-Larsen B, Nordestgaard BG, Steffensen R, Jensen G, Tybjaerg-Hansen A. Elevated HDL cholesterol is a risk factor for ischemic heart disease in white women when caused by a common mutation in the cholesteryl ester transfer protein gene [In Process Citation]. Circulation 2000;101:1907–1912.

48. Tenkanen H, Koshinen P, Kontula K, et al. Polymorphisms of the gene encoding cholesterol ester transfer protein and serum lipoprotein levels in subjects with and without coronary heart disease. Hum Genet 1991;87:574–578.

49. van Venrooij FV, Stolk RP, Banga JD, et al. Common cholesteryl ester transfer protein gene polymor-phisms and the effect of atorvastatin therapy in type 2 diabetes. Diabetes Care 2003;26:1216–1223.
50. Fumeron F, Betoulle D, Luc G, et al. Alcohol intake modulates the effect of a polymorphism of the cholesteryl ester transfer protein gene on plasma high density lipoprotein and the risk of myocardial infarction. J Clin Invest 1995;96:1664–1671.
51. Kuivenhoven JA, Kastelein JJP. Polymorphism of the Cholesteryl Ester Transfer Protein Gene [let-ter]. N Engl J Med 1998;338:1625–1626.
52. Freeman DJ, Samani NJ, Wilson V, et al. A polymorphism of the cholesteryl ester transfer protein gene predicts cardiovascular events in non-smokers in the West of Scotland Coronary Prevention Study. Eur Heart J 2003;24:1833–1842.
53. Blankenberg S, Bickel C, Jiang XC, et al. Common genetic variation of the cholesteryl ester transfer protein gene strongly predicts future cardiovascular death in patients with coronary artery disease. J Am Coll Cardiol 2003;41:1983–1989.
54. Ye S, Eriksson P, Hamsten A, Kurkinen M, Humphries S, Henney AM. Progression of coronary atherosclerosis is associated with a common genetic variant of the human stromelysin-1 promotor which results in reduced gene expression. J Biol Chem 1996;271:13055–13060.
55. Nikkari ST, O'Brien KD, Ferguson M, et al. Interstital Collagenase (MMP-1) expression in human carotid atherosclerosis. Circulation 1995;92:1393–1398.
56. Galis ZS, Sukhova GK, Kranzhofer R, Clark S, Libby P. Macrophage foam cells from experimental atheroma constitutively produce matrix-degrading proteinases. Proc Natl Acad Sci USA 1995;92:402–406.
57. Brown DL, Hibbs MS, Kearney M, Loushin C, Isner JM. Identification of 92-kD gelatinase in human coronary atherosclerotic lesions. Association of active enzyme synthesis with unstable angina. Cir-culation 1995;91:2125–2131.
58. Humphries SE, Luong LA, Talmud PJ, et al. The 5A/6A polymorphism in the promoter of the stromelysin-1 (MMP-3) gene predicts progression of angiographically determined coronary artery disease in men in the LOCAT gemfibrozil study. Lopid Coronary Angiography Trial. Atherosclerosis 1998;139:49–56.
59. de Maat MP, Jukema JW, Ye S, et al. Effect of the stromelysin-1 promoter on efficacy of pravastatin in coronary atherosclerosis and restenosis. Am J Cardiol 1999; 83:852–856.
60. Meade TW, Mellows S, Brozovic M, et al. Haemostatic function and ischaemic heart disease: prin-cipal results of the Northwick Park Heart Study [see comments]. Lancet 1986;2:533–537.
61. Kannel WB, Wolf PA, Castelli WP, D'Agostino RB. Fibrinogen and risk of cardiovascular disease. The Framingham Study. JAMA 1987;258:1183–1186.
62. Yarnell JW, Baker IA, Sweetnam PM, et al. Fibrinogen, viscosity, and white blood cell count are major risk factors for ischemic heart disease. The Caerphilly and Speedwell collaborative heart disease studies. Circulation 1991;83:836–844.
63. Cremer P, Nagel D, Labrot B, et al. Lipoprotein Lp(a) as predictor of myocardial infarction in com-parison to fibrinogen, LDL cholesterol and other risk factors: results from the prospective Gottingen Risk Incidence and Prevalence Study (GRIPS). Eur J Clin Invest 1994;24:444–53.
64. Heinrich J, Balleisen L, Schulte H, Assmann G, van de Loo J. Fibrinogen and factor VII in the prediction of coronary risk. Results from the PROCAM study in healthy men. Arterioscler Thromb 1994;14:54–59.
65. Thompson SG, Kienast J, Pyke SD, Haverkate F, van de Loo JC. Hemostatic factors and the risk of myocardial infarction or sudden death in patients with angina pectoris. European Concerted Action on Thrombosis and Disabilities Angina Pectoris Study Group. N Engl J Med 1995;332:635–641.
66. Resch KL, Ernst E, Matrai A, Paulsen HF. Fibrinogen and viscosity as risk factors for subsequent cardiovascular events in stroke survivors. Ann Intern Med 1988;19:634–636.
67. de Maat MP, Kastelein JJP, Jukema JW, et al. –455G/A polymorphism of the beta-fibrinogen gene is associated with the progression of coronary atherosclerosis in symptomatic men: proposed role for an acute-phase reaction pattern of fibrinogen. REGRESS group. Arterioscler Thromb Vasc Biol 1998;18:265–271.
68. Henry I, Uzan G, Weil D, et al. The genes coding for A alpha-, B beta-, and gamma-chains of fibrinogen map to 4q2. Am J Hum Genet 1984;36:760–768.
69. Zannis VI, Breslow JL, SanGiacomo TR, Aden DP, Knowles BB. Characterization of the major apolipoproteins secreted by two human hepatoma cell lines. Biochemistry 1981;20:7089–7096.
70. Schaefer EJ, Lamon-Fava S, Johnson S, et al. Effects of gender and menopausal status on the asso-ciation of apolipoprotein E phenotype with plasma lipoprotein levels. Results from the Framingham Offspring Study. Arterioscler Thromb 1994;14:1105–1113.

71. Corbo RM, Scacchi R. Apolipoprotein E (APOE) allele distribution in the world. Is APOE*4 a 'thrifty' allele? Ann Hum Genet 1999;63:301–310.

72. Sanllehy C, Casals E, Rodriguez-Villar C, et al. Lack of interaction of apolipoprotein E phenotype with the lipoprotein response to lovastatin or gemfibrozil in patients with primary hypercholesterolemia. Metabolism 1998;47:560–565.

73. Ballantyne CM, Herd JA, Stein EA, et al. Apolipoprotein E genotypes and response of plasma lipids and progression-regression of coronary atherosclerosis to lipid-lowering drug therapy. J Am Coll Cardiol 2000;36:1572–1578.

74. Ordovas JM, Lopez-Miranda J, Perez-Jimenez F, et al. Effect of apolipoprotein E and A-IV phenotypes on the low density lipoprotein response to HMG CoA reductase inhibitor therapy. Atherosclerosis 1995;113:157–166.

75. Nestel P, Simons L, Barter P, et al. A comparative study of the efficacy of simvastatin and gemfibrozil in combined hyperlipoproteinemia: prediction of response by baseline lipids, apo E genotype, lipoprotein(a) and insulin. Atherosclerosis 1997;129:231–239.

76. Carmena R, Roederer G, Mailloux H, Lussier-Cacan S, Davignon J. The response to lovastatin treatment in patients with heterozygous familial hypercholesterolemia is modulated by apolipoprotein E polymorphism. Metabolism 1993;42:895–901.

77. Ojala JP, Helve E, Ehnholm C, Aalto-Setala K, Kontula KK, Tikkanen MJ. Effect of apolipoprotein E polymorphism and XbaI polymorphism of apolipoprotein B on response to lovastatin treatment in familial and non-familial hypercholesterolaemia. J Intern Med 1991;230:397–405.

78. Marques-Vidal P, Bongard V, Ruidavels JB, Fauve, J, Perret B, Ferrieres J. Effect of apolipoprotein E alleles and angiotensin converting enzyme insertion/deletion polymorphisms on lipid and lipoprotein markers in middle aged men and in patients with stable angina pectoris or healed myocardial infarction. Am J Cardiol 2003;92:1102–1105.

79. Berglund L, Wiklund O, Eggertsen G, et al. Apolipoprotein E phenotypes in familial hypercholesterolaemia: importance for expression of disease and response to therapy. J Intern Med 1993;233:173–738.

80. De Knijff P, Stalenhoef AF, Mol MJ, et al. Influence of apo E polymorphism on the response to simvastatin treatment in patients with heterozygous familial hypercholesterolemia. Atherosclerosis 1990;83:89–97.

81. Gerdes LU, Gerdes C, Kervinen K, et al. The apolipoprotein epsilon4 allele determines prognosis and the effect on prognosis of simvastatin in survivors of myocardial infarction : A substudy of the scandinavian simvastatin survival study [In Process Citation]. Circulation 2000;101:1366–1371.

82. O'Malley JP, Illingworth DR. The influence of apolipoprotein E phenotype on the response to lovastatin therapy in patients with heterozygous familial hypercholesterolemia. Metabolism 1990;39:150–154.

83. Pedro-Botet J, Schaefer EJ, Bakker-Arkema RG, et al. Apolipoprotein E genotype affects plasma lipid response to atorvastatin in a gender specific manner. Atherosclerosis 2001;158:183–193.

84. Maitland-van der Zee AH, Jukema JW, Zwinderman AH, et al. Influence of apolipoprotein E polymorphisms on coronary artery disease and on the efficacy of HMG-CoA reductase inhibitors in men. Circulation Suppl 2003;108:IV-771.

85. Maitland-van der Zee AH, Stricker BH, Klungel OH, et al. The effectiveness of hydroxy-methylglutaryl coenzyme A reductase inhibitors (statins) in the elderly is not influenced by apolipoprotein E genotype. Pharmacogenetics 2002;12:647–653.

86. Maitland-van der Zee AH, Stricker BH, Klungel OH, et al. Adherence to and dosing of beta-hydroxy-beta-methylglutaryl coenzyme A reductase inhibitors in the general population differs according to apolipoprotein E-genotypes. Pharmacogenetics 2003;13:219–223.

87. Medh JD, Bowen SL, Fry GL, et al. Lipoprotein lipase binds to low density lipoprotein receptors and induces receptor-mediated catabolism of very low density lipoproteins in vitro. J Biol Chem 1996;271:17,073–17,080.

88. Mulder M, Lombardi P, Jansen H, van Berkel TJ, Frants RR, Havekes LM. Low density lipoprotein receptor internalizes low density and very low density lipoproteins that are bound to heparan sulfate proteoglycans via lipoprotein lipase. J Biol Chem 1993;268:9369–9375.

89. Clee SM, Bissada N, Miao F, et al. Plasma and vessel wall lipoprotein lipase have different roles in atherosclerosis. J Lipid Res 2000;41:521–531.

90. Mailly F, Tugrul Y, Reymer PW, et al. A common variant in the gene for lipoprotein lipase (Asp9Asn). Functional implications and prevalence in normal and hyperlipidemic subjects. Arterioscler Thromb Vasc Biol 1995;15:468–478.

91. Jukema JW, van Boven AJ, Groenemeijer B, et al. The Asp9 Asn mutation in the lipoprotein lipase gene is associated with increased progression of coronary atherosclerosis. Circulation 1996;94:1913–1918.

92. Gagne SE, Larson MG, Pimstone SN, et al. A common truncation variant of lipoprotein lipase (Ser447X) confers protection against coronary heart disease: the Framingham Offspring Study. Clin Genet 1999;55:450–454.

93. Fisher RM, Humphries SE, Talmud PJ. Common variation in the lipoprotein lipase gene: effects on plasma lipids and risk of atherosclerosis. Atherosclerosis 1997;135:145–159.

94. Wittrup HH, Tybjaerg-Hansen A, Nordestgaard BG. Lipoprotein lipase mutations, plasma lipids and lipoproteins, and risk of ischemic heart disease. A meta-analysis. Circulation 1999;99:2901–2907.

95. Rigat B, Hubert C, Alhenc-Gelas F, Cambien F, Corvol P, Soubrier F. An insertion/deletion polymorphism in the angiotensin I-converting enzyme gene accounting for half the variance of serum enzyme levels. J Clin Invest 1990;86:1343–1346.

96. Gardemann A, Fink M, Stricker J, et al. ACE I/D gene polymorphism: presence of the ACE D allele increases the risk of coronary artery disease in younger individuals. Atherosclerosis 1998;139:153–159.

97. Beohar N, Damaraju S, Prather A, et al. Angiotensin-I converting enzyme genotype DD is a risk factor for coronary artery disease. J Investig Med 1995;43:275–280.

98. Cambien F, Poirier O, Lecerf L, et al. Deletion polymorphism in the gene for angiotensin-converting enzyme is a potent risk factor for myocardial infarction. Nature 1992;359:641–644.

99. Staessen JA, Wang JG, Ginocchio G, et al. The deletion/insertion polymorphism of the angiotensin converting enzyme gene and cardiovascular-renal risk. J Hypertens 1997;15:1579–1592.

100. Bray PF, Cannon CP, Goldschmidt-Clermont P, et al. The platelet Pl(A2) and angiotensin-converting enzyme (ACE) D allele polymorphisms and the risk of recurrent events after acute myocardial infarction. Am J Cardiol 2001;88:347–352.

101. Marian AJ, Safavi F, Ferlic L, Dunn JK, Gotto AM, Ballantyne CM. Interactions between angiotensin-I converting enzyme insertion/deletion polymorphism and response of plasma lipids and coronary atherosclerosis to treatment with fluvastatin: the lipoprotein and coronary atherosclerosis study. J Am Coll Cardiol 2000;35:89–95.

102. van Geel P, Pinto Y, Zwinderman A, et al. The angiotensin-converting enzyme deletion-type gene is associated with ischemic events and a blunted effect of lipid-lowering treatment on angiographically defined coronary atherosclerosis (Abstr). Eur Heart J 1997;IS:1.

103. Maitland-van der Zee AH, Stricker BH, Klungel OH, et al. Effectiveness of HMG-CoA reductase inhibitors is affected by ACE insertion/deletion polymorphism. PDS 2002;11:s10–s11.

104. Fornage M, Amos CI, Kardia S, Sing CF, Turner ST, Boerwinkle E. Variation in the region of the angiotensin-converting enzyme gene influences interindividual differences in blood pressure levels in young white males. Circulation 1998;97:1773–1779.

105. O'Donnell CJ, Lindpaintner K, Larson MG, et al. Evidence for association and genetic linkage of the angiotensin-converting enzyme locus with hypertension and blood pressure in men but not women in the Framingham Heart Study. Circulation 1998;97:1766–1772.

106. Deeb SS, Peng R. The C-514T polymorphism in the human hepatic lipase gene promoter diminishes its activity. J Lipid Res 2000;41:155–158.

107. Austin MA, Breslow JL, Hennekens CH, Buring JE, Willett WC, Krauss RM. Low-density lipoprotein subclass patterns and risk of myocardial infarction. JAMA 1988;260:1917–1921.

108. Zambon A, Deeb SS, Brown BG, Hokanson JE, Brunzell JD. Common hepatic lipase gene promoter variant determines clinical response to intensive lipid-lowering treatment. Circulation 2001;103:792–798.

109. Hoffmann R, Mintz GS, Dussaillant GR, et al. Patterns and mechanisms of in-stent restenosis. A serial intravascular ultrasound study. Circulation 1996;94:1247–1254.

110. Walter DH, Schachinger V, Elsner M, et al. Statin therapy is associated with reduced restenosis rates after coronary stent implantation in carriers of the Pl(A2)allele of the platelet glycoprotein IIIa gene. Eur Heart J 2001;22:587–595.

111. Dornbrook-Lavender KA, Pieper JA. Genetic polymorphisms in emerging cardiovascular risk factors and response to statin therapy. Cardiovasc Drugs Ther 2003;17:75–82.

112. Ross R. Atherosclerosis—an inflammatory disease. N Engl J Med 1999;340:115–126.

113. Wiedermann CJ, Kiechl S, Dunzendorfer S, et al. Association of endotoxemia with carotid atherosclerosis and cardiovascular disease: prospective results from the Bruneck Study. J Am Coll Cardiol 1999;34:1975–1981.

114. Goto T, Eden S, Nordenstam G, Sundh V, Svanborg-Eden C, Mattsby-Baltzer I. Endotoxin levels in sera of elderly individuals. Clin Diagn Lab Immunol 1994;1:684–688.

115. Arbour NC, Lorenz E, Schutte BC, et al. TLR4 mutations are associated with endotoxin hyporesponsiveness in humans. Nat Genet 2000;25:187–191.

116. Kiechl S, Lorenz E, Reindl M, et al. Toll-like receptor 4 polymorphisms and atherogenesis. N Engl J Med 2002;347:185–192.

117. Boekholdt SM, Agema WR, Peters RJ, et al. Variants of toll-like receptor 4 modify the efficacy of statin therapy and the risk of cardiovascular events. Circulation 2003;107:2416–2421.

118. Lehtimaki T, Laaksonene R, Janatuinen T, et al. Interleukin-1B genotype modulates the improvement of coronary artery reactivity by lipid-lowering therapy with pravastatin: a placebo-controlled positron emission tomography study in young healthy men. Pharmacogenetics 2003;13:633–639.

119. Goldstein MR. Polymorphism of the cholesteryl ester transfer protein gene. N Engl J Med 1998;338:1624–1625.

120. Roses AD. Pharmacogenetics and future drug development and delivery. Lancet 2000;355:1358–1361.

121. Poirier J, Delisle MC, Quirion R, et al. Apolipoprotein E4 allele as a predictor of cholinergic deficits and treatment outcome in Alzheimer disease. Proc Natl Acad Sci USA 1995;92:12,260–12,264.

122. Maitland-van der Zee AH, Klungel OH, Stricker BH, et al. Economic evaluation of testing for angiotensin converting enzyme (ACE) genotype before starting HMG-CoA reductase therapy in men. Pharmacogenetics 2004;14:1–8.

7

Monogenic Causes of Heart Failure

Familial Dilated Cardiomyopathy

Hideko Kasahara, MD, PhD

SUMMARY

Dilated cardiomyopathy (DCM) without an established causative factor for the damage to the myocardium is termed "idiopathic DCM," and it is the cause of approximately one-fourth of the cases of congestive heart failure in the United States. Familial occurrence accounts for 20% or more of idiopathic DCM, and recently a considerable number of genes associated with DCM have been identified. This review will focus on 18 genes currently known as *DCM response genes* because of their pathological involvement in this disease. The incidence of DCM caused by each gene is relatively small; however, the study of these genes has led us to understand the specific disease pathways of DCM, which may ultimately lead to understanding the more common condition of heart failure.

Key Words: Dilated cardiomyopathy; (DCM); gene; cardiomyocytes; familial; sarcomere; Z-disc; desmosome; costamere; adherens junction.

INTRODUCTION

Heart failure defined by Braunwald is the pathophysiological state in which the heart is unable to pump blood at a rate commensurate with the requirement of the metabolizing tissues (*1*). It is usually, but not always, caused by a defect in myocardial contraction. A number of adaptive mechanisms for maintenance of pumping function occur both rapidly and slowly: the Frank–Starling mechanism, in which an increased preload helps to sustain cardiac performance; activation of neurohumoral systems, especially the release of

From: *Contemporary Cardiology: Cardiovascular Genomics*
Edited by: M. K. Raizada, et al. © Humana Press Inc., Totowa, NJ

the norepinephrine, which augments myocardial contractility; and the activation of the renin–angiotensin–aldosterone system, which maintains arterial pressure and perfusion of vital organs. Myocardial remodeling develops over weeks to months, and plays an important role in long-term adaptation to hemodynamic overload. If compensatory responses are adequate to match the work demands, a period of relative stability ensues. However, if the extent or form of myocardial remodeling is insufficient, or if the magnitude of the overload increases, there is further deterioration in myocardial function leading to advanced heart failure *(1)*.

Approximately 400,000 new cases of heart failure occur annually, and its prevalence demonstrates the enormous burden exacted on the public: 4.7 million patients and their direct health care cost $17.8 billion in 1993 *(2)*. Primary cardiovascular diseases including coronary atherosclerosis, hypertension, myocarditis, diabetes, valvular and congenital heart malformations, and cardiomyopathy lead to the common final pathway of heart failure. The cardiomyopathies constitute a group of diseases in which the dominant feature is direct involvement of the heart muscle, not the result of hypertensive, valvular and congenital heart malformations, or ischemic diseases. Dilated cardiomyopathy (DCM) is characterized by dilation and impaired contraction of the left or both ventricles, and is caused by a variety of cytotoxic, metabolic, immunological, infectious, and familial mechanisms. DCM without an established causative factor that damages the myocardium is termed "idiopathic DCM." About one-fourth of the cases of congestive heart failure in the United States are the result of idiopathic DCM. Although the causes remain unclear, interest has been centered on three possible basic mechanisms: (1) familial and genetic factors, (2) viral myocarditis and other cytotoxic insults, and (3) immunological abnormalities *(1)*.

Familial occurrence accounts for 20% or more of idiopathic DCM *(1)*, and recently a considerable number of genes have been identified as causative factors for DCM. Although the detailed disease mechanisms caused by each mutation have not been be elucidated, current general agreement is that familial DCM is likely a disease of the cytoskelton leading to inadequate force transmission *(3–6)*. In this review, 18 genes, currently known as DCM responsive genes, are focused on for their pathological involvement in DCM. The incidence of DCM caused by each gene is relatively small; however, these studies have led to a great understanding of the specific disease pathways of DCM that may ultimately lead to understanding the more common condition of heart failure.

STRUCTURES OF THE CARDIAC CYTOSKELETON, CELL ADHESION, AND THE SARCOMERE

The major function of cardiomyocytes is in the cardiac contraction–relaxation cycle. The contractile proteins in cardiomyocytes constitute about 75% of the total volume of the myocardium, although only about one-third of the number of all the cells in the myocardium are cardiomyocytes. About half of each ventricular cell is occupied by myofibers, and about one-fourth to one-third by mitochondria. The major proteins involved in contraction and relaxation are the thin filament (composed of actin, tropomyosin, and C-, I-, and T-troponin) and the thick myosin filament. During contraction, the filaments slide over each other (A band) without the individual molecules of actin or myosin actually shortening, leading to a pulling together of the two ends of the fundamental contractile unit called the sarcomere (Fig. 1A,B). The sarcomere is limited on either side by the Z-disc ("Z" is an abbreviation for the German "Zückung", meaning "contraction") to which the actin filaments are attached. Conversely, the myosin filaments extend from the center of the sarcomere (M-line) in either direction toward, but not actually reaching the Z-discs.

The third component, titin (or connectin), is anchored in the Z-disc and extends to the M-line region of the sarcomere (Fig. 1A,B). Titin is an extraordinarily long, flexible, and slender myofibrillar protein that tethers myosin to the Z-disc to maintain the precise structural arrangement of thick and thin filaments (7,8). Titin's I-band region appears to function as a molecular spring. When the sarcomere is stretched, this region is also extended and held away from the Z-disc, giving rise to the passive force that pulls Z-discs toward each other. When the sarcomere shortens, the thick filament moves into titin's near the Z-disc region, leading to titin's spring region being stretched in an opposite direction and generating the force that pushes the Z-disc away (Fig. 1B).

Contractile force generated within cardiac sarcomeres transmits to adjacent sarcomeres via the Z-disc (Fig. 1A,B), to neighboring myocytes via intercalated discs (desmosome, adherens junction) (Fig. 2A), and to the extracellular matrix via costameres (Fig. 2B). In DCM, it is likely that the structural integrity of force-transmitting proteins is compromised, leading to nonuniform myocyte contraction and increased vulnerability to myocellular injury and death under physiological mechanical stress.

GENES IDENTIFIED AS RESPONSIBLE FOR IDIOPATHIC DCM

The genes that cause familial DCM are summarized in Table 1 according to their intracellular localization: Z-disc localizing proteins (α-actinin-2, muscle LIM protein [MLP], Z-disc alternatively spliced PDZ motif [ZASP]/cypher, titin-cap [T-cap]/telethonin); costameres, adherens junctions, desmosomes, and interemediate filaments (vinculin/metavinculin, desmoplakin, plakoglobin, desmin, lamin A/C, α-actinin-2, MLP, dystrophin, δ-sarcoglycan); sarcomere proteins (cardiac α-actin, β-myosin heavy chain, cardiac troponin T, α-tropomyosin, titin); sarcoplasmic reticulum proteins (phospo-lamban); and ion channel (SUR2A).

Titin and Z-Disc Proteins (α-actinin-2, MLP, ZASP/Cypher, T-Cap/Telethonin)

Both thin filaments (actin) and thick filaments (myosin through a titin) anchor at Z-discs. Therefore, the Z-disc is considered a sensor of contraction with other Z-disc localizing proteins to keep the normal integrity of the cardiac muscle (9).

TITIN

A giant protein, titin (or connectin) is the third most abundant protein of vertebrate striated muscle after myosin and actin (7,8). The titin molecule is a flexible filament that is more than 1 μm long, spanning half the sarcomere from the Z-disc (amino terminus of titin) to the M-line (carboxyl terminus of titin) (Fig. 1B). The molecule is formed as a single polypeptide with a molecular weight of up to 3 MDa, and is the largest polypeptide found so far in nature (10). The titin molecule is predominantly composed of nearly 300 immunoglobulin-like domains and fibronectin type III repeats. An additional kinase domain near the carboxyl terminus and several potential phosphorylation sites have also been identified. Within the Z-disc, titin interacts with other Z-disc proteins: T-cap/telethonin at two amino terminal immunoglobulin-like domains and α-actinin at the repeated unique 45 amino acid residues (Z-repeats), which crosslinks antiparallel thin

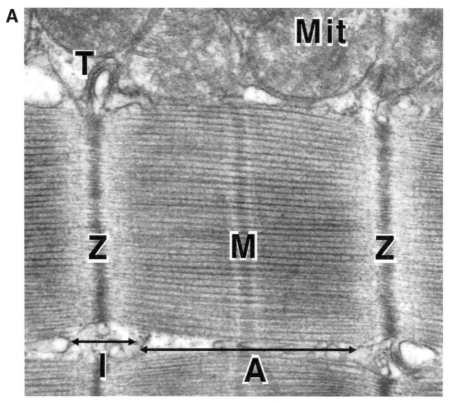

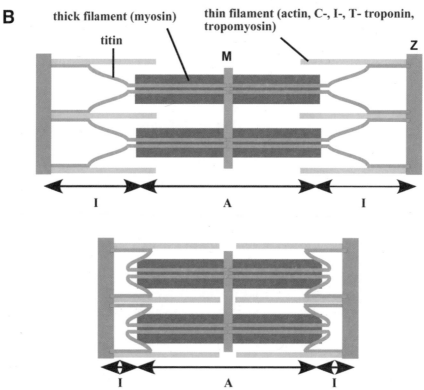

thick filament (myosin)

thin filament (actin, C-, I-, T- troponin, tropomyosin)

titin

filaments from adjacent sarcomeres. The two immunoglobulin-like domains located carboxyl terminus to the Z-repeats associate with obscurin, a giant multimodular protein that probably has a signaling function. The relationship between titin and actin within the Z-disc region is not yet clear, but it is known that near the edge of the Z-disc, titin attaches to the thin filaments (Fig. 2C). The Z-disc part of titin is also likely to be physically linked to intracellular membrane systems, T-tubules, and the sarcoplasmic reticulum (SR). Association with the T-tubule is likely through T-cap/telethonin, which binds to T-tubule potassium channels (MinK). Links with the SR could involve either direct interactions between titin and ankyrin, or indirect interactions through obscurin, which could link titin with ankyrin.

The carboxyl end of titin binds to M protein and myomesin at the M-line. The I-band region of titin contains only immunoglobulin domains and has a unique sequence, whereas the A band contains immunoglobulin-like domains and fibronectin type III repeats in long-range patterns.

Two mutations of titin proteins have been identified in autosomal dominant DCM without cardiac conduction defects or clinically detectable skeletal muscle disease *(11)*. One 2-basepair (bp) insertion mutation in exon 326 causes a frameshift, generating a premature stop codon. However, tissue lysates prepared from skeletal muscle of an affected individual demonstrated that the mutant protein is smaller than the predicted molecular weight and only proteolytic digested mutant proteins near the PEVK segment (enriched with proline [P], glutamate [E], valine [V], and lysine [K] residues), which is important for titin's spring in the I-band region of titin, are stably expressed. The other mutation, a single nucleotide substitution in exon 18, alters tryptophane to arginine within an immunoglobulin domain located near the Z-disc to I-band transition zone *(11)*. Clear explanations for the functions of mutant proteins that dominantly affect only cardiac myocytes remain to be found, but these mutant proteins may disrupt the assembly of contractile filaments or decrease the elasticity of titin molecules.

T-cap/Telethonin

Nineteen-kDa of T-cap, or telethonin *(12,13)*, interacts with the amino terminus of immunoglobulin-like domain of titin (Fig. 2C). T-cap/telethonin function has been suggested as important for organizing myofibrils because overexpression of T-cap/telethonin protein results in myofibril disruption, likely through inhibiting endogenous titin-T-cap/telethonin interaction at Z-discs.

T-cap/telethonin mutation was identified in a single DCM patient (Arg87Gln mutation). This mutation disrupts a stable complex formation with MLP *(14)*. T-cap/telethonin

---

Fig. 1. Structure of the sarcomere. **(A)** Thick filament myosin is attached to M line (M), and thin filament (composed with actin, tropomyosin, and C-, I-, and T-troponin) is attached to Z-disc (Z). Thin filaments and thick filaments overlap at A band (A) but no myosin at I band (I). T tubules (T) penetrate into the muscle at the level of the Z-line. Mit, mitochondria. EM from adult mouse heart. **(B)** The third component, titin (or connectin) anchors in the Z-disc and extends to the M-line region of the sarcomere. The titin's I-band region appears to function as a molecular spring. When the sarcomere is stretched (top panel), this region is also extended and held away from the Z-disc, giving rise to the passive force that pulls Z-discs toward each other. When the sarcomere shortens (bottom panel), the thick filament moves into titin's near Z-disc region leading to the titin's spring region being stretched in an opposite direction and generating the force that pushes the Z-disc away.

A Intercalated Disc: Desmosome and Adherens Junction

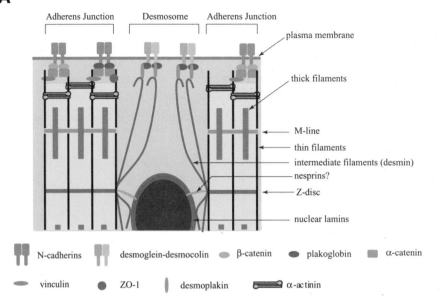

B Costamere: Dystrophin-glycoprotein complex, Integrin-based focal adhesion, Spectrin-based membrane cytoskeleton

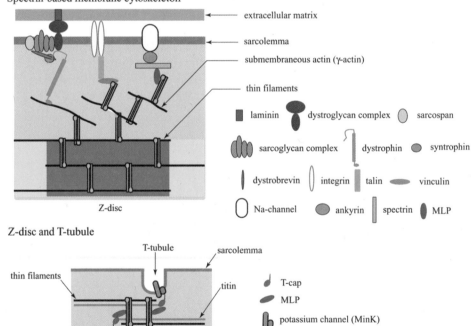

C Z-disc and T-tubule

Fig. 2. Structure of desmosome and intermediate filaments, adherens junction, and costamere. (**A**) Two cells are attached at adherens junction and desmosome. Adherens junction is composed of transmembrane protein. (N-cadherin) and intracellular attachment proteins (including β-catenin, γ-catenin, vinculin, 201 and α-actinin). Actin filaments are attached to the adherens junction. Desmosome is composed of transmembrane protein, desmosomal cadherin, desmoglein, and desmocolin, and intracellular attachment proteins (including desmoplakin and plakoglobin). Thick intermediate

mutations were also identified in autosomal recessive limb-girdle muscular dystrophies type 2G in which some patients show a cardiac phenotype *(15)*.

In addition, T-cap/telethonin associates with MinK, β-subunit of slow activating component of the delayed rectifier potassium current channel (I_{Ks}) *(16)*. This interaction may contribute to a stretch-dependent regulation of potassium flux in cardiac muscle, providing a mechano-electrical feedback system. The T-tubule is located at the Z-disc in cardiomyocytes, whereas it is located at the A–I junction in mammalian skeletal muscle. The different T-tubule localization between cardiac and skeletal muscle may indicate the importance of physical interactions between ion channels on the T-tubule and Z-disc proteins in cardiomyocytes.

MUSCLE LIM PROTEIN

MLP is a striated muscle-specific factor of the cysteine-rich protein (CRP) family that enhances myogenic differentiation and is critical for maintaining structural integrity. MLP protein is composed of two tandem LIM domains followed by a glycine-rich region. Each LIM domain contains double zinc finger-like structures that serve as a protein-binding interface. The first LIM domain seems to be important for binding to α-actinin *(14)*, the second LIM motif of MLP can associate with β-spectrin (Fig. 2B) *(17)*, and the short fragment (5 amino acids) at the amino terminus of MLP is critical for interactions with T-cap/telethonin *(14)*. In addition to Z-disc accumulation, MLPs are localized in the nucleus and regulate transcription as a cofactor of transcription factors, including myoD in the skeletal myocytes *(18,19)*.

Among 536 DCM patients, 10 patients show an autosomal dominant mutation at the amino terminus of MLP (Trp4Arg) that abolish the interaction with T-cap/telethonin (Fig. 2C) *(14)*. In normal neonatal cardiomyocytes, both mechanical stretch as well as the α-adrenergic agonist phenylephrine induce expression of the hypertropnic gene marker, brain natriuretic peptide (BNP). In MLP-null cardiomyocytes, phenylephrine induced BNP expression, whereas mechanical stretch failed to induce BNP expression, suggesting specific defects in mechanosensing pathways for BNP induction in MLP-null cardiomyocytes. DCM mutations in T-cap/telethonin and in MLP are found in the region critical for interaction of the two proteins, indicating that the T-cap/telethonin-MLP interaction is important for a mechanical stress sensor pathway *(14)*. Another mutation in MLP (Lys69Arg) adjacent to the first LIM domain was found in DCM patients *(20)*. This mutation abolished the interaction with α-actinin; however, three other MLP mutations identified in hypertrophic cardiomyopathy (HCM) patients were within the same LIM domain that is critical for binding to α-actinin *(21)*. Because MLP-knockout mice

---

Fig. 2. *(continued from opposite page)* filaments (desmin) are attached to the desmosomes, which will connect to sarcomere at the Z-disc. Another intermediate filament comprising inner nuclear membrane, nuclear lamins are also connecting to Z-disc through nesprin proteins. Nuclear membrane structure is composed of nuclear pore complex, outer nuclear membrane, and inner nuclear membrane, to which heterochromatin is attached. **(B)** Cell–substrate interactions are mediated by costameres at the sarcolemma overlying the Z-discs. At costameres, multiple unique protein complexes link among the extracellular matrix, sarcolemma, and intracellular cytoskeleton, including actin and intermediate filaments. Three major protein complexes at the costameres are known: integrin–talin–vinculin–α-actinin complex **(1–4)**, Na-channel–ankyrin–spectrin–α-MLP-actinin complex, and dystrophin–glycoproteins complexes. **(C)** Protein interactions among titin, T-cap/telethonin, MLP, α-actinin, and potassium channel (MinK) at Z-disc and T-tubule.

Table 1
Genes Causing Familial DCM

Group	Gene/protein	Chromosomal locus	OMIM no.	Inheritance pattern	Additional phenotype
Z-disc proteins	ZASP/cypher	10q22.3-q23.2	605906	AD	Isolated noncompaction of the left-ventricular myocardium
	α-actinin-2	1q42-q43	102573	AD	
	MLP	11p15.1	607482	AD	
	T-cap/telethonin	17q12	604488	AR	LGMD 2G
Costameres and adherens junction	Metavinculin/vinculin	10q22.1-q23	193065	AD	
Desmosome and intermediate filaments	α-actinin-2	1q42-q43	102573	AD	
Dystrophin–sarcoglycan	MLP	11p15.1	607482	AD	
	Desmoplakin	6p24	125647	AR	Woolly hair, keratoderma, ARVD/C
	Plakoglobin	17q21	601214	AR	Naxos disease, ARVD/C, woolly hair, keratoderma
	Desmin	2q35	125660	AD, AR, *de novo*	Desmin myopathy
	Lamin A/C	1q21.2	607920, 150330	AD	Conduction disease, skeletal myopathy
	Dystrophin	Xp21	300377, 302045	X	Skeletal myopathy
	δ-sarcoglycan	5q33	601411, 606685	AD	LGMD 2F
Sarcomeric proteins	Cardiac α-actin	15q14	102540	AD	
	Cardiac troponin T	1q32	601494, 191045	AD	
	β-myosin heavy chain	14q12	160760	AD	
	α-tropomyosin	15q2	191010	AD	
	Titin	2q31	18840	AD	Familial HCM; tibial muscular dystrophy
Sarcoplasmic reticulum protein	Phospholamban	6q22.1	172405	AD	
Ion channel	SUR2A	12p12.1	601439	AD	Ventricular tachycardia

DCM, dilated cardiomyopathy; OMIM, Online Mendelian Inheritance in Man; LGMD, limb-girdle muscular dystrophy; HCM, hypertrophic cardiomyopathy; MLP, major latex protein; ZASP, Z-band alternatively spliced PD2 motif.

show both hypertrophic and dilated cardiomyopathic features *(22)*, MLP mutations may cause both DCM and HCM at different stages.

Additional potential MLP functions can be observed by interacting with β-spectrin through the second LIM domain of MLP. β-spectrin is localized both at the sarcomere and costamere *(17)*. Costameres, submembranous transverse ribs found in many cardiac muscle cells, are thought to anchor the Z-discs of the peripheral myofibrils to the sarcolemma (Fig. 2B). It has been postulated that costameres provide mechanical linkage between the cells' internal contractile machinery and the extracellular matrix *(23)*.

α-ACTININ-2

α-actinin is an actin-binding protein with multiple roles in different cell types. In nonmuscle cells, the cytoskeletal isoforms (α-actinin-1 and -4) are found along microfilament bundles and adherens junctions, where actinin is involved in actin and membrane interactions. In contrast, skeletal, cardiac, and smooth muscle isoforms (α-actinin-2 and -3) are localized to the Z-disc, where they help anchor the myofibrillar actin filaments (Fig. 2A). In humans, α-actinin-2 is widely expressed in skeletal and cardiac myocytes, whereas α-actinin-3 is expressed only in skeletal muscle and is absent in 18% of normal human populations *(24)*.

One mutation identified in DCM patient substitutes glutamine 9 to arginine. Wild-type α-actinin-2 binds to MLP, whereas it was abolished in Gln9Arg mutants. This result suggests the importance of α-actinin-2 and MLP interaction in forming mechano-sensing complexes *(20)*.

ZASP/CYPHER

ZASP, or cypher, is a member of ALP-enigma family containing one amino terminal PDZ domain, and one or three carboxyl-terminal LIM domains. Most of the members including enigma, ENH, ALP, and Ril associate with the cytoskeleton, such as α-actinin and/or β-tropomyosin with their PDZ domain, and are localized at the Z-disc *(25,26)*. ZASP/cypher-null mice showed congenital myopathy resulting in a gasping respiratory pattern, limb weakness, and a limited range of motion, and the majority of mice die within 24 h *(27)*. Cardiac muscle ZASP/cypher-null mice display fragmented and disorganized Z-discs, suggesting that ZASP/cypher is essential to support Z-disc structure by linking with α-actinin.

ZASP/cypher mutations are found in human patients with DCM with or without isolated noncompaction of the left ventricular myocardium. Vatta et al. reported 6 ZASP/cypher mutations among 100 patients *(28)*, in which five are missense mutations within the linker between PDZ and LIM domain, likely to form different secondary structures. Indeed, C2C12 cells transfected with ZASP/cypher with one mutation, Asp117Asn, showed abnormal ZASP/cypher and actin staining. Arimura et al. reported 1 among 96 patients *(29)*. The mutation was in the third LIM domain, which increases the interaction with protein kinase C, suggesting the involvement of intracellular signaling in disease mechanisms.

Desmosome, Adherens Junction, Costamere, and Interemediate Filaments

In the heart, cell–cell and cell–substrate interactions are mediated by specific structures: desmosome, adherens junction, and costamere (Fig. 2A,B). These structures are important for holding cells together under the influences of the extracellular matrix and for their development, migration, proliferation, shape, and function. Desmosomal cell–cell junctions are found predominantly in the heart and skin. In the heart, desmosomes are localized at the intercalated disc. They link the intermediate-size filament networks (such as desmin in the heart) to the cell membrane to maintain tissue architecture and integrity. The desmosome consists of several proteins, which can be divided into two groups: the urea-insoluble "core" and the urea-soluble "plaque" components. The main proteins of the plaque comprise the desmoplakins and plakoglobins (γ-catenin) that are responsible for connecting the cytoskeleton to the transmembrane adhesion proteins, desmoglein and desmocolin which belong to the cadherin family and fractionate into the urea-insoluble "core" *(30)*.

Adherens junctions are localized at the intercalated disc and contain the "classical" cadherin cell adhesion molecules, N-cadherin, of which the extracellular domains mediate Ca^{2+}-dependent homophilic adhesion (Fig. 2A). Cytoplasmic domains of N-cadherin binds to β-catenin or plakoglobin (γ-catenin) and mediate the anchorage of the cadherin–β-catenin/plakoglobin complex to the actin cytoskeleton through α-actinin, either directly interacting with F-actin or indirectly through the actin-binding proteins vinculin, α-actinin, and ZO1 *(30)*.

Costameres are rib-like bands at the sarcolemma overlying the Z-discs (Fig. 2B). At costameres, multiple unique protein complexes link among the extracellular matrix, sarcolemma, and intracellular cytoskeleton, including actin and intermediate filaments. Three major protein complexes at the costameres are known: integrin–talin–vinculin–α-actinin complex, Na-channel–ankyrin–spectrin–MLP-α-actinin complex, and dystrophin–glycoproteins complexes *(31)*.

Intermediate filaments are tough and durable protein fibers found in the cytoplasm of most cells. They are called "intermediate" because in electron micrographs their apparent diameter (8–10 nm) is between that of the thin actin filaments and the thick myosin filaments of muscle cells, where they were first described (they are also intermediate in diameter between actin filaments and microtubules). In most animal cells, an extensive network of intermediate filaments connects among the nucleus, contractile proteins (by surrounding the Z-discs), sarcolemma (Fig. 2A), and extracellular matrix via costameres (Fig. 2B). They also have the potential to associate with other organelles including mitochondria, and the SR.

VINCULIN/METAVINCULIN

Vinculin and metavinculin are components of adherens junctions as well as costermeres (Fig. 2A,B). Vinculin and metavinculin contain binding domains for multiple cytoskeletal proteins, including actin, α-actinin, talin, paxillin, vasodilator-stimulated phosphoprotein, ponsin, vinexin, and protein kinase C. Their head and tail regions physically interact in a resting state to mask most binding sites. By exposure to phosphatidylinositol *(4,5)-bis*-phosphate (PIP2), the open "activated" conformation of vinculin exposes all binding sites *(32)*. The vinculin gene is located on chromosome 10q22.1-q23 and comprises 22 exons. Exon 19 is alternatively spliced in a tissue-specific manner, and the smaller isoform with a shorter tail, vinculin (116 kDa), is ubiquitously expressed, whereas metavinculin, the larger isoform with a longer tail containing an additional 68 amino acids, is expressed exclusively in cardiac and smooth muscle. In cardiac myocytes, vinculin and metavinculin are coexpressed at intercalated discs and costameres.

An absence of metavinculin transcripts and protein combined with normal vinculin expression was detected in one DCM patient *(33)*. Another study showed two mutations, a single missense mutation (Arg975Trp), and a 3-bp deletion (Leu954del), in the metavinculin-specific exon 19 among 350 DCM patients *(34)*. A Z-disc abnormality was detected in both cases, suggesting a metavinculin-specific role in maintaining Z-disc structure uncompensated by vinculin. The tail domains of vinculin and metavinculin both bind to F-actin. Vinculin forms large needle-like structures with actin, whereas metavinuclin form viscous webs with actin. Different actin organization may arise as a result of a longer tail domain of metavinculin, making it more flexible to bind at crossover points of actin filaments and preventing parallel arrangements seen in vinculin *(35)*.

DESMOPLAKIN, PLAKOGLOBIN (γ-CATENIN)

Desmoplakin and plakoglobin are components of desmosome (Fig. 2A). Recessive mutations in the desmoplakin gene cause a generalized striated keratoderma, particularly affecting the palmoplantar epidermis, resulting in woolly hair and leading to a dilated left ventricular cardiomyopathy that progresses to heart failure in the teenage years *(36)*. The mutation identified in three families produces a premature stop codon, leading to a truncated desmoplakin protein missing the carboxyl-terminal domain which is important for interacting with the intermediate filaments network. Homozygous desmoplakin-null mice die in early embryogenesis (E 6.5) *(37)*, whereas human recessive mutations (homozygous mutations) in the desmoplakin gene are not embryonically lethal, suggesting that the truncated desmoplakin molecule has some residual desmosomal function that is able to maintain the intermediate filament network without the desmoplakin tail domain unless it is stressed. However, in the restricted areas, such as the epidermal sites prone to pressure or in the continuously beating heart, the mutant desmoplakin may not be able to maintain tissue architecture.

In contrast, an autosomal dominant mutation at the aminoterminus domain of desmoplakin was found in arrhythmogenic right ventricular cardiomyopathy (ARVD/C), a progressive disease characterized by degeneration of the right ventricular myocardium, followed by fibrous-fatty replacement *(38)*. ARVD/C usually clinically presents with arrhythmias of right ventricular origin, ranging from isolated premature ventricular beats to sustained ventricular tachycardia or to ventricular fibrillation leading to sudden death. The aminoterminus region of desmoplakin is required for localization of desmoplakin to the desmosomal plaque by binding to desmoplakin itself, desmocolin, and plakoglobin. Plakoglobin gene is also mapped to the ARVD/C disease locus (Naxos disease). The involvement of two desmosomal proteins in ARVD/C suggests that some ARVD/C might result from defects in intercellular connections.

Plakoglobin (γ-catenin) is a component of desmosome, as well as the adherens junction (Fig. 2A) at which the cadherin–catenin complex anchors to actin filaments. Plakoglobin-null mice die around E12–16 due to defects in heart function often associated with ventricular rupture and blood floods in the pericardium *(39)*. Hearts from plakoglobin-null mice demonstrate no desmosome formation, instead extended adherens junctions develop, which contain desmosomal proteins such as desmoplakin. These results suggest that plakoglobin is not only essential for the formation of stable cardiac desmosomes, but is also critically involved in the segregation and/or sorting of the molecules into desmosome and adherens junction.

INTERMEDIATE FILAMENT

Intermediate filament, desmin *(40,41)*, and nuclear lamin A/C mutations (Fig. 2A) are also identified in DCM patients *(40,41)*.

DESMIN

Desmin is encoded by a single copy gene located in chromosome 2q35. A 53-kDa protein interacts with other intermediate filament proteins to form an intracytoplasmic network that maintains spatial relationships between the contractile apparatus and other structural elements of the cell. Twenty-one pathogenic mutations have been identified in desmin, and the current understanding of disease mechanisms is that mutant desmin proteins are unable to properly assemble into normal filaments. The desmin-null mice are viable and fertile. However, these mice demonstrated a multisystem disorder involving cardiac, skeletal, and smooth muscle. Histological and electron microscopic analyses in both heart and skeletal muscle revealed severe disruptions of muscle architecture and degeneration. Structural abnormalities included loss of lateral alignment of myofibrils and abnormal mitochondrial organization *(42)*.

LAMIN *A/C*

The nuclear envelope consisting of the inner membrane, outer membranes, and nuclear pore complexes organizes nuclear architecture and separates the chromosomes from the cytoplasm. The inner membrane is a network of an intermediate filament protein, lamins, that faces the chromosomes and anchors several membrane proteins such as the lamin B receptor, lamin-associated protein-1(LAP-1), and emerin (Fig. 2A). At least three lamin genes—*A, B1,* and *B2*—identified in humans are differentially expressed during development. B-type lamins are expressed widely, whereas lamin A protein is expressed primarily, but not exclusively, in differentiated nonproliferating cells. Lamins *A* and *C* are the alternatively spliced forms encoded by a single gene, and both contain the identical first 566 amino acids with 98 unique carboxyl-terminal amino acids for lamin A and 6 unique amino acids for lamin C *(43)*.

Fatkin et al. first reported five missense mutations among 11 families with autosomal dominant DCM with conduction defects *(44)*. Since then, up to 40 mutations have been reported *(45)*. Lamin *A/C* mutations are identified in several different inherited diseases, including cardiomyopathy with variable skeletal muscle dystrophy (dilated cardiomyo-pahty with conduction defects, autosomal dominant and recessive Emery–Dreifuss muscular dystrophy, limb-girdle dystrophy type 1B), peripheral neuropathy (Charcot–Marie–Tooth disorder type 2B1), and partial lipodystrophy syndromes *(46)*. Lamin A has two globular domains (N- and C-terminus) and a central α-helical region. The positions of mutation-causing DCM are scattered in lamin A protein and a broad spectrum in the severity of phenotypes within family members carrying the same mutation are observed *(47–49)*.

The disease mechanisms of lamin *A/C* mutations have been explained by two nonexclusive hypotheses: the "mechanical stress" hypothesis, and the "gene expression" hypothesis *(46)*. The mechanical stress hypothesis states that abnormalities in nuclear structure resulting from lamin mutations lead to increased susceptibility to cellular damage by physical stress, based on the abnormalities in nuclear morphology observed in both human patients and animal models. The gene expression hypothesis states that the nuclear envelope plays a role in tissue-specific gene expression that can be altered by mutations in lamins, primarily based on known interactions between the nuclear envelope and chromatin components.

Animal models of lamin *A/C* mutations have been examined in both lamin *A/C*-null mice and Leu 530 Pro knock-in mice, a mutation identical to that which causes autosomal dominant Emery–Dreifuss muscular dystrophy *(50,51)*. Heterozygous Leu 530 Pro knock-in mice do not show signs of muscular dystrophy; however, homozygous Leu 530 Pro mice show growth retardation and death by 4 wk, with premature aging. Mutant hearts are smaller with decreased number of cardiomyocytes, suggesting either incomplete heart development or loss of muscle mass. Lamin *A/C*-null mice also show growth retardation and muscular dystrophy, and die by 8 wk.

Recently, a connection between lamin A and the cytoskeleton has been reported through a newly identified protein, nesprin-1 and -2 (Syne-1/myne-1, Syne-2), nesprin is a large protein containing actin-binding calponin homology at its amino-terminus and many spectrin repeats at the central region. Specific antibodies against the amino-terminus region (residue 5470–5485) revealed a predominantly cytoplasmic distribution with localization to the Z-discs, whereas the antibody against the carboxyl-terminus region (residue 8689–8704) revealed a strong localization at the nuclear envelope in association with lamin A and emerin *(52)*. Mutations in the *Caenorhabditis elegans* homolog of nesprin, ANC-1 resulted in freely floating nuclei within the cytoplasm and nuclei formed clusters in the hypodermal cells that contain more than 100 nuclei, which are normally uniformly spaced. This study suggests an important role of nesprin in the process of nuclear positioning in the cytoskelton *(46,53–55)*.

DYSTROPHIN–SARCOGLYCAN COMPLEX

Dystrophin is a large, rod-shaped protein with a molecular weight of 427 kDa that comprises four domains. The amino-terminal domain has homology with α-actinin, and contains between 232 and 240 amino acid residues depending on the isoform. The central rod domain is a succession of 25 triple-helical repeats similar to spectrin, and contains about 3000 residues and a cysteine-rich domain of 280 residues which bind to β-dystroglycan. The last carboxyl-terminal domain comprises 420 residues, which bind to syntrophin and α-dystrobrevin. The protein is associated with the plasma membrane of cardiac and skeletal muscle (sarcolemma), and its main role at the sarcolemma is to interact with integral membrane proteins (sarcoglycans, dystroglycans, syntrophins, and dystrobrevin complexes) that are assembled in the dystrophin–glycoprotein complex (Fig. 2B) *(56)*. This complex forms a bridge across the sarcolemma and flexibly connects the basal lamina to the extracellular matrix to the inner cytoskeleton, F-actin. The main roles of the dystrophin–glycoprotein complex are to stabilize the sarcolemma and to protect muscle fibers from long-term, contraction-induced damage and necrosis, and to have a role in cellular communication by acting as a transmembrane signaling complex *(57)*.

Mutations in the dystrophin gene cause Duchenne and Becker muscular dystrophies. Although cardiac involvement is invariably associated with Duchenne and Becker muscular dystrophies, rare mutations cause an almost exclusive cardiac involvement. According to Ferlini et al., the pathogenesis underlying the selective cardiac muscle impairment in the X-linked dilated cardiomyopathy families is not clear, although two main regions of the dystrophin gene appeared to be most commonly involved in X-linked dilated cardiomyopathy: the 5' end of the gene and the central hot-spot region, centered around exon 48–49 among a total of 79 exons *(58)*. Mutations in the 5' end of the dystrophin gene likely affect splicing, leading to cardiac-specific transcriptional regulation of the dystrophin gene. On the other hand, mutations surrounding exons 48–49, including intron 48, may contain sequences very relevant for dystrohpin function or expression mainly in the heart.

The sarcoglycan complex is a group of single-pass transmembrane proteins (α-, β-, γ-, and δ-sarcoglycan) expressed in skeletal and cardiac muscle. The sarcoglycans are typically found in a heterodimeric complex including at least four different sarcoglycans. Although the exact function of the sarcoglycan complex is not known, it is well established that mutations in any of α-, β-, γ-, and δ-sarcoglycan genes result in distinct forms of muscular dystrophy *(59)*.

δ-sarcoglycan mutations cause autosomal recessive limb-girdle type muscular dystrophy *(60)*. In contrast, autosomal dominant single missense mutations in δ-sarcoglycan were reported in familial DCM without skeletal muscle abnormalities *(61,62)*. Involvement of δ-sarcoglycan in cardiomyopathy has been studied for several decades in the BIO14.6 Syrian cardiomyopathic hamsters, which have an approx 30-kb deletion in the regulatory region of the δ-sarcoglycan gene leading to loss of δ-sarcoglycan expression in cardiac and skeletal muscle *(63,64)*. The BIO14.6 hamster carries a recessive mutation that leads to a degenerative disease of both heart and skeletal muscle. Although there are several sublineages of cardiomyopathic hamsters bred to have either dilated or hypertrophic cardiomyopathy, the pathogenetic mutation in δ-sarcoglycan gene is identical. Hypertrophy in HCM hamsters is considered a compensatory reaction, and DCM hamsters might have another generic defect in this hypertrophic compensatory mechanism *(63)*.

Recently, vascular spasm, especially in the coronary artery, resulting in focal cardiac ischemia has been reported in both hamsters and γ- and δ-sarcoglycan knock-out mice *(65,66)*. Transgenic expression of γ- or δ-sarcoglycan using the α-myosin heavy chain promoter, restoring cardiomyocyte expression of these proteins, rescued vascular spasm in γ- or δ-sarcoglycan knockout mice, whereas SM-22-driven transgenic protein in vascular smooth muscle cells did not rescue vascular spasm. These observations suggest that cytokine release (presumably from vascular smooth muscle cells) accompanied by cardiomyocyte degeneration from lack of γ- or δ-sarcoglycan can produce vascular spasm, which can lead to further cardiomyocyte damage resulting from focal cardiac ischemia.

Sarcomeric Proteins/α-Tropomyosin, β-Myosin Heavy Chain, Cardiac Troponin T, Cardiac α-Actin

Another group of DCM-responsive genes are sarcomeric proteins, including α-tropomyosin, β-myosin heavy chain, cardiac troponin T, and cardiac α-actin, which are all well-established causes of HCM rather than DCM. Many detailed reviews are available in HCM *(6,67–69)*, therefore only the underlying pathological differences between HCM and DCM will be discussed here.

HCM mutations in sarcomere proteins were identified as early as 1990 *(70)*. In addition, approx 60% of HCM populations are associated with mutations in sarcomeric proteins. Therefore, genotype–phenotype relations, as well as pathophysiology, are better understood in HCM than DCM. The pathogenesis of HCM has been explained by incorporation of mutant sarcomeric proteins, resulting in contractile dysfunction and subsequent activation of neuroendocrine and mechanical responses leading to compensatory hypertrophy. However, recent studies demonstrate that mutant sarcomeric proteins have enhanced motor activity with inefficient sarcomeric adenosine triphosphate (ATP) utilization, leading to a new energy-depletion hypothesis *(69,71)*. Several animal models of reduced myocardial energy production reveal HCM phenotypes, including mitochondrial tRNA mutations, fatty acid uptake defects in CD36 deficiency, mitochondrial fatty acid oxidation defects in acyl-CoA dehydrogenase deficiency, adenine nucleotide translocator-1 knockout, which disrupts ATP export from mitochondria, as well as knockout of AMP-activated protein kinase (AMPK), which is both a sensor and critical orchestrator of cellular energy homeostasis.

In contrast, mutations found in sarcomere proteins in DCM in many respects oppose the data presented for HCM. For example, Arg92Gln troponin T mutation found in HCM patients shows increased Ca^{2+} sensitivity, ATPase activity, and thin-filament sliding velocity. In contrast, 3 nucleotides-deletion leading to a single amino acid deletion in Lys210 (Δ210) of troponin T mutation found in DCM patients is in the region responsible for Ca^{2+}-sensitive troponin C binding *(72)*. This mutation is expected to reduce Ca^{2+}-stimulated actomyosin ATPase activity leading to reduced contractility, which was proven at least in vitro *(73)*.

Four β-myosin heavy chain gene mutations were identified in DCM patients— Ala223Thr, Ser532Pro, Ser642Leu, or Phe764Leu amino acid substitutions—and none of them were found in HCM patients *(72,74)*. Myosin–actin interactions for sliding movement occur with the head portion of myosin protein. Ser532 and Ser642, located in the head portion of myosin protein, contribute to the tight binding of actin; therefore, Ser532Pro and Ser642Leu mutations are expected to disrupt interactions between myosin and actin that are critical for initiating the power stroke of contraction. Phe764 locates in the hinge between the myosin head and rod part, suggesting its role for determining the magnitude or polarity of the head movement, and Phe764Leu mutation is suspected to reduce the efficiency of contraction. Ala223Thr mutation, locating close to the ATP-binding site, may decrease thermostability or affect the protein folding to change protein motility *(74)*.

HCM mutation in the actin gene is involved in the direct actin–myosin interface, whereas in DCM, a Glu361Gly mutation in the actin gene is located at the actinin-binding domain important for force transmission to adjacent sarcomeres and neighboring myocytes *(75)*.

Tropomyosin is one of five proteins comprising thin filaments of sarcomeres. Thin filaments play a dual role in force dynamics by regulating contractile force generation through thick filament (myosin) interactions and transmitting force through filament ends anchored to Z-bands and intercalated discs. Two missense mutations in the *α-tropomyosin* gene, *Glu40Lys* and *Glu54Lys*, were reported as DCM-causative mutations that are different from HCM tropomyosin mutations (Ala63Val, Lys70Thr, Asp175Asn, Glu180Gly) *(76)*. Because the surface of tropomyosin is dominated by negative charge, altered electrical charge resulting from a glutamate-to-lysine mutation observed in DCM patients may change electrostatic interactions between actin and tropomyosin filaments *(76)*.

Sarcoplasmic Reticulum Proteins

Phospholamban

Phospholamban, a small, 6-kDa pentameric protein, comprises polypeptide subunits 52 amino acids in length. The nonphoshorylated form of phospholamban is an inhibitor of sarcoendoplasmic reticulum calcium pump (SERCA) 2a, but inhibition is relieved upon phosphorylation of phospholamban by β-adrenergic stimuli through cAMP-dependent protein kinase and Ca^{2+}-dependent calmodulin kinase. The subsequent activation of SERCA leads to enhanced muscle relaxation rates and an increased cardiac contraction rate and force by releasing Ca^{2+} from SR through the ryanodine receptor.

Two different types of phospholamban mutations were identified in DCM patients. Schmitt et al. reported an autosomal dominant DCM with C25T point mutation (causing Arg9Cys substitution). Arg9Cys mutant phospholamban appears to sequester protein kinase A from wild-type phospholamban, leading to increased levels of unphosphorylated forms of phospholamban *(77)*. Haghighi et al. reported T116G point mutation (causing early termination Leu39-stop) in two independent families. Patients with heterozygous mutation of Leu39-stop exhibited hypertrophy without diminished contractile performance, whereas patients with homozygous mutations developed dilated cardiomyopathy and heart failure *(78)*.

Accordingly, two mutations will cause opposite effects: an Arg9Cys mutation will increase the level of dephosphorylated phospholamban, therefore SERCA 2a function should be inhibited; whereas a Leu39-stop mutation will cause a loss of phospholamban, therefore SERCA 2a function should be disinhibited (that is, activated). The consequent phenotype was not explained clearly, but these studies suggest the importance of balanced SERCA 2a activity that is both inhibited as well as augmented by phospholamban activity for normal heart function. Of note, phospholamban-null mice with increased SERCA 2a activity display chronically increased basal cardiac contractile function without developing heart failure even with advanced age, which is radically different from the DCM phenotype in human patients *(79)*.

Ion Channel

A recent study demonstrated a new DCM-causing mutant protein of sulfornylurea receptor-2 ([SUR2A]; sulfonylureas are widely used as oral hypoglycemic reagents in the treatment of noninsulin-dependent diabetes mellitus), a catalytic subunit of K_{ATP} ion channel protein *(80)*. Cardiac K_{ATP} channels are composed of Kir6.2 and a regulatory subunit, SUR2A. One frameshift and one missense mutation were identified at the carboxyl-terminus of SUR2A, and are predicted to distort ATP-dependent channel pore regulation. Kir6.2-null mice developed arrhythmia and sudden death following sympathetic stimulation, which was preventable with calcium-channel blockers. The aderenergic stimuli enhance cardiac performance by increased Ca^{2+} handling, both inward and outward flow, which appears defective in K_{ATP}-null hearts *(81)*.

Frequency of the Genetic Mutations in Familial and Sporadic DCM

Although the prevalence of mutations in DCM described previously will be influenced by the patient population, several studies show that the causes of DCM are heterogenetic. Defects in δ-sarcoglycan were found in two among 50 young DCM patients (aged 3 d–18 yr) *(61)*, and two among 52 DCM patients (mean aged 50, age 11–71 yr) in Finnish patients. In the later study, the desmin gene and the metavinculin-specific exon of the vinculin gene were also examined in the same group, but no mutations were identified in these two genes *(62)*. Also, the same author reported that no actin gene mutations were detected in 32 DCM patients *(82)*. Apparently, only some of the known genes were screened in these studies, making it difficult to estimate the contribution of the known gene in DCM patients without screening all of the genes.

A recent study by Mohapatra et al. examined a total of 291 individuals with DCM, including 110 probands for the mutations in a total of 9 genes including cardiac actin, desmin, δ-sarcoglycan, lamin A/C, troponin T, metavinculin, α-dystrobrevin *(83)*, MLP, and α-actinin-2 *(20)*. The contribution of these nine known genes in DCM patients seems relatively small; MLP mutations were found in two families, and α-actinin mutations were found in one family.

OVERVIEW

According to the list of DCM-related genes, three major categories of genes are dominant in the disease mechanism: Z-disc proteins, cell–cell or cell–substrate complex and associated intracellular cytoskeltons, and sarcomere components. These proteins, when mutated, are likely to disrupt force-transmission within a single cardiomyocyte as well as in neighboring cardiomyocytes. However, two newly identified genes, phospholamban and SUR2, a subunit of K_{ATP} channel, do not fit into this hypothesis. It is highly likely that more genes will be identified as causative factors in DCM after detailed genetic screening. Combination with systemic screening of the known gene mutations in familial DCM patients and their disease phenotype will lead to a better understand of pathogenesis and prevalence of the monogenic causes of DCM.

ACKNOWLEDGMENT

I thank E. O. Weinberg and N. Sato for critical reading of the manuscript and valuable suggestions. Apologies to many researchers for omitting their important contributions to this research field in order to keep this review brief.

REFERENCES

1. Braunwald E, Zipes DP, Libby P, eds. Heart disease: a textbook of cardiovascular medicine. 6th ed. W.B. Saunders, Philadelphia: 2001.
2. Cohn JN, Bristow MR, Chien KR, et al. Report of the National Heart, Lung, and Blood Institute Special Emphasis Panel on Heart Failure Research. Circulation 1997;95:766–770.
3. Chien KR. Stress pathways and heart failure. Cell 1999;98:555–558.
4. Hein S, Kostin S, Heling A, Maeno Y, Schaper J. The role of the cytoskeleton in heart failure. Cardiovasc Res 2000;45:273–278.
5. Schonberger J, Seidman CE. Many roads lead to a broken heart: the genetics of dilated cardiomyopathy. Am J Hum Genet 2001;69:249–260.
6. Towbin JA, Bowles NE. The failing heart. Nature 2002;415:227–233.
7. Tskhovrebova L, Trinick J. Titin: properties and family relationships. Nat Rev Mol Cell Biol 2003;4:679–689.
8. Granzier HL, Labeit S. The giant protein titin: a major player in myocardial mechanics, signaling, and disease. Circ Res 2004;94:284–295.
9. Pyle WG, Solaro RJ. At the crossroads of myocardial signaling: the role of Z-discs in intracellular signaling and cardiac function. Circ Res 2004;94:296–305.
10. Bang ML, Centner T, Fornoff F, et al. The complete gene sequence of titin, expression of an unusual approximately 700-kDa titin isoform, and its interaction with obscurin identify a novel Z-line to I-band linking system. Circ Res 2001;89:1065–1072.
11. Gerull B, Gramlich M, Atherton J, et al. Mutations of TTN, encoding the giant muscle filament titin, cause familial dilated cardiomyopathy. Nat Genet 2002;30:201–24.
12. Valle G, Faulkner G, De Antoni A, et al. Telethonin, a novel sarcomeric protein of heart and skeletal muscle. FEBS Lett 1997;415:163–168.
13. Gregorio CC, Trombitas K, Centner T, et al. The NH2 terminus of titin spans the Z-disc: its interaction with a novel 19-kD ligand (T-cap) is required for sarcomeric integrity. J Cell Biol 1998;143:1013–1027.
14. Knoll R, Hoshijima M, Hoffman HM, et al. The cardiac mechanical stretch sensor machinery involves a Z disc complex that is defective in a subset of human dilated cardiomyopathy. Cell 2002;111:943–955.
15. Moreira ES, Wiltshire TJ, Faulkner G, et al. Limb-girdle muscular dystrophy type 2G is caused by mutations in the gene encoding the sarcomeric protein telethonin. Nat Genet 2000;24:163–166.
16. Furukawa T, Ono Y, Tsuchiya H, et al. Specific interaction of the potassium channel beta-subunit minK with the sarcomeric protein T-cap suggests a T-tubule-myofibril linking system. J Mol Biol 2001;313:775–784.

17. Flick MJ, Konieczny SF. The muscle regulatory and structural protein MLP is a cytoskeletal binding partner of betaI-spectrin. J Cell Sci 2000;113(Pt 9):1553–164.

18. Kong Y, Flick MJ, Kudla AJ, Konieczny SF. Muscle LIM proteins promotes myogenesis by enhancing the activity of MyoD. Mol Cell Biol 1997;17:4750–4760.

19. Weiskirchen R, Gunther K. The CRP/MLP/TLP family of LIM domain proteins: acting by connecting. Bioessays 2003; 25:152–162.

20. Mohapatra B, Jimenez S, Lin JH, et al. Mutations in the muscle LIM protein and alpha-actinin-2 genes in dilated cardiomyopathy and endocardial fibroelastosis. Mol Genet Metab 2003;80:207–215.

21. Geier C, Perrot A, Ozcelik C, et al. Mutations in the human muscle LIM protein gene in families with hypertrophic cardiomyopathy. Circulation 2003;107:1390–1395.

22. Arber S, Hunter JJ, Ross J, Jr., et al. MLP-deficient mice exhibit a disruption of cardiac cytoarchitectural organization, dilated cardiomyopathy, and heart failure. Cell 1997;88:393–403.

23. Danowski BA, Imanaka-Yoshida K, Sanger JM, Sanger JW. Costameres are sites of force transmission to the substratum in adult rat cardiomyocytes. J Cell Biol 1992;118:1411–1420.

24. Mills M, Yang N, Weinberger R, et al. Differential expression of the actin-binding proteins, alpha-actinin-2 and -3, in different species: implications for the evolution of functional redundancy. Hum Mol Genet 2001;10:1335–1346.

25. Faulkner G, Pallavicini A, Formentin E, et al. ZASP: a new Z-band alternatively spliced PDZ-motif protein. J Cell Biol 1999;146:465475.

26. Zhou Q, Ruiz-Lozano P, Martone ME, Chen J. Cypher, a striated muscle-restricted PDZ and LIM domain-containing protein, binds to alpha-actinin-2 and protein kinase C. J Biol Chem 1999;274:19,807–19,813.

27. Zhou Q, Chu PH, Huang C, et al. Ablation of cypher, a PDZ-LIM domain Z-line protein, causes a severe form of congenital myopathy. J Cell Biol 2001;155:605–612.

28. Vatta M, Mohapatra B, Jimenez S, et al. Mutations in Cypher/ZASP in patients with dilated cardiomyopathy and left ventricular non-compaction. J Am Coll Cardiol 2003;42:2014–2027.

29. Arimura T, Hayashi T, Terada H, et al. A Cypher/ZASP mutation associated with dilated cardiomyopathy alters the binding affinity to protein kinase C. J Biol Chem 2004;279:6746–6752.

30. Alberts B, Johnson A, Lewis J, Raff M, Roberts K, Walter P. Molecular biology of the cell, 4th ed. Garland Publishing, New York, NY:2002.

31. Clark KA, McElhinny AS, Beckerle MC, Gregorio CC. Striated muscle cytoarchitecture: an intricate web of form and function. Ann Rev Cell Dev Biol 2002;18:637–706.

32. Bailly M. Connecting cell adhesion to the actin polymerization machinery: vinculin as the missing link? Trends Cell Biol 2003;13:163–165.

33. Maeda M, Holder E, Lowes B, Valent S, Bies RD. Dilated cardiomyopathy associated with deficiency of the cytoskeletal protein metavinculin. Circulation 1997;95:17–20.

34. Olson TM, Illenberger S, Kishimoto NY, Huttelmaier S, Keating MT, Jockusch BM. Metavinculin mutations alter actin interaction in dilated cardiomyopathy. Circulation 2002;105:431–437.

35. Rudiger M, Korneeva N, Schwienbacher C, Weiss EE, Jockusch BM. Differential actin organization by vinculin isoforms: implications for cell type-specific microfilament anchorage. FEBS Lett 1998;431:49–54.

36. Norgett EE, Hatsell SJ, Carvajal-Huerta L, et al. Recessive mutation in desmoplakin disrupts desmoplakin-intermediate filament interactions and causes dilated cardiomyopathy, woolly hair and keratoderma. Hum Mol Genet 2000;9:2761–2766.

37. Gallicano GI, Kouklis P, Bauer C, et al. Desmoplakin is required early in development for assembly of desmosomes and cytoskeletal linkage. J Cell Biol 1998;143:2009–2022.

38. Rampazzo A, Nava A, Malacrida S, et al. Mutation in human desmoplakin domain binding to plakoglobin causes a dominant form of arrhythmogenic right ventricular cardiomyopathy. Am J Hum Genet 2002;71:1200–1206.

39. Ruiz P, Brinkmann V, Ledermann B, et al. Targeted mutation of plakoglobin in mice reveals essential functions of desmosomes in the embryonic heart. J Cell Biol 1996;135:215–225.

40. Goldfarb LG, Vicart P, Goebel HH, Dalakas MC. Desmin myopathy. Brain 2004;127:723–734.

41. Goldfarb LG, Park KY, Cervenakova L, et al. Missense mutations in desmin associated with familial cardiac and skeletal myopathy. Nat Genet 1998;19:402–403.

42. Milner DJ, Weitzer G, Tran D, Bradley A, Capetanaki Y. Disruption of muscle architecture and myocardial degeneration in mice lacking desmin. J Cell Biol 1996;134:1255–1270.

43. Wilson KL. The nuclear envelope, muscular dystrophy and gene expression. Trends Cell Biol 2000;10:125–129.

44. Fatkin D, MacRae C, Sasaki T, et al. Missense mutations in the rod domain of the lamin A/C gene as causes of dilated cardiomyopathy and conduction-system disease. N Engl J Med 1999;341:1715–1724.
45. Taylor MR, Fain PR, Sinagra G, et al. Natural history of dilated cardiomyopathy due to lamin A/C gene mutations. J Am Coll Cardiol 2003;41:771–780.
46. Worman HJ, Courvalin JC. How do mutations in lamins A and C cause disease? J Clin Invest 2004;113:349–351.
47. Mounkes LC, Burke B, Stewart CL. The A-type lamins: nuclear structural proteins as a focus for muscular dystrophy and cardiovascular diseases. Trends Cardiovasc Med 2001;11:280–285.
48. Mounkes L, Kozlov S, Burke B, Stewart CL. The laminopathies: nuclear structure meets disease. Curr Opin Genet Dev 2003;13:223–230.
49. Brodsky GL, Muntoni F, Miocic S, Sinagra G, Sewry C, Mestroni L. Lamin A/C gene mutation associated with dilated cardiomyopathy with variable skeletal muscle involvement. Circulation 2000;101:473-6.
50. Sullivan T, Escalante-Alcalde D, Bhatt H, et al. Loss of A-type lamin expression compromises nuclear envelope integrity leading to muscular dystrophy. J Cell Biol 1999;147:913–920.
51. Mounkes LC, Kozlov S, Hernandez L, Sullivan T, Stewart CL. A progeroid syndrome in mice is caused by defects in A-type lamins. Nature 2003;423:298–301.
52. Zhang Q, Ragnauth C, Greener MJ, Shananan CM, Roberts RG. The nesperins are giant actin-binding protein, orthologous to *Drosophilia* melanogaster muscle protein MSP-300. Genomics 2002;80:473–481.
53. Starr DA, Han M. Role of ANC-1 in tethering nuclei to the actin cytoskeleton. Science 2002; 298:406–409.
54. Hedgecock EM, Thomson JN. A gene required for nuclear and mitochondrial attachment in the nematode *Caenorhabditis elegans*. Cell 1982;30:321–330.
55. Starr DA, Han M. ANCnors away: an actin-based mechanism of nuclear positioning. J Cell Sci 2003;116:211–216.
56. Yoshida M, Hama H, Khikawa-Sakurai M, et al. Biochemical evidence for association of dystrobrevin with the sarcoglycan–sarcospan complex as a basis for understanding sarcoglycanopathy. Hum Mol Genet 2000;9:1033–1040.
57. Muntoni F, Torelli S, Ferlini A. Dystrophin and mutations: one gene, several proteins, multiple phenotypes. Lancet Neurol 2003;2:731–740.
58. Ferlini A, Sewry C, Melis MA, Mateddu A, Muntoni F. X-linked dilated cardiomyopathy and the dystrophin gene. Neuromuscul Disord 1999;9:339–346.
59. Durbeej M, Campbell KP. Muscular dystrophies involving the dystrophin-glycoprotein complex: an overview of current mouse models. Curr Opin Genet Dev 2002;12:349–361.
60. Nigro V, de Sa Moreira E, Piluso G, et al. Autosomal recessive limb-girdle muscular dystrophy, LGMD2F, is caused by a mutation in the delta-sarcoglycan gene. Nat Genet 1996;14:195–198.
61. Tsubata S, Bowles KR, Vatta M, et al. Mutations in the human delta-sarcoglycan gene in familial and sporadic dilated cardiomyopathy. J Clin Invest 2000;106:655–662.
62. Karkkainen S, Miettinen R, Tuomainen P, et al. A novel mutation, Arg71Thr, in the delta-sarcoglycan gene is associated with dilated cardiomyopathy. J Mol Med 2003;81:795–800.
63. Sakamoto A, Ono K, Abe M, et al. Both hypertrophic and dilated cardiomyopathies are caused by mutation of the same gene, delta-sarcoglycan, in hamster: an animal model of disrupted dystrophin-associated glycoprotein complex. Proc Natl Acad Sci USA 1997;94:13,873–13,878.
64. Sakamoto A, Abe M, Masaki T. Delineation of genomic deletion in cardiomyopathic hamster. FEBS Lett 1999;447:124–128.
65. Shimizu T, Okamoto H, Watanabe M, et al. Altered microvasculature is involved in remodeling processes in cardiomyopathic hamsters. Jpn Heart J 2003;44:111–126.
66. Wheeler MT, Allikian MJ, Heydemann A, Hadhazy M, Zarnegar S, McNally EM. Smooth muscle cell-extrinsic vascular spasm arises from cardiomyocyte degeneration in sarcoglycan-deficient cardiomyopathy. J Clin Invest 2004;113:668–675.
67. Seidman JG, Seidman C. The genetic basis for cardiomyopathy: from mutation identification to mechanistic paradigms. Cell 2001;104:557–567.
68. Arad M, Seidman JG, Seidman CE. Phenotypic diversity in hypertrophic cardiomyopathy. Hum Mol Genet 2002;11:2499–2506.
69. Ashrafian H, Redwood C, Blair E, Watkins H. Hypertrophic cardiomyopathy: a paradigm for myocardial energy depletion. Trends Genet 2003;19:263–268.
70. Geisterfer-Lowrance AA, Kass S, Tanigawa G, et al. A molecular basis for familial hypertrophic cardiomyopathy: a beta cardiac myosin heavy chain gene missense mutation. Cell 1990;62:999–1006.
71. Schwartz K, Mercadier JJ. Cardiac troponin T and familial hypertrophic cardiomyopathy: an energetic affair. J Clin Invest 2003;112:652–654.

72. Kamisago M, Sharma SD, DePalma SR, et al. Mutations in sarcomere protein genes as a cause of dilated cardiomyopathy. N Engl J Med 2000;343:1688–1696.

73. Robinson P, Mirza M, Knott A, et al. Alterations in thin filament regulation induced by a human cardiac troponin T mutant that causes dilated cardiomyopathy are distinct from those induced by troponin T mutants that cause hypertrophic cardiomyopathy. J Biol Chem 2002;277:40,710–40,716.

74. Daehmlow S, Erdmann J, Knueppel T, et al. Novel mutations in sarcomeric protein genes in dilated cardiomyopathy. Biochem Biophys Res Commun 2002;298:116–120.

75. Olson TM, Michels VV, Thibodeau SN, Tai YS, Keating MT. Actin mutations in dilated cardiomyopathy, a heritable form of heart failure. Science 1998;280:750–752.

76. Olson TM, Kishimoto NY, Whitby FG, Michels VV. Mutations that alter the surface charge of alpha-tropomyosin are associated with dilated cardiomyopathy. J Mol Cell Cardiol 2001;33:723–732.

77. Schmitt JP, Kamisago M, Asahi M, et al. Dilated cardiomyopathy and heart failure caused by a mutation in phospholamban. Science 2003;299:1410–1413.

78. Haghighi K, Kolokathis F, Pater L, et al. Human phospholamban null results in lethal dilated cardiomyopathy revealing a critical difference between mouse and human. J Clin Invest 2003;111:869–876.

79. Slack JP, Grupp IL, Dash R, et al. The enhanced contractility of the phospholamban-deficient mouse heart persists with aging. J Mol Cell Cardiol 2001;33:1031–1040.

80. Bienengraeber M, Olson TM, Selivanov VA, et al. ABCC9 mutations identified in human dilated cardiomyopathy disrupt catalytic K(ATP) channel gating. Nat Genet 2004;36:382–387.

81. Zingman LV, Hodgson DM, Bast PH, et al. Kir6.2 is required for adaptation to stress. Proc Natl Acad Sci USA 2002;99:13,278–13,283.

82. Karkkainen S, Peuhkurinen K, Jaaskelainen P, et al. No variants in the cardiac actin gene in Finnish patients with dilated or hypertrophic cardiomyopathy. Am Heart J 2002;143:E6.

83. Ichida F, Tsubata S, Bowles KR, et al. Novel gene mutations in patients with left ventricular noncompaction or Barth syndrome. Circulation 2001;103:1256–1263.

II GENE TRANSFER FOR COMBATING CARDIOVASCULAR DISEASE

8   Gene Therapy vs Pharmacotherapy

Ryuichi Morishita, MD, PhD

CONTENTS

SUMMARY

Recent progress in molecular and cellular biology has developed numerous effective cardiovascular drugs. However, there are still number of diseases for which no known effective therapy exists, such as peripheral arterial disease, ischemic heart disease, restenosis after angioplasty, vascular bypass graft occlusion, and transplant coronary vasculopathy. Currently, gene therapy is emerging as a potential strategy for the treatment of cardiovascular disease to treat such diseases despite this limitation. The first human trial in cardiovascular disease started in 1994 to treat peripheral vascular disease, using vascular endothelial growth factor (VEGF). Since then, many different potent angiogenic growth factors have been clinically tested to treat peripheral arterial disease. In addition, therapeutic angiogenesis using *VEGF* gene was applied to treat ischemic heart disease from 1997. The results from these clinical trials appear to exceed expectations. Improvement of clinical symptoms in peripheral arterial disease and ischemic heart disease has been reported. Many different potent angiogenic growth factors have been tested in clinical trials to treat peripheral arterial disease or ischemic heart disease. In addition, another strategy for combating disease processes, to target to transcriptional process, has been tested in a human trial. Transfection of *cis*-element double-stranded (ds) oligodeoxynucleotides (ODN) (decoy) is an especially powerful tool in a new class of antigene strategies for gene therapy. Transfection of ds ODN, corresponding to the *cis* sequence, will result in the attenuation of authentic *cis*-trans interaction, leading to the removal of transfactors from the endogenous *cis*-elements with subsequent modulation of gene expression. Genetically modified vein grafts transfected with decoy against E2F, an essential transcription factor in cell cycle progression, revealed apparent long-term potency

From: *Contemporary Cardiology: Cardiovascular Genomics*
Edited by: M. K. Raizada, et al. © Humana Press Inc., Totowa, NJ

in human patients. This review focuses on the future potential of gene therapy for the treatment of cardiovascular disease.

Key Words: *cis*-element decoy; antisense; angiogenesis; VEGF; HGF.

INTRODUCTION

Somatic gene therapy consists of the introduction of normal genes into the somatic cells of patients to correct an inherited or acquired disorder through the synthesis of specific gene products in vivo. In general, there are three methods of gene modification: (1) gene replacement, (2) gene correction, and (3) gene augmentation. Gene augmentation is the most promising technique for the modification of targeted cells in therapy for cardiovascular disease. For this purpose, many in vivo gene transfer methods have been developed. In vivo gene transfer techniques for cardiovascular applications include: (1) viral gene transfer—retrovirus, adenovirus, adeno-associated virus (AAV) or hemagglutinating virus of Japan (HVJ, or Sendai virus); (2) liposomal gene transfer using cationic liposomes; and (3) naked plasmid DNA transfer. These in vivo gene transfer techniques have different advantages and disadvantages. Although current in vivo methods for cardiovascular gene transfer are still limited by the lack of efficiency and potential toxicity, recent advances in in vivo gene transfer may provide the opportunity to treat cardiovascular diseases, such as peripheral arterial disease by manipulating angiogenic growth factor genes.

Simple comparison of gene therapy vs pharmacotherapy may not be appropriated. The present promising gene therapy is mainly by locally administrated agents, whereas most of pharmacotherapy is based on oral drug administration. To consider the advantage of gene therapy, one might compare it with recombinant therapy, because both concepts are relatively close. There are at least three advantages of gene therapy. First, it has the potential to maintain an optimally high and local concentration over time. This issue may be critical in the case of arterial gene therapy. In order to avoid side effects in the case of therapeutic angiogenesis, however, it may be preferable to deliver a lower dose over a period of several days or more from an actively expressed transgene in the iliac artery, rather than a single or multiple bolus doses of recombinant protein. Indeed, our initial trial using HGF did not demonstrate the increase in serum hepatocyte growth factor (HGF) level. Second, regarding economics, one must consider which therapy would ultimately cost more to develop, implement, and reimburse, particularly for those indications requiring multiple or even protracted treatment. Third, the feasibility of a clinical trial of recombinant protein is currently limited by the lack of approved or available quantities of human-quality recombinant protein. This may be due, in large part, to the nearly prohibitive cost of scaling up from research grade to human quality recombinant protein. Indeed, the report that compared the effectiveness of fibroblast growth factor-2 (FGF-2) as protein and as naked plasmid DNA, in a porcine model of chronic myocardial ischemia, demonstrated that intramyocardial injection of FGF-2 plasmid was more effective than that of FGF-2 protein in improving regional perfusion and contractility compared to untreated ischemia *(1)*. In contrast, gene therapy also has disadvantages, such as safety aspects, and local and limited effects.

GENE THERAPY FOR VASCULAR DISEASES

Gene Therapy to Treat Peripheral Arterial Disease Using Therapeutic Angiogenesis

Critical limb ischemia, which is estimated to develop in 500 to 1000 individuals per million per year, is considered one of most suitable diseases for gene therapy. In a large proportion of these patients, the anatomical extent and the distribution of arterial occlusive disease make the patients unsuitable for operative or percutaneous revascularization. Thus, the disease frequently follows an inexorable downhill course. Of importance, there is no optimal medical therapy for critical limb ischemia, as the Consensus Document of the European Working Group on Critical Limb Ischemia concluded. Thus, in patients with critical limb ischemia, amputation, despite its associated morbidity, mortality, and functional implications, is often recommended as a solution to the disabling symptoms, particularly in the case of excruciating ischemic rest pain. Indeed, a second major amputation is required in nearly 10% of such patients. Consequently, the need for alternative treatment strategies in patients with critical limb ischemia is compelling. Therefore, novel therapeutic modalities are needed to treat these patients. In the pathophysiology of the disease, in the presence of obstruction of a major artery, blood flow to the ischemic tissue is often dependent on collateral vessels. When spontaneous development of collateral vessels is insufficient to allow normal perfusion of the tissue at risk, ischemia occurs. Recently, the efficacy of therapeutic angiogenesis using vascular endothelial growth factor (VEGF) gene transfer has been reported in human patients with critical limb ischemia *(2–5)*. Thus, the strategy for therapeutic angiogenesis using angiogenic growth factors should be considered for the treatment of patients with critical limb ischemia. Most of the initial studies have used VEGF, also known as vascular permeability factor, as well as a secreted endothelial cell mitogen. The endothelial cell specificity of VEGF has been considered to be an important advantage for therapeutic angiogenesis, as endothelial cells represent the critical cellular element responsible for new vessel formation *(2,3)*.

A human clinical trial using *VEGF* gene started in 1994 by Professor Isner at Tufts University. An initial trial was performed using a hydrogel catheter with naked $VEGF_{165}$ plasmid. Although this procedure seems to be effective to stimulate collateral formation in patients with peripheral arterial disease (PAD) *(2–5)*, it is not ideal to treat many patients, as most patients lack an appropriate target vascular lesion for catheter delivery. Thus, his group applied intramuscular injection of naked plasmid encoding $VEGF_{165}$ gene (Fig. 1). Exceeding expectations, this clinical trial demonstrated clinical efficacy for treatment of PAD *(2–5)*. Since then, numerous angiogenic growth factors, such as $VEGF_{121}$, VEGF-2, and basic-fibroblast growth factor (bFGF) have been tested in clinical trials *(6,7)*. In addition to intramuscular injection of naked plasmid DNA, adenoviral delivery, liposomal delivery of angiogenic growth factors, was also utilized in these trials *(2–9)*, despite an unfortunate accident using adenoviral vector reported at the University of Pennsylvania *(10)*. In addition to the success to the intramuscular injection of $VEGF_{165}$ and VEGF2 plasmid DNA, local catheter-mediated $VEGF_{165}$ gene therapy in ischemic lower-limb arteries after percutaneous transluminal angioplasty (PTA) was also success-

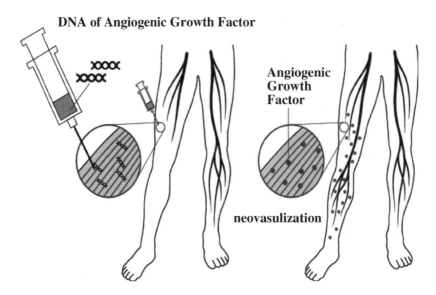

Fig. 1. Concept of therapeutic angiogenesis using DNA of angiogenic growth factors.

ful *(7)*. Follow-up digital subtraction angiography revealed increased vascularity in the VEGF-treated groups distally to the gene transfer site and the region of the most clinically severe ischemia *(7)*. A recent report, using adenovirus-encoding VEGF$_{121}$, demonstrated the improvement of endothelial dysfunction in response to acetylcholine or nitroglycerine *(8)*. However, a high incidence of edema has been reported as side effect in the VEGF trial. The recent results from the Regional Angiogenesis with Vascular Endothelial growth factor (RAVE) trial demonstrated that adenoviral *VEGF$_{121}$* gene transfer was not successful in subjects with intermittent claudication *(9)*. The selection of the agent (VEGF$_{121}$ vs $_{165}$), patient population (intermittent claudication vs critical limb ischemia), and outcome measures (peak walking time vs ulcer size) should be considered in the quest for optimal angiogenic strategies that result in the growth of functional blood vessels and improvement in clinical symptoms.

The safety and efficacy of increasing single and repeated doses of intramuscular naked plasmid DNA encoding for *FGF* type 1 administered to patients with unreconstructible end-stage PAD was also reported *(6)*. A significant reduction in pain and aggregate ulcer size was detected after *FGF* gene transfer associated with an increased transcutaneous oxygen pressure and Ankle Pressure Index (ABI) as compared with baseline pretreatment values *(6)*. We also identified HGF as a novel candidate for therapeutic angiogenesis. HGF is a mesenchyme-derived pleiotropic factor that regulates cell growth, cell motility, and morphogenesis of various types of cells, and is thus considered a humoral mediator of epithelial–mesenchymal interactions responsible for morphogenic tissue interactions during embryonic development and organogenesis. We and others previously reported that HGF stimulated angiogenesis in a rabbit ischemic hindlimb model, a rat ischemia model, and mouse ischemia models *(11–18)*. In addition, the angiogenic activity of HGF is more potent than VEGF or bFGF in vitro as well as in vivo *(11,19)*. Moreover, transfection of the human *HGF* gene by naked plasmid DNA or HVJ-liposome method resulted in a significant increase in blood flow *(14)*. The angiogenic property of transfection of the *HGF* gene was also proven in a diabetic and a high lipoprotein (a) models *(15,16)*.

Based upon these findings, we planned a human clinical trial using intramuscular injection of naked human HGF plasmid (0.5 mg × 4 sites) two times. Currently, *HGF* gene transfer has been performed in six patients with PAD (*n* = 3) or Buerger disease (*n* = 3) of Fontaine grade III or IV who had failed conventional therapy. Reduction of pain scale (1 cm in visual analog scale) was observed in five of six patients (efficacy rate approx 80%). Increase in ABI to greater than 0.1 was observed in five of five patients (efficacy rate 100%), whereas in one patient we failed to measure ABI before gene therapy because of severe calcification. Importantly, the serum level of human HGF protein did not change during gene therapy. No acute severe complications or allergic events were observed in any patient. Two-month follow-up studies showed no evidence of the development of neoplasm or hemangioma. Although these results are still preliminary, gene therapy using *HGF* may have therapeutic value to treat PAD. It is noteworthy that there was no evidence of edema in patients that were transfected with the human *HGF* gene. This finding is in marked contrast to the VEGF trial in which 60% of patients developed moderate or severe edema in a phase I/IIa trial. Currently, there is a phase III trial to treat PAD underway in Japan and a phase II trial in the United States.

We believe that one of the distinguishing features of HGF is that it stimulates the migration of vascular smooth muscle cells (VSMC) without the replication of VSMC, whereas VEGF does not stimulate either the migration or proliferation of VSMC because of the lack of its receptors in VSMC *(20)*. As shown in Fig. 2A, the initial event in angiogenesis induced by VEGF is the migration of endothelial cells, leading to the sprouting of blood vessels. Later, the migration of VSMC occurs as a result of the release of platelet-derived growth factor, followed by the migration of endothelial cells. However, a delay in the maturation of blood vessels might exist in the case of angiogenesis induced by VEGF. In contrast, HGF simultaneously stimulated the migration of both endothelial cells and VSMC (Fig. 2B). Thus, the blood vessels may mature at an earlier time point, thereby avoiding the release of blood-derived cells into the extracellular space, although further studies might be necessary to examine the angiogenic properties among various angiogenic growth factors including HGF, VEGF, and FGF. Although these trials are not complete, the feasibility of gene therapy using angiogenic growth factors to treat peripheral arterial disease seems obtainable in near future. Based upon these properties, it is assumed that the first gene therapy drug may be commercial available in 2005.

Gene Therapy to Treat Myocardial Ischemic Disease Using Therapeutic Angiogenesis

Similar ideas have been applied to treat coronary artery disease. A human gene therapy trial to treat coronary artery disease using $VEGF_{165}$ gene has been started by Professor Isner and colleagues *(21,22)*. His group performed intramuscular injection of naked plasmid encoding *VEGF* gene into ischemic myocardium through mini-operation. Similar to human trials in PAD, transfection of *VEGF* gene resulted in a marked increase in blood flow and improved clinical symptoms without apparent toxicity *(21)*. More recently, the results from 13 consecutive patients with chronic stable angina have been reported *(22)*. Although all of them had failed conventional therapy (drugs, percutaneous transluminal coronary angioplasty, and/or coronary artery bypass graft), reduction in the size of the defects documented by serial single-photon emission computed tomography imaging was observed after direct myocardial injection of $phVEGF_{165}$ via a minithoraco-tomy *(22)*.

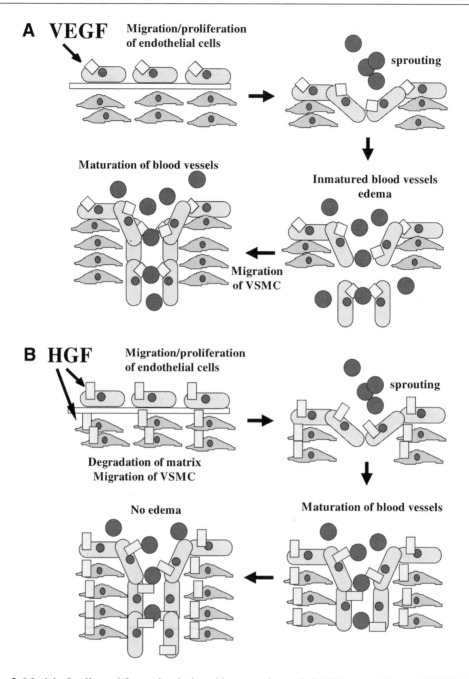

Fig. 2. Model of collateral formation induced by vascular endothelial growth factor (VEGF) (**A**) and hepatocyte growth factor (HGF) (**B**). HGF stimulated the growth and migration of endothelial cells together with the migration, but not proliferation, of vascular smooth muscle cells (VSMC) through c-met. In contrast, VEGF only stimulated the growth and migration of endothelial cells without the migration or proliferation of VSMC, because of the lack of receptors in VSMC.

These data clearly suggest that *phVEGF₁₆₅* gene therapy may successfully rescue foci of hibernating myocardium. In addition, the recent report summarized the anesthetic management of 30 patients with class 3 or 4 angina, enrolled in a phase 1 clinical trial of direct myocardial gene transfer of naked DNA-encoding VEGF165, as sole therapy for refractory angina. Twenty-nine of 30 patients experienced reduced angina (56.2 ± 4.1 episodes/week preoperatively vs 3.8 ± 1.6 postoperatively) and reduced sublingual nitroglycerin consumption (60.1 ± 4.4 tablets/week preoperatively vs 2.9 ± 1.1 postoperatively) *(23)*. Even at 1-yr follow-up, the average number of angina episodes per week and average number of nitroglycerin tablets used per week significantly improved at all measured time points after gene transfer *(24)*. This observation persisted at a 12-mo follow-up, when the average number of anginal episodes was 10 ± 19 and average weekly nitroglycerin tablet usage was 3 ± 8 ($p < 0.05$ vs baseline for both). Following this success, gene therapy using $VEGF_{121}$ gene was performed by intramuscular injection of adenoviral vector *(25)*. A phase I study using adenovirus-mediated transfection of $VEGF_{121}$ gene demonstrated clinical safety *(25)*. It is noteworthy that no evidence of systemic or cardiac-related adverse events related to vector administration was observed up to 6 mo after therapy *(26)*. Intracoronary gene transfer of $VEGF_{165}$ resulted in a significant increase in myocardial perfusion, although no differences in clinical restenosis rate or minimal lumen diameter were present after the 6-mo follow-up *(27)*. More recently, intracoronary infusion of adenovirus encoding *FGF* gene was performed in a multicenter trial as phase I/IIa. The report documented that intracoronary infusion of *FGF* gene improved cardiac dysfunction without severe toxicity *(28)*. Seventy-nine patients with chronic stable angina Canadian Cardiovascular Society class 2 or 3 underwent double-blind randomization (1:3) to placebo ($n = 19$) or Ad5-FGF4 ($n = 60$). Excitingly, a protocol-specified, subgroup analysis showed the greatest improvement in patients with baseline exercise tolerance test ≤ 10 min (1.6 vs 0.6 min, $p = 0.01$, $n = 50$). In addition, the report documented that treatment of 52 patients with stable angina and reversible ischemia with FGF4 adenoviral injection resulted in a significant reduction of ischemic defect size *(29)*. Currently, the phase IIb/III trials using adenoviral delivery of FGF4 are now underway.

In addition to these angiogenic growth factors, overexpression of HGF was also reported to stimulate angiogenesis and collateral formation in a rat myocardial infarction model *(30)*. Moreover, it was reported that intramuscular injection of HGF gene into the ischemic myocardium resulted in a significant increase in blood flow and prevention of cardiac dysfunction in a canine model *(31)*. The molecular mechanisms of the angiogenic activity of HGF seem to be largely dependent on the ets pathway (an essential transcription factor for angiogenesis), because members of the ets family play important roles in regulating gene expression in response to the multiple developmental and mitogenic signals. The ets family of transcription factors has a DNA-binding domain in common that binds to a core GGA (A/T) DNA sequence. *In situ* hybridization studies have revealed that the proto-oncogene c-ets 1 is expressed in endothelial cells at the start of blood vessel formation, under normal and pathological conditions. Thus, the ets family may activate the transcription of genes encoding collagenase 1, stromelysine 1, and urokinase plasminogen activator, which are proteases involved in extracellular matrix degradation. It is believed that the ets family takes part in regulating angiogenesis by controlling the transcription of these genes, whose activity is necessary for the migration of endothelial cells from pre-existing capillaries. Our previous study demonstrated that HGF upregulated ets activity and ets-1 protein in a myocardial infarction model *(30)*. In addition, exogenously expressed HGF also stimulated endogenous HGF expression through induction of ets activity *(32)* (Fig. 3), because the promoter region of the *HGF* gene contains a number of putative regulatory elements, such as a B cell- and a macrophage-specific transcription factor binding site (PU.1/ETS),

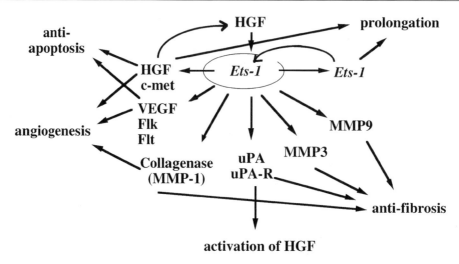

Fig. 3. Molecular mechanisms of angiogenesis induced by hepatocyte growth factor (HGF) through ets-1. HGF stimulated various actions on collateral formation through ets-1, revealing that HGF plays a pivotal role as a master gene in the cascade of angiogenesis.

as well as an interleukin (IL)-6 response element (IL-6 RE), a transforming growth factor (TGF)-β inhibitory element, and a cAMP response element *(33)*. Severe ischemic heart disease may also be curable using therapeutic angiogenesis by HGF, as a result of the autoinduction of the endogenous HGF system.

Recently, an antifibrotic action of HGF has been identified, as HGF inhibited collagen synthesis through TGF-β and stimulated collagen degradation through upregulation of matrix metalloproteinase (MMP-1) and urinary plasminogen activator (uPA) *(34)*. Although the mechanisms through which HGF inhibited TGF-β synthesis are not clear, HGF stimulated various metallo-proteases, such as MMP-1 through induction of ets-1 activity *(35)*. Prevention of fibrosis by HGF was confirmed by previous studies in which administration of human rHGF or gene transfer of human HGF prevented and/or regressed fibrosis in liver and pulmonary injury models *(36,37)*. Thus, HGF may also provide a new therapeutic strategy to treat fibrotic cardiovascular disease, e.g., cardiomyopathy. Our group has also applied to start a human gene therapy protocol using intracardiac muscular injection of HGF plasmid DNA through surgical operation. Overall, the treatment for coronary artery disease may also be curable using therapeutic angiogenesis by gene therapy.

Gene Therapy Into the Brain: A New Era for Cardiovascular Gene Therapy

In addition, gene therapy may be used to treat cerebrovascular disease. Cerebral occlusive disease caused by atherosclerosis of the cerebral arteries or Moyamoya disease often causes chronic hypoperfusion of the brain. Such a condition leads to not only cerebral ischemic events, but also neuropathological changes including dementia. Currently, an effective treatment to improve hypoperfusion has not yet been established. It is known that ischemic stroke induces active angiogenesis, particularly in the ischemic penumbra, which correlates with longer survival in humans. However, the natural course of angiogenesis is not sufficient to compensate for the hypoperfusion state. In the pathophysiology of the disease, in the presence of the obstruction of a major artery, blood flow to the ischemic tissue is often dependent on collateral vessels. When spontaneous development of collateral vessels is insufficient to allow normal perfusion of the tissue at risk, residual ischemia occurs. From this viewpoint, therapeutic angiogenesis must be an effective therapy for cerebral ischemia, resulting in the prevention of future stroke. Angiogenesis can be promoted in the rat brain using adenoviral vectors containing cDNA from bFGF *(38)*. After intraventricular administration of the viral vector, bFGF gene transfer induced angiogenesis in normal rat brain accompanied by an extremely high concentration of bFGF in the brain. In addition to bFGF and VEGF, HGF might be useful to treat ischemic cerebrovascular disease. Our preliminary data revealed that transfection of the HGF gene into the subarachnoid space immediately after occlusion of the bilateral carotid arteries induced angiogenesis on the brain surface and had a significant protective effect against the impairment of cerebral blood flow by carotid occlusion. Moreover, HGF has been the center of interest in neuroprotective substances, because HGF is both a chemoattractant and a survival factor for embryonic motor neurons *(39)*. Sensory and sympathetic neurons and their precursors also respond to HGF with increased differentiation, survival, and axonal outgrowth *(39)*. The broad spectrum of HGF activities suggests that the major role of HGF is to potentiate the response of developing neurons to specific signals. Our recent study demonstrated that gene transfer of HGF into the subarachnoid space has a profound neuroprotective effect against postischemic delayed neuronal death in the hippocampus *(40)*. Stimulation of new vessel formation and prevention of neuronal death by HGF is likely to create new therapeutic options in angiogenesis-dependent conditions, such as stroke, Moyamoya disease, and dementia, although a number of important issues, such as safety and side effects, have not yet been addressed. Our recent report demonstrated that gene transfer into the brain by injection of human *HGF* gene with HVJ-envelope vector into the cerebrospinal fluid via the cisterna magna resulted in a significant decrease in the infarcted brain area without cerebral edema or destruction of the blood–brain barrier *(41)*. Reduction of brain injury by HGF may provide a new therapeutic option to treat cerebrovascular disease.

Gene Therapy for Restenosis After Angioplasty

Another important cardiovascular disease potentially amenable to gene therapy is restenosis after angioplasty, because the long-term effectiveness of this procedure is limited by the development of restenosis in over 40% of patients. Balloon angioplasty is one of the major therapeutic approaches to coronary artery stenosis. However, restenosis occurs in 30–40% of patients after angioplasty. Intimal hyperplasia develops in large part as a result of VSMC proliferation and migration induced by a complex interaction of multiple growth factors that are activated by vascular "injury." The process of VSMC proliferation is dependent on the coordinated activation of a series of cell cycle regulatory genes that results in mitosis. Therefore, inhibition of the cell cycle using nonphosphorylated retinoblastoma *(Rb)* gene or antioncogenes, such as *p53* and *p21* has been reported in several animal models *(42–45)*. Recently, overexpression of inducible nitric oxide synthase gene has been tested in human subjects, although the results are not yet published.

Alternatively, it has been hypothesized that rapid regeneration of endothelial cells without replication of VSMC may also modulate vascular growth, because multiple antiproliferative endothelium-derived substances (PGI_2, NO, CNP) are secreted from endothelial cells. This concept was first tested by overexpression of $VEGF_{165}$ gene *(46)*. Asahara et al. reported a significant inhibition of neointimal formation by acceleration of endothelial cells replication by *VEGF* gene transfer *(46)*. Based on this finding, a human trial using $VEGF_{165}$ gene by hydrogel catheter delivery of naked $VEGF_{165}$ plasmid DNA has been started for restenosis after angioplasty in a peripheral artery *(47)*. Although the final results have not yet been reported, the preliminary results documented the successful inhibition of restenosis after angioplasty *(48)*. A similar trial using $VEGF_{165}$ gene has been started in Finland. In this trial, *VEGF* gene was transfected by cationic liposome or adenovirus with a catheter into the coronary artery *(49)*. A recent report demonstrated the clinical safety of *VEGF* gene transfer with cationic liposome or adenovirus *(49)*. Although gene transfer with *VEGF* using adenovirus during PTCA and stenting shows that intracoronary gene transfer can be performed safely (no major gene transfer-related adverse effects were detected), no differences in clinical restenosis rate or minimal lumen diameter were present after the 6-mo follow-up *(27)*. Nevertheless, a significant increase was detected in myocardial perfusion in the VEGF-treated patients *(27)*. Further studies are necessary to prove the efficacy of re-endothelialization strategy to treat restenosis. In addition, we also reported preclinical experiments in which overexpression of *HGF* gene in balloon-injured arteries could accelerate re-endo-thelialization, thereby attenuating intimal hyperplasia *(50)*. In this study, we also found that re-endothelialized balloon-injured arteries showed impairment of endothelial dys-function *(50)*. Further studies are necessary to clarify the utility of gene therapy to treat restenosis after angioplasty.

GENE THERAPY FOR CARDIOVASCULAR DISEASE USING OLIGONUCLEOTIDE-BASED STRATEGY

General Concept

Recent progress in molecular biology has provided new techniques to inhibit target gene expression. The application of DNA technology, such as antisense strategy to regu-late the transcription of disease-related genes in vivo has especially important therapeu-tic potential. Antisense oligodeoxynucleotides (ODN) are widely used as inhibitors of specific gene expression, because they offer the exciting possibility of blocking the expression of a particular gene without any change in function of other genes (*see* Fig. 4). Therefore, antisense ODN are useful tools in the study of gene function and may be potential therapeutic agents. The second approach is the use of ribozymes, a unique class of RNA molecules that not only store information but also process catalytic activity. Ribozymes are known to catalytically cleave specific target RNA, leading to degradation, whereas antisense ODN inhibit translation by binding to mRNA sequences on a stoichio-metric basis. Theoretically, ribozymes are more effective to inhibit target gene expres-sion. Conversely, we recently have found a novel molecular strategy in which synthetic double-stranded DNA with high affinity for a target transcription factor may be intro-duced into target cells as a "decoy" *cis* element to bind the transcription factor and alter gene transcription *(51)*.

Antisense or Ribozyme-Based Gene Therapy

As discussed earlier, angioplasty is limited by the development of restenosis in over 40% of patients. Intimal hyperplasia develops in large part as a result of VSMC prolif-eration and migration induced by the complex interaction of multiple growth factors. First, the effectiveness of antisense ODN against a proto-oncogene, c-myb, was reported for the treatment of restenosis *(52)*. Accordingly, inhibition of other proto-oncogenes,

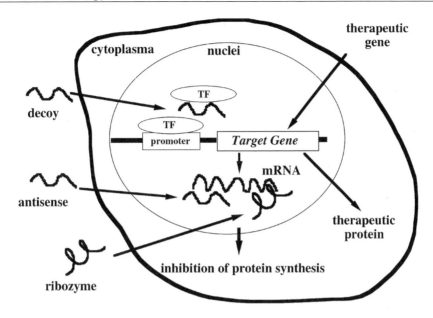

Fig. 4. Target sites for antisense, ribozyme and decoy strategies. Antisense, antisense ODN; ribozyme, ribozyme ON; decoy, decoy ODN; TF, transcription factor.

such as c-myc by antisense ODN, was also reported to inhibit neointimal formation in several animal models *(53)*. Currently, a phase II trial using antisense c-myc to treat restenosis is underway, although its results have not been reported. However, as this trial utilized intracoronary infusion of antisense c-myc ODN, several issues, such as low transfection efficiency may limit the efficacy of this strategy.

On the other hand, the process of VSMC proliferation is dependent on the coordinated activation of a series of cell cycle regulatory genes that results in mitosis. Our previous data revealed that a single administration of antisense ODN against proliferating cell nuclear antigen (PCNA) and cdc 2 kinase genes inhibited neointimal formation after angioplasty for up to 8 wk after transfection *(54)*. In addition, a single administration of cyclin B_1/cdc 2 antisense ODN combination significantly inhibited the extent of neointimal formation for a period of 8 wk after transfection *(55,56)*. Similar trials have been employed for other vascular diseases, e.g., restenosis after vein grafting and vasculopathy in transplanted heart. This proliferative vascular disease may also be an ideal target for antisense ODN-based strategy. Mann et al. reported that transfection of antisense ODN against proliferating cell nuclear antigen (PCNA) and cdc 2 kinase resulted in the inhibition of hyperplasia at 2 wk after transfection in a vein graft model *(52)*. Moreover, the prevention of neointimal formation in the balloon injury model by the cell cycle inhibition strategy was sustained long-term over the period of antisense survival *(54–57)*. This may relate to the vascular remodeling induced by the inhibition of cell cycle progression. Indeed, administration of antisense PCNA and cdc 2 kinase ODN into a vein graft model improved the resistance to diet-induced atherogenesis *(58)*. In addition to the prevention of restenosis after vein grafting, the inhibition of hyperplasia in transplanted hearts has also been reported by Suzuki et al. Transfection of antisense cdk2 kinase ODN resulted in significant inhibition of VSMC growth in the transplanted heart *(59)*. The first antisense drug appeared on the market in the United States at the end of 1999 as a novel drug to treat cytomegaloviral-mediated retinopathy.

Another strategy for combating disease processes by targeting to the transcriptional process is the use of ribozymes. We demonstrated the utility of ribozyme oligonucleotides against TGF-β by targeting the common sequence of *TGF-β* genes among humans, rats, and mice to treat restenosis in a balloon injury carotid artery model *(60)*. In addition, we also reported inhibition of production of lipoprotein (a) (Lp [a]), which is a risk factor for atherosclerosis, restenosis after angioplasty, cardiac disease, and stroke, without affecting plasminogen level using a ribozyme strategy *(61)*. Nevertheless, similar to antisense strategy, application of ribozyme technology to human gene therapy may require enhancement of the efficiency of cellular uptake and the stability of ribozyme oligonucleotides, because ribozyme oligonucleotides are easily degraded by nucleases because of their RNA backbone.

Decoy-Based Gene Therapy

Transfection of *cis*-element ds ODN (decoy) has been reported as a powerful tool in a new class of antigene strategies for gene therapy *(49)*. Transfection of ds ODN corresponding to the *cis* sequence will result in the attenuation of authentic *cis*-trans interaction, leading to the removal of transfactors from the endogenous *cis*-element, with subsequent modulation of gene expression. Therefore, the decoy approach may also enable us to treat diseases by modulation of endogenous transcriptional regulation. Recently, several studies have demonstrated application of the "decoy" ODN strategy as in vivo gene therapy *(62–64)*, and provide evidence of in vivo application of this novel molecular approach as a therapeutic strategy against cardiovascular disease. Many researchers have employed antisense technology as a "loss-of-function" approach at the transcriptional and translational levels, whereas the *cis*-element decoy strategy is also applicable as a "loss-of-function" approach at the pretranscriptional and transcriptional levels to study transcription factors.

As discussed above, the process of VSMC proliferation is dependent on the coordinated activation of a series of cell cycle regulatory genes, which results in mitosis. A critical element of cell-cycle progression regulation involves the complex formed by E2F, cyclin A, and cdk 2. The dissociation of the transcription factor E2F from the Rb gene product is proposed to play a pivotal role in the regulation of cell proliferation by inducing coordinated transactivation of genes involved in cell-cycle regulation including c-*myc*, c-*myb*, cdc 2, PCNA, and thymidine kinase. Accordingly, we hypothesized that transfection of VSMC with a sufficient quantity of decoy ODN containing the E2F *cis* element (consensus sequence "TTTTCGGCGC") would effectively bind E2F, prevent it from transactivating the gene expression of essential cell cycle regulatory proteins and thereby inhibit VSMC proliferation and neointimal formation. Transfection of E2F decoy ODN into rat balloon-injured carotid arteries resulted in almost complete inhibition of neointimal formation at 2 wk after balloon injury, accompanied by a reduction in mRNA of PCNA and cdc 2 kinase, but not β-actin *(62)*. Of importance, sustained inhibition of neointimal formation by a single administration of E2F decoy ODN was observed for at least 8 wk after treatment. Inhibition of neointimal formation by E2F decoy with hydrogel catheter delivery was also demonstrated using a porcine coronary artery model *(65)*. Modification of the delivery of ODN by a hydrogel catheter may overcome issues, such as the low transfection efficiency observed with coronary infusion. Based on these results, we started a clinical trial using hydrogel catheter delivery of E2F decoy to treat restenosis after angioplasty in April 2000. As of March 2002, we have treated five patients with E2F decoy ODN. We did not observe any side effects up to 6 mo, although the clinical outcome has not yet been evaluated.

In addition, in 1996, clinical application of "decoy" against E2F by Dr. Dzau at Harvard University was also approved by the FDA to treat neointimal hyperplasia in vein bypass grafts, which results in failure in up to 50% of grafts within a period of 10 yr. A proof-of-concept study, the Project in Ex-Vivo Vein Graft Engineering Via Transfection (PREVENT I) study, was the first clinical trial using genetic engineering techniques to inhibit cell-cycle activation in vein grafts *(66)*. This prospective, randomized, controlled trial demonstrated the safety and biological efficacy of intraoperative transfection of human bypass vein grafts with E2F decoy oligonucleotides in a high-risk human patient population with peripheral arterial occlusion. They demonstrated successful inhibition of graft occlusion, accompanied by selective inhibition of PCNA and c-myc expression *(66)*. More recently, similar results were obtained in PREVENT II, a randomized, double-blind, placebo-controlled trial investigating the safety and feasibility of E2F decoy oligonucleotides in preventing autologous vein graft failure after coronary artery bypass surgery *(67)*. The interim results confirmed the safety and feasibility of using this product. Analysis of the secondary end points using quantitative coronary angiography and three-dimensional intravascular ultrasound demonstrated increased patency and positive vascular remodeling (inhibition of neointimal size and volume) in the treated group at 12 mo. Patients examined at follow-up were found to have, on average, a 40% reduction in critical stenosis. Further assessment of this encouraging therapeutic approach should be completed by 2005 in adequately powered phase III studies in coronary and peripheral vessel disease, to determine definitively the extent and duration of clinical benefit. Because E2F has been postulated to play an important role in the pathogenesis of numerous diseases, e.g., vasculopathy after transplantation *(68)*, the development of the E2F decoy strategy may provide a useful therapeutic tool for treating these proliferative diseases.

On the other hand, the transcription factor NFκB also plays a pivotal role in the coordinated transactivation of cytokine and adhesion molecule genes whose activation has been postulated to be involved in numerous diseases, such as myocardial infarction. These diseases are, importantly, potentially amenable to ODN-based gene therapy, because treatment of these diseases is extremely difficult because of the lack of effective pharmacological agents. The pathophysiology of myocardial infarction is quite complicated. Numerous cytokines including interleukin-1, -2, -6, -8, and TNF-α, to name a few, regulate this process. However, gene regulation of many cytokines is relatively simple, because the transcription factor NFκB has been reported to upregulate these cytokines. Interestingly, adhesion molecules such as VCAM and ICAM are also known to be upregulated by NFκB. Accordingly, we hypothesized that myocardial infarction and glomerulonephritis could be prevented by the blockade of genes regulating cell inflammation—the final common pathway that is induced by NFκB binding (*see* Fig. 5). The necessity to block cytokine and adhesion molecule genes at more than one point to achieve maximum inhibitory effects may be a result of the redundancy and complexity of the interactions of these genes.

Importantly, increased NFκB binding activity has been confirmed in balloon-injured blood vessels *(69)*. Our recent study provided the first evidence of the feasibility of a decoy strategy against NFκB in treating restenosis *(69)*. Transfection of NFκB decoy ODN into balloon-injured carotid artery or porcine coronary artery markedly reduced

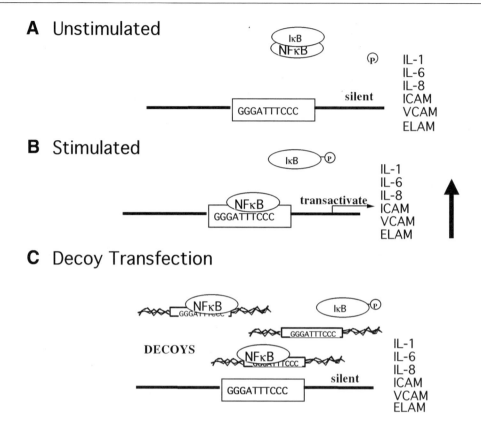

Fig. 5. Mechanisms of NFκB decoy ODN.

neointimal formation, whereas no difference was observed between scrambled decoy ODN-treated and untransfected blood vessels *(69,70)*. Based on the therapeutic efficacy of this strategy, we obtained permission for a second clinical trial using the decoy strategy to treat restenosis from 2001. In addition, the inhibition of VSMC replication was confirmed by the observation that transfection of NFκB decoy ODN inhibited the progression of vasculopathy in cardiac transplantation models *(71,72)*. Blockade of NFκB is also effective in treating reperfusion myocardial injury *(63,64)*. Transfection of NFκB decoy ODN into rat coronary artery prior to left-ascending artery (LAD) occlusion markedly reduced the area of damaged myocytes 24 h after reperfusion. The therapeutic efficacy of this strategy via intracoronary administration immediately after reperfusion, similar to the clinical situation, was also examined. NFκB decoy ODN reduced the damage of myocytes resulting from reperfusion, in contrast with rats treated with scrambled control decoy or vehicle.

Because NFκB has been postulated to play an important role in the pathogenesis of numerous diseases, e.g., cancer and arthritis, the development of a NFκB decoy strategy may provide a useful therapeutic tool for treating these diseases. Furthermore, modifications of ODN composition to prolong decoy stability in vivo and/or development of a delivery system into the cardiovascular organs/tissues will be critical to enhance potential therapeutic efficacy *(73,74)*. Despite these limitations, development of this technology offers great promise as a new tool for defining biological processes and treating pathological conditions. Overall, this approach is particularly attractive for several reasons: (1) the potential drug targets (transcription factors) are plentiful and readily identifiable; (2) the synthesis of sequence-specific decoys is relatively simple and can be targeted to specific tissues; (3) knowledge of the exact molecular structure of the targeted transcription factor is unnecessary; and (4) decoy ODN may be more effective than antisense ODN in blocking constitutively expressed factors as well as multiple transcription factors that bind to the same *cis* element. Thus, the decoy strategy may be useful for treating a broad range of human diseases. In contrast, because an important concern regarding the decoy strategy revolves around the potential inhibition of normal physiological responses, the application of decoy strategy as gene therapy may be limited to treatment of acute conditions, namely transcription factor-driven diseases.

Unresolved Issues in ODN-Based Gene Therapy

ODN-based gene therapy still has many unsolved problems, such as the short half-life, low efficiency of uptake, and degradation by endocytosis and nucleases. Therefore, many groups currently are focusing on modifications of the gel approach using a catheter delivery system. Further modification of ODN pharmacokinetics will facilitate the potential clinical utility of the agents by: (1) allowing a shorter intraluminal incubation time to preserve organ perfusion; (2) prolonging the duration of biological action; and (3) enhancing efficacy, such that the nonspecific effects of high doses of ODN can be avoided. Regarding the ODN-based strategy as gene therapy, one of the major concerns is nonspecific effects, particularly those of phosphorothioate-substituted ODN *(75–78)*. To overcome these issues, carefully controlled experiments must be performed to eliminate the potential nonspecific effects of ODN-mediated therapy. For gene therapy using an ODN-based strategy, the toxicity of phosphorothioate ODN may also be important. Although low-dosage administration does not seem to cause any toxicity, bolus infusions may be dangerous. Higher doses over prolonged periods of time may cause kidney damage, as evidenced by proteinuria and leukocytes in the urine in animals *(77)*. Liver enzymes may also be increased in animals treated with moderate to high doses. Several phosphorothioate ODN have been shown to cause acute hypotensive events in monkeys *(79,80)*, probably as a result of complement activation *(81)*. These effects are transient, if managed appropriately, and relatively uncommon. This toxicity can be avoided by giving intravenous infusions rather than bolus injections. More recently, prolongation of prothrombin, partial thromboplastin, and bleeding times has been reported in monkeys *(82)*. Alternatively, we recently developed new modification of decoy ODN in order to increase their stability against nucleases. Although the chemical modifications of ODN, such as phosphorothioation and methylphosphonation, were employed, problems with these modified ODNs became apparent including insensitivity to RNaseH, lack of sequence specificity, and immune activation, as described previously. To overcome these limitations, covalently modified ODN were developed by enzymatically ligating two identical molecules, thereby preventing their degradation by exonucleases (Fig. 6) *(83)*. In fact, the transfection of novel AP-1 decoy ODN with circular ribbon structure, prior to the balloon injury procedure, prevented neointimal formation in the rat balloon-injured artery more effectively than nonmodified decoy ODN *(83)*.

PERSPECTIVES IN GENE THERAPY

Gene therapy in the field of cardiovascular disease would be useful for the treatment of many diseases, including PAD, myocardial infarction, restenosis after angioplasty,

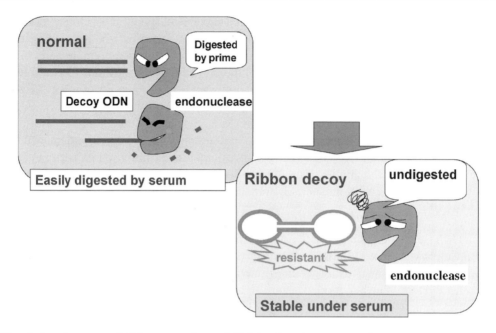

Fig. 6. Development of ribbon-type decoy ODN that has the potent resistance to endonuclease.

and rejection in heart transplantation. The first federally approved human gene therapy protocol started on September 14, 1990 for adenosine deaminase deficiency patients. Ten years since the commencement of the first trial, over 4000 patients have been treated by gene therapy. The objectives are generally to evaluate: (1) the in vivo efficacy of the gene transfer method; (2) the safety of the gene transfer method, and (3) the possible therapeutic efficacy. Although there are still many unresolved issues in the clinical application of gene therapy, gene therapy for cardiovascular disease now appears to be not far from reality and it is time to take a hard look at practical issues that will determine the real clinical potential. These include: (1) further innovations in gene transfer methods, (2) well-defined disease targets, (3) cell-specific targeting strategies, and (4) effective and safe delivery systems.

REFERENCES

1. Heilmann C, von Samson P, Schlegel K, et al. Comparison of protein with DNA therapy for chronic myocardial ischemia using fibroblast growth factor-2. Eur J Cardiothorac Surg 2002;22:957–964.
2. Isner JM, Pieczek A, Schainfeld R, et al. Clinical evidence of angiogenesis after arterial gene transfer of phVEGF165 in patient with ischaemic limb. Lancet 1996;348:370–374.
3. Baumgartner I, Pieczek A, Manor O, et al. Constitutive expression of phVEGF165 after intramuscular gene transfer promotes collateral vessel development in patients with critical limb ischemia. Circulation 1998;97:1114–1123.
4. Isner JM, Baumgartner I, Rauh G, et al. Treatment of thromboangiitis obliterans (Buerger's disease) by intramuscular gene transfer of vascular endothelial growth factor: preliminary clinical results. J Vasc Surg 1998;28:964–973.
5. Baumgartner I, Rauh G, Pieczek A, et al. Lower-extremity edema associated with gene transfer of naked DNA encoding vascular endothelial growth factor. Ann Intern Med 2000;132:880–884.
6. Makinen K, Manninen H, Hedman M, et al. Increased vascularity detected by digital subtraction angiography after VEGF gene transfer to human lower limb artery: a randomized, placebo-controlled, double-blinded phase II study. Mol Ther. 2002;6:127–133.

7. Comerota AJ, Throm RC, Miller KA, et al. Naked plasmid DNA encoding fibroblast growth factor type 1 for the treatment of end-stage unreconstructible lower extremity ischemia: preliminary results of a phase I trial. J Vasc Surg 2002;35:930–936.
8. Rajagopalan S, Shah M, Luciano A, Crystal R, Nabel EG.. Adenovirus-mediated gene transfer of VEGF(121) improves lower-extremity endothelial function and flow reserve. Circulation 2001;104:753–755
9. Rajagopalan S, Mohler ER 3rd, Lederman RJ, et al. Regional angiogenesis with vascular endothelial growth factor in peripheral arterial disease: a phase II randomized, double-blind, controlled study of adenoviral delivery of vascular endothelial growth factor 121 in patients with disabling intermittent claudication. Circulation 2003;108:1933–1938.
10. Marshall E. Gene therapy death prompts review of adenovirus vector. Science 1999;286:2244–2245.
11. Morishita R, Nakamura S, Hayashi S, et al. Therapeutic angiogenesis induced by human recombinant hepatocyte growth factor in rabbit hind limb ischemia model as "cytokine supplement therapy." Hypertension 1999;33:1379–1384.
12. Belle EV, Witzenbichler B, Chen D, et al. Potentiated angiogenic effect of scatter factor/hepatocyte growth factor via induction of vascular endothelial growth factor: the case for paracrine amplification of angiogenesis. Circulation 1998;97:381–390.
13. Hayashi S, Morishita R, Nakamura S, et al. Potential role of hepatocyte growth factor, a novel angiogenic growth factor, in peripheral arterial disease: down-regulation of HGF in response to hypoxia in vascular cells. Circulation 1999;100:II301–II308.
14. Taniyama Y, Morishita R, Aoki M, et al. Therapeutic angiogenesis induced by human hepatocyte growth factor gene in rat and rabbit hind limb ischemia models: preclinical study for treatment of peripheral arterial disease. Gene Ther 2001;8:181–189.
15. Taniyama Y, Morishita R, Hiraoka K, et al. Therapeutic angiogenesis induced by human hepatocyte growth factor gene in rat diabetic hind limb ischemia model: molecular mechanisms of delayed angiogenesis in diabetes. Circulation 2001;104:2344–2350.
16. Morishita R, Sakaki M, Yamamoto K, et al. Impairment of collateral formation in Lp(a) transgenic mice: therapeutic angiogenesis induced by human hepatocyte growth factor gene. Circulation 2002;105:1491–1496.
17. Hiraoka K, Koike H, Yamamoto S, et al. Enhanced therapeutic angiogenesis by co-transfection of prostacyclin synthase gene or optimization of intramuscular injection of naked plasmid DNA. Circulation 2003;108:2689–2696.
18. Koike H, Morishita R, Iguchi S, et al. Enhanced angiogenesis and improvement of neuropathy by co-transfection of human hepatocyte growth factor and prostacyclin synthase gene. FASEB J 2003;17:779–781.
19. Nakamura Y, Morishita R, Nakamura S, et al. A vascular modulator, hepatocyte growth factor, is associated with systolic pressure. Hypertension 1996;28:409–413.
20. Nakamura Y, Morishita R, Higaki J, et al. Hepatocyte growth factor (HGF) ia a novel member of endothelium-specific growth factors: additive stimulatory effect of HGF with basic fibroblast growth factor, but not vascular endothelial growth factor. J Hypertens 1996;14:1067–1072.
21. Losordo DW, Vale PR, Symes JF, et al. Gene therapy for myocardial angiogenesis: initial clinical results with direct myocardial injection of phVEGF165 as sole therapy for myocardial ischemia. Circulation 1998;98:2800–2804.
22. Vale PR, Losordo DW, Milliken CE, et al. Left ventricular electromechanical mapping to assess efficacy of phVEGF165 gene transfer for therapeutic angiogenesis in chronic myocardial ischemia. Circulation 2000;102:965-974.
23. Lathi KG, Vale PR, Losordo DW, et al. Gene therapy with vascular endothelial growth factor for inoperable coronary artery disease: anesthetic management and results. Anesth Analg 2001;92:19–25.
24. Fortuin FD, Vale P, Losordo DW, et al. One-year follow-up of direct myocardial gene transfer of vascular endothelial growth factor-2 using naked plasmid deoxyribonucleic acid by way of thoracotomy in no-option patients. Am J Cardiol 2003;92:436–439.
25. Rosengart TK, Lee LY, Patel SR, et al. Angiogenesis gene therapy: phase I assessment of direct intramyocardial administration of an adenovirus vector expressing VEGF121 cDNA to individuals with clinically significant severe coronary artery disease. Circulation 1999;100:468–474.
26. Rosengart TK, Lee LY, Patel SR, et al. Six-month assessment of a phase I trial of angiogenic gene therapy for the treatment of coronary artery disease using direct intramyocardial administration of an adenovirus vector expressing the VEGF121 cDNA. Ann Surg 1999;230:466–470.

27. Hedman M, Hartikainen J, Syvanne M, et al. Safety and feasibility of catheter-based local intracoronary vascular endothelial growth factor gene transfer in the prevention of postangioplasty and in-stent restenosis and in the treatment of chronic myocardial ischemia: phase II results of the Kuopio Angiogenesis Trial (KAT). Circulation 2003;107:2677–2683.

28. Grines CL, Watkins MW, Helmer G, et al. Angiogenic Gene Therapy (AGENT) trial in patients with stable angina pectoris. Circulation 2002;105:1291–1297.

29. Grines CL, Watkins MW, Mahmarian JJ, et al. Angiogene GENe Therapy (AGENT-2) Study Group. A randomized, double-blind, placebo-controlled trial of Ad5FGF-4 gene therapy and its effect on myocardial perfusion in patients with stable angina. J Am Coll Cardiol 2003;42:1339–1347.

30. Aoki M, Morishita R, Taniyama Y, et al. Angiogenesis induced by hepatocyte growth factor in non-infarcted myocardium and infarcted myocardium: up-regulation of essential transcription factor for angiogenesis, ets. Gene Ther 2000;7:417–427.

31. Ueda H, Sawa Y, Matsumoto K, et al. Gene transfection of hepatocyte growth factor attenuates reperfusion injury in the heart. Ann Thorac Surg 1999;67:1726–1731.

32. Tomita N, Morishita R, Taniyama Y, et al. Angiogenic property of hepatocyte growth factor is dependent on up-regulation of essential transcription factor for angiogenesis, ets-1. Circulation 2003;107:1411–1417.

33. Liu Y, Michalopoulos GK, Zarnegar R. Structural and functional characterization of the mouse hepatocyte growth factor gene promoter. J Biol Chem 1994;269:4152–4160.

34. Taniyama Y, Morishita R, Nakagami H, et al. Potential contribution of a novel antifibrotic factor, hepatocyte growth factor, to prevention of myocardial fibrosis by angiotensin II blockade in cardiomyopathic hamsters. Circulation 2000;102:246–252.

35. Taniyama Y, Morishita R, Aoki M, et al. Angiogensis and anti-fibrotic action by hepatocyte growth factor in cardiomyopathic hamster. Hypertension 2002;40:47–53.

36. Ueki T, Kaneda Y, Tsutsui H, et al. Hepatocyte growth factor gene therapy of liver cirrhosis in rats. Nat Med 1999;5:226–230.

37. Nakamura T, Sakata R, Ueno T, Sata M, Ueno H. Inhibition of transforming growth factor beta prevents progression of liver fibrosis and enhances hepatocyte regeneration in dimethylnitrosamine-treated rats. Hepatology 2000;32:247–255.

38. Yukawa H, Takahashi JC, Miyatake SI, et al. Adenoviral gene transfer of basic fibroblast growth factor promotes angiogenesis in rat brain. Gene Ther 2000;7:942–949.

39. Maina F, Klein R. Hepatocyte growth factor, a versatile signal for developing neurons. Nat Neurosci 1999;2:213–217.

40. Hayashi K, Morishita R, Nakagami H, et al. Gene therapy for preventing neuronal death using hepatocyte growth factor: in vivo gene transfer of HGF to subarachnoid space prevents delayed neuronal death in gerbil hippocampal CA1 neurons. Gene Ther 2001;8:1167–1173.

41. Shimamura M, Sato N, Oshima K, et al. A novel therapeutic strategy to treat brain ischemia: over-expression of hepatocyte growth factor gene reduced ischemic injury without cerebral edema in rat model. Circulation 2004;109:424–431.

42. Chang MW, Barr E, Seltzer J, et al. Cytostatic gene therapy for vascular proliferative disorders with a constitutively active form of the retinoblastoma gene product. Science 1995;267:518–522.

43. Chang MW, Barr E, Liu MM, Barton K, Leiden JM. Adenovirus-mediated over-expression of the cyclin/cyclin-dependent kinase inhibitor, p21 inhibits vascular smooth muscle cell proliferation and neointima formation in the rat carotid artery model of balloon angioplasty. J Clin Invest 1995;96;2260–2268.

44. Yonemitsu Y, Kaneda Y, Tanaka S, et al. Transfer of wild-type p53 gene effectively inhibits vascular smooth muscle cell proliferation in vitro and in vivo. Circ Res 1998;82:147–156.

45. Taniyama Y, Tachibana K, Hiraoka K, et al. Local delivery of plasmid DNA into rat carotid artery using ultrasound. Circulation 2002;105:1233–1239.

46. Asahara T, Bauters C, Pastore C, et al. Local delivery of vascular endothelial growth factor accelerates reendothelialization and attenuates intimal hyperplasia in balloon-injured rat carotid artery. Circulation 1995;91:2793–2801.

47. Isner JM, Walsh K, Rosenfield K, et al. Clinical protocol: arterial gene therapy for restenosis. Hum Gene Ther 1996;7:989–1011.

48. Vale PR, Wuensch DI, Rauh GF, Rosenfield KM, Schainfeld RM, Isner JM. Arterial gene therapy for inhibiting restenosis in patients with claudication undergoing superficial femoral artery angioplasty. Circulation 1998;98:I–66.

49. Laitinen M, Hartikainen J, Hiltunen MO, et al. Catheter-mediated vascular endothelial growth factor gene transfer to human coronary arteries after angioplasty. Hum Gene Ther 2000;11:263–270.

50. Hayashi K, Nakamura S, Morishita R, et al. In vivo transfer of human hepatocyte growth factor gene accelerates re-endothelialization and inhibits neointimal formation after balloon injury in rat model. Gene Ther 2000;7:1664–1671

51. Morishita R, Higaki J, Tomita N, Ogihara T. Application of transcription factor "decoy" strategy as means of gene therapy and study of gene expression in cardiovascular disease. Circ Res 1998;82:1023–1028.

52. Simons M, Edelman ER, DeKeyser J-L, Langer R, Rosenberg RD. Antisense c-myb oligonucleotides inhibit intimal arterial smooth muscle cell accumulation in vivo. Nature 1992;359:67–80.

53. Shi Y, Fard A, Galeo A, et al. Transcatheter delivery of c-myc antisense oligomers reduces neointimal formation in a porcine model of coronary artery balloon injury. Circulation 1994;90:944–951.

54. Morishita R, Gibbons GH, Ellison KE, et al. Single intraluminal delivery of antisense cdc 2 kinase and PCNA oligonucleotides results in chronic inhibition of neointimal hyperplasia. Proc Natl Acad Sci USA 1993;90:8474–8479.

55. Morishita R, Gibbons GH, Ellison KE, et al. Intimal hyperplasia after vascular injury is inhibited by antisense cdk 2 kinase oligonucleotides. J Clin Invest 1994;1458–1464.

56. Morishita R, Gibbons GH, Kaneda Y, Ogihara T, Dzau VJ. Pharmacokinetics of antisense oligonucleotides (cyclin B1 and cdc 2 kinase) in the vessel wall: enhanced therapeutic utility for restenosis by HVJ-liposome method. Gene 1994;149:13–19.

57. Mann MJ, Gibbons GH, Kernoff RS, et al. Genetic engineering of vein grafts resistant to atherosclerosis. Proc Natl Acad Sci USA 1995;92:4502–4506.

58. Mann MJ, Gibbons GH, Tsao PS, et al. Cell cycle inhibition preserves endothelial function in genetically engineered rabbit vein grafts. J Clin Invest 1997;99:1295–1301.

59. Suzuki J, Isobe M, Morishita R, et al. Prevention of graft coronary arteriosclerosis by antisense cdk 2 kinase oligonucleotides. Nat Med 1997;3:900–903.

60. Yamamoto K, Morishita R, Tomita N, et al. Ribozyme oligonucleotides against transforming growth factor-β inhibited neointimal formation after vascular injury in rat model: potential application of ribozyme strategy to treat cardiovascular disease. Circulation 2000;102:1308–1314.

61. Morishita R, Yamada S, Yamamoto K, et al. Novel therapeutic strategy for atherosclerosis: ribozyme oligonucleotides against apolipoprotein (a) selectively inhibit apolipoprotein (a), but not plasminogen, gene expression. Circulation 1998;98:1898–1904.

62. Morishita R, Gibbons GH, Horiuchi M, et al A novel molecular strategy using *cis* element "decoy" of E2F binding site inhibits smooth muscle proliferation in vivo. Proc Natl Acad Sci USA 1995;92:5855–5859.

63. Morishita R, Sugimoto T, Aoki M, et al. In vivo transfection of cis element "decoy" against NFκB binding site prevented myocardial infarction as gene therapy. Nat Med 1997;3:894–899.

64. Sawa Y, Morishita R, Suzuki K, et al. A novel strategy for myocardial protection using in vivo transfection of cis element "decoy" against NFκB binding site: evidence for a role of NFκB in ischemic-reperfusion injury. Circulation 1997;965:II-280–285.

65. Nakamura T, Morishita R, Asai T, et al. Molecular strategy using *cis*-element "decoy" of E2F binding site inhibits neointimal formation in porcine balloon-injured coronary artery model. Gene Ther 2002;9:488–494.

66. Mann MJ, Whittemore AD, Donaldson MC, et al. Ex-vivo gene therapy of human vascular bypass grafts with E2F decoy: the PREVENT single-centre, randomised, controlled trial. Lancet 1999;354:1493–1498.

67. Dzau VJ. Predicting the future of human gene therapy for cardiovascular diseases: what will the management of coronary artery disease be like in 2005 and 2010? Am J Cardiol 2003;92:32N–35N.

68. Kawauchi M, Suzuki J, Morishita R, et al. Gene therapy for attenuating cardiac allograft arteriopathy using ex vivo E2F decoy transfection by HVJ-AVE-liposome method in mice and nonhuman primates. Circ Res 2000;87:1063–1068.

69. Yoshimura S, Morishita R, Hayashi K, et al. Inhibition of intimal hyperplasia after balloon injury in rat carotid artery model using *cis*-element "decoy" of nuclear factor-κB binding site as a novel molecular strategy. Gene Ther 2001;8:1635–1642.

70. Yamasaki K, Asai T, Shimizu M, et al. Inhibition of NFκB activation using *cis*-element "decoy" of NFκB binding site reduces neointimal formation in porcine balloon-injured coronary artery model. Gene Therapy 2003;10:356–364.

71. Suzuki J, Morishita R, Amano J, Kaneda Y, Isobe M. Decoy against nuclear factor-kappa B attenuates myocardial cell infiltration and arterial neointimal formation in murine cardiac allografts. Gene Ther 2000;7:1847–1852.

72. Yokoseki O, Suzuki J, Kitabayashi H, et al. *Cis* element decoy against nuclear factor-kappaB attenuates development of experimental autoimmune myocarditis in rats. Circ Res 2001;89:899–906.
73. Chu BC, Orgel LE. The stability of different forms of double-stranded decoy DNA in serum and nuclear extracts. Nucleic Acids Res 1992;20:5857–5858.
74. Kaneda Y, Iwai K, Uchida T. Increased expression of DNA cointroduced with nuclear protein in adult rat liver. Science 1989;243:375–378.
75. Gibson I. Antisense approaches to the gene therapy of cancer—'Recnac'. Cancer Metastasis Rev 1996;15:287–299.
76. Khaled Z, Benimetskaya L, Zeltser R, et al. Multiple mechanisms may contribute to the cellular anti-adhesive effects of phosphorothioate oligodeoxynucleotides. Nucleic Acids Res 1996;24:737–775.
77. Henry SP, Bolte H, Auletta C, Kornbrust DJ. Evaluation of the toxicity of ISIS 2302, a phosphorothioate oligonucleotide, in a four-week study in cynomolgus monkeys. Toxicology 1997;120:145–155.
78. Burgess TL, Fisher EF, Ross SL, et al. The antiproliferative activity of c-myb and c-myc antisense oligonucleotides in smooth muscle cells is caused by a nonantisense mechanism. Proc Natl Acad Sci USA 1995;92:4051–4055.
79. Srinivasan SK, Iversen P. Review of in vivo pharmacokinetics and toxicology of phosphorothioate oligonucleotides. J Clin Lab Anal 1995;9:129–137.
80. Cornish KG, Iversen P, Smith L, Arneson M, Bayever E. Cardiovascular effects of a phosphorothioate oligonucleotide with sequence antisense to p53 in the conscious rhesus monkey. Pharmacol Commun 1993;3:239.
81. Henry SP, Giclas PC, Leeds J, et al. Activation of the alternative pathway of complement by a phosphorothioate oligonucleotide: potential mechanism of action. J Pharmacol Exp Ther 1997;281:810–816.
82. Crooke ST. Progress in antisense therapeutics. Hematol Pathol 1995;9:59–72.
83. Ahn JD, Morishita R, Kaneda Y, et al. Inhibitory effects of novel AP-1 decoy oligodeoxynucleotides on vascular smooth muscle cell proliferation in vitro and neointimal formation in vivo. Circ Res 2002;90:1325–1332.
84. Chu BCF, Orgal L. The stability of different forms of double-stranded decoy DNA in serum and nuclear extracts. Nucleic Acids Res 1992;20:5857–5858.
85. Abe T, Takai K, Nakada S, Yokota T, Takaku H. Specific inhibition of influenza virus RNA polymerase and nucleoprotein gene expression by circular dumbbell RNA/DNA chimeric oligonucleotides containing antisense phosphodiester oligonucleotides. FEBS Lett 1998;425:91–96.

9 Molecular Therapeutic Approaches for Myocardial Protection

Alok S. Pachori, PhD,
Luis G. Melo, PhD,
and Victor J. Dzau, MD

CONTENTS

SUMMARY

Heart failure associated with coronary artery disease is a major cause of morbidity and mortality. Recent developments in the understanding of the molecular mechanisms of heart failure have led to the identification of novel therapeutic targets which, combined with the availability of efficient gene delivery vectors, offer the opportunity for the design of gene therapies for protection of the myocardium. Viral and cell-based therapies have been developed to treat polygenic and complex diseases such as myocardial ischemia, hypertension, atherosclerosis, and restenosis. In addition, cell-based therapies may have potential application in neovascularization and regeneration of ischemic and infarcted myocardium. The recent isolation of regeneration-competent endothelial precursor cells from adult bone marrow provides a novel opportunity for repair of the failing heart using autologous cell transplantation. In this chapter we will focus on the latest advances in the field of gene- and cell-based therapies for treatment of heart failure, and their clinical applications.

Key Words: Gene therapy; cell-based therapy; myocardial protection.

INTRODUCTION

Despite significant advances in the clinical management of cardiovascular disease, acute myocardial infarction (MI), and heart failure (HF) resulting from coronary artery disease (CAD), cardiomyopathy and systemic vascular disease remain the prevalent

From: *Contemporary Cardiology: Cardiovascular Genomics*
Edited by: M. K. Raizada, et al. © Humana Press Inc., Totowa, NJ

causes of premature death across all age and racial groups *(1)*. The epidemiological impact of heart disease imposes a severe physical and financial strain on health delivery systems. The complexity of the pathological processes leading to heart disease and the lack of specific predictive markers has been a major impediment to the development of effective preventive therapies, despite the identification of various risk factors and sensitive risk assessment technologies *(2–4)*. Consequently, the focus has been on the design of "rescue" treatments for overt symptoms of the disease, such as hyperlipidemia, myocardial ischemia, left-ventricular pump failure, and hemodynamic overload *(5)*. Although these therapies have improved the clinical outlook for patients afflicted by MI and HF, morbidity and mortality associated with these diseases remain high, indicating the need for more effective treatments.

The current availability of efficient vector systems, such as adeno-associated virus (AAV) *(6,7)* and the recent identification of several gene targets associated with heart disease *(8,9)* offer opportunities for the design of gene therapies for myocardial protection and rescue. The ability of AAV to confer long-term and stable protein expression with a single administration of the therapeutic gene *(10–12)* renders them ideally suited for delivery of therapeutic genes. In addition, the repair and vascularization of injured myocardium using autologous cell transplantation may be possible with the recent identification and isolation of cardiomyocyte and endothelial progenitor cells from adult bone marrow and peripheral blood *(13–16)*.

In this chapter we review the major advances in gene- and cell-based therapies for heart disease, with emphasis on strategies for protection and rescue of the heart from failure, their clinical feasibility, and a perspective on future developments in the field. We will highlight the breakthroughs, the challenges in making the transition from preclinical studies to clinical application, and the opportunities ahead in this exciting and growing field.

STRATEGIES AND TOOLS FOR GENETIC MANIPULATION OF THE MYOCARDIUM

Strategies for Genetic Manipulation of the Myocardium

A wide selection of therapeutic strategies, vectors, and delivery methods are available for genetic manipulation of the myocardium with variable degrees of efficiency *(6,17–19)*. The most common gene therapy strategy for the myocardium involves the exogenous delivery and expression of genes whose endogenous activity may either be defective or attenuated as a result of a mutation or a pathological process. Such "gain-of-function" gene transfer strategies have been widely used with a variety of therapeutic genes, including proangiogenic and survival factors *(21,22)*, antioxiadant enzymes *(22)*, and antiinflammatory cytokines *(23)*. On the other hand, strategies have also been devised for inhibition of genes that may be involved in the development of heart disease. Acute inhibition of transcription and translation can be achieved by treatment with short single-stranded antisense oligdeoxynucleotides, ribozymes, and more recently, using RNA interference technology *(12,18,24–26)*. Inhibition of transcription factor DNA binding using double-stranded "decoy" oligonucleotides for several transcriptional factors has also been employed to inhibit the transactivating activity of target transcription factors *(19,27,28)*. In many instances, the acute inhibition (loss-of-function) of a pathogenic gene is sufficient to prevent the development of disease. For example, the inhbition of cell-cycle regulatory proteins using decoy oligonucleotides was shown to prevent neointimal hyperplasia and subsequent restenosis following balloon angioplasty or bypass grafting *(27)*.

Selection of Therapeutic Target, Vector, and Delivery Strategy

The choice of therapeutic target, vector, and delivery strategy is, to a large extent, governed by the pathological features of the disease, the putative role of the target gene(s) in the pathophysiological process, and the timing of intervention *(29)*. The efficiency of gene transfer to the myocardium is highly dependent on the type of vector, route, dosage, volume of delivery of the genetic material, and the ability to transduce dividing or nondividing cells *(30,31)*. Other vector characteristics, such as the capacity to accommodate the transgene, ability to integrate into the host genome, and immunogenicity should also be taken into consideration. The characteristics of the disease dictate whether transient or long-term transgene expression is warranted. Thus, vector systems capable of integrating into the genome of the host and providing sustained transgene expression should be used for gene transfer in conditions requiring prolonged transgene expression, whereas nonintegrating vectors should be used for conditions requiring transient transgene expression.

With regard to the route of administration, intracoronary delivery of the therapeutic material is favored for global myocardial diseases such as HF and cardiomyopathy. The selectivity of coronary endothelium may, however, restrict the diffusion of some vectors, thus limiting distribution and uptake of the therapeutic transgene. In contrast, localized delivery of the therapeutic material by intramyocardial injection may be the preferred method for regional myocardial diseases, such as coronary ischemia or myocardial infarction. This approach has been used for delivery of angiogenic and cytoprotective genes to ischemic myocardium *(32)*. The major shortcoming of direct injection is the fact that transgene expression is restricted to the area surrounding the site of injection. In some cases, this may require multiple injections to adequately cover the affected area. The overall safety and specificity of gene transfer protocols may be enhanced by incorporating regulatory elements that can direct tissue-specific expression of the transgene in response to underlying pathophysiological cues, such as hypoxia, oxidative stress, or inflammation *(33–35)*. This degree of physiological control of transgene expression would allow spatial and temporal control over gene expression and could avert potential biological and ethical problems associated with nonregulated constitutive transgene expression, such as cytotoxicity and germ cell line transmission *(36)*.

Nonviral Vectors

Gene transfer vectors may be classified under three broad categories—nonviral, viral, and cell-based. Nonviral vectors include naked plasmids, cationic liposome and hybrid formulations, synthetic peptides, and several physical methods *(31,37–41)*. However, myocardial gene transfer efficiency using nonviral vectors is low as a result of rapid degradation of the vector, resulting in transient transgene expression. Nevertheless, there have been reports where naked plasmid-mediated gene transfer into the myocardium led to a sustained therapeutic effect *(20,42)*. The efficiency of plasmid gene transfer can be increased by encapsulating the plasmid in neutral liposomes fused to the viral coat of the Sendai virus (hemagglutinating virus of Japan [HVJ]) *(43)*, but transgene expression with this vector system is transient, rendering it unsuitable for use in chronic heart disease.

Electroporation has been used for transfer of naked DNA into embryonic chick hearts ex vivo with moderate efficiency *(40)*, but this protocol is impractical for myocardial gene transfer in humans. Application of nondistending pressure in an enclosed environment has been used to deliver oligonucleotides ex vivo to the heart *(41)* and vein grafts *(44)*, highlighting a potential application of this technique for genetic engineering of blood vessels and other organs in preparation for transplantation. Other nonviral methods of gene transfer, such as cationic liposomes, calcium phosphate, and particle bombardment, have shown limited efficacy in myocardial gene therapy *(17)*. A promising new delivery technology uses synthetic peptide carriers containing a nuclear localization signal to facilitate nuclear uptake of the target cDNA *(39)*. These peptide–DNA heteroplexes are recognized by intracellular receptor proteins and imported into the nucleus, where the target cDNA is transcribed.

Viral Vectors

Recombinant viruses have become the preferred vectors for myocardial gene transfer because they can deliver genetic material into cells with higher efficiency than nonviral vectors *(6)* and are capable of sustaining expression of the therapeutic gene for extended periods of time. However, in some instances, a robust immune reaction may be triggered by the host in response to the viral proteins synthesized by the vector. This may reduce the efficiency of gene transfer and the sustainability of transgene expression *(45)*. Furthermore, although the viral vectors used in gene therapy are replication-deficient, there is the possibility, albeit remote, that these vectors may revert to replication proficiency, thus raising safety concerns about biological hazards such as oncogenesis and insertional mutagenesis *(46)*.

Adenoviruses are the most widely used viral vectors *(45)*. These viruses can transduce a wide variety of myocardial cell types and can accommodate large DNA inserts. The vector infects both dividing and terminally differentiated cells. However, the cytotoxicity associated with induction of the immune response and the episomal localization of the viral genomes results in rapid loss of transgene expression even in the absence of cell division *(45)*. A new generation of "gutted" adenoviral vectors has been developed in which the host inflammatory response is highly attenuated by removing all of the adenoviral coding sequences *(47)*. These adenoviral vectors can accommodate very large DNA fragments and may be useful for delivering multiple genes.

AAV has emerged as the vector of choice for myocardial gene transfer because of its high myocardial tropism and ability to stably transduce terminally differentiated myocytes with high efficiency *(10,11)*. Intramyocardial delivery of AAV is usually more efficient than intracoronary delivery; however, the efficiency of the latter method can be improved by transient permeabilization of the endothelium with histamine. The vector is poorly immunogenic *(48)*, thus minimizing inflammatory damage. The major limitation of the vector is its inability to accommodate large DNA inserts (transgene size is restricted to 4 Kb or less) *(7);* however, trans-splicing between two separate AAV vectors has recently been used as a strategy for delivery of genes greater than 4Kb *(49)*.

RNA-based retroviral and lentiviral vectors have not found widespread application in myocardial gene transfer protocols for several biological and technical reasons *(50,51)*. These vectors integrate into the host genome leading to the possibility of long-term transgene expression *(50)*. However, retroviral integration requires cell division, rendering these vectors inefficient in transduction of adult cardiomyocytes. Furthermore, retrovirally delivered transgenes are prone to transcription silencing, which may significantly shorten the duration of transgene expression. Production of high-titer retrovirus preparations is difficult; however, recent improvements in packaging systems, such as the use of pseudotypcd viral coats incorporating the vesicular stomatitis virus G protein (VSV-G) has greatly improved the stability of the viral particles and has allowed transduction of a wider spectrum of cell types with relatively high efficiency *(51)*. In contrast with the oncoretroviruses, the human immunodeficiency virus (HIV-1)-related retroviruses can infect both dividing and quiescent cells. Moderate transgene expression has been observed in the heart following transduction with a pseudotyped lentivirus *(52,53)*.

Other viral vector systems currently used for gene transfer, such as herpes simplex viruses (HSV) and alphaviruses, have had limited application in myocardial gene transfer. The ability of HSV-based vectors to accommodate very large DNA fragments provide an advantage for the transfer of very large genes, such as dystrophin or sarcoglycans for treatment of inherited cardiomyopathies *(54)*. Alphaviruses are positive-strand RNA viruses based on the Semliki Forest virus (SFV) and Sendibis virus *(55)*. These viruses have recently been used for very rapid and efficient transduction of several cells and tissues in vitro *(56)*. These viruses are capable of expressing transgenes within 24 h of transduction in the heart with minimal cytoxicity, suggesting their potential application for gene manipulation in acute myocardial disease such as MI.

Cell-Mediated Gene Delivery

A number of cell types have also been used as vectors for delivery of genetic material to tissues. The recent identification and isolation of endothelial and cardiomyocyte precursor stem cells from adult bone marrow and peripheral blood *(13,15)* provides a nondepleting, self-renewing autologous cell source that can simultaneously be used as substrate for regeneration and reconstruction of injured myocardium and blood vessels, and as vehicles for delivery of therapeutic genes. For example, the cells could be engineered ex vivo to express cytoprotective and/or proangiogenic genes that would promote survival of the grafted cells and neovascularization of the infarcted myocardium *(57)*. Macrophages, erythrocytes, and vascular endothelial cells have also been successfully transduced ex vivo with retroviral vectors for efficient delivery of therapeutic genes into tissues *(58,59)*. Macrophages genetically engineered to express protective genes under endogenous regulation by hypoxia may have potential application for targeted delivery of genes in myocardial ischemia.

GENE THERAPY FOR MYOCARDIAL PROTECTION

Pathogenesis of Heart Disease and Targets for Gene Therapy

Myocardial ischemia associated with CAD is the primary cause of myocardial failure *(60)*. Systemic hypertension, disorders of lipid metabolism, and diabetes are the predominant predisposing factors for CAD *(2)*. Acute ischemic events, if sufficiently prolonged, will lead to irreversible damage and infarction, underlined by alterations in membrane fluidity, intracellular hydrogen ion concentration and metabolic activity, and eventual cell death, resulting in arrhythmia and impaired pump function *(61)*. Paradoxically, reoxygenation of the ischemic myocardium induces a robust increase in reactive oxygen species (ROS), which triggers a profound inflammatory response that may exacerbate the damage initiated during ischemia *(61–63)*. In time, the left ventricle undergoes a process of remodeling characterized by myocyte hypertrophy, interstitial fibrosis, chamber dilatation, and increased propensity for contractile dysfunction that ultimately leads to ventricular failure *(64)*. The remodeling process is complex and highly dependent on the activity of matrix metalloproteinases (MMPs), a group of zinc-dependent proteases that are involved in extracellular matrix degradation *(65)*. Chronic ischemic heart disease is also characterized by heightened inflammatory state and oxidative stress *(66,67)*. The increased levels of proinflammatory cytokines depress myocardial contractility and activate neurohormonal systems such as the renin-angiotensin system, which promote ventricular fibrosis and remodeling.

Gene Therapy for Myocardial Ischemia

The vascular endothelium usually remains in a quiescent, nonproliferative state, and with the exception of the female reproductive tract and neoplastic disease, postnatal neovascularization is rare *(68)*. However, injury, inflammation, and oxidative stress activate the endothelium, resulting in cell proliferation, migration, and formation of new vascular networks by angiogenesis *(68)*. In patients and animal models with ischemic heart disease, the progressive occlusion of the coronary artery leads to a chronic imbalance in myocardial oxygen supply and demand, which stimulates the development of collateral vessels aimed at maintaining tissue perfusion and oxygenation *(69)*. This native adaptive response of the myocardium, however, does not provide adequate compensation in face of severe ischemia, and depression of cardiac function ensues, which in time leads to heart failure.

Evidence of enhanced neovascularization and functional recovery of ischemic myocardium has been reported in several animal and human studies after exogenous supplementation of proangiogenic cytokines by gene transfer *(70–76)*. This novel strategy, commonly known as therapeutic angiogenesis, offers a potentially efficacious method for treatment of coronary artery disease in clinical cases where percutaneous angioplasty or surgical revascularization has been excluded. Proof-of-principle for therapeutic angiogenesis has been demonstrated in several animal models of hindlimb and myocardial ischemia by gene transfer of vascular endothelial growth factor (VEGF) *(36,72,73,75,77)* and hepatocyte growth factor (HGF) *(74,78,79)*. In all cases, improvement in tissue perfusion was accompanied by morphological and angiographic evidence of new vessel formation, thus establishing a relationship between improved tissue viability and neovascularization. For example, Mack et al. *(71)* showed that intramyocardial delivery of $VEGF_{121}$ by adenovirus led to an improvement in regional myocardial perfusion and left-ventricular function in response to stress in an ameroid constrictor model of chronic myocardial ischemia in pigs. Using intracoronary injection of an adenovirus vector encoding human fibroblast growth factor (FGF)-5, Giordano et al. *(72)* also showed a significant improvement in blood flow and a reduction in stress-induced functional abnormalities as early as 2 wk after ameroid placement around the proximal left circumflex coronary artery in pigs, in association with an increase in capillary-to-fiber ratios.

Several phase I and II clinical trials of angiogenic gene therapy have been carried out with patients suffering from myocardial and limb ischemia *(32,75,80–82)*. These safety trials, although they consist of small, nonrandomized patient samples, nevertheless demonstrate, the potential of angiogenic gene therapy for treatment of ischemic heart disease. Losordo et al. *(20)* carried out a phase I study in five male patients aged 53–71 yr with angiographic evidence of CAD who did not respond to conventional antianginal therapy. The authors reported that direct intramyocardial delivery of naked plasmid encoding VEGF$_{165}$ into the ischemic myocardium resulted in significant reduction of anginal symptoms and modest improvement in left-ventricular function concomitant with reduced ischemia and improved Rentrop score. Vale and colleagues *(80)* carried out a randomized, single-blinded placebo-controlled phase I trial in patients with chronic myocardial ischemia using catheter-based delivery of naked VEGF$_{165}$ assisted by electromechanical NOGA mapping of the left ventricle. The results of this study indicated significant reductions in weekly anginal attacks for as long as 1 yr after gene delivery in the treated patients, in contrast with the patients receiving placebo. The reduction in anginal episodes was accompanied by improved myocardial perfusion as evidenced by SPECT-sestamibi perfusion scanning and electromechanical mapping. Recently, Grines and colleagues *(81)* completed the Angiogenic GENE Therapy (AGENT) double-blinded randomized, placebo-controlled trial using dose-escalating adenovirus-mediated intracoronary delivery of FGF-4 in patients with angina, in order to evaluate the safety an efficacy of this protocol in reducing ischemic symptoms. The authors reported increased exercise tolerance and improved stress echocardiograms at 4 and 12 wk after gene transfer in the patients that received FGF-4 gene therapy compared with the patients receiving placebo. The long-term outcome beyond 12 wk, however, has not been followed.

The success of these initial small-scale phase I and phase II trials warrant larger and more adequately controlled later phase trials. However, several issues relating to feasibility, safety, and sustainability require further investigation before therapeutic angiogenesis may be envisaged as a viable therapeutic option for treatment of ischemic heart disease. The broad issue of safety of the approach requires systematic evaluation. This is particularly relevant in light of recent evidence that transplantation of myoblasts constitutively expressing VEGF under a retroviral promoter into mouse hearts led to intramural angiomas followed by heart failure and death *(36)*.

Gene Therapy for Protection From Ischemia and Reperfusion Injury

The continuum of myocardial injury that is initiated by a coronary ischemic event and perpetuated by reperfusion (I/R injury) may be clinically manifested in patients undergoing thrombolytic therapy following an acute coronary episode. The increase in ROS formation during reperfusion of the ischemic myocardium may eventually deplete the buffering capabilities of endogenous antioxidant systems, thereby exacerbating the cytotoxic effects of these reactive species *(83)*. The development of gene therapies for acute myocardial infarction has been difficult because the time required for transcription and translation of therapeutic genes with the current generation of vectors exceeds the time window for successful intervention. An alternative gene therapy for myocardial protection is to "prevent" I/R by the transfer of cytoprotective genes into the myocardium of high-risk patients prior to ischemia using a gene delivery method that could confer long-term therapeutic gene expression. This novel concept of "preventive" gene therapy would protect the heart from future I/R injury, thereby minimizing the need for acute intervention. Given the prominent role of oxidative stress in I/R injury, a therapeutic approach aimed at increasing endogenous antioxidant reserves should, in principle, be a useful strategy for prevention/protection in patients at risk of acute MI. This strategy would potentiate the native protective response of the myocardium *(84)*, rendering it resistant to future ischemic insults.

We have evaluated the feasibility of antioxidant enzyme gene transfer as a long-term first line of defence against I/R-induced oxidative injury, using an recombinant AAV vector for intramyocardial delivery of heme oxygenase-1 *(HO-1)* gene in a rat model of myocardial I/R injury *(22)*. Our findings show that *HO-1* gene delivery to the left-ventricular risk area several weeks in advance of myocardial infarction results in approx 80% reduction in infarct size. The reduction in myocardial injury in the treated animals is accompanied by decreases in oxidative stress, inflammation, and interstitial fibrosis. Consistent with the histopathology, echocardiographic assessment showed post-infarction recovery of left-ventricular function in the *HO-1* treated animals, whereas the untreated control animals presented evidence of ventricular enlargement and significantly depressed fractional shortening and ejection fraction. Thus, these findings suggest that AAV-mediated delivery of *HO-1* may be a viable therapeutic option for long-term myocardial protection from I/R injury in patients with CAD. Comparable findings were found with extracellular superoxide dismutase *(ecSOD)* gene transfer *(85,86)*. This secreted metalloenzyme plays an essential role in maintenance of redox homeostasis by dismutating the oxygen free radical superoxide. Our findings showed that long-term survival after acute MI is improved in the *ecSOD*-treated animals relative to the animals treated with the control vector, in parallel with smaller infarcts and decreased myocardial inflammation *(87)*. Efficient protection from I/R injury has also been achieved by overexpression of other major antioxidant enzyme systems, such as ec-SOD *(88)*, catalase *(89)*, and glutathione peroxidase *(90)*, stress-induced heat shock proteins (HSP), such as HSP 70 *(91)* and HSP 27 *(92)*, survival genes *(Bcl-2, Akt) (21,93)*, as well as immunosuppressive cytokines *(23)*, adenosine A_1 and A_3 receptors *(94)*, kallikrein *(95)*, caspase inhibitor *(96)*, and HGF *(74)*.

The inhibition of proinflammatory genes involved in the pathogenesis of I/R injury offers another option for cardioprotection. Morishita et al. *(28)* showed that pretreatment with a decoy oligonucleotide capable of inhibiting the transactivating activity of the proinflammatory transcription factor NFκB reduces MI after coronary artery ligation in rats. Similarly, intravenous administration of antisense oligonucleotide against angiotensin converting enzyme mRNA *(97)* or angiotensin AT_1 receptor *(94)* significantly reduces myocardial dysfunction and injury following ischemia and reperfusion. Although the rapid in vivo degradation of oligonucleotides would preclude their use in long-term myocardial protection, they may be useful in treatment of acute myocardial ischemia and cardiac transplantation *(98)* by providing a tool for inhibiting of prooxidant, proinflammatory and immunomodulatory genes activated by ischemia and reperfusion. For example, treatment with antisense oligonucleotide directed against intercellular adhesion molecule-1 (ICAM-1) was shown to prolong cardiac allograft tolerance and long-term survival when administered ex vivo prior to transplantation into the host *(99)*. Such an approach could be beneficial in the preparation of donor hearts for transplantation. For example, oligonucleotide-mediated inhibition of anti-inflammatory genes and adhesion molecules in donor organs in advance of transplantation could be used to suppress the acute inflammatory response that ensues upon reperfusion of the transplanted organ in the recipient.

Gene Therapy for Myocardial Hypertrophy and Remodeling

The progression of HF resulting from hemodynamic overload, chronic myocardial ischemia, or acute MI is invariably accompanied by hypertrophy and remodelling of the left ventricle *(100)*. This process, which usually begins as an adaptive physiological mechanism aimed at normalizing wall stress in response to the increased load or myocyte death from infarction, eventually becomes maladaptive, resulting in alteration in ventricular geometry, mechanical decompensation, and contractile failure. Following MI, the left ventricle undergoes an early healing phase during which the infarcted area expands, resulting in wall thinning and ventricular dilation that leads to increased wall stress. This is followed by long-term dilation of the noninfarcted region, and myocyte hypertrophy and interstitial fibrosis leading to ventricular chamber distortion and enlargement *(100,101)*.

Inhibition of ventricular remodelling is a prime target in the treatment of HF, and the long-term survival benefits of therapies such as ACE inbition and β-blockade in patients suffering from MI or HF are attributed, at least in part, to a decrease in left ventricle remodeling. Pharmacological inhibtion of these pathways attenuates the hypertrohpic and remodeling process and delay the progression of disease *(5)*. More recently, treatment with MMP inhibitors was shown to effectively attenuate post-infarction LV dilation *(102)*, suggesting that this could be a potential therapeutic strategy for HF. Genetic manipulation of these targets may prove to be an effective alternate therapy to current pharmacological approaches for treatment of HF. Gene therapies aimed at inhbiting hypertrophic and profibrotic pathways should be useful in limiting the extent of remodeling. For example, inhibition of AT_1-receptor signaling by antisense reduces cardiac hypertrophy in a renin-overexpressing transgenic rat independently of systemic effects *(103)*, suggesting a role of local ANG II in inducing the hypertrophic phenotype. A similar approach could be used for inhibtion of cardiotrophic factors, such as calcineurin and protein kinases *(104)*. Antisense inhibition of myocardial transforming growth factor (TGF)-β1 factor signaling and metalloproteinase activity could be employed as strategies to reduce fibrosis and remodeling. Conversely, myocardial overexpression of antihypertrophic factors may be used as a strategy to reverse hypertrophy in failing hearts. Li et al. *(105)* demonstrated that cardiac specific overexpression of insulin-like growth factor-1 in mice prevented myocyte death in the viable myocardium and attenuated ventricular dilation and hypertrophy after MI. Similarly, cardiac overexpression of glycogen synthase-3β, an endogenous antagonist of calcineurin action, was reported to inhibit hypertrophy in response to chronic β-adrenergic stimulation and pressure overload *(106)*. Overexpression of cyclin-dependent kinase inhibitor p16 has also been shown to reduce cardiac hypertrophy in response to endothelin-1 (ET-1) *(107)*, in agreement with findings that cyclin-dependent kinase inhibitors play an essential role in inhibition of pressure-induced hypertrophy *(108)*. Systemic overexpression of vasodilatory genes such as NOS *(109)*, ANP *(110)*, and kallikrein *(111)* were effective in reducing cardiac hypertrophy and fibrosis in hypertensive rat models.

Cell-Based Therapy for Myocardial Ischemia

More recently, cell-based therapy has emerged as an exciting alternative strategy for therapeutic angiogenesis and involves the use of endothelial precursor cells as angiogenic susbtrate. Several reports have documented the existence of blood-borne endothelial progenitor cells (EPC) originating from a common hemangioblast precursor in adult bone marrow *(13,112,113)*. These endothelial lineage cells have the properties of an endothelial progenitor (CD34[+], Flk-1[+]) and are recruited to foci of neovascularization, such as ischemic muscle *(114)* and the myocardium *(115)*, where they differentiate into functional endothelial cells, indicating that they may play a role in postembryonic vasculogenesis in ischemic tissues. The therapeutic potential of these cells as vehicles for tissue salvage and/or regeneration from ischemia has been demonstrated. Local implantation of autologous bone marrow-derived cells in rat *(116)* and mouse *(117,118)* ischemic hindlimb induces angiogenesis and partially restores blood flow and exercise capacity in the ischemic limb. Similarly, transplantation of ex vivo-expanded human EPC into nude rats *(114,115)* and pigs *(119)* with myocardial ischemia led to increased capillary density and improved ventricular function. More recently it was reported that the number of circulating EPC increases in patients with acute myocardial infarction *(114)* and is lower in patients with coronary artery disease *(120)*, indicating that these cells may play an essential role in neovascularization of the myocardium in response to ischemia.

The ability to culture and genetically engineer EPC ex vivo with vectors expressing therapeutic genes suggests that these cells may be ideally suited as a substrate for cell-based gene therapy for neovascularization of ischemic tissues. In this scheme, EPC genetically modified to express angiogenic growth factors could serve as a cell substrate for new vessel growth by vasculogenesis, driven by local proliferation and differentiation of the transplanted cells, and as a source of proangiogenic growth factors for growth of preexisting vessels by sprouting. This concept was recently validated by Iwaguro et al. *(57)*. Using athymic mice with hindlimb ischemia, they showed that transplantion of murine EPC transduced ex vivo with an adenoviral vector expressing VEGF resulted in more efficient neovascularization and blood flow recovery compared to treatment with nontransduced EPC. The improved neovascularization in the animals treated with VEGF-transduced EPC appeared to be, at least in part, the result of enhanced EPC proliferation and adhesion. A potential noninvasive approach for angiogenesis of ischemic myocardium in CAD may involve the mobilization of EPC to the ischemic region using conventional pharmacological therapeutic agents used in treatment of CAD, such as statins. Recently, several groups showed that statin administration increased the number of EPC in patients with stable CAD *(1) 20,121*, suggesting that the beneficial therapeutic effect of these drugs may be mediated via mobilization of EPC and subsequent neovascularization of ischemic myocardium. In addition, Walter et al. *(122)* showed that statin therapy accelerates re-endothelization of balloon-injured arterial segments in rats, leading to reduction in neointimal thickening.

Cell-Based Therapy for Myocardial Regeneration

Despite evidence of myocyte replication in the heart *(123)*, the vast majority of adult cardiomyocytes are terminally differentiated, and are thus unable to divide *(124)*. Consequently, the regenerative capacity of the infarcted myocardium is limited *(125)*. Hypertrophy and, possibly, hyperplasia of the surviving myocytes may provide initial structural and functional compensation, but in time these processes lead to maladaptive remodeling of the ventricle and heart failure *(100)*. Cell transplantation (cellular cardiomyoplasty) may offer a potential alternative for reconstitution of infarcted myocardium and recuperation of cardiac function *(126)*. The basic premise of this approach is that repopulation of the necrotic myocardium with replication-competent cells capable of generating force should rescue contractile function and the structural integrity that is disrupted by MI. Several cell-based regenerative strategies have evolved using a variety of substrates, such as skeletal muscle myoblasts *(127)*, fetal *(105)* and embryonic *(128)* cardiomyocytes, and autologous marrow-derived mesenchymal cardiomyocyte progenitors *(129)*. The therapeutic efficacy of cellular cardiomyoplasty has, however, been inconsistent, and several technical and safety issues remain to be resolved. The optimal time for grafting after injury, the source and availability of cellular substrate, the delivery method, and the immunetolerance of the host to the grafted cells are important technical and safety considerations. The use of an adult self-regenerating autologous source of progenitor cells with the potential for differentiation into cardiomyocytes that would graft and electrically couple to the native myocardium would appear ideal. Mesenchymal cells from the bone marrow stroma of long bones may provide the best option for cellular cardiomyoplasty using autologous cells *(130)*. These cells are multipotent and have been shown to differentiate into functional cardiomyocytes under specific culture conditions *(16,131)*. MSCs can also be induced to differentiate into cardiomyocytes in vitro after treatment with the cytosine analog 5-azacytidine *(15,129)*. The differentiated cells display genetic and biophysical characteristics of fetal ventricular myocytes—namely, the expression of a fetal cardiac gene profile and prolonged action potentials *(15)*, as well as expression of functional adrenergic and muscarinic receptors *(130)*. Administration of mononuclear cell preparations harvested from bone marrow has been reported to improve cardiac function in various models of myocardial injury *(16,129,132)*.

Bone marrow mobilization with cytokines is being investigated as a potential strategy for treatment of acute MI. Treatment with stem cell factor and granulocyte-colony stimulating prior and immediately following infarction led to significant regeneration of infarcted myocardium and improvement in ventricular function, chamber dimensions, and long-term survival in mice *(133)*. These findings suggest that mobilization and "homing" of bone-marrow-derived cardiogenic precursors to sites of injury in the heart may constitute a natural repair mechanism that complements native reparative processes *(134,135)*. The mobilization of cardiogenic precursors could potentially be a therapeutic approach for potentiating this indigenous repair mechanism. The regenerative capability of this cardiac "self-repair" mechanism has, however, recently been questioned by several groups *(136,137)*, who have argued that the number of extracardiac progenitors that are capable of migrating to the heart is too small to induce effective long-term regeneration of the myocardium.

From a clinical perspective, the effectiveness and simplicity of bone marrow mobilization protocols is attractive and may hold therapeutic potential as a noninvasive strategy for treatment of acute MI. However, further work is required to establish the lineage of these precursors, the nature of the migratory and homing signals, the mechanism of transdifferentiation, and the optimal timing for therapeutic intervention. Despite these outsanding issues, one group recently demonstrated the feasibility of using unfractionated bone marrow for treatment of acute MI *(138)*. The authors reported that intracoronary delivey of autologous mononuclear bone marrow cells 6 d after infarction led to a reduction in infarct size and improvement in ventricular function and chamber geometry assessed at 10 wk after transplantation. Although this study illustrates the therapeutic potential of bone marrow stem cell transplantation for treatment of MI in humans, the general consensus of those working in the field is that further characterization of the biology of these cells is required before larger clinical trials are undertaken.

PERSPECTIVES AND FUTURE DIRECTIONS

Several molecular mechanisms underlying many of the most common cardiovascular diseases have recently been identified. This has led to the development of an array of gene and cell-based strategies with potential therapeutic value for treatment of these diseases. Some of these strategies have already made the transition from the preclinical phase into clinical trial and are now being considered for use in human patients, whereas several others are currently undergoing safety and feasibility evaluation in early phase trials. Notwithstanding these significant advances, there is still need for further developments in several aspects of cardiovascular gene therapy. Progress in vector and delivery technologies have not kept pace with the identification of novel therapeutic targets. All vectors currently in use for transfer of genetic material do not meet the criteria of the "ideal" vector. Emphasis must be placed on the development of vectors that are amenable to endogenous regulation and with the capability of conferring tissue specificity of transgene expression. Such a degree of spatial and temporal control over transgene expression will enhance the safety of human gene therapy protocols and potentially overcome many of the potential ethical issues that can arise as a result of nonspecific transgene expression, such as germ cell line transmission. Much of this development can be carried out using current vector platforms. Rigorous systematic evaluation of the safety and efficacy of delivery strategies and improvement of delivery devices are also essential prerequisites for human gene therapy protocols.

The optimal genetic therapy for complex diseases, such as CAD and MI may require a combination of cell transplantation and proangiogenic gene therapy for long-term sustenance of the regenerated myocardium. Such potentially synergistic combinatorial approaches have seldom been considered in the design of cardiovascular gene therapy strategies, which have traditionally been developed around a single therapeutic target. Genomic profiling and screening is being employed for molecular phenotyping of patients and will permit the detection of disease-causing polymorphisms and the design of individualized therapies. The convergence of gene transfer technology and genomic technology will facilitate the elucidation of novel genes and may help uncover new roles for previously known genes, thereby leading to the discovery of novel therapeutic targets and approaches for myocardial protection.

ACKNOWLEDGMENTS

Dr. Melo is a New Investigator of the Heart and Stroke Foundation of Canada and is supported by grants from the Canadian Institutes of Health Research, Canadian Foundation of Innovation, and the Health and Services Utilization and Research Commission of Saskatchewan. Dr. Dzau is supported by grants from the National Institutes of Health and is the recipient of a MERIT award from NIH. Dr. Pachori is the recipient of a postdoctoral fellowship from the American Heart Association.

REFERENCES

1. Kannel WB, Belanger AJ. Epidemiology of heart failure. Am Heart J 1991;12:951–957.
2. Stein EA. Identification and treatment of individuals at high risk of coronary artery disease. Am J Med 2002;112(8A).
3. Wilson PWF, D'Agostino RB, Levy D, Belanger, AJ, Silbershatz H, Kannel WB. Prediction of coronary heart disease using risk factor categories. Circulation 1998;97:1837–1847.
4. D'Agostino RB, Russel MW, Huse DM, et al. Primary and subsequent coronary risk appraisal: new results from the Framingham study. Am Heart J 2000;139:272–281.
5. McMurray JC, Pfeffer MA. New therapeutic options in congestive heart failure. Circulation 2002;105:2099–2106.

6. Robbins PD, Ghivizzani SC. Viral vectors for gene therapy. Pharmacol Ther 1998;80:35–47.
7. Monahan PE, Samulski RJ. Adeno-associated virus vectors for gene therapy: more pros than cons? Mol Med Today 2000;6:433–440.
8. Colucci WS. Molecular and cellular mechanisms of myocardial failure. Am J Cardiol 1997;80(11A):15L–25L.
9. Givertz MM, Colucci WS. New targets for heart failure therapy: endothelin, inflammatory cytokines, and oxidative stress. Lancet 1998;352(Suppl 1):S134–S138.
10. Svensson EC, Marshall DJ, Woodard K, et al. Efficient and stable transduction of cardiomyocytes after intramyocardial injection or intracoronary perfusion with recombinant adeno-associated virus vectors. Circulation 1999;99:201–205.
11. Kaplitt MG, Xiao X, Samulski RJ, et al. Long term gene transfer in porcine myocardium after coronary infusion of and adeno-associated virus vector. Ann Thorac Surg 2000;62:1669–1676.
12. Kimura B, Mohuczy D, Tang X, Phillips MI. Attenuation of hypertension and heart hypertrophy by adeno-associated virus delivering angiotensin antisense. Hypertension 2001;37:376–380.
13. Asahara T, Murohara T, Sullivan A, et al. Isolation of putatitve progenitor endothelial cells for angiogenesis. Science 1997;275:964–967.
14. Kocher AA, Schuster MD, Szabolcs MJ, et al. Neovascularization of ischemic myocardium by human bone marrow-derived angioblasts prevents cardiomyocyte apoptosis, reduces remodeling and improves cardiac function. Nature Med 2001;4:430–436.
15. Makino S, Fukuda K, Miyoshi S, et al. Cardiomyocytes can be generated from marrow stromal cells in vitro. J Clin Invest 1999;103:697–705.
16. Jackson K, Majka SM, Wang H, et al. Regeneration of ischemic cardiac muscle and vascular endothelium by adult stem cells. J Clin Invest 2001;107:1395–1402.
17. Li S, Huang L. Nonviral gene therapy: promises and challenges. Gene Ther 2000;7:31–34.
18. Akhtar S, Hughes MD, Khan A, et al. The delivery of antisense therapeutics. Adv Drug Del Rev 2000;44:3–21.
19. Morishita R, Higaki J, Tomita N, Ogihara T. Application of transcription factor "decoy strategy" strategy as a means of gene thereapy and study of gene expression in cardiovascular disease. Circ Res 1998;82:1023–1028.
20. Losordo DW, Vale PR, Symes JF, et al. Gene therapy for myocardial angiogenesis. Initial clinical results with direct myocardial injection of phVEGF$_{165}$ as sole therapy for myocardial ischemia. Circulation 1998;98:2800–2804.
21. Matsui T, Li L, Del Monte F, et al. Adenoviral gene transfer of activated phosphatidylinositol 3'-kinase and Akt inhibits apoptosis of hypoxic cardiomyocytes in vitro. Circulation 1999;100:2373–2379.
22. Melo LG, Agrawal R, Zhang L, et al. Gene Therapy strategy for long term myocardial protection using adeno-associated virus-mediated delivery of heme oxygenase gene. Circulation 2002;105:602–607.
23. Brauner R, Nonoyama M, Laks H, et al. Intracoronary adenovirus-mediated transfer of immunosuppressive cytokine genes prolongs allograft survival. J Thorac Cardiovasc Surg 1997;114:923–933.
24. Simons M, Edeelman ER, DeKeyser JL, Langer R, Rosenberg RD Antisense c-myb oligonucleotides inhibit intimal arterial smooth muscle accumulation in vivo. Nature 1992;359:67–70.
25. Mann MJ, Gibbons GH, Tsao PS, et al. Cell cycle inhibition preserves endothelial function in genetically-engineered rabbit vein grafts. J Clin Invest 1997;99:1295–1301.
26. Hannon GJ. RNA interference. Nature 2002;418:244–251.
27. Morishita R, Gibbons GH, Ellison KE, et al. A gene therapy strategy using a transcription factor decoy of the E2F binding site inhibits smooth muscle proliferation in vivo. Proc Natl Acad Sci USA 1995;92:5855–5859.
28. Morishita R, Sugimoto T, Aoki M, et al. In vivo transfection of cis element "decoy" against nuclear factor factor κB binding sites prevents myocardial infarction. Nat Med 1997;3:894–899.
29. Isner JM. Myocardial gene therapy. Nature 2002;415:234–239.
30. Alexander MY, Webster KA, McDonald PH, Prentice HW. Gene transfer and models of gene therapy for the myocardium. Clin Exp Pharnacol Physiol 1999;26:661–668.
31. Wright MJ, Wightman LML, Lilley C, et al. In vivo myocardial gene transfer: Optimization, evaluation and direct comparison of gene transfer vectors. Bas Res Cardiol 2001;96:227–236.
32. Losordo DW, Vale PR, Isner JM. Gene therapy for myocardial angiogenesis. Am Heart J 1999;138:S132–S141.
33. Prentice H, Bishopric N, Hicks MN, et al. Regulated expression of a foreign gene targeted to the ischemic myocardium. Cardiovasc Res 1997;35:567–574.

34. Shibata T, Giaccia AJ, Brown JM. Development of a hypoxia-responsive vector for tumour-specific gene therapy. Gene Ther 2000;7:493–498.

35. Nicklin SA, Buening H, Dishart KL, et al. Efficient and selective AAV-2 mediated gene transfer directed to human vascular endothelial cells. Mol Ther 2001;4:174–181.

36. Lee LY, Patel SR, Hackett NR, et al. Focal angiogen therapy using intramyocardial delivery of an adenovirus vector coding for vascular endothelial growth factor 121. Ann Thorac Surg 2000;69:14–24.

37. Song YK, Liu F, Chu S, Liu D. Characterization of cationic liposome-mediated gene transfer in vivo by intravenous administration. Human Gene Ther 1997;8:1585–1594.

38. Labhasetwar V, Bonadio J, Goldstein S, Chen W, Levy RJ. A DNA controlled-release coating for gene transfer: transfection in skeletal and cardiac muscle. J Pharm Sci 1998;87:1347–1350.

39. Cartier R, Reszka R. Utilization of synthetic peptides containing nuclear localization signals for non viral gene transfer systems. Gene Ther 2002;9:157–167.

40. Harrison RL, Byrne BJ, Tung L. Electroporation-mediated gene transfer in cardiac tissue. FEBS Lett 1998;435:1–5.

41. Mann DL. Mechanisms and models in heart failure. A combinatorial approach. Circulation 1999;100:999–108.

42. Shyu KG, Wang MT, Wang BW, et al. Intrmyocardial injection of naked DNA encoding HIF-1α/VP16 hybrid to enhnance angiogenesis in an acute myocardial infarction model in the rat. Caridovasc Res 2002;54:576–583.

43. Dzau VJ, Mann MJ, Morishita R, Kaneda Y. Fusigenic viral liposome for gene therapy in cardiovascular diseases. Proc Natl Acad Sci USA 1996;93:11,421–11,425.

44. Poston RS, Tran KP, Mann MJ, Hoyt EG, Dzau VJ, Robbins RC. Prevention of ischemically-induced neointimal hyperplasia using ex vivo antisense oligodeoxynucleotides. J Heart Lung Transplant 1998;17:349–355.

45. Krasnykh VN, Douglas JT, van Beusechem VW. Gene targeting of adenoviral vectors. Mol Ther 2000;1:391–405.

46. Mah C, Byrne BJ, Flotte TR. Virus-based gene delivery systems. Clin Pharmacokinet 2002;41:901–911.

47. Hartigan-O'Connor D, Amalfitano A, Chamberlain JS. Improved production of gutted adenovirus in cells expressing adenovirus preterminal protein and DNA polymerase. J Virol 1999;73:7835–7841.

48. Chirmule N, Propert K, Magosin S, Qian Y, Qian R, Wilson JM. Immune response to adenovirus and adenoassociated virus in humans. Gene Ther 1999;6:1574–1583.

49. Yan Z, Zhang Y, Duan D, Engelheardt JF. Trans-splicing vectors expand the utility of adeno-associated virus for gene therapy. Proc Natl Acad Sci USA 2000;97:6716–6721.

50. Hu W-S, Pathak VK. Design of retroviral vectors and helper cells for gene therapy. Pharmacol Rev 2000;52:493–511.

51. Daly G, Chernajovski Y. Recent developments in retroviralk-mediated gene transduction. Mol Ther 2000;2:423–434.

52. Sakoda T, Kasahara N, Hamamori Y, Kedes L. A high titer lentiviral production system mediates transduction of differentiated cells including beating cardiac myocytes. J Mol Cell Cardiol 1999;31:2037–2047.

53. Zhao J, Pettigrew GJ, Thomas J, et al. Lentiviral vectors for delivery of genes into neonatal and adult ventricular cardiac myocytes in vitro and in vivo. Basic Res Cardiol 2002;97:348–358.

54. Coffin RS, Howard MK, Cummings DV, et al. Gene delivery to the heart in vivo and to cardiac myocytes and vascular smooth muscle cells in vitro using herpes virus vectors. Gene Ther 1996;3:560–566.

55. Schlesinger S. Alphavirus vectors: development and potential therapeutic applications. Expert Opin Biol Ther 2001;1:177–191.

56. Datwyler DA, Eppenberger HM, Koller D, Bailey JE, Magyar JP. Efficient gene delivery into adult cardiomyocytes by recombinant Sindis virus. J Mol Med 1999;77:859–864.

57. Iwaguro H, Yamaguchi J, Kalka C, et al. Endothelial progenitor cell vascular endothelial growth factor gene transfer for vascular regeneration. Circulation 2002;105:732–738.

58. Griffiths I, Binley K, Iqball S, et al. The macrophage—a novel system to deliver gene therapy to pathological hypoxia. Gene Ther 2000;7:255–262.

59. Magnani M, Rossi L, Fraternale A, et al. Erythrocyte-mediated delivery of drugs, peptides and modified oligonucleotides. Gene Ther 2002;9:749–751.

60. Funk M, Krumholz HM. Epidemiologic and economic impact of advanced heart failure. J Cardiovasc Nurs 1996;10:1–10.

61. Carden DL, Granger DN. Pathophysiology of ischemia-reperfusion injury. Am J Pathol 2000;190:255–266.

62. Yellon DM, Baxter GF. Reperfusion injury revisited. Is there a role for growth factor signalling in limiting lethal reperfusion injury? Trends Cardiovasc Med 2000;9:245–249.
63. Braunwald E, Kloner RA. Myocardial reperfusion: a double edged sword. J Clin Invest 1985;76:1713–1719.
64. Pfeffer JM, Pfeffer MA, Fletcher PJ, Braunwald E. Progressive ventricular remodelling in rat myocardial infarction. Am J Physiol 1991;260:H1406–H1414.
65. Peterson JT, Li H, Dillon L, Bryant JW. Evolution of metlloprotease and tissue inhibitor expression during heart failure progression in the infarcted heart. Cardiovasc Res 2000;46:307–315.
66. Mehta JL, Li DY. Inflammation in ischemic heart disease: Response to tissue injury or a pathogenic villain? Cardiovasc Res 1999;43:291–299.
67. Singal PK, Khaper N, Palace V, Kumar D. The role of oxidative stress in the genesis of heart disease. Cardiovasc Res 1998;40:436–442.
68. Carmeliet P. Mechanisms of angiogenesis and arteriogenesis. Nat Med 2000;6:389–395.
69. Ware JH, Simons M. Angiogenesis in ischemic heart disease. Nat Med 1997;3:158–164.
70. Tio RA, Tkebuchava T, Scheurermann TH, et al. Intramyocardial gene therapy with naked DNA encoding vascular endothelial growth factor improves collateral blood flow to ischemic myocardium. Human Gene Ther 1999;10:2953–2960.
71. Mack CA, Patel SA, Schwarz EA, et al. Biological bypass with the use of adenovirus-mediated transfer of the complementary deoxyribonucleic acid for vascular endothelial growth factor 121 improves myocardial perfusion and function in the ischemic porcine heart. J Thorac Cardiovasc Surg 1998;115:168–177.
72. Giordano FJ, Ping P, McKirnan MD, et al. Intracoronary gene transfer of fibroblast growth factor-5 increases blood flow and contractile function in an ischemic region of the heart. Nat Med 1996;2:534–539.
73. Ueno H, Li JJ, Masuda S, Qi Z, Yamamoto H, Takeshita A. Adenovirus-mediated expression of the secreted form of basic fibroblast growth factor (FGF-2) induces cellular proliferation and angiogenesis in vivo. Arterioscler Thromb Vasc Biol 1997;17:2453–2460.
74. Ueda H, Sawa Y, Matsumoto K, et al. Gene transfection of hepatocyte growth factor attenuates reperfusion injury in the heart. Ann Thorac Surg 1999;67:1726–1731.
75. Symes JF, Losordo DW, Vale PR, et al. Gene therapy with vascular endothelial growth factor for inoperable coronary artery disease. Ann Thorac Surg 1999;68:830–837.
76. Hammond HK, McKirnan MD. Angiogenic gene therapy for heart disease: a review of animal studies and clinical trials. Cardiovasc Res 2001;49:561–567
77. Tabata H, Silver M, Isner JM. Arterial gene transfer of acidic fibroblast growth factor for therapeutic angiogenesis in vivo: critical role of secretion signal in use of naked DNA. Cardiovasc Res 1997;25:470–479.
78. Taniyama Y, Morishita R, Aoki M, et al. Angiogenesis and antifibrotic action by hepatocyte growth factor in cardiomyopathy. Hypertension 2002;40:47–53.
79. Aoki M, Morishita R, Taniyama Y, Kaneda Y, Ogihara T. Therapeutic angiogenesis induced by hepatocyte growth factor: potential gene therapy for ischemic diseases. J Atheroscler Thromb 2000;7:71–76.
80. Vale PR, Losordo DW, Milliken CE, et al. Randomized, single-blind, placebo-controlled pilot study of catheter-based myocardial gene transfer for therapeutic angiogenesis using left ventricular electromechanical mapping in patients with chronic myocardial ischemia. Circulation 2001;103:2138–2143.
81. Grines CL, Watkins MW, Helmer G, et al. Angiogenic gene therapy (AGENT) trial in patients with stable angina pectoris. Circulation 2002;105:1291–1297.
82. Bashir R, Vale PR, Isner JM, Losordo DW. Angiogenic gene therapy: pre-clinical studies and phase I clinical data. Kideny Int 2002;61(Suppl 1):110–114.
83. Park JL, Lucchesi BR. Mechanisms of myocardial reperfusion injury. Ann Thorac Surg 1999;68:1905–1912.
84. Williams RS, Benjamin IJ. Protective responses of the ischemic myocardium. J Clin Invest 2000;106:813–818.
85. Li Q, Bolli R, Qiu Y, Tang X-L, Guo Y, French BA. Gene therapy with extracellular superoxide dismutase protects conscious rabbits against myocardial infarction. Circulation 2001;103:1893–1898.
86. Chen EP, Bittner HB, Davis RD, Van Trigt P, Folz RJ. Physiological effects of extracellular superoxide dismutase transgene overexpression on myocardial function after ischemia and reperfusion injury. J Thorac Cardiovasc Surg 1998;115:450–458.

87. Agrawal RS, Muangman S, Melo LG, et al. Recombinant adeno-associated virus mediated antioxidant enzyme delivery as preventive gene therapy against ischemia-reperfusion injury of the rat myocardium. Mol Ther 2001;3:A837.
88. Li Q, Bolli R, Qiu Y, Tang XL, Murphree SS, French BA. Gene therapy with extracellular superoxide dismutase attenuates myocardial stunning in conscious rabbits. Circulation 1998;98:1438–1448.
89. Zhu HL, Stewart AS, Taylor MD. Blocking free radical production via adenoviral gene transfer decreases cardiac ischemia-reperfusion injury. Mol Ther 2000;2:470–475.
90. Yoshida T, Watanabe M, Engelman DT, et al. Transgenic mice overespressing glutathione peroxidase are resistant to myocardial reperfusion injury. J Mol Cell Cardiol 1996;28:1759–1767.
91. Suzuki K, Sawa Y, Kaneda Y. In vivo gene transfer of heat shock protein 70 enhances myocardial tolerance to ischemia-reperfusion injury in rat. J Clin Invest 1997;99:1645–1650.
92. Vander Heide RS. Increased expression of HSP27 protects canine myocytes from simulated ischemia-reperfusion injury. Am J Physiol 2002;282:H935–H941.
93. Chatterjee S, Stewart AS, Bish LT, et al. Viral gene transfer of the antiapoptotic factor Bcl-2 protects against chronic ischemic heart failure. Circulation 2002;106(Suppl):I212–I217.
94. Yang Z, Cerniway RJ, Byford AM. Cardiac overexpression of A1-adenosine receptor protects intact mice against myocardial infarction. Am J Physiol 2002;282:H949–H955.
95. Agata J, Chao L, Chao J. Kallikrein gene delivery improves cardiac reserve and attenuates remodeling after myocardial infarction. Hypertension 2002;40:653–659.
96. Holly TA, Drincic A, Byun Y, Nakamura S, Kloche FJ, Cryns VL. Caspase inhibition reduces myocyte cell death induced by myocardial ischemia and reperfusion in vivo. J Mol Cell Cardiol 1999;31:1709–1715.
97. Chen H, Mohuczy D, Li D, et al. Protection against ischemia/reperfusion injury and myocardial dysfunction by antisense-oligodeoxyynucleotide directed at angiotensin-converting enzyme mRNA. Gene Ther 2001;8:804–810.
98. Stepkowski SM. Development of antisense oligodeoxynucleotides for transplantation. Curr Opin Mol Ther 2000;2:304–317.
99. Poston RS, Mann MJ, Hoyt EG, Ennen M, Dzau VJ, Robbins RC. Antisense oligodeoxynucleotides prevent acute cardiac allograft rejection via a novel, non-toxic, highly efficient transfection method. Transplantation 1999;68:825–832.
100. St. John Sutton MG, Sharpe N. left ventricular remodeling after myocardial infarction. Pathophysiology and therapy. Circulation 2000;101:2981–2988.
101. Swynghedauw B. Molecular mechanisms of myocardial remodeling. Physiol Rev 1999;79:215–262.
102. Asakura M, Kitakaze M, Taskashima S, et al. Cardiac hypertrophy is inhibited by antagonism of ADAM12 processing of HB-EGF: Metalloproteinase inhibitors as a new therapy. Nature Med 2002;8:35–40.
103. Pachori AS, Numan MT, Ferrario CM, Diz DM, Raizada MK, Katovich MJ. Blood pressure-independent attenuation of cardiac hypertrophy by AT(1)R-AS gene therapy. Hypertension 2002;20:969–975.
104. Taigen T, Windt LJ, Lim HW, Molkentin JD. Targeted inhibition of calcineurin prevents agonist-induced cardiomyocyte hypertrophy. Proc Natl Acad Sci USA 2000;97:1196–1201.
105. Li Q, Li B, Wang X, et al. Overexpression of insulin-like growth factor-1 in mice protects from myocyte death after infarction, attenuating ventricular dilation, wall stress, and cardiac hypertrophy. J Clin Invest 1997;100:1991–1999.
106. Antos CL, McKinsey TA, Frey N, et al. Activated glycogen synthase kinase 3-β suppresses cardiac hypertrophy in vivo. Proc Natl Acad Sci USA 2002;99:907–912.
107. Nozato T, Ito H, Watanabe M, et al. Overexpression of Cdk inhibitor p16 by adenovirus vector inhibits cardiac hypertrophy in vitro and in vivo: a novel strategy for the gene therapy of cardiac hypertrophy. J Mol Cell Cardiol 2001;33:1493–1504.
108. Tamamori M, Ito H, Hiroe M, Terada Y, Marumo F, Ikeda M. Essential roles for G1 cyclin-dependent kinase activity in development of cardiomyocyte hypertrophy. Am J Physiol 1998;275:H2036–H2040.
109. Lin KF, Chao L, Chao J. Prolonged reduction of high blood pressure with human nitric oxide synthase delivery. Hypertension 1997;30:307–3113.
110. Lin KF, Chao J, Chao L. Atrial natriuretic peptide gene delivery attenuates hypertension, cardiac hypertrophy and renal injury in salt-sensitive rats. Hum Gene Ther 1998;9:1429–1438.
111. Yoshida H, Zhang JJ, Chao L, Chao J. Kallikrein gene delivery attenuates myocardial infarction and apoptosis after myocardial ischemia and reperfusion. Hypertension 2000;35:25–31.
112. Shi Q, Raffi S, Wu MH, et al. Evidence for circulating bone marrow derived endothelial cells. Blood 1998;92:362–367.

113. Asahara T, Masuda H, Takahashi T, et al. Bone marrow origin of endothelial progenitor cells responsible for postnatal vasculogenesis in physiological and pathological neovascularization Circ Res. 1999;85:221–228.

114. Shintani S, Murohara T, Ikeda H, et al. Augmentation of postnatal neovascularization with autologous bone marrow transplantation. Circulation 2001;103:897–903.

115. Kawamoto A, Gwon H-C, Iwaguro H, et al. Therapeutic potential of ex vivo expanded endothelial progenitor cells for myocardial ischemia. Circulation 2001;103:634–637.

116. Ikenaga S, Hamano K, Nishida M, et al. Autologous bone marrow implantation induced angiogenesis and improved deteriorated exdercise capacity in a rat ischemic hindlimb model. J Surg Res 2001;96:277–283.

117. Murohara T, Ikeda H, Duan J, et al. Transplanted chord blood-derived endothelial precursor cells augment postnatal neovascularization. J Clin Invest 2000;105:1527–1536.

118. Kalka C, Masuda H, Takahashi T, et al. Transplantation of ex vivo expanded endothelial progenitor cells foe therapeutic neovascularization. Proc Natl Acad Sci USA 2000;97:3422–3427.

119. Fuchs S, Baffour R, Zhou YF, et al. Transendocardial delivery of autologous bone marrow enhances collateral perfusion and regional function in pigs with chronic experimental myocardial ischemia. J Am Coll Cardiol 2001;37:1726–1732.

120. Vasa M, Fichtscherer S, Aicher A, et al. Number and migratory activity of circulating endothelial progenitor cells inversely correlate with risk factors for coronary artery disease. Circ Res 2001;89:E1–E7.

121. Dimmeler S, Aicher A, Vasa M, et al. HMG-CoA reductase inhibitors (statins) increase endothelial progenitor cells via the PI3-kinase/Akt pathway. J Clin Invest 2001;108:391–397.

122. Walter DH, Rittig K, Bahlmann FH, et al. Statin therapy accelerates reendothelialization: a novel effect involving mobilization and incorporation of bone marrow-derived endothelial progenitor cells. Circulation 2002;105:3017–3024.

123. Beltrami AP, Urbanek K, Kajstura J, et al. Evidence that human cardiac myocytes divide after myocardial infarction. New Engl J Med 2001;344:175–1757.

124. Soonpaa MH, Field L. Survey of studies examining mammalian cardiomyocyte DNA synthesis. Circ Res 1998;83:15–26.

125. Li F, Wang X, Capasso JM, Gerdes AM. Rapid transition of cardiac myocytes from hyperplasia to hypertrophy during postnatal development. J Mol Cell Cardiol 1996;28:1737–1746.

126. Reinlib L, Field L. Cell transplantation as future therapy for cardiovascular disease? Circulation 2000;101:e192–e197.

127. Taylor DA, Atkins BZ, Hungspreugs P, et al. Regenerating functional myocardium: improves performance after skeletal myoblast transplantation. Nat Med 1998;4:929–933.

128. Min JY, Yang Y, Converso KL, et al. Transplantation of embryonic stem cells improves cardiac function in postinfarcted rats. J Appl Physiol 2002;92:288–296.

129. Tomita S, Li RK, Weisel RD, et al. Autologous transplantation of bone marrow cells improves damaged heart function. Circulation 1999;100(Suppl):II247–II256.

130. Jiang Y, Jahagirdar BN, Reinhardt RL, et al. Pluripotency of mesenchymal stem cells derived from adult marrow. Nature 2002;418:41–49.

131. Hakuno D, Fukuda K, Makino S, et al. Bone marrow-derived regenerated cardiomyocytes (CMG cells) express functional adrenergic and muscarinic receptors. Circulation 2002;105:380–386.

132. Orlic D, Kajstura J, Chimenti S, et al. Bone marrow cells regenerate infarcted myocardium. Nature 2001;410:710–705.

133. Orlic D, Kajstura J, Chimenti S, et al. Mobilized bone marrow cells repair the infarcted heart, improving function and survival. Proc. Natl Acad Sci USA 2001;98:10,344–10,349.

134. Quaini F, Urbanek K, Beltrami AP, et al. Chimerism of the transplanted heart. N Engl J Med 2002;346:5–15.

135. Muller P, Pfeiffer P, Koglin J, et al. Cardiomyocytes of non cardiac origin in myocardial biopsies of human transplanted hearts Circulation 2002;106:31–35.

136. Taylor DA, Hruban R, Rodriguez R, Goldschmidt-Clermont PJ. Cardiac chimerism as a mechanism for self-repair. Does it happen and if so to what degree. Circulation 2002;106:2–4.

137. Laflamme MA, Myerson D, Saffitz JE, Murry CE. Evidence for cardiomyocyte repopulation by extracardiac progenitors in transplanted human hearts. Circ Res 2002;90:634–640.

138. Strauer BE, Brehm M, Zeus T, et al. Myocardial regeneration after intracoronary transplantation of human autologous stem cells following acute myocardial infarction. Dtsch Med Wochenschr 2001;126:932–938.

Gene Transfer and the Cardiovascular System

William H. Miller, PhD,
Stuart A. Nicklin, PhD,
Andrew H. Baker, PhD,
and Anna F. Dominiczak, PhD

CONTENTS

SUMMARY

The cardiovascular application of gene transfer and therapy has three overlapping goals. First, it can be seen as a molecular tool to probe pathways and mechanisms that are difficult to elucidate by other means. Second, it is widely used in preclinical studies and a variety of cardiovascular disease models to find the most efficient and safe clinical applications. Lastly, it is increasingly being used in clinical trial settings, for example to attenuate restenosis and vascular graft failure in coronary and peripheral vascular disease. We provide a critical overview of all three spheres of gene therapy-related strategies in cardiovascular disease research.

Key Words: Cardiovascular disease; gene therapy; adenovirus; AAV; targeting; vascular; tropism.

INTRODUCTION

A wide variety of cardiovascular pathologies are potentially amenable to treatment using gene therapy. Examples include myocardial ischemia, vein graft failure, atherosclerosis, hypercholesterolemia, peripheral ischemia, and hypertension. Gene transfer offers the potential for overexpression of candidate therapeutic genes in these conditions, with the ultimate aim of prevention, improvement, or regression of the condition.

From: *Contemporary Cardiology: Cardiovascular Genomics*
Edited by: M. K. Raizada, et al. © Humana Press Inc., Totowa, NJ

Gene therapy has two distinct modes of use. In monogenic disorders, in which a single mutated or absent gene has been identified as being causal, the aim of gene therapy would be to insert the corrected form of the gene into the appropriate target cell type to restore normal function. A number of monogenic cardiovascular diseases have been well documented, for example, in conditions such as hypertension *(1)* or hypercholesterolemia *(2)*. However, the majority of cardiovascular conditions are complex, polygenic disorders, in which environmental factors, such as diet, lifestyle, smoking, exercise, and so on also play a highly important role. In such conditions, elucidating causative genes is difficult. Therefore, the potential for gene therapy is not so much to replace malfunctioning genes in these disorders, but to offer an alternative or adjunct to conventional pharmacological approaches. Thus gene therapy may be aimed at manipulating molecular pathways that have been identified as being crucial in the pathogenesis of a disease—for example, the overexpression of antioxidant genes to combat vascular oxidative stress in hypertension.

Rapid progress has been made in gene therapy research in a number of fields, including cardiovascular disease, to the extent that a number of potential therapies are now undergoing extensive clinical trials. This has led to greater understanding of the requirements for optimal gene transfer, and it has become apparent that an idealized gene delivery system should meet a number of criteria. These include provision of efficient gene delivery, selectivity for the target tissue or cell type, nontoxicity and nonimmunogenicity, in vivo stability, and appropriate regulation of transgene expression in vivo, which may be inducible under pathophysiological conditions. Moreover, the desired vector system should be economical to construct and propagate to high titers, and possess targeting capabilities, thus allowing systemic administration directed at target tissues or show minimal dissemination after local application.

Although it is highly unlikely that any vector will ever meet all of these idealized criteria, a great deal of progress has been made toward attaining many of them. This chapter discusses the current strategies and vectors utilized for gene transfer studies and outlines the techniques used to tailor and specifically target these vectors for cardiovascular use, before describing some key cardiovascular disorders in which gene therapy research is becoming increasingly well characterized.

MODES OF TRANSGENE DELIVERY

The disparate diseases and conditions potentially amenable to gene therapy results in a number of differing approaches for delivery of gene transfer vectors, each with their own advantages and drawbacks. The main approaches for gene transfer used in current studies—cell-based gene transfer, local in vivo and ex vivo delivery, and systemic in vivo delivery—are outlined in this section.

Cell-Based Gene Transfer

In cell-based gene transfer, a patient's autologous cells are harvested, transduced in vitro with the appropriate vector, and reintroduced. As with other gene transfer methods, this approach offers both advantages and disadvantages. The use of autologous cells reduces the likelihood of immune responses. Furthermore, the in vitro phase of the procedure allows for the generation of a homogeneous population of transduced cells that can easily be assessed for transfection and expression efficiencies. However, the in vitro techniques utilized cause an unavoidable delay resulting from the harvest of the cells, genetic modification, screening, propagation, and reintroduction. Additionally, phenotypical changes in cells can occur during culture, the harvest and implantation steps each require individual invasive techniques, and the implantation step may in itself result in damage to the target site. Taken together, these drawbacks may underlie the relative paucity of clinical studies based on this approach. Nonetheless, cell-based gene transfer has been successfully used in a rodent model of vascular injury *(3)* and a murine model of hypercholesterolemia and atherosclerosis *(4)*. Moreover, a pilot study utilizing cell-based gene transfer of the low-density lipoprotein (LDL) receptor in humans found a significant reduction in total cholesterol levels in individuals who have familial hypercholesterolemia *(5)*. Thus it may be the case that further optimization of the techniques involved in cell-based genetic modification may yet result in more widespread use of this approach as a gene therapy tool.

Localized Gene Transfer

Ex Vivo Delivery

Gene transfer to tissue ex vivo offers an almost idealized approach to gene therapy, as it allows transduction of the target tissue in an isolated manner, making manipulation and access easier, while also circumventing potential problems caused by systemic leakage of the vector. The ready access of the target tissue makes this approach useful in combination with any of the vectors outlined below in the section titled "Vectors for Cardiovascular Gene Therapy." Clinical applications of this approach are limited to those in which the target tissue is accessible. It has been predominantly investigated in gene therapy for coronary artery bypass vein graft failure *(6–9)*. During the coronary artery bypass procedure there is a window of opportunity following harvest of the vein that allows for direct transduction ex vivo, prior to the grafting of the vein to the aorta. Thus, gene therapy vectors can be applied directly to the graft tissue in a manner that avoids systemic administration, and at a lower total dose. A number of candidate transgenes have shown promise in this area, and are discussed in the section titled "Application of Gene Transfer to Cardiovascular Disease."

In Vivo Delivery

The inaccessibility of most target sites for ex vivo gene transfer, coupled with a need for refinement of systemic gene delivery approaches, has led to the development of local in vivo gene transfer strategies. Such techniques generally rely on the use of modified intravascular delivery catheters or impregnated stents. These are initially introduced at a distal site before being advanced to the target area prior to transgene or vector infusion, or deployment of the stent. A number of specialized devices are now available for this purpose, and have been the subject of review *(10)*. Studies of coronary vessels in both animal models *(11)* and in humans *(12)* indicate that, with further refinement, localized gene delivery may hold promise as a means to improve longevity and patency of both stent and bypass approaches to coronary artery disease.

Systemic In Vivo Gene Transfer

Systemic administration of gene transfer vectors in vivo offers an idealized approach toward the treatment of a number of cardiovascular conditions. Optimization of this approach would potentially allow infusion of a targeted vector into a peripheral vessel, representing a minimally invasive approach, which may also result in less accessible target tissues (e.g., the pulmonary vasculature) becoming amenable to gene therapy.

However, a key characteristic of systemically infused vectors is their high level of sequestration and destruction by the liver. This has been demonstrated for a number of systems, including adenovirus *(13,14)*, adeno-associated virus (AAV) *(15)*, lentivirus *(16)*, and liposomes *(17)*. This dramatically limits systemic administration of gene therapy vectors for use in cardiovascular disease. A great deal of effort is currently being devoted to modifying the natural tropism of viral vectors to circumvent this problem (*see* Section entitled "Targeted Gene Transfer"). However, even in the absence of vector modification, it is still possible to utilize the liver as a "factory" for transgene production if the gene product is soluble and can be secreted into the bloodstream to exert an effect at an extrahepatic site. It is also possible to utilize the hepatic tropism to direct gene transfer to the liver *per se*, with the aim of modifying lipid metabolism *(18)*.

VECTORS FOR CARDIOVASCULAR GENE THERAPY

Whereas a variety of diseases are potentially suitable targets for gene therapy, most cell types resist the uptake of foreign DNA. This has lead to the development of various vehicles or vectors, each with advantages and disadvantages, in order to facilitate efficient gene transfer (Table 1).

Adenovirus

In cardiovascular research, the adenovirus serotype 5 (Ad5) is the most commonly studied and best characterized of the gene transfer vectors. Deletion of the *E1* and *E3* viral genes has produced a replication deficient system, which generates transgene expression in an episomal manner. Ad5 allows packaging of a relatively large transgene (up to 36kb in helper-dependent adenoviral vectors) and can be propagated to high titers using straightforward methods. Furthermore, adenovirus can infect both dividing and non-dividing cells. The ability to transfect vascular cells, coupled with high efficiency of gene transfer, positions adenovirus as a strong candidate vector for cardiovascular gene therapy. It has been demonstrated that adenovirus can transduce up to 100% of endothelial cells in vitro *(19–21)*, however, this is lower in vivo, reflecting the high tropism for hepatic tissue of adenoviruses *(13)*. Administration of higher doses of adenoviral vector does not improve the therapeutic potential of this system, but instead leads to toxic effects *(22)*. A further limitation to the use of adenoviral vectors is the relatively transient nature of gene expression. Trans-activation of viral genes can result in "leaky" expression, instigating a cytotoxic T-lymphocyte mediated response against infected cells. However, recent studies using "gutless" vectors *(18,23)* in which the coding sequences for viral structural proteins have been deleted, suggest that it possible to overcome this problem and produce stable, long-term expression.

Adeno-Associated Virus

In contrast with the nonintegrating adenovirus, AAV can integrate into the host genome at a specific position on chromosome 19 *(24)*. For specific integration to occur, the *rep* protein must be present—integration otherwise occurs semirandomly, with a preference for active genes *(25)*. Chromosomal integration may help to promote long-term transgene expression, a key advantage over other vector systems, such as adenovirus, although recent studies now suggest that virally-mediated, long-term expression mainly occurs from episomal vectors *(26,27)*. AAV is a human parvovirus, which can be stripped of all viral coding sequences, allowing inserts of up to 4.5 kb to be packaged. AAV is a

Table 1
Characteristics of Common Gene Transfer Vectors

Technique	Advantages	Disadvantages
Adenovirus	Broad tropism	Broad tropism
	Only infects nonreplicating cells	Transient expression limits applicability
	Relatively large cloning capacity	Can invoke immune and inflammatory responses
	High levels of transgene expression	
	Transient expression increases safety	
	Can be grown to high titers	
	Amenable to retargeting techniques	
Adeno-associated virus	Integration into host genome at specific site	Possible removal and dissemination of vector after wild-type adenovirus infection
	No immune responses	Cloning capacity is limited to 5 kb
	Infects dividing and nondividing cells	
	Can be grown to high titers	
Retrovirus	Integration into host genome offers longevity of transgene expression	Integration can be random
	Hold relatively large DNA inserts	Only infect replicating cells
		Difficult to propagate to high titer
Naked DNA	Nonpathogenic and easy to construct	Very low efficiency
	Can deliver large DNA constructs	
Liposomes	Can hold large inserts	Low efficiency in comparison to viral gene transfer
	Can be used in wide range of cells	Nonspecific targeting
	Nonpathogenic	

179

replication-deficient system—lytic infection of host cells requires coinfection with a helper virus, such as adenovirus or herpes simplex virus type I. Greater than 90% of the human population is thought to be infected with AAV, although this infection is asymptomatic in nature. These features—stable and long-term transgene expression and low levels of immunogenicity—position AAV as a promising vector system for cardiovascular gene therapy. Two obvious disadvantages in using AAV as a vector for gene transfer, in comparison with others, such as adenovirus, are the relatively small size of insert (4.5 kb) and the markedly reduced efficiency of transduction of vascular tissue. However, it has been shown that AAV can transduce primary cultures of both endothelial and vascular smooth muscle cells from a number of mammalian species, including human *(28)*. The same study further reported in vivo transduction of primate carotid arteries. Moreover, transgene expression in excess of 18 mo has been shown using AAV *(29)*, whereas AAV-mediated gene transfer restored normal heart function and increased life expectancy in a hamster model of congenic cardiomyopathy *(30)*. Delivery of vascular endothelial growth factor (VEGF) using AAV has shown benefit in animal models of ischemia *(31)*. Moreover, clinical trials of AAV-mediated gene therapy for cystic fibrosis are underway *(32)*, while initial studies of AAV-2 mediated gene therapy for hemophilia B in man *(33)* have so far demonstrated the safety profile of this vector. Although development of this approach in the setting of common cardiovascular diseases in humans lags a little behind, longevity of expression coupled with the ability to deliver potentially therapeutic genes in a low-toxicity manner would suggest that AAV will continue to attract attention as a potential gene therapy vector in this field.

Retroviruses

The retroviruses were the first group of viral vectors to be studied for the purposes of gene transfer, starting in the mid-1980s. Research into this class of vector continues, because of their chromosomal integration (resulting in long-term transgene expression) and high efficiency of gene transfer. However, a number of factors limit the applicability of these vectors. First, they are difficult to grow to sufficiently high titers that are required for systemic in vivo administration. Second, chromosomal integration occurs randomly, presenting the possibility of mutational events occurring. The requirement that the host cells be replicating for efficient infection to occur *(34)* further limits the use of these vectors in vascular tissue, as normal vascular smooth muscle cells divide only once in a lifetime. The main application of retrovirus has been in ex vivo transduction of cells prior to reimplantation *(3)*. However, the recent development of leukemia in patients treated for severe combined immunodeficiency disease using retrovirally-mediated transduction of bone marrow cells, through insertion of retroviral DNA into the LMO2 proto-oncogene, led to the halting of clinical trials using this vector *(35)*. Currently, trials using retrovirus are continuing on a case-by-case basis. Ultimately, the future of this vector platform (as with other interventions) will depend on the balance between benefit and risk

The retrovirus-derived lentivirus, which *can* infect nondividing cells, has shown promise in a number of cardiovascular studies in animal models and has been demonstrated to transfer therapeutic genes into human tissue *(36)*, although clinical trials using this vector have not yet been undertaken. Although concerns exist about the use of HIV-derived lentivirus *(37)*, further development of this vector, e.g., through retargeting strategies to alter tropism *(38)* and potentially improve biosafety, may lead to its more widespread use in cardiovascular research.

Nonviral

Whereas the focus of much of the current research into gene transfer relies on refinement of virally based vectors, a good deal of progress has also been made utilizing nonviral vectors. Indeed, of ongoing cardiovascular gene therapy trials in 2001, just under half used either naked plasmid DNA or liposomal carriers.

The most simple of the nonviral approaches is the direct injection of naked DNA into the target site, or into a site such as skeletal muscle if the intended target is inaccessible. The latter of these methods requires that the gene product be secreted, non-toxic, and easily transported via the blood stream. A variation of this method utilizes a balloon catheter that has been coated with the plasmid DNA to deliver it to the required vascular site. More recently, it has been shown that ultrasound can dramatically enhance the efficiency of transfection of naked DNA to vascular smooth muscle cells and endothelial cells in culture *(39,40)*, and to rat carotid arteries in vivo *(41)*. Liposomal carriers have also been shown to improve transfection efficiency of plasmid DNA *(42)*; however, such systems are at least 20-fold less efficient than viral vectors, such as adenovirus.

A key advantage of the use of nonviral delivery is the reduction in the likelihood of immune responses or toxic effects, which can be seen after administration of viral vectors. However, the relatively low efficiency of gene transfer, further compounded by a lack of nuclear targeting, represents a significant disadvantage in comparison with viral vectors. Despite such drawbacks, transfer of naked plasmid DNA and liposome-mediated transfer have proved promising in a number of studies, for example, of vascular balloon injury *(43)* and ischemia *(44)*. In particular, clinical trials utilizing the ex vivo hydrodynamic transfer of decoy oligonucleotides against the cell cycle transcription factor E2F have shown benefit in vein graft occlusion *(6)*, resulting in fewer graft occlusions, revisions, or critical stenoses at a 12-mo time point. Indeed, so promising are the results from these initial trials that E2F decoy is currently being evaluated in two ongoing phase III trials, PREVENT III, and PREVENT IV.

TARGETED GENE TRANSFER

Although relatively more efficient than other vector systems in terms of vascular gene transfer, the natural tropism for adenovirus has been shown to be the liver and spleen in rodent and primate models *(14)* and the lung in porcine studies *(45)* following systemic administration. Thus, there is a need for efficient vascular gene transfer that does not result in high levels of transgene expression in nontarget tissues. Strategies for retargeting of adenoviral, AAV, and other vectors have been developed, forming the basis of a vast body of ongoing research in this field. Optimal targeting of vectors would enable the lowering of the total dose of vector used, thus improving safety profiles, whereas at the same time improving transductional efficiency in the target tissue. The techniques outlined in this section will focus on Ad5 and AAV-2, the most widely characterized systems.

Targeting of Adenoviral Vectors

The process of infection of the Ad5 serotype has been well documented (*see* Fig. 1), and occurs as a two-stage process. In the first phase, attachment to the host cell occurs via an interaction between the knob domain of the capsid fiber and the Coxsackie–adenovirus receptor (CAR) *(46,47)*. Following this, internalization occurs via the activation of $\alpha_v\beta_3$ or $\alpha_v\beta_5$ integrins by the penton base of the adenoviral capsid *(48,49)*. Dechecchi et al. showed that Ad5 binding could be inhibited by the presence of heparin, suggesting the

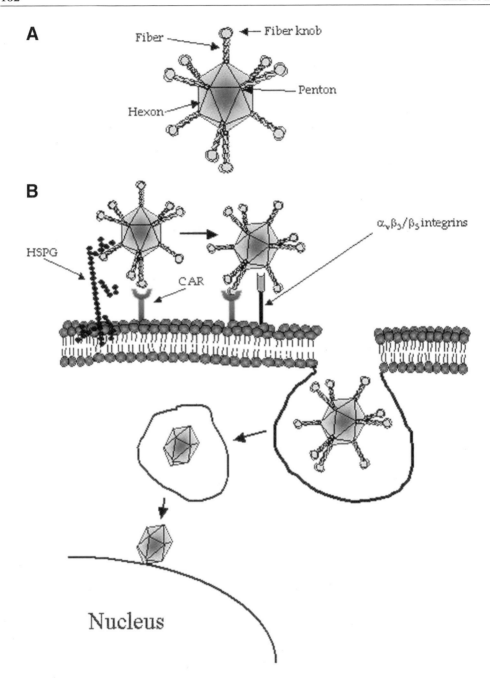

Fig. 1. Ad5 structure and infection route. **(A)** Ad5 has an icosahedral capsid consisting of three main proteins: the fiber, penton base, and hexon, which protects the viral core. **(B)** Ad5 tethers to the cell surface primarily via interaction of the fiber knob domain with Coxsackie–adenovirus receptor and is then internalized through activation of α_v integrins by the RGD motif in penton base. Recent data has also demonstrated a role for the Ad5 fiber shaft binding heparin sulphate proteoglycans at the cell surface. The virion then triggers endosomal lysis and trafficks to the nucleus, where it delivers its genome for episomal maintenance. Ad5, adenovirus serotype 5; CAR, Coxsackie–adenovirus receptor; HSPG, heparan sulfate proteoglycans.

presence of a heparan sulphate proteoglycan binding domain *(50)*. More recently, this domain has been defined and localized to the fiber shaft, and its importance in liver transduction demonstrated *(51)*. Thus, strategies aimed at modifying targeting of Ad5 vectors can do so via either ablation or modification of the binding regions within these domains. Such transductional retargeting can be carried out at a genetic or nongenetic level by altering either the coding sequences for structural proteins of the virus or by direct modification of the adenoviral capsid *per se*. Furthermore, retargeting at a transcriptional level via the incorporation of cell-specific promoters to drive transgene expression in target tissues may only further enhance the effects of transductional targeting.

NONGENETIC RETARGETING OF ADENOVIRAL VECTORS

Nongenetic retargeting usually relies on the use of antigen-binding fragments (Fab), single-chain antibody variable fragments (scFv)/fusion protein constructs, or bispecific antibodies to neutralize the binding domain on the Ad5 knob protein. For example, a bispecific antibody was designed that bound to and neutralized the knob domain of the Ad fiber while simultaneously redirecting it to E-selectin, producing a 300-fold increase in transduction of tumor necrosis factor (TNF)-α-activated porcine endothelium, relative to nontargeted vector *(52)*. Further refinement of this approach has seen the fusion of specific novel targeting peptides (isolated using random phage display *[53]*) to scFv fragments, resulting in 15-fold increases in transduction of human endothelial cells *(54)*. The same approach has been used to increase transduction of endothelial cells using preexisting markers, such as endoglin *(55)*. The use of bispecific antibodies is potentially extremely powerful. Systemic administration of Ad5 vectors preincubated with a bispecific antibody with affinity for both the Ad5 capsid and angiotensin-converting enzyme (which is expressed at relatively high levels in the pulmonary vasculature) produced a 20-fold increase in transduction levels in rat lung, with an 80% decrease in hepatic transgene expression *(56)*. The effect was further enhanced in subsequent experiments in which this transductional targeting approach was combined with transcriptional targeting, using the endothelial-specific promoter *fms*-like tyrosine kinase (FLT)-1 *(57,58)*. A key set of experiments based on this system by Reynolds et al. resulted in the first study to successfully combine transductional and transcriptional targeting *(58; see also* Fig. 2), one of the most significant demonstrations of detargeting and retargeting approaches. The combination of the endothelial-specific FLT-1 promoter and lung-specific targeting of the adenovirus resulted in a 300,000-fold increase in lung:liver targeting ratio following systemic administration in rats. Whereas this system offers great potential in pulmonary pathologies *per se*, it further acts as striking proof of the concept and potential of dual transductional/transcriptional strategies. These findings suggest that the "holy grail" of a systemically injectable, specifically targeted gene transfer vector may well be tangible, and indeed further study is underway to utilize this system to deliver potentially therapeutic genes (*see* section titled "Hypertension").

GENETIC RETARGETING OF ADENOVIRAL VECTORS

A further refinement of transductional retargeting of adenoviral vectors has been the introduction of genetic modification to the capsid. Such single-component systems may offer a number of distinct advantages over the binary systems described previously, in terms of manufacture and quality control. Genetic retargeting strategies are based around the direct insertion of modified ligands (increasingly novel peptide sequences derived from biopanning of random phage libraries), pseudotyping (in which an element of the

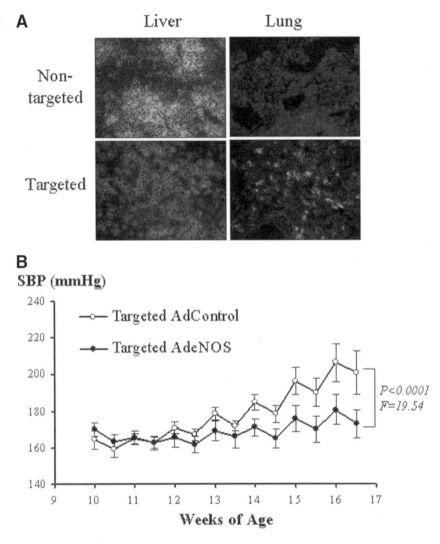

Fig. 2. Retargeting of adenovirus tropism in vivo. (**A**) Combined transductional and transcriptional targeting of Ad5. Retargeting was carried out by using a bispecific antibody, to direct the vector to the pulmonary vasculature, and FLT-1, an endothelium-specific promoter. Systemic infusion of retargeted reporter vector in rats resulted in a significant shift in the ratio of lung:liver transgene expression, visible as bright immunofluorescence *(58)*. (**B**) Using the same bispecific antibody system, systemic in vivo infusion at 11 wk of age of a targeted AdeNOS vector resulted in a significant and sustained reduction in systolic blood pressure relative to a similarly targeted control vector in the stroke prone spontaneously hypertensive rat (unpublished data from our group). AdeNOS, adenovirus-encoding endothelial nitric oxide synthase; SBP, systolic blood pressure.

viral capsid is replaced by a corresponding element of a different serotype), or genetic ablation of native tropism by disruption of ligand binding motifs. These techniques are often used in varying combinations with each other.

PSEUDOTYPING

In pseudotyping, the main approach has been to replace the Ad5 fiber shaft or knob domain with that of another serotype that does not bind to CAR. Studies utilizing this method have shown improved gene transfer to endothelial cells, vascular smooth muscle cells, and blood vessels ex vivo *(59–61)* using particular pseudotyped Ad5 variants. It has also been noted that interspecies differences exist in transduction levels produced by pseudotyped vectors *(62)*, suggesting differences in biodistribution of receptors for these modified viruses across species and providing a note of caution as to the extrapolation of results from animal studies to human disease.

RETARGETING BY TROPISM ABLATION AND LIGAND INSERTION

The majority of studies aimed at incorporation of retargeting ligands now utilize a structural feature of the fiber protein, known as the HI loop *(63)*, as a point of insertion. This loop is not important in maturation of the virus or in molecular interactions of the fiber with other domains *(64)*, and has been demonstrated to be amenable to targeting peptide insertion in a number of studies. Many of these studies have utilized incorporation into the HI loop of the integrin-binding arginine–glycine–aspartate (RGD)–4C motif, originally isolated by in vivo phage display *(65)*. This results in enhanced transduction of a number of cell and tissue types, including endothelial cells *(66)* and rabbit jugular vein grafts *(67)*. Incorporation of the RGD motif into the hexon base of the Ad5 capsid produced a significantly increased level of transduction of human vascular smooth muscle cells *(68)*. However, despite markedly more efficient gene transfer in vectors engineered to incorporate the RGD motif, a key limitation of this system is a lack of selectivity. This has led to the development of vectors engineered to include specific targeting sequences (typically identified using biopanning of random phage libraries) in the HI loop. This has been shown to be successful in a number of studies *(69–72)*. In particular, it has been demonstrated that it is feasible to incorporate retargeting peptides, as well as mutations aimed at ablation of the natural tropism of the vector, resulting in selective and efficient transgene delivery into vascular endothelial cells *(71*; *see also* Fig. 3) and vascular smooth muscle cells *(70)* in vitro.

Intriguingly, the in vivo profile of modified vectors can be complex, often showing increased transgene expression in target tissues but unaltered natural tropism (i.e., high levels of hepatocyte transduction), in contrast with in vitro studies *(72–74)*. Thus, it appears that yet further elucidation of the molecular basis for Ad5 binding and internalization is required in order to significantly ablate liver uptake and facilitate cardiovascular-specific targeting of this vector following systemic administration.

Targeting of AAV

Although fewer targeting strategies based on the AAV system are reported in the literature, parallel advances to those in Ad5 retargeting are being developed. Long-term expression and the ability to transduce nondividing cells makes the AAV-2 platform an attractive option for gene therapy in a number of particular pathologies. This is despite a significantly decreased ability, relative to adenovirus, to transduce endothelial cells, which are a key target in cardiovascular disease *(36)*. The development of pseudotyping strategies or the adoption of alternative serotypes may eventually prove fruitful methods by which to retarget AAV-2. This observation is based in part on the range of different AAV serotypes, many of which exhibit variations in tropism *(75)*. However, determination of the binding characteristics and infection pathways of these individual serotypes has yet to be described in detail, limiting the applicability of this approach. Some studies have begun to unravel this complexity of tropism in individual isoforms, demonstrating for example enhanced transduction of human endothelial and vascular smooth muscle

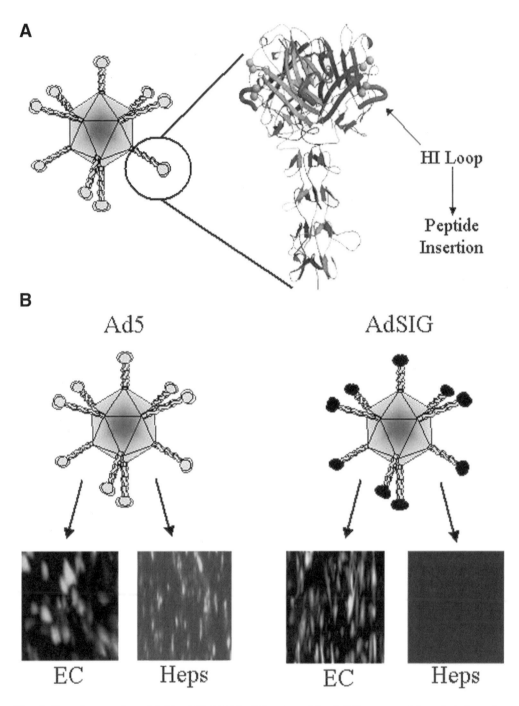

Fig. 3. Genetic targeting of Ad5 to EC. **(A)** Modification of the Ad fiber was achieved via insertion of the peptide SIGYPLP into the HI loop in combination with two amino acid substitutions in the fiber AB loop to ablate fiber: Coxsackie-adenovirus receptor interaction creating AdSIG*(71)*. **(B)** Transduction of EC and hepatocytes (Heps) by AdSIG in comparison to Ad5. Viruses express enhanced green fluorescent protein as a reporter gene. Image of Ad5 fiber crystal structure courtesy of Vijay Reddy, The Scripps Research Institute, CA. Ad5, adenovirus serotype5.

cells in AAV-2 relative to AAV-3, -4, -5, and -6 *(36)*. Further elucidation of the native tropism of these isoforms may eventually lead to the identification of serotypes specific for particular target cells.

Genetic modification of the AAV-2 capsid has also been described in the literature, and offers promise in the specific targeting of this vector. Since the identification of a site at position 587 on the AAV-2 capsid by Girod *(76)*, which is optimal for the insertion of targeting peptides, this approach has been demonstrated to successfully enable targeting to a range of cell types, including human vascular endothelial *(77)* and smooth muscle *(70)* cells. The publication of the crystal structure of AAV-2 *(78)* has already led to the identification of a heparan-binding motif that contributes to cell binding *(79)*. Subsequent studies seem likely to reveal further specific capsid epitopes and potential sites for modification of AAV-2 tropism.

APPLICATION OF GENE TRANSFER TO CARDIOVASCULAR DISEASE

A wide variety of cardiovascular pathologies are potential targets for gene therapy intervention. The majority of cardiovascular gene therapy studies are still based on preclinical models, although a number of clinical trials have begun to show promise. Some of the most frequently studied and clinically important cardiovascular diseases and gene therapy strategies aimed at overcoming them are outlined in this section.

Hypertension

Primary systemic hypertension is a chronic elevation of blood pressure that is thought to be the result of interplay between polygenic and numerous environmental factors. Hypertension is a well established risk factor for secondary conditions, such as stroke, atherosclerosis, peripheral vascular disease, cardiac failure, and others *(1)*. Although current pharmacological interventions are able to offer effective blood pressure control, such treatments are relatively short-acting, have a propensity for side effects, and rely heavily on good patient compliance for optimum benefit. In practice, these problems can mean that hypertension is often poorly controlled. Thus, gene therapy for the various features of hypertension has become increasingly explored as an alternative or adjunct to established pharmacological approaches.

The role of the renin-angiotensin system and its relationship with vascular oxidative stress have become well characterized features in the pathophysiology of hypertension. For example, it is now well established that reduced nitric oxide bioavailability and increased superoxide levels (via the actions of NADPH oxidase and uncoupled endothelial nitric oxide synthase [eNOS], among others) may underlie the vascular dysfunction that is a prominent feature of both human hypertension and animal models of the disease *(80–82)*. Thus, various elements of this system are potential targets for gene transfer intervention and form the basis for the majority of gene therapy studies in relation to hypertension *(83)*. However, probably resulting in part from the multifactorial nature of hypertension, clinical study of gene therapy for this condition has yet to be undertaken. Nonetheless, increasing experimental studies have shown much promise in this area. For example, it has been shown that local in vivo administration of adenoviral vectors encoding either eNOS (*see* Fig. 4) or extracellular superoxide dismutase (EC-SOD) can improve nitric oxide bioavailability and vascular function in the stroke-prone, spontaneously hypertensive rat (SHRSP) model *(84,85)*. Similarly, eNOS overexpression was able to

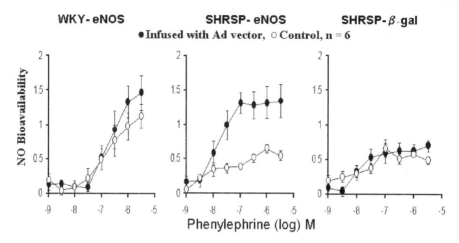

Fig. 4. Improving vascular function in hypertensive rats using gene transfer. Adenoviral vectors encoding for endothelial nitric oxide synthase (eNOS) or the control reporter gene, β-galactosidase, were infused locally in vivo into the carotid artery of spontaneously hypertensive rat, stroke prone (SHRSP), or the normotensive reference strain, Wistar Kyoto (WKY). Basal nitric oxide (NO) bioavailability was determined as a function of the difference in contractile responses to phenylephrine in the presence and absence of the NOS inhibitor L-NAME. Overexpression of eNOS, but not β-galactosidase, in the carotid artery of SHRSP caused a significant augmentation in basal NO bioavailability, to levels comparable to the normotensive WKY strain. (Adapted from ref. *85.*)

restore endothelial function in aortic rings in a model of angiotensin II-induced hypertension *(86)*. Encouraging systemic hypotensive effects of gene transfer have also been demonstrated. For example, AdeNOS delivery into the rostral ventral medulla significantly lowered blood pressure in the spontaneously hypertensive rat (SHR) strain, as well as in the normotensive Wistar Kyoto strain *(87)*. Intramuscular injection of adenoviral vector encoding tissue kallikrein inhibited the normal developmental increase in spontaneously hypertensive rat (SHR) blood pressure for a period of 5 wk *(88)*, whereas infusion of naked human eNOS plasmid DNA reduced blood pressure for 6 wk in rats *(89)*. More recently, systemic administration of AdEC-SOD was shown to significantly lower blood pressure in the SHR *(90)*. Intriguingly, a heparin-binding domain-deleted version of this transgene—which should in theory produce a secreted product that is able to have more widely disseminated effects—did not affect blood pressure in this latter study, showing that further understanding of the molecular activity of putative therapeutic agents may be required. Recent work from our own group has shown that systemic administration of a retargeted adenovirus expressing eNOS (based on the previous work of Reynolds and others *[56–58]*) can lower systolic blood pressure in the SHR, stroke prone model (*see* Fig. 2). A more novel approach has been the use of AAV-mediated delivery of antisense angiotensin 1 receptor into cardiac tissue of SHR, producing a reduction in blood pressure of 30 mmHg *(91)*. As the fine details of the molecular pathways involved in maintaining vascular function become increasingly well defined, so the number of potential gene therapy targets increases *(92)*. For example, it has recently been demonstrated that gene transfer of human guanosine 5'-triphosphate cyclohydrolase I, which is the initial and rate-limiting step in the generation of the essential eNOS cofactor tetrahydrobiopterin, can correct vascular superoxide levels in a rat model of hypertension *(93)*. Furthermore, the identification of putative candidate genes involved in the development of hypertension using congenic breeding strategies and gene microarray techniques *(94)* has been the subject of recent studies, and is now beginning to prove fruitful *(95)*. Further characterization of such candidates will present further targets for hypertension gene therapy.

Late Vein Graft Failure

Coronary artery bypass grafting (CABG) is a procedure that successfully alleviates angina pectoris and increases life expectancy in patients with coronary artery disease. However, the vein graft undergoes adaptive responses to transplantation into the arterial circulation, with early thrombus formation occurring in 10% of grafts, and patency dropping to 50% at 10 yr postprocedure. Vein graft failure is associated with progressive intimal thickening, atheroma development, and neointima formation *(96)*, with associated affects on morbidity and mortality after CABG. Drug treatments (typically antiplatelet agents) can slow and reduce this process, but can be associated with hemorrhagic events. However, vein grafting is particularly amenable to gene transfer, as the vein graft itself is isolated and able to undergo genetic modification during the surgical procedure. This concept was demonstrated clearly in a clinical trial in which vein grafts transduced during the procedure with vectors expressing decoy oligodeoxynucleotides against the transcription factor E2F showed significantly reduced postoperative occlusion *(6)*. While research into E2F decoy administration continues, the majority of transgenes investigated in other studies have been chosen for their antiproliferative, antiinflammatory, proapoptotic, or antimigratory agents *(97)*.

A key component in the remodeling of the failing vessel is the migration and proliferation of smooth muscle cells, a feature partly determined by the activity of the matrix metalloproteinases. Adenovirally mediated overexpression of the endogenous tissue inhibitors of MMPs has shown beneficial effects, such as reduction of neointima and inhibition of lesion development in a number of studies of vein graft failure, including porcine in vivo and human ex vivo models *(7–9)*. Other transgenes that have shown promise include nitric oxide synthase *(98)*, p53 *(99)*, retinoblastoma gene product *(100)* and natriuretic peptide *(101)*. The majority of these studies have examined endpoints measured in days or weeks, although significantly reduced neointima and increased vessel patency at 3 mo was recently demonstrated in a porcine model following adenovirally mediated p53 overexpression *(102)*. However, the long-term nature of vein graft failure requires gene therapy capable of producing long-lasting effects, a feature that remains to be fully demonstrated in this setting.

Hypercholesterolemia and Atherosclerosis

Familial hypercholesterolemia is caused by the absence of or a defect in the LDL receptor. This results in an inability to clear LDL from the bloodstream, leading to severe hypercholesterolemia and accelerated atherosclerosis. Various models of this condition have been studied. Gene transfer of the corrected LDL receptor has been shown to be beneficial in both murine and human studies *(5,103–106)*. Furthermore, it has been shown that delivery of the very low-density lipoprotein (VLDL) receptor (using modified helper-dependent adenoviral vectors) into the LDL receptor-deficient mouse model *(107)* could produce sustained lipid-lowering effects for up to 6 mo. Even more promising, in an *ApoE*-deficient mouse model, delivery of the *ApoE* gene using a helper-dependent adenoviral vector *(18)* resulted in decreased serum lipid concentrations and virtually complete absence of aortic lesions for the lifetime of the animals (approx 2.5 yr). This was in contrast with complete coverage of control aortae by atherosclerotic plaque. Although such studies are very encouraging (and indeed also highlight the choice of appropriate vector), it remains to be determined how these findings may relate to the clinical situation, where atherosclerotic plaque development may already be well advanced before treatment is commenced.

The multifactorial nature of the development of atherosclerosis, and in particular the inextricable interaction between environmental and genetic factors, make utilization of gene therapy approaches a difficult challenge. This may underlie, in part, the relatively few successful studies of gene therapy approaches as an intervention for established atherosclerosis, with many studies instead focusing on primary conditions, such as hypercholesterolemia. It has been suggested that low gene-transfer efficiency across atherosclerotic plaques and atheroma may be as a result of the high level of connective tissue and the low number of transducible cells (108). Nonetheless, there are reports of potentially beneficial results utilizing gene transfer for expression of a number of proteins involved in lipid metabolism, including apolipoprotein AI, lecithin-cholesterol acyltransferase (109), and heme oxygenase (110).

Ischemic Disease and Reperfusion Injury

Ischemic disease can affect both the peripheral and coronary circulations, and is manifest as reduced blood flow resulting from the presence of thrombus, atherosclerotic plaque, or vascular spasm. This has the effect of starving tissues distal to the narrowing of oxygen and other nutrients. Although surgical bypass and angioplasty are able to provide symptomatic relief, this tends to be temporary in nature and is not suitable for all patients. Thus, the only long-term solution in some cases may ultimately be the amputation of affected limbs or heart transplantation. Gene therapy may therefore offer a promising alternative for treatment of these conditions (111,112). Most studies in this area have focused on delivery of VEGF and fibroblast growth factor (FGF), two angiogenic growth factors, to the ischemic areas. Furthermore, because VEGF is a secreted protein, its physiological effect may extend beyond transduced cells, reducing the requirement to transduce as many cells as possible.

Intramuscular injection of adenoviral (113) and AAV (31) vectors expressing VEGF has been shown to induce angiogenesis, improve peripheral blood flow, and also be protective in animal models of limb ischemia. Furthermore, adenovirally mediated delivery of VEGF was shown to improve endothelial function and lower extremity blood flow in humans with peripheral artery disease (114). Similar effects have been observed in ischemic heart disease in humans—for example, alleviation of angina and angiographic improvement of vessel narrowing—following direct myocardial injection of VEGF vectors (115). Clinical trials of adenoviral delivery of FGF-4 improved patient exercise tolerance, with an absence of adverse effects (116) and increased myocardial perfusion, while reducing ischemic defect size (117).

Although these preclinical and early clinical studies of gene therapy for ischemia show promise, concerns still exist over the safety of overexpression of angiogenic factors, such as VEGF. For example, it has been suggested that VEGF may enhance the development of atherosclerosis (118), stimulate the generation of dysfunctional vessels (119), and promote formation of vascular tumours (120). More recently, it has been shown that the microenvironment concentration of VEGF, rather than the overall dose, is of extreme importance in determining whether its effects are normal or abberant *(121)*. Specific targeting of vectors and tight regulation of transgene expression, therefore, seem necessary to further improve the safety profile of these vectors. Following an ischemic episode, reperfusion of the myocardium can itself lead to further injury of the ischemic zone, in a process that has been shown to involve oxidative stress. Gene therapy strategies utilizing expression of antioxidants and other agents, including superoxide dismutase *(122)* and heme oxygenase *(123)*, have shown promise in animal models. Refinement of such approaches to include a myocardium-specific promoter and a hypoxia-regulatory element (to switch on transgene expression only under hypoxic conditions), has also been described *(124)*.

CONCLUSIONS

The past decade has seen an explosion in gene therapy studies, and it is now clear that this field offers promise in terms of new approaches to molecular medicine. Application of gene transfer as an approach to cardiovascular disease is a complex matter, because of the multifactorial nature of such diseases. It is therefore clear that further elucidation of the pathophysiology of cardiovascular diseases, and thus identification of key molecular genetic targets, coupled with the further development of safe, efficient, targeted gene transfer vectors, are key requirements. Further development of methods of gene suppression, such as antisense technology and RNA interference, and their incorporation into gene therapy vectors will offer an alternative to overexpression as a means of intervention. Progress in these areas will ultimately determine if the promise shown in both laboratory studies of gene therapy and in initial clinical trials is to translate into a standard therapeutic approach for cardiovascular disease.

REFERENCES

1. Staessen JA, Wang J, Bianchi G, Birkenhager WH. Essential hypertension. Lancet 2003;361:1629–1641.
2. Rader DJ, Cohen J, Hobbs HH. Monogenic hypercholesterolemia: new insights in pathogenesis and treatment. J Clin Invest 2003;111:1795–1803.
3. Forough R, Koyama N, Hasenstab D, et al. Overexpression of tissue inhibitor of matrix metalloproteinase-1 inhibits vascular smooth muscle cell functions in vitro and in vivo. Circ Res 1996;79:812–820.
4. Cioffi L, Sturtz FG, Wittmer S, et al. A novel endothelial cell-based gene therapy platform for the in vivo delivery of apolipoprotein E. Gene Ther 1999;6,1153–1159.
5. Grossman M, Rader DJ, Muller DW, et al. A pilot study of ex vivo gene therapy for homozygous familial hypercholesterolaemia. Nat Med 1995;1:1148–1154.
6. Mann MJ, Whittemore AD, Donaldson MC, et al. *Ex-vivo* gene therapy of human vascular bypass grafts with E2F decoy: the PREVENT single-centre randomised, controlled trial. Lancet 1999;354:1493–1498.
7. Hu T, Baker AH, Zou Y, Newby AC, Xu Q. Local gene transfer of tissue inhibitor of metalloproteinase-2 influences vein graft remodeling in a mouse model. Arterioscler Thromb Vasc Biol 2001;21:1275–1280.
8. George SJ, Lloyd CT, Angelini GD, Newby AC, Baker AH. Inhibition of late vein graft neointima formation in human and porcine models by adenovirus-mediated overexpression of tissue inhibitor of metalloproteinase-3. Circulation 2000;101:296–304.
9. George SJ, Johnson JL, Angelini GD, Newby AC, Baker AH. Adenovirus-mediated gene transfer of the human TIMP-1 gene inhibits smooth muscle cell migration and neointimal formation in human saphenous vein. Hum Gene Ther 1998;9:867–877.
10. Yla-Herttuala S, Martin JF. Cardiovascular gene therapy. Lancet 2000;355:213–222.
11. Pancetta CJ, Miyauchi K, Berry D, et al. A tissue-engineered stent for cell-based vascular gene transfer. Hum Gene Ther 2002;13:433–441.

12. Baim DS, Wahr D, George B, et al. Randomized trial of a distal embolic protection device during percutaneous intervention of saphenous vein aorto-coronary bypass grafts. Circulation 2002;105:1285–1290.

13. Tao N, Gao GP, Parr M, et al. Sequestration of adenoviral vector by Kupffer cells leads to a nonlinear dose response of transduction in liver. Mol Ther 2001;3:28–35.

14. Huard J, Lochmuller H, Acsadi G, Jani A, Massie B, Karpati G. The route of administration is a major determinant of the transduction efficiency of rat tissues by adenoviral recombinants. Gene Ther 1995;2:107–115.

15. Koeberl DD, Alexander IE, Halbert CL, Russell DW, Miller AD. Persistent expression of human clotting factor IX from mouse liver after intravenous injection of adeno-associated virus vectors. Proc Natl Acad Sci USA 1997;94:1426–1431.

16. Ohashi K, Park F, Kay MA. Role of hepatocyte derived hyperplasia in lentivirus-mediated liver transduction in vivo. Hum Gene Ther 2002;13:653–663.

17. Kamps JAAM, Morslet HWM, Swart PJ, Meijer DKF, Scherphof GL. Massive targeting of liposomes, surface modified with anionized albumins, to hepatic endothelial cells. Proc Natl Acad Sci USA 1997;94:11,681–11,685.

18. Kim I, Jozkowicz A, Piedra PA, Oka K, Chan L. Lifetime correction of genetic deficiency in mice with a single injection of helper-dependent adenoviral vector. Proc Natl Acad Sci USA 2001;98:13,282–13,287.

19. Merrick AF, Shewring LD, Sawyer GJ, Gustafsson KT, Fabre JW. Comparison of adenovirus gene transfer to vascular endothelial cells in cell culture, organ culture, and in vivo. Transplantation 1996;62:1085–1089.

20. Lemarchand P, Jaffe HA, Danel C, et al. Adenovirus-mediated transfer of a recombinant human alpha 1-antitrypsin cDNA to human endothelial cells. Proc Natl Acad Sci USA 1992;89:6482–6486.

21. Lemarchand P, Jones M, Yamada I, Crystal RG. In vivo gene transfer and expression in normal uninjured blood vessels using replication-deficient recombinant adenovirus vectors. Circ Res 1993;72:1132–1138.

22. Channon KM, Qian H, Youngblood S A, et al. Acute host-mediated endothelial injury after adenoviral gene transfer in normal rabbit arteries: impact on transgene expression and endothelial function. Circ Res 1998;82:1253–1262.

23. Kochanek S, Clemens PR, Mitani K, Chen HH, Chan S, Caskey CT. A new adenoviral vector: replacement of all viral coding sequences with 28 kb of DNA independently expressing both full-length dystrophin and beta-galactosidase. Proc Natl Acad Sci USA 1996;93:5731–5736.

24. Kotin RM, Siniscalco M, Samulski RJ, et al. Site-specific integration by adeno-associated virus. Proc Natl Acad Sci USA 1990;87:2211–2215.

25. Nakai H, Montini E, Fuess S, Storm TA, Grompe M, Kay MA. AAV serotype 2 vectors preferentially integrate into active genes in mice. Nat Genet 2003;34:297–302.

26. Kreppel F, Kochanek S. Long-term transgene expression in proliferating cells mediated by episomally maintained high-capacity adenovirus vectors. J Virol 2004;78:9–22.

27. Ehrhardt A, Xu H, Kay MA. Episomal persistence of recombinant adenoviral vector genomes during the cell cycle in vivo. J Virol 2003;77:7689–7695.

28. Lynch CM, Hara PS, Leonard JC, Williams JK, Dean RH, Geary RL. Adeno-associated virus vectors for vascular gene delivery. Circ Res 1997;80:497–505.

29. Xiao X, Li J, Samulski RJ. Efficient long-term gene transfer into mouse tissue of immunocompetent mice by adeno-associated virus vector. J Virol 1996;70:8098–8108

30. Kawada T, Nakazawa M, Nakauchi S, et al. Rescue of hereditary form of dilated cardiomyopathy by rAAV-mediated somatic gene therapy: amelioration of morphological findings, sarcolemmal permeability, cardiac performances, and the prognosis of TO-2 hamsters. Proc Natl Acad Sci USA 2002;99:901–906.

31. Shimpo M, Ikeda U, Maeda Y, et al. AAV-mediated VEGF gene transfer into skeletal muscle stimulates angiogenesis and improves blood flow in a rat hindlimb ischemia model. Cardiovasc Res 2002;53:993–1001.

32. Wagner JA, Nepomuceno IB, Messner AH, et al. A phase II, double-blind, randomized, placebo-controlled clinical trial of tgAAVCF using maxillary sinus delivery in patients with cystic fibrosis with antrostomies. Hum Gene Ther 2002;13:1349–1359.

33. Manno CS, Chew AJ, Hutchison S, et al. AAV-mediated factor IX gene transfer to skeletal muscle in patients with severe hemophilia B. Blood 2003;101:2963–2972.

34. Miller DG, Adam MA, Miller AD. Gene transfer by retrovirus vectors occurs only in cells that are actively replicating at the time of infection. Mol Cell Biol 1990;10:4239–4242.
35. Hacein-Bey-Abina S, Von Kalle C, Schmidt M, et al. LMO2-associated clonal T cell proliferation in two patients after gene therapy for SCID-X1. Science 2003;302:415–419.
36. Dishart KL, Denby L, George SJ, et al. Third-generation lentivirus vectors efficiently transduce and phenotypically modify vascular cells: implications for gene therapy. J Mol Cell Cardiol 2003;35:739–748.
37. Roy I. Ethical considerations in the use of lentiviral vectors for genetic transfer. Somat Cell Mol Genet 2001;26:175–191.
38. Sandrin V, Russell SJ, Cosset FL. Targeting retroviral and lentiviral vectors. Curr Top Microbiol Immunol 2003;281:137–178.
39. Lawrie A, Brisken AF, Francis SE, et al. Ultrasound enhances reporter gene expression after transfection of vascular cells in vitro. Circulation 1999;99:2617–2620.
40. Lawrie A, Brisken AF, Francis SE, et al. Microbubble-enhanced ultrasound for vascular gene delivery. Gene Ther 2000;7:2023–2027.
41. Taniyama Y, Tachibana K, Hiraoka K, et al. Local delivery of plasmid DNA into rat carotid artery using ultrasound. Circulation 2002;105:1233–1239.
42. Stephan DJ, Yang ZY, San H, et al. A new cationic liposome DNA complex enhances the efficiency of arterial gene transfer in vivo. Hum Gene Ther 1996;7:1803–1812.
43. Asahara T, Chen D, Tsurumi Y, et al. Accelerated restitution of endothelial integrity and endothelium-dependent function after phVEGF$_{165}$ gene transfer. Circulation 1996;94:3291–3302.
44. Tsurumi Y, Takeshita S, Chen D, et al. Direct intramuscular gene transfer of naked DNA encoding vascular endothelial growth factor augments collateral development and tissue perfusion. Circulation 1996;94:3281–3290.
45. Hackett NR, El Sawy T, Lee LY, et al. Use of quantitative TaqMan real-time PCR to track the time-dependent distribution of gene transfer vectors in vivo. Mol Ther 2000;2:649–656.
46. Bergelson JM, Cunningham JA, Droguett G, et al. Isolation of a common receptor for Coxsackie B viruses and adenoviruses 2 and 5. Science 1997;275:1320–1323.
47. Tomko RP, Xu R, Philipson L. HCAR and MCAR: the human and mouse cellular receptors for subgroup C adenoviruses and group B coxsackieviruses. Proc Natl Acad Sci USA 1997;94:3352–3356.
48. Wickham TJ, Mathias P, Cheresh DA, Nemerow GR. Integrins alpha v beta 3 and alpha v beta 5 promote adenovirus internalization but not virus attachment. Cell 1993;73:309–319.
49. Wickham TJ, Filardo EJ, Cheresh DA, Nemerow GR. Integrin alpha v beta 5 selectively promotes adenovirus mediated cell membrane permeabilization. J Cell Biol 1994;127:257–264.
50. Dechecchi MC, Tamanini A, Bonizzato A, Cabrini G. Heparan sulfate glycosaminoglycans are involved in adenovirus type 5 and 2-host cell interactions. Virology 2000;268:382–390.
51. Smith TA, Idamakanti N, Rollence ML, et al. Adenovirus serotype 5 fiber shaft influences in vivo gene transfer in mice. Hum Gene Ther 2003;14:777–787.
52. Harari OA, Wickham TJ, Stocker CJ, et al. Targeting an adenoviral gene vector to cytokine-activated vascular endothelium via E-selectin. Gene Ther 1999;6:801–807.
53. Watkins SJ, Mesyanzhinov VV, Kurochkina LP, Hawkins RE. The 'adenobody' approach to viral targeting: specific and enhanced adenoviral gene delivery. Gene Ther 1997;4:1004–1012.
54. Nicklin SA, White SJ, Watkins SJ, Hawkins RE, Baker AH. Selective targeting of gene transfer to vascular endothelial cells by use of peptides isolated by phage display. Circulation 2000;102:231–237.
55. Nettelbeck DM, Miller DW, Jerome V, et al. Targeting of adenovirus to endothelial cells by a bispecific single-chain diabody directed against the adenovirus fiber knob domain and human endoglin (CD105). Mol Ther 2001;3:882–891.
56. Reynolds PN, Zinn KR, Gavrilyuk VD, et al. A targetable, injectable adenoviral vector for selective gene delivery to pulmonary endothelium in vivo. Mol Ther 2000;2:562–578.
57. Nicklin SA, Reynolds PN, Brosnan MJ, et al. Analysis of cell-specific promoters for viral gene therapy targeted at the vascular endothelium. Hypertension 2001;38:65–70.
58. Reynolds PN, Nicklin SA, Kaliberova L, et al. Combined transductional and transcriptional targeting improves the specificity of transgene expression in vivo. Nat Biotechnol 2001;19:838–842.
59. Su EJ, Stevenson SC, Rollence M, Marshall-Neff J, Liau G. A genetically modified adenoviral vector exhibits enhanced gene transfer of human smooth muscle cells. J Vasc Res 2001;38:471–478.
60. Havenga MJ, Lemckert AA, Grimbergen JM, et al. Improved adenovirus vectors for infection of cardiovascular tissues. J Virol 2001;75:3335–3342.
61. Chillon M, Bosch A, Zabner J, et al. Group D adenoviruses infect primary central nervous system cells more efficiently than those from Group C. J Virol 1999;73:2537–2540.

62. Havenga MJ, Lemckert AA, Ophorst OJ, et al. Exploiting the natural diversity in adenovirus tropism for therapy and prevention of disease. J Virol 2002;76:4612–4620.

63. Xia D, Henry L, Gerard RD, Deisenhofer J. Structure of the receptor binding domain of adenovirus type 5 fiber protein. Curr Top Microbiol Immunol 1995;199:39–46.

64. Krasnykh V, Dmitriev I, Mikheeva G, Miller CR, Belousova N, Curiel DT. Characterization of an adenovirus vector containing a heterologous peptide epitope in the HI loop of the fiber knob. J Virol 1998;72:1844–1852.

65. Pasqualini R, Koivunen E, Ruoslahti E. A peptide isolated from phage display libraries is a structural and functional mimic of an RGD-binding site on integrins. J Cell Biol 1995;130:1189–1196.

66. Dmitriev I, Krasnykh V, Miller CR, et al. An adenovirus vector with genetically modified fibers demonstrates expanded tropism via utilization of a coxsackievirus and adenovirus receptor-independent cell entry mechanism. J Virol 1998; 72:9706–9713.

67. Hay CM, De Leon H, Jafari JD, et al. Enhanced gene transfer to rabbit jugular veins by an adenovirus containing a cyclic RGD motif in the HI loop of the fiber knob. J Vasc Res 2001;38:315–323.

68. Vigne E, Mahfouz I, Dedieu JF, Brie A, Perricaudet M, Yeh P. RGD inclusion in the hexon monomer provides adenovirus type 5-based vectors with a fiber knob-independent pathway for infection. J Virol 1999;73:5156–5161.

69. Xia H, Anderson B, Mao Q, Davidson BL. Recombinant human adenovirus: targeting to the human transferrin receptor improves gene transfer to brain microcapillary endothelium. J Virol 2000;74:11,359–11,366.

70. Work LM, Nicklin SA, Brain NJ, et al. Development of efficient viral vectors selective for vascular smooth muscle cells. Mol Ther 2004;9:198–208.

71. Nicklin SA, Von Seggern DJ, Work LM, Pek DC, Dominiczak AF, Nemerow GR, Baker AH. Ablating adenovirus type 5 fiber-CAR binding and HI loop insertion of the SIGYPLP peptide generate an endothelial cell-selective adenovirus. Mol Ther 2001;4:534–542.

72. Nicklin SA, White SJ, Nicol CG, Von Seggern DJ, Baker AH. In vitro and in vivo characterisation of endothelial cell selective adenoviral vectors. J Gene Med 2004;6:300–308.

73. Leissner P, Legrand V, Schlesinger Y, et al. Influence of adenoviral fiber mutations on viral encapsidation, infectivity and in vivo tropism. Gene Ther 2001;8:49–57.

74. Alemany R, Curiel DT. CAR-binding ablation does not change biodistribution and toxicity of adenoviral vectors. Gene Ther 2001;8:1347–1353.

75. Gao GP, Alvira MR, Wang L, Calcedo R, Johnston J, Wilson JM. Novel adeno-associated viruses from rhesus monkeys as vectors for human gene therapy. Proc Natl Acad Sci USA 2002;99:11,854–11,859.

76. Girod A, Ried M, Wobus C, et al. Genetic capsid modifications allow efficient re-targeting of adeno-associated virus type 2. Nat Med 1999;5:1052–1056.

77. Nicklin SA, Buening H, Dishart KL, et al. Efficient and selective AAV2-mediated gene transfer directed to human vascular endothelial cells. Mol Ther 2001;4:174–181.

78. Xie Q, Bu W, Bhatia S, et al. The atomic structure of adeno-associated virus (AAV-2), a vector for human gene therapy. Proc Natl Acad Sci USA 2002;99:10,405–10,410.

79. Kern A, Schmidt K, Leder C, et al. Identification of a heparin-binding motif on adeno-associated virus type 2 capsids. J Virol 2003;77:11,072–11,081.

80. Channon KM, Guzik TJ. Mechanisms of superoxide production in human blood vessels: relationship to endothelial dysfunction, clinical and genetic risk factors. J Physiol Pharmacol 2002;53:515–524.

81. Kerr S, Brosnan MJ, McIntyre M, Reid JL, Dominiczak AF, Hamilton CA. Superoxide anion production is increased in a model of genetic hypertension: role of the endothelium. Hypertension 1999;33:1353–1358.

82. Berry C, Hamilton CA, Brosnan MJ, et al. Investigation into the sources of superoxide in human blood vessels: angiotensin II increases superoxide production in human internal mammary arteries. Circulation 2000;101:2206–2212.

83. Hamilton CA, Miller WH, Al-Benna S, et al. Strategies to reduce oxidative stress in cardiovascular disease. Clin Sci (Lond) 2004;106:219–234.

84. Alexander MY, Brosnan MJ, Hamilton CA, et al. Gene transfer of endothelial nitric oxide synthase but not Cu/Zn superoxide dismutase restores nitric oxide availability in the SHRSP. Cardiovasc Res 2000;47:609–617.

85. Fennell JP, Brosnan MJ, Frater AJ,. Adenovirus-mediated overexpression of extracellular superoxide dismutase improves endothelial dysfunction in a rat model of hypertension. Gene Ther 2002;9:110–117

86. Nakane H, Miller FJ, Faraci FM, Toyoda K, Heistad DD. Gene transfer of endothelial nitric oxide synthase reduces angiotensin II-induced endothelial dysfunction. Hypertension 2000;35:595–601

87. Kishi T, Hirooka Y, Ito K, Sakai K, Shimokawa G, Takeshita A. Cardiovascular effects of overexpression of endothelial nitric oxide synthase in the rostral ventrolateral medulla in stroke-prone spontaneously hypertensive rats. Hypertension 2002;39:264–268.
88. Zhang JJ, Wang C, Lin KF, Chao L, Chao J. Human tissue kallikrein attenuates hypertension and secretes into circulation and urine after intramuscular gene delivery in hypertensive rats. Clin Exp Hypertens 1999;21:1145–1160.
89. Lin KF, Chao L, Chao J. Prolonged reduction of high blood pressure with human nitric oxide synthase gene delivery. Hypertension 1997;30:307–313.
90. Chu Y, Iida S, Lund DD, et al. Gene transfer of extracellular superoxide dismutase reduces arterial pressure in spontaneously hypertensive rats: role of heparin-binding domain. Circ Res 2003;92:461–468.
91. Phillips MI, Mohuczy D, Coffey M, et al. Prolonged reduction of high blood pressure with an in vivo, nonpathogenic, adeno-associated viral vector delivery of AT1-R mRNA antisense. Hypertension 1997;29:374–380
92. Dominiczak AF, Negrin DC, Clark JS, Brosnan MJ, McBride MW, Alexander MY. Genes and hypertension: from gene mapping in experimental models to vascular gene transfer strategies. Hypertension 2000;35:164–172.
93. Zheng JS, Yang XQ, Lookingland KJ, et al. Gene transfer of human guanosine 5'-triphosphate cyclohydrolase I restores vascular tetrahydrobiopterin level and endothelial function in low rennin hypertension. Circulation 2003;108:1238–1245.
94. Lee WK, Padmanabhan S, Dominiczak AF. Genetics of hypertension: from experimental models to clinical applications. J Hum Hypertens 2000;14:631–647.
95. McBride MW, Carr FJ, Graham D, et al. Microarray analysis of rat chromosome 2 congenic strains. Hypertension 2003;41:847–853.
96. Baker AH, Mehta D, George SJ, Angelini GD. Prevention of vein graft failure: potential applications for gene therapy. Cardiovasc Res 1997;35:442–450.
97. Kibbe MR, Billiar TR, Tzeng E. Gene therapy for restenosis. Circ Res 2000;86:829–833.
98. West NEJ, Qian H, Guzik TJ, et al. Nitric oxide synthase (nNOS) gene transfer modifies venous bypass graft remodeling. Effects on vascular smooth muscle cell differentiation and superoxide production. Circulation 2001;104:1526–2532.
99. George SJ, Angelini GS, Capogrossi MC, Baker AH. Wild-type p53 gene transfer inhibits neointima formation in human saphenous vein by modulation of smooth muscle cell migration and induction of apoptosis. Gene Ther 2001;8:668–676.
100. Schwartz LB, Moawad J, Svensson EC, et al. Adenoviral-mediated gene transfer of a constitutively active form of the retinoblastoma gene product attenuates neointimal thickening in experimental vein grafts. J Vasc Surg 1999;29:874–881.
101. Ohno N, Itoh H, Ikeda T, et al. Accelerated reendothelialization with suppressed thrombogenic property and neointimal hyperplasia of rabbit jugular vein grafts by adenovirus-mediated gene transfer of C-type natriuretic peptide. Circulation 2002;105:1623–1626.
102. Wan S, George SJ, Nicklin SA, Yim APC, Baker AH. Overexpression of p53 increases lumen size and blocks neointima formation in porcine interposition vein grafts. Mol Ther 2004;9:689–698.
103. Herz J, Gerard RD. Adenovirus-mediated transfer of low density lipoprotein receptor gene acutely accelerates cholesterol clearance in normal mice. Proc Natl Acad Sci USA 1993;90:2812–2816.
104. Kozarsky KF, Jooss K, Donahee M, Strauss JF 3rd, Wilson JM. Effective treatment of familial hypercholesterolaemia in the mouse model using adenovirus-mediated transfer of the VLDL receptor gene. Nat Genet 1996;13:54–62.
105. Stevenson SC, Marshall-Neff J, Teng B, Lee CB, Roy S, McClelland A. Phenotypic correction of hypercholesterolemia in apoE-deficient mice by adenovirus-mediated in vivo gene transfer. Arterioscler Thromb Vasc Biol 1995;15:479–84.
106. Grossman M, Raper SE, Kozarsky K, et al. Successful ex vivo gene therapy directed to liver in a patient with familial hypercholesterolaemia. Nat Genet 1994;6:335–341.
107. Oka K, Pastore L, Kim IH, Merched A, Nomura S, Lee HJ, Merched-Sauvage M, Arden-Riley C, Lee B, Finegold M, Beaudet A, Chan L. Long-term stable correction of low-density lipoprotein receptor-deficient mice with a helper-dependent adenoviral vector expressing the very low-density lipoprotein receptor. Circulation 2001;103:1274–1281.
108. Laitinen M, Makinen K, Manninen H, et al. Adenovirus-mediated gene transfer to lower limb artery of patients with chronic critical leg ischemia. Hum Gene Ther 1998;9:1481–1486.
109. Fan L, Drew J, Dunckley MG, Owen JS, Dickson G. Efficient coexpression and secretion of anti-atherogenic human apolipoprotein AI and lecithin-cholesterol acyltransferase by cultured muscle cells using adeno-associated virus plasmid vectors. Gene Ther 1998;5:1434–1440.

110. Juan SH, Lee TS, Tseng KW, et al. Adenovirus-mediated heme oxygenase-1 gene transfer inhibits the development of atherosclerosis in apolipoprotein E-deficient mice. Circulation 2001;104:1519–1525.
111. Losordo DW, Vale PR, Symes JF, et al. Gene therapy for myocardial angiogenesis—initial clinical results with direct myocardial injection of phVEGF(165) as sole therapy for myocardial ischaemia. Circulation 1998;98:2800–2804.
112. Baumgartner I, Pieczek A, Manor O, et al. Constitutive expression of phVEGF$_{165}$ after intramuscular gene transfer promotes collateral vessel development in patients with critical limb ischemia. Circulation 1998;97:1114–1123.
113. Gowdak LHW, Poliakova L, Wang X, et al. Adenovirus-mediated VEGF$_{121}$ gene transfer stimulates angiogenesis in normoperfused skeletal muscle and preserves tissue perfusion after induction of ischemia. Circulation 2000;102:565–571.
114. Rajagopalan S, Shah M, Luciano A, Crystal R, Nabel EG. Adenovirus-mediated gene transfer of VEGF$_{121}$ improves lower-extremity endothelial function and flow reserve. Circulation 2001;104:753–755.
115. Rosengart TK, Lee LY, Patel SR, et al. Angiogenesis gene therapy. Phase I assessment of direct intramyocardial administration of an adenovirus vector expressing VEGF121 cDNA to individuals with clinically significant severe coronary artery disease. Circulation 1999;100:468–474.
116. Grines CL, Watkins MW, Helmer G, et al. Angiogenic gene therapy (AGENT) trial in patients with stable angina pectoris. Circulation 2002;105:1291–1297.
117. Grines CL, Watkins MW, Mahmarian JJ, et al., Angiogene GENe Therapy (AGENT-2) Study Group. A randomized, double-blind, placebo-controlled trial of Ad5FGF-4 gene therapy and its effect on myocardial perfusion in patients with stable angina. J Am Coll Cardiol 2003;42:1339–1347.
118. Celletti, FL, Waugh JM, Amabile PG, Brendolan A, Hilfiker PR, Dake MD. Vascular endothelial growth factor enhances atherosclerotic plaque progression. Nat Med 2001;7:425–429.
119. Springer ML, Chen AS, Kraft PE, Bednarski M, Blau HM. VEGF gene delivery to muscle: potential role for vasculogenesis in adults. Mol Cell 1998;2:549–548.
120. Lee RJ, Springer ML, Blanco-Bose WE, Shaw R, Ursell PC, Blau HM. VEGF gene delivery to myocardium. Deleterious effects of unregulated expression. Circulation 2000;102:898–901.
121. Ozawa CR, Banfi A, Glazer NL, et al. Microenvironmental VEGF concentration, not total dose, determines a threshold between normal and aberrant angiogenesis. J Clin Invest 2004;113:516–527.
122. Wheeler MD, Katuna M, Smutney OM, et al. Comparison of the effect of adenoviral delivery of three superoxide dismutase genes against hepatic ischaemia-reperfusion injury. Hum Gene Ther 2001;12:2167–2177.
123. Melo LG, Agrawal R, Zhang LN, et al. Gene therapy strategy for long-term myocardial protection using adeno-associated virus-mediated delivery of heme oxygenase gene. Circulation 2002;105:602–607.
124. Phillips MI, Tang Y, Schmidt-Ott K, Qian KP, Kagiyama S. Vigilant vector: heart-specific promoter in an adeno-associated virus vector for cardioprotection. Hypertension 2002;39:651–655.

11

Kallikrein Gene Transfer in Hypertension, Cardiovascular and Renal Disease, and Stroke

Julie Chao, PhD and Lee Chao, PhD

CONTENTS

From: *Contemporary Cardiology: Cardiovascular Genomics*
Edited by: M. K. Raizada, et al. © Humana Press Inc., Totowa, NJ

SUMMARY

Tissue kallikrein cleaves low-molecular-weight kininogen substrate to produce the potent vasodilator kinin peptide, which binds to kinin receptors and triggers a wide spectrum of biological effects. Tissue kallikrein levels are reduced in humans and animal models with hypertension and cardiovascular and renal disease. We investigated the role of the tissue kallikrein–kinin system in the cardiovascular, renal, and central nervous systems by systemic and local delivery of the human tissue kallikrein gene using a plasmid DNA or an adenovirus vector. Enhanced kallikrein/kinin levels following kallikrein gene transfer reduce blood pressure in several pressure- and volume-overload hypertensive animal models. Kallikrein gene transfer also exerts beneficial effects in protection against cardiac remodeling, renal fibrosis, restenosis, cerebral infarction, and neurological deficits. The improvement in cardiovascular, renal, and neurological function following kallikrein gene transfer is independent of kallikrein's ability to lower blood pressure. Kallikrein gene transfer has pleiotropic effects on apoptosis, inflammation, proliferation, hypertrophy, fibrosis, and angiogenesis in the heart, blood vessel, kidney, and brain. These effects are blocked by icatibant, a bradykinin B2 receptor antagonist, indicating a kinin-mediated event. Mechanistically, kallikrein gene transfer leads to increased nitric oxide (NO) levels and decreased oxidative stress and inflammatory response. These novel findings indicate that kallikrein/kinin, through NO formation, may act as an antioxidant and anti-inflammatory agent in protection against cardiovascular and renal disease in animal models, and may uncover new drug targets for the prevention and treatment of heart failure, end-stage renal disease, and stroke in humans.

Key Words: Tissue kallkrein; kinin; gene therapy; hypertension; oxidative stress; heart; kidney; blood vessel; brain.

THE TISSUE KALLIKREIN–KININ SYSTEM COMPONENTS

Tissue kallikreins (E.C. 3.4.21.35) belong to a subgroup of serine proteinases that process kininogen substrates and release vasoactive kinin peptides (1). The well-recognized function of tissue kallikrein is mediated by lysyl-bradykinin (Lys-BK or kallidin) and bradykinin (BK), which consist of 10 and 9 amino acid peptides, respectively. Kinins are then degraded by enzymes, such as kininases I and II and neutral endopeptidase to produce a number of kinin metabolites or inactive fragments. Intact kinins bind to BK B2 receptors, whereas kinin metabolites, such as Des-Arg^9-BK or Des-Arg^{10}-Lys-BK, bind to BK B1 receptors. The physiological functions of the tissue kallikrein–kinin system (KKS) are mediated by the constitutively expressed B2 receptor. Unlike the B2 receptor, the B1 receptor is expressed at low levels in the heart, vasculature, and kidney and is induced by trauma or inflammation (2). The binding of kinins to their respective receptors activates second messengers, such as nitric oxide (NO), cyclic adenosine monophosphate (cAMP), prostacyclin, and cyclic guanosine monophosphate (cGMP), which trigger a broad spectrum of biological effects including vasodilation, smooth muscle contraction and relaxation, inflammation, and pain (3,4).

Regulation of the KKS exists through system-specific inhibitors, kininases, and antagonists, as well as through a kininase shared with the renin–angiotensin system (RAS) (Fig. 1). The KKS can be blocked by tissue kallikrein inhibitors (kallistatin or aprotinin), icatibant (Hoe 140, a specific B2 receptor antagonist), or Des-Arg^9-[Leu^8]BK (a specific B1 receptor antagonist) (1,3). Kallistatin is a serine proteinase inhibitor (serpin) that forms a covalently linked complex with tissue kallikrein, resulting in inhibition of tissue kallikrein activity (5–7). The KKS and RAS are linked by angiotensin-converting enzyme (ACE), a dipeptidase, which is the same enzyme as kininase II. ACE has dual

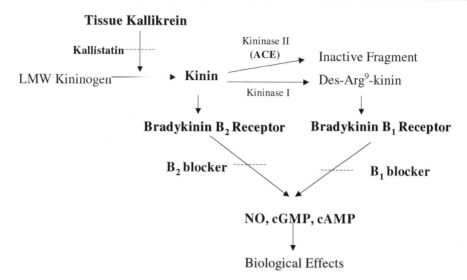

Fig. 1. The tissue kallikrein–kinin system. ACE, angiotensin-converting enzyme; LMW, low-molecular-weight; NO, nitric oxide; cGMP, cyclic guanosine monophosphate; cAMP, cyclic adenosine monophosphate.

functions: it not only converts angiotensin I to vasoconstrictor peptide angiotensin II (Ang II), but also degrades kinin to release a dipeptide fragment, Phe-Arg, from the carboxyl end of the kinin peptide, rendering kinin inactive. Therefore, the beneficial effects of ACE inhibition in hypertension and cardiovascular and renal disease can also be attributed to kinin accumulation, as icatibant can partially abolish these effects (8–10). Thus, the vasodilator action of the KKS can counter-regulate the vasoconstrictive action of the RAS.

TISSUE KALLIKREIN IN HYPERTENSION

Hypertension is a major disease that affects approx 25% of the population in the United States. African Americans are more likely to develop salt-sensitive hypertension. A previous study suggested that 50–75% of the hypertensive population demonstrates salt sensitivity, as blood pressure can be altered in response to changes in dietary salt intake (11). Moreover, hypertensive individuals are more likely to develop other cardiovascular and renal disorders, such as peripheral vascular disease, coronary heart disease, congestive heart failure, and renal disease. Hypertension could result from either an excess of vasoconstrictor substances or a deficiency in vasodilator substances. Abnormality of renal kallikrein levels has long been documented in the pathogenesis of hypertension (12,13). Epidemiological studies have identified an inverse relationship between urinary or renal kallikrein levels and blood pressure in patients with essential hypertension (14–16). Because urinary kallikrein originates in the kidney, reduced urinary kallikrein levels would suggest impaired renal function. An association between reduced excretion of kallikrein and human hypertension has been reported both in Caucasian and African-American individuals (13–15). It has been shown that the influence of both race and dietary sodium intake upon kallikrein excretion in hypertensive patients is greater than that of normotensive individuals (13–15). Furthermore, a study aimed at identifying genetic factors associated with cardiovascular risks using highly informative family pedigrees indicated that a dominant gene expressed as renal or urinary kallikrein may be associated with a reduced risk of hypertension *(16)*. This finding suggests that high urinary kallikrein may have a protective effect against the development of high blood pressure.

Reduced urinary kallikrein excretion has also been described in a number of genetically hypertensive rat models such as spontaneously hypertensive rats (SHR), New Zealand rats, Fawn-Hooded rats, and Dahl salt-sensitive (DSS) hypertensive rats *(17–21)*. Kinin appears to play a role in blood pressure regulation in SHR fed a salt-deficient diet, because the administration of a BK antagonist caused an increase in blood pressure *(22)*. Furthermore, kininogen-deficient (Brown Norway–Katholiek) rats, which cannot generate kinin, are susceptible to the development of salt-induced hypertension *(23)*. Several restriction fragment length polymorphisms have been mapped in the rat tissue kallikrein gene, and their regulatory regions have been identified in the SHR model *(24)*. These findings indicate a possible difference in the tissue kallikrein gene locus between SHR and normotensive Wistar–Kyoto rats. Moreover, a tissue kallikrein RFLP has been shown to cosegregate with high blood pressure in the F2 offspring of SHR and normotensive Brown Norway–Katholiek crosses *(25)*, suggesting a close linkage between the kallikrein gene locus and the hypertensive phenotype in SHR.

We have shown that transgenic mice and rats overexpressing human tissue kallikrein were permanently hypotensive throughout their lifetime compared with their control littermates *(26–29)*. Administration of aprotinin or icatibant to the transgenic mice raised their blood pressures to normal levels *(26,27)*. These results indicate that the expression of functional human tissue kallikrein can permanently alter the blood pressure setting in the transgenic animals, and that the effect is mediated by the BK B2 receptor. This conclusion is further reinforced by a study showing that transgenic mice overexpressing human BK B2 receptor are hypotensive when compared with their control littermates *(30)*. Moreover, ablation of the B2 receptor gene in mice causes salt-sensitive hypertension *(31)*. Taken together, these findings provide the first direct evidence demonstrating the role of the KKS in blood pressure regulation in vivo and lend support to the hypothesis that elevated levels of tissue kallikrein may offer a protective effect in preventing the development of hypertension and cardiovascular and renal complications.

SOMATIC GENE DELIVERY OF TISSUE KALLIKREIN IN HYPERTENSIVE ANIMAL MODELS

One strategy to study the potential role of kallikrein/kinin in hypertension is via protein or gene delivery. Oral administration of purified pig pancreatic kallikrein has been used to temporarily lower the blood pressure of hypertensive patients *(32,33)*. This hypotensive effect requires repeated administrations of the enzyme, and the antihypertensive effect disappears shortly after the treatment is discontinued *(32,33)*. Somatic gene delivery results in continuous expression of the gene of interest for an extended period of time, and is a potential therapeutic tool in treating cardiovascular and renal disease. To investigate the impact of supplying tissue kallikrein by gene delivery, we generated a series of human tissue kallikrein gene constructs under the control of the metallothionein metal response element, the albumin promoter, the Rous sarcoma virus 3' long terminal repeat, or the cytomegalovirus (CMV) promoter *(28)*. Injection of these plasmid cDNA constructs into SHR caused a prolonged reduction of systemic blood pressure for several weeks *(34–36)*. The extent of blood pressure reduction was dependent on the dose of DNA injected, the gender of the animals, the promoter used in the gene construct, and the route of injection *(34–36)*.

To achieve high-efficiency expression of tissue kallikrein in animal models, a transgene expression cassette containing the human tissue kallikrein cDNA under the control of the CMV promoter and 4F2 enhancer was inserted into an adenovirus vector and then transfected into human embryonic kidney 293 cells. Expression of human tissue kallikrein was detected in the culture media by a specific enzyme-linked immunosorbent assay (ELISA). We have shown that a single intravenous injection of adenovirus encoding the human tissue kallikrein gene resulted in a rapid and profound reduction of blood pressure for weeks in SHR, DSS, deoxycorticosterone-acetate (DOCA)-salt, 2 kidney 1 clipped (2K1C), and 5/6 nephrectomy rats *(37–41)*, compared with rats injected with control adenovirus. Kallikrein gene transfer was also effective in causing a prolonged reduction of blood pressure using several nonsystemic delivery routes, including intramuscular, intraportal vein, and intracerebroventricular injections *(34,36,42)*. The expression of recombinant human tissue kallikrein in rats following systemic or local gene delivery was detected by specific ELISA and immunohistochemistry, as well as by reverse transcription-polymerase chain reaction followed by Southern blot analysis. Immunoreactive human tissue kallikrein levels in rat sera or urine were highest at 3–5 d after adenovirus-mediated gene delivery, and were still detectable at 24 d after injection *(37)*. However, no human tissue kallikrein was detected in the urine or sera of rats injected with control virus. The kallikrein inhibitor aprotinin reversed the blood pressure-lowering effect in SHR receiving kallikrein gene transfer *(35)*. These results indicate that the hypotensive effect of kallikrein gene delivery is mediated by the expression of functional kallikrein. The effect of kallikrein on blood pressure reduction can also be reversed by icatibant, suggesting that the effect is dependent on a BK B2 receptor-signaling event *(29)*.

KALLIKREIN/KININ AND CARDIAC PROTECTION

The KKS has been demonstrated to play a vital part in cardiac protection in a variety of animal models. Studies using ACE inhibitors clearly showed a protective effect of endogenous kinins in the development of cardiac hypertrophy and neointimal vascular injury *(43,44)*. By employing transgenic and somatic gene transfer approaches, we demonstrated that the KKS plays an important role in cardiac protection. Overexpression of human tissue kallikrein in transgenic rats resulted in reduction of isoproterenol-induced cardiac hypertrophy and fibrosis, and these effects were abolished by icatibant *(29)*. In addition, ablation of the B2 receptor gene in mice caused dilated cardiomyopathy followed by cardiac failure *(45)*. Moreover, systemic delivery of adenovirus containing the tissue kallikrein gene led to blood pressure reduction and attenuation of cardiac hypertrophy and fibrosis in pressure- and volume-overload hypertensive rat models, such as SHR, 2K1C, DSS, and DOCA-salt rats *(37–40)*. Our recent studies also showed that kallikrein gene transfer attenuated cardiac hypertrophy and fibrosis in normotensive rats after myocardial infarction and in genetically hypertensive rats without apparently affecting blood pressure *(46,47)*. These results indicate that kallikrein/kinin not only plays an important role in the regulation of blood pressure homeostasis, but also in cardiovascular function.

KALLIKREIN/KININ ATTENUATES CARDIAC REMODELING AFTER MYOCARDIAL INFARCTION

ACE inhibition has been shown to improve the survival of rats with coronary ligation-induced myocardial infarction and with congestive heart failure *(9,10)*. ACE inhibitors have many beneficial effects in respect to the reduction of morbidity and mortality rates and improvement of the quality of life for patients with heart disease *(48,49)*. Ang II formation in the heart increases after myocardial infarction *(50)*, and elevation of Ang II levels causes cardiac hypertrophy, fibrosis, and apoptosis, leading to cardiac remodeling and heart failure *(50–53)*. A continuous supply of kallikrein/kinin may counteract the action of Ang II and thus protect against cardiac remodeling and heart failure. Our studies showed that kallikrein gene transfer improved cardiac and endothelial function and attenuated myocardial infarction in normotensive animals with acute ischemic and chronic heart disease *(46,54)*. Kallikrein gene delivery reduced cardiac remodeling and apoptosis after myocardial infarction and delayed the progression of heart failure without changes in blood pressure *(46,54)*. The cardioprotective effects mediated by kallikrein gene transfer include: (1) improved cardiac function and cardiac reserve in response to stress; (2) reduced cardiac hypertrophy, fibrosis, and left-ventricular enlargement; (3) improved endothelial function by increasing blood flow and decreasing vascular resistance; (4) increased capillary density in the heart; (5) reduced oxygen consumption; and (6) reduced myocardial apoptosis. This study indicates that the KKS plays an important role in preventing the progression of heart failure after myocardial infarction in chronic heart disease.

INHIBITION OF CARDIOMYOCYTE APOPTOSIS IN ISCHEMIC MYOCARDIUM BY KALLIKREIN GENE DELIVERY

In rats subjected to acute ischemia/reperfusion (I/R), systemic delivery of the tissue kallikrein gene exerts cardiac protection by reducing myocardial infarction, the incidence of ventricular fibrillation, and apoptosis *(54,55)*. Icatibant abolished these beneficial effects, indicating a kinin-mediated event. To achieve a high level of heart-specific expression of recombinant proteins, we employed a catheter-based gene delivery technique to deliver the kallikrein or reporter gene locally into the left ventricle *(55)*. The expression and localization of immunoreactive human tissue kallikrein was identified throughout the left ventricle after local delivery of the kallikrein gene. No specific staining was found in rats injected with control adenovirus *(55)*. In addition, local delivery of adenovirus harboring the green fluorescent protein gene showed homogenous distribution of green fluorescence in the left ventricle, whereas the control left ventricle showed little background fluorescence *(56)*. Moreover, after injection of the adenovirus encoding the luciferase gene, the highest level of luciferase activity was found in the left ventricle with very low levels in the right ventricle, aorta, and other tissues, indicating left ventricle-specific expression *(56)*. Similar to systemic gene delivery, local kallikrein gene delivery significantly reduced I/R-induced myocardial apoptosis in the left ventricle, as detected by both the terminal deoxynucleotidyl transferase-mediated nick end-labeling (TUNEL) staining and DNA laddering.

Akt is a serine/threonine kinase that has been shown to be a key player in promoting cell survival and suppressing apoptosis. Akt promotes survival of cardiomyocytes in vitro, and protects against I/R-induced injury in the mouse heart *(57,58)*. Akt inhibits apoptosis by phosphorylating Bad, leading to increased Bcl-2 and Bcl-xL levels and cell survival *(59,60)*. We showed that kallikrein gene transfer inhibited I/R-induced cardiomyocyte apoptosis, which was accompanied by activation of Akt, Bad, and increased Bcl-2 levels, indicating a role for Akt-Bad-Bcl-2 signaling in kallikrein-mediated protection against myocardial apoptosis *(55)*. Moreover, glycogen synthase kinase-

3β (GSK-3β) is also a downstream target of Akt signaling. Phosphorylation of GSK-3β by Akt inhibits its activity in insulin-mediated signal transduction *(61)*. Kallikrein gene transfer led to increased phosphorylation of GSK-3β and reduced GSK-3β activity, as well as decreased caspase-3 activation in the ischemic myocardium and in primary cultured cardiomyocytes subjected to hypoxia/reoxygenation. Kallikrein's protective effect on apoptosis was blocked by icatibant and by a dominant-negative Akt construct *(55)*. These results indicate that kallikrein/kinin protects against cardiomyocyte apoptosis via activation of Akt-Bad and Akt-GSK-3β signaling pathways.

PROTECTION OF VASCULAR INJURY BY KALLIKREIN GENE DELIVERY

We have shown that transfection of the kallikrein gene or kinin peptide inhibited the proliferation of cultured vascular smooth muscle cells *(62)*. Transfection of the kallikrein gene into isolated aortic segments resulted in a time-dependent secretion of recombinant human tissue kallikrein, which coincided with significant increases in NO and cGMP levels *(63)*. To further investigate the role of kallikrein/kinin in vascular injury, human tissue kallikrein gene was delivered locally into the rat's left common carotid artery after balloon angioplasty. Kallikrein gene delivery resulted in a significant reduction in intima/media ratio at the injured vessel compared with the rats receiving control virus *(62,63)*. The inhibitory effect of kallikrein on neointima formation was blocked L-NAME, a NO synthase inhibitor, and by icatibant, indicating a kinin-B2-receptor-NO-dependent event *(62,63)*. Moreover, systemic delivery of the kallikrein gene into a mouse model of arterial remodeling induced by permanent alteration in shear-stress conditions resulted in a reduction of neointima formation *(64)*. The protective action of kallikrein gene transfer was significantly reduced in kinin B2 knockout mice, but amplified in transgenic mice overexpressing human kinin B2 receptor, compared with wild-type mice *(64)*. In streptozotocin-induced diabetic mice, local delivery of the human tissue kallikrein gene halted the progression of microvascular rarefaction in hindlimb skeletal muscle by inhibiting apoptosis and promoting vascular regeneration *(65)*. Taken together, these results provide new insights into the role of the KKS in the vasculature and may have significant implications for a therapeutic application to treat restenosis and atherosclerosis.

RENAL PROTECTION BY TISSUE KALLIKREIN AND KININ

The link between renal function and the KKS has been demonstrated by several studies. Renal kallikrein excretion has been reported to be significantly reduced in patients with mild renal disease, and more markedly reduced in patients with severe renal failure *(66,67)*. Genetic linkage analysis has shown that a polymorphic site in the proximal promoter region of the human tissue kallikrein gene is associated with the development of end-stage renal disease and hypertension *(68,69)*. Additionally, the kallikrein promoter polymorphism participates in regulating gene expression and modifies blood pressure in response to dietary salt intake *(70)*. These findings suggest that expression of the kallikrein gene may serve as a powerful marker for linkage analysis in populations with salt-sensitive hypertension and renal disease. A variety of studies, including our own, indicate a direct protective effect of the KKS in the kidney. A previous report by other investigators showed that intravenous infusion of kallikrein protein via an osmotic minipump reduces renal damage without affecting the blood pressure of DSS rats fed a high-salt diet *(71)*. Renal protection by kallikrein infusion was abolished by icatibant, indicating a role of the KKS in protection against salt-induced renal injury through mechanisms independent of blood pressure reduction. Using a somatic gene transfer approach, we demonstrated that expression of human tissue kallikrein resulted in enhanced renal function by increasing the glomerular filtration rate and renal blood flow, and reducing glomerular sclerosis, tubular dilatation, and luminal protein cast accumulation *(72)*. These beneficial effects were in conjunction with a partial reduction of blood pressure. Moreover, kallikrein gene transfer also reduced gentamicin-induced nephropathy in a normotensive animal model without affecting hemodynamic parameters *(73)*. These results indicate that the KKS could protect against renal injury through mechanisms independent of its ability to lower blood pressure.

TISSUE KALLIKREIN PROTECTS AGAINST SALT-INDUCED RENAL INJURY

Progressive renal injury is the consequence of a process of destructive fibrosis. High salt intake induces hypertension, cardiac hypertrophy, and progressive renal damage. DSS rats represent a model of progressive and sclerotic renal lesions and have been regarded as the closest model of human salt-sensitive hypertension. After high salt intake, DSS rats develop hypertension, severe renal damage, cerebral infarction, and hemorrhage *(38,72,74)*. An increase in apoptosis in the glomerular and tubular compartments has also been observed in DSS rats *(75)*. This event occurred at a time when renal function was markedly impaired and irreversible changes in renal morphology had developed, indicating a pathological role for apoptosis in renal dysfunction and fibrosis. We have shown that kallikrein gene transfer reduced salt-induced hypertension, glomerular sclerosis, and tubulointerstitial damage in DSS rats *(38,72)*. In addition, we recently demonstrated that kallikrein gene delivery in DSS rats attenuated glomerular and tubular fibrosis scores, interstitial collagen accumulation, renal cell proliferation, glomerular hypertrophy, and apoptosis induced by high salt intake. These effects correlated with increased NO bioavailability and suppression of oxidative stress and transforming growth factor (TGF)-$\beta 1$ expression. Based on these observations, kallikrein gene transfer appears to exert pleiotropic effects on the kidney of DSS rats.

KALLIKREIN/KININ PROTECTS AGAINST GENTAMICIN-INDUCED NEPHROTOXICITY

Gentamicin is an aminoglycoside antibiotic commonly used in treating life-threatening Gram-negative bacterial infections. However, gentamicin treatment causes serious complications, such as nephrotoxicity and ototoxicity. Gentamicin treatment has been reported to cause apoptosis in both cultured renal proximal tubules and auditory hair cells *(76,77)*, as well as inflammation in the kidney *(78)*. We have demonstrated that kallikrein gene transfer enhances renal function and reduces blood urea nitrogen in gentamicin-induced nephrotoxic rats *(73)*. Moreover, kallikrein gene transfer significantly attenuated gentamicin-induced glomerular sclerosis and tubular dilatation, inflammatory cell (macrophage/monocyte) infiltration, and TUNEL-positive apoptotic cells in both the cortex and medulla. These protective effects were accompanied by increased NO formation and reduced nicotinamide adenine dinucleotide oxidase activity, superoxide formation, intercellular adhesion molecule-1, and TGF-β levels, as well as c-jun N-terminal kinase phosphorylation. Kallikrein's effects on these signaling events were blocked by icatibant, indicating a kinin-mediated event. This study indicates that kallikrein/kinin protects against gentamicin-induced nephrosclerosis by inhibiting inflammatory cell recruitment, and against apoptosis through suppression of oxidative stress-mediated signaling pathways.

KALLIKREIN GENE DELIVERY PROTECTS AGAINST PRESSURE-BASED STROKE

Hypertension is critical in the development of stroke in humans. In stroke-prone, spontaneously hypertensive rats (SHRSP), high salt intake accelerates the development of malignant hypertension *(79)*. In the brains of SHRSP, fibrinoid necrosis and associated thrombosis primarily affect cerebral arterioles, leading to their obstruction and infarction, whereas cerebral hemorrhage is caused by microaneurysms *(80)*. In addition, a lethal form of hypertension has been shown to develop in DSS rats fed a high-salt diet at an early age *(81)*. Pathological changes in the brain of DSS rats affected by stroke include hemorrhage, edema, and infarction. We showed that a single injection of adenovirus carrying the human tissue kallikrein gene significantly reduced hypertension, stroke-induced mortality, aortic hypertrophy, and cerebral hemorrhage in DSS rats on a high-salt diet *(74)*. These findings indicate that kallikrein/kinin may play a protective role in pressure-based stroke.

KALLIKREIN GENE DELIVERY PROTECTS AGAINST ISCHEMIC STROKE

Stroke is the third leading cause of death, and the most common cause of long-term disability, in the United States *(82)*. Currently, therapeutic options for the treatment of ischemic stroke are limited primarily to agents that block platelet aggregation or the coagulation cascade *(83)*. However, these antiplatelet agents are only effective in decreasing the incidence of ischemic stroke, and not in reducing cerebral infarct size *(83)*. Stroke-induced neurological deficits and mortality are often associated with timing of treatment after the onset of stroke. The therapy approved for the treatment of acute ischemic stroke is intravenous recombinant tissue-type plasminogen activator initiated within 3 h of symptom onset *(84)*. Focal brain ischemia is the most common event leading to stroke in humans. To prevent or reduce irreversible ischemic brain damage, it is necessary to develop new interventions for acute stroke therapies to meet the large need for this important and undertreated disorder.

To determine the potential protective role of kallikrein/kinin in ischemic stroke, we employed a focal cerebral ischemic rat model with middle cerebral artery occlusion. Intracerebroventricular injection of adenovirus containing the human tissue kallikrein gene significantly reduced ischemia-induced locomotor deficits and cerebral infarction after focal cerebral ischemia. Expression of recombinant human tissue kallikrein in rat ischemic brain was identified by both immunohistochemistry and ELISA. Kallikrein gene transfer improved neurological function and enhanced the survival and migration of glial cells into the ischemic penumbra and core *(85)*. Neuroprotection after kallikrein gene transfer was accompanied by markedly increased cerebral NO levels, phosphorylated Akt and Bcl-2 levels, and reduced nicotinamide adenine dinucleotide phosphate oxidase activity and caspase-3 activation *(85)*. These results indicate that local delivery of the kallikrein gene provides neuroprotection against focal ischemic brain injury by enhancing glial cell survival and inhibiting neuronal apoptosis through suppression of oxidative stress and activation of the Akt-Bcl-2 signaling pathway.

We also employed a more practical approach to further investigate the potential therapeutic time window for ischemic stroke by intravenous injection of the human tissue kallikrein gene. It has been reported that cerebral ischemia disrupts the blood–brain barrier and allows increased vascular permeability for up to 46 h *(86)*. By taking advantage of this increased permeability, adenovirus containing the kallikrein gene was delivered intravenously to determine whether the kallikrein gene could reach damaged brain tissues to exert protection against I/R-induced cerebral injury. We showed that systemic delivery of the kallikrein gene before or after cerebral ischemia was effective in reducing locomotor deficit scores and cerebral infarction. Similar to local gene delivery, systemic delivery of the kallikrein gene attenuated neuronal apoptosis and promoted glial cell survival in the ischemic penumbra and core. In addition, kallikrein gene transfer promoted angiogenesis and neurogenesis in the brain after cerebral I/R. Icatibant blocked the kallikrein-mediated effects. These results indicate that systemic delivery of the tissue kallikrein gene after the onset of acute ischemic stroke can still provide protection against ischemia-induced brain injury. Taken together, our findings provide new and significant insights into potentially extending the time window for the treatment of ischemic stroke by kallikrein/kinin using a convenient delivery method.

POTENTIAL ROLE OF KALLIKREIN/KININ AS AN ANTIOXIDANT IN PROTECTION AGAINST CARDIOVASCULAR AND RENAL DISEASE AND STROKE

Reduced tissue kallikrein levels could result in reduced NO formation, as a result of lower kinin receptor activation. NO is a potent vasodilator and inhibitor of the formation of reactive oxygen species *(87)*. Therefore, reduced NO bioavailability may lead to increased oxidative stress. Oxidative stress causes the activation of the signaling molecules and results in inflammation, apoptosis, proliferation, hypertrophy, and fibrosis eventually leading to cardiovascular and renal disease. Therefore, a continuous supply of tissue kallikrein by gene transfer or kallikrein protein infusion could reduce oxidative stress, leading to inhibition of inflammation, apoptosis, proliferation, and hypertrophy, and thus protect against cardiovascular and renal disease and stroke (Fig. 2).

MULTIPLE ROLES OF KALLIKREIN/KININ IN CARDIOVASCULAR AND RENAL DISEASE AND STROKE

Using transgenic and somatic gene transfer approaches to achieve a continuous supply of kallikrein/kinin in vivo, we have shown that the KKS exhibits protective effects in hypertension and cardiovascular, renal, and central nervous systems. Our studies demonstrated that kallikrein gene delivery exhibits multiple beneficial effects in the heart, kidney, blood vessel, and brain in various animal models (Fig. 3). These include blood

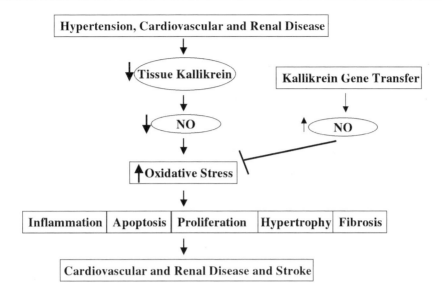

Fig. 2. The protective role of tissue kallikrein as an antioxidant in cardiovascular and renal disease and stroke. NO, nitric oxide.

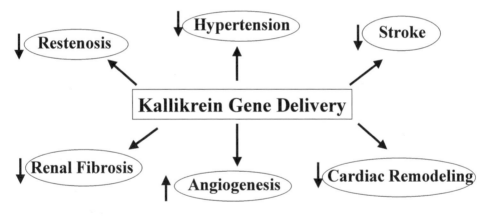

Fig. 3. Multiple functions of tissue kallikrein in the heart, blood vessel, and brain.

pressure reduction; attenuation of renal injury, cardiac infarction and cardiac remodeling; inhibition of neointimal formation in blood vessels after balloon angioplasty; and reduction of stroke-induced mortality, cerebral infarction, and neurological dysfunction. Enhanced kallikrein/kinin levels contribute to these pleiotropic effects by reducing apoptosis, inflammation, hypertrophy, fibrosis, and vascular smooth muscle and renal cell proliferation, and increasing angiogenesis (Table 1). Taken together, our results indicate that kallikrein gene transfer may have significant therapeutic potential for treating cardiovascular and renal diseases and stroke.

Table 1
Pleitropic Effects of Kallikrein Gene Delivery on the Heart,
Kidney, Blood Vessels, and Brain in Various Animal Models

Organ	Effects
Heart	↑ Cardiac function
	↓ Hypertrophy
	↓ Fibrosis
	↑ Capillary density
	↓ Apoptosis
Kidney	↑ Renal function
	↓ Glomerular hypertrophy
	↓ Fibrosis
	↓ Cellular proliferation
	↓ Apoptosis
Blood vessels	↓ VSMC proliferation
	↓ Neointima formation
	↑ Reendothelialization
	↑ Angiogenesis
Brain	↓ Cerebral infarct size
	↓ Cerebral hemorrhage
	↓ Neurological deficits
	↑ Glial cell migration and survival
	↓ Apoptosis
	↑ Angiogenesis

ACKNOWLEDGMENTS

This work was supported by National Institutes of Health grants HL-29397 and DK-66350.

REFERENCES

1. Bhoola KD, Figueroa CD, Worthy K. Bioregulation of kinins: kallikreins, kininogens, and kininases. Pharmacol Rev 1992;44:1–80.
2. Marceau F. Kinin B1 receptors: a review. Immunopharmacology 1995;30:1–26.
3. Regoli D, Gobeil F, Nguyen QT, et al. Bradykinin receptor types and B2 subtypes. Life Sci 1994;55:735.749.
4. Regoli D, Rhaleb, NE, Drapeau G, Dion S. Kinin receptor subtypes. J Cardiovasc Pharmacol 1990;15:S30–S38.
5. Chao J, Tillman DM, Wang MY, Margolius HS, Chao L. Identification of a new tissue kallikrein-binding protein. Biochem J 1986;239:325–331.
6. Zhou GX, Chao L, Chao J. Kallistatin: a novel human tissue kallikrein inhibitor. Purification, characterization, and reactive center sequence. J Biol Chem 1992;267:25,873–25,880.
7. Chao J, Chai KX, Chen LM, et al. Tissue kallikrein-binding protein is a serpin. I. Purification, characterization, and distribution in normotensive and spontaneously hypertensive rats. J Biol Chem 1990;265:16,394–16,401.
8. Linz W, Scholkens BA. Role of bradykinin in the cardiac effects of angiotensin-converting enzyme inhibitors. J Cardiovasc Pharmacol 1992;20:S83–S90.

9. Martorana PA, Kettenbach B, Breipohl G, Linz W, Scholkens BA. Reduction of infarct size by local angiotensin-converting enzyme inhibition is abolished by a bradykinin antagonist. Eur J Pharmacol 1990;182:395-396.

10. Liu YH, Yang XP, Sharov VG, et al. Effects of angiotensin-converting enzyme inhibitors and angiotensin II type 1 receptor antagonists in rats with heart failure. J Clin Invest 1997;99:1926–1935.

11. Weinberger MH, Miller JZ, Luft FC, Grim CE, Fineberg NS. Definitions and characteristics of sodium sensitivity and blood pressure resistance. Hypertension 1986;8:II127–II134.

12. Elliot R, Nuzum F. Urinary excretion of a depressor substance (kallikrein of Frey and Kraut) in arterial hypertension. Endocrinology 1934;18:462–474.

13. Margolius HS. Tissue kallikreins and kinins: regulation and roles in hypertensive and diabetic diseases. Ann Rev Pharmacol Toxicol 1989;29:343–364.

14. Zinner SH, Margolius, HS, Rosner B, Kass, EH. Stability of blood pressure rank and urinary kallikrein concentration in childhood. Circulation 1978;58:908–915.

15. Zinner SH, Margolius HS, Rosner B, Keiser HR, Kass EH. Familial aggregation of urinary kallikrein concentration in childhood: relation to blood pressure, race and urinary electrolytes. Am J Epidemiol 1976;104:124–132.

16. Berry TD, Hasstedt SJ, Hunt SC, et al. A gene for high urinary kallikrein may protect against hypertension in Utah kindreds. Hypertension 1989;13:3–8.

17. Favaro S, Baggio B, Antonello A, et al. Renal kallikrein content of spontaneously hypertensive rats. Clin Sci Mol Med 1975;49:69–71.

18. Powers CA, Baer PG, Nasjletti A. Reduced glandular kallikrein-like activity in the anterior pituitary of the New Zealand genetically hypertensive rat. Biochem Biophys Res Commun 1984;119:689–693.

19. Gilboa N, Rudofsky UH, Phillips MI, Magro AM. Modulation of urinary kallikrein and plasma renin activities does not affect established hypertension in the Fawn-Hooded rat. Nephron 1989;51:61–66.

20. Maddedu P, Varoni MV, Demontis MP, et al. Kallikrein-kinin system and blood pressure sensitivity to salt. Hypertension 1997;29:471–477.

21. Bouhnik J, Richoux JP, Huang H, et al. Hypertension in Dahl salt-sensitive rats: biochemical and immunohistochemical studies. Clin Sci 1992;83:13–22.

22. Gavras I, Gavras H. Anti-hormones and blood pressure: Bradykinin antagonists in blood pressure regulation. Kidney Int 1988;34:S60–S62.

23. Majima M, Mizogami S, Kuribayashi Y, Katori M, Oh-ishi S. Hypertension induced by a nonpressor dose of angiotensin II in kininogen-deficient rats. Hypertension 1994;24:111–119.

24. Woodley-Miller C, Chao J, Chao L. Restriction fragment length polymorphisms mapped in spontaneously hypertensive rats using kallikrein probes. J Hypertens 1989;7:865–871.

25. Pravenec M, Kren V, Kunes J, et al. Cosegregation of blood pressure with a kallikrein gene family. Hypertension 1991;17:242–246.

26. Wang J, Xiong W, Yang Z, et al. Human tissue kallikrein induces hypotension in transgenic mice. Hypertension 1994;23:236–243.

27. Song Q, Chao J, Chao L. High level of circulating human tissue kallikrein induces hypotension in a transgenic mouse model. Clin Exper Hypertens 1996;18:975–993.

28. Chao J, Chao L. Functional analysis of human tissue kallikrein in transgenic mouse models. Hypertension 1996;27:491–494.

29. Silva JA Jr, Araujo RC, Baltatu O, et al. Reduced cardiac hypertrophy and altered blood pressure control in transgenic rats with the human tissue kallikrein gene. FSAEB J 2000;14:1858–1860.

30. Wang D, Chao J, Chao L. Hypotension in transgenic mice overexpressing human bradykinin B2 receptor. Hypertension 1997;29:488–493.

31. Alfie ME, Yang X, Hess F, Carretero OA. Salt-sensitive hypertension in bradykinin B2 receptor knockout mice. Biochem Biophys Res Commun 1996;224:625–630.

32. Overlack A, Stumpe KO, Ressel C, Kolloch R, Zywzok W, Kruck F. Decreased urinary kallikrein activity and elevated blood pressure normalized by orally applied kallikrein in essential hypertension. Klin Wochenschr 1980;58:37–42.

33. Overlack A, Stumpe KO, Kolloch R, Ressel C, Krueck F. Antihypertensive effect of orally administered glandular kallikrein in essential hypertension. Results of double blind study. Hypertension 1981;3:I18–I21.

34. Chao J, Jin L, Chen LM, Chen VC, Chao L. Systemic and portal vein delivery of human kallikrein gene reduces blood pressure in hypertensive rats. Hum Gene Ther 1996;7:901–911.

35. Wang C, Chao L, Chao J. Direct gene delivery of human tissue kallikrein reduces blood pressure in spontaneously hypertensive rats. J Clin Invest 1995;95:1710–1706.
36. Xiong W, Chao J, Chao L. Muscle delivery of human tissue kallikrein gene reduces blood pressure in hypertensive rats. Hypertension 1995;25:715–719.
37. Jin L, Zhang JJ, Chao L, Chao J. Gene therapy in hypertension: adenovirus-mediated kallikrein gene delivery in hypertensive rats. Hum Gene Ther 1997;8:1753–1761.
38. Chao J, Zhang J, Lin KF, Chao L. Adenovirus-mediated kallikrein gene delivery attenuates hypertension, cardiac hypertrophy and renal injury in Dahl salt-sensitive rats. Hum Gene Ther 1998;9:21–31.
39. Dobrzynski E, Yoshida H, Chao J, Chao L. Adenovirus-mediated kallikrein gene delivery attenuates hypertension and protects against renal injury in deoxycorticosterone-salt rats. Immunopharmacology 1999;44:57–65.
40. Yayama K, Wang C, Chao L, Chao J. Kallikrein gene delivery attenuates hypertension and cardiac hypertrophy and enhances renal function in Goldblatt hypertensive rats. Hypertension 1998;31:1104–1110.
41. Wolf WC, Yoshida H, Agata J, Chao L, Chao J. Human tissue kallikrein gene delivery attenuates hypertension, renal injury, and cardiac remodeling in chronic renal failure. Kidney Int 2000;58:730–739.
42. Wang C, Chao C, Madeddu P, Chao L, Chao J. Central delivery of human tissue kallikrein gene reduces blood pressure in hypertensive rats. Biochem Biophys Res Commun 1998;244:449–454.
43. Linz W, Schölkens BA. Role of bradykinin in the cardiac effects of angiotensin-converting enzyme inhibitors. J Cardiovas Pharmacol 1992;20:S83–S90.
44. Farhy RD, Carretero OA, Ho KL, Scicli AG. Role of kinins and nitric oxide in the effects of angiotensin converting enzyme inhibitors on neointima formation. Circ Res 1993;72:1202–1210.
45. Emanueli C, Maestri R, Corradi D, et al. Dilated and failing cardiomyopathy in bradykinin B(2) receptor knockout mice. Circulation 1999;100:2359–2365.
46. Agata J, Chao L, Chao J. Kallikrein gene delivery improves cardiac reserve and attenuates remodeling after myocardial infarction. Hypertension 2002;40:653–659.
47. Bledsoe G, Chao L, Chao J. Kallikrein gene delivery attenuates cardiac remodeling and promotes neovascularization in spontaneously hypertensive rats. Am J Physiol Heart Circ Physiol 2003;285:H1479–488.
48. Richer C, Mulder P, Fornes P, Domergue V, Heudes D, Giudicelli JF. Long-term treatment with trandolapril opposes cardiac remodeling and prolongs survival after myocardial infarction in rats. J Cardiovasc Pharmacol 1992;20:147–156.
49. Mulder P, Devaux B, Richard V, et al. Early versus delayed angiotensin-converting enzyme inhibition in experimental chronic heart failure: effects on survival, hemodynamics, and cardiovascular remodeling. Circulation 1997;95:1314–1319.
50. Sadoshima J, Izumo S. Molecular characterization of angiotensin II-induced hypertrophy of cardiomyocytes and hyperplasia of cardiac fibroblasts: critical role of AT1 receptor subtype. Circ Res 1993;73:413–423.
51. Brilla CG, Zhou G, Matsubara L, Weber KT. Collagen metabolism in cultured adult rat cardiac fibroblasts: response to angiotensin II and aldosterone. J Mol Cell Cardiol 1994;26:809–820.
52. Cigola E, Kajstura J, Li B, Meggs LG, Anversa P. Angiotensin II activates programmed myocyte cell death in vitro. Exp Cell Res 1997;231:363–371.
53. Leri A, Claudio PP, Li Q, et al. Stretch-mediated release of angiotensin II induces myocyte apoptosis activation of p53 that enhances the local renin-angiotensin system and decreases the Bcl-2-to-Bax protein ratio in the cell. J Clin Invest 1998;101:1326–1342.
54. Yoshida H, Zhang JJ, Chao L, Chao J. Kallikrein gene delivery attenuates myocardial infarction and apoptosis after myocardial ischemia and reperfusion. Hypertension 2000;35:25–31.
55. Yin H, Chao L, Chao J. Kallikrein-kinin protects against myocardial apoptosis after ischemia and reperfusion via activation of Akt-Bad-14-3-3 and Akt-GSK-3 signaling pathways. High Blood Pressure Council, September 23–26, 2003 Washington, DC: p. 66, abstract #P75.
56. Yin H, Chao L, Chao J. Adrenomedullin protects against myocardial apoptosis after ischemia/reperfusion through activation of Akt-GSK signaling. Hypertension 2004;43:452–459.
57. Mehrhof FB, Muller FU, Bergmann MW, et al. In cardiomyocyte hypoxia, insulin-like growth factor-I-induced antiapoptotic signaling requires phosphotidylinositol-3-OH-kinase-dependent and mitogen-activated protein kinase-dependent activation of the transcription factor cAMP response element-binding protein. Circulation 2001;104:2088–2094.

58. Matsui T, Tao J, del Monte F, et al. Akt activation preserves cardiac function and prevents injury after transient cardiac ischemia in vivo. Circulation 2001;104:330–334.

59. Shimamura H, Terada Y, Okado T, Tanaka H, Inoshita S, Sasaki S. The PI3-kinase-Akt pathway promotes mesangial cell survival and inhibits apoptosis in vitro via NF-kappa B and Bad. J Am Soc Nephrol 2003;14:1427–1434.

60. Henshall DC, Araki T, Schindler CK, et al. Activation of Bcl-2-associated death protein and counter-response of Akt within cell populations during seizure-induced neuronal death. J Neurosci 2002;22:8458–8465.

61. Moule SK, Welsh GI, Edgell NJ, Foulstone EJ, Proud CG, Denton RM. Regulation of protein kinase B and glycogen synthase kinase-3 by insulin and beta-adrenergic agonists in rat epididymal fat cells. Activation of protein kinase B by wortmannin-sensitive and -insensitive mechanisms. J Biol Chem 1997;272:7713–7719.

62. Murakami H, Yayama K, Miao RQ, Wang C, Chao L, Chao J. Kallikrein gene delivery inhibits vascular smooth muscle cell growth and neointima formation in the rat artery after balloon angioplasty. Hypertension 1999;34:164–170.

63. Murakami H, Miao RQ, Chao L, Chao J. Adenovirus-mediated kallikrein gene transfer inhibits neointima formation via increased production of nitric oxide in rat artery. Immunopharmacology 1999;44:137–43.

64. Emanueli C, Salis MB, Chao J, et al. Adenovirus-mediated human tissue kallikrein gene delivery inhibits neointima formation induced by interruption of blood flow in mice. Arterioscler Thromb Vasc Biol 2000;20:1459–1466.

65. Emanueli C, Salis MB, Pinna A, et al. Prevention of diabetes-induced microangiopathy by human tissue kallikrein gene transfer. Circulation 2002;106:993–999.

66. Price RG. Urinary enzymes, nephrotoxicity and renal disease. Toxicology 1982;23:99–134.

67. Naicker S, Naidoo S, Ramsaroop R, Moodley D, Bhoola K. Tissue kallikrein and kinins in renal disease. Immunopharmacology 1999;44:183–192.

68. Yu H, Song Q, Freedman BI, et al. Association of the tissue kallikrein gene promoter with ESRD and hypertension. Kidney Int 2002; 61:1030–1039.

69. Sterzel RB, Luft FC, Gao Y, et al. Renal disease and the development of hypertension in salt-sensitive Dahl rats. Kidney Int 1988;33:1119–1129.

70. Song Q, Hunt SC, Zheng D, Willams GH, Chao J, Chao L. A promoter polymorphism of human tissue kallikrein gene is associated with the response of blood pressure to dietary salt restriction. Circulation, to be submitted, 2003.

71. Uehara Y, Hirawa N, Kawabata Y, et al. Long-term infusion of kallikrein attenuates renal injury in Dahl salt-sensitive rats. Hypertension 1994;24:770–778.

72. Chao J, Zhang JJ, Lin KF, Chao L. Adenovirus-mediated kallikrein gene delivery reverses salt-induced renal injury in Dahl salt-sensitive rats. Kidney Int 1998;54:1250–1260.

73. Murakami H, Yayama K, Chao L, Chao J. Human kallikrein gene delivery protects against gentamycin-induced nephrotoxicity in rats. Kidney Int 1998;53:1305–1313.

74. Zhang JJ, Chao L, Chao J. Adenovirus-mediated kallikrein gene delivery reduces aortic thickening and stroke-induced death rate in Dahl salt-sensitive rats. Stroke 1999;30:1925–1931.

75. Ying WZ, Wang PX, Sanders PW. Induction of apoptosis during development of hypertensive nephrosclerosis. Kidney Int 2000;58:2007–2017.

76. El Mouedden M, Laurent G, Mingeot-Leclercq MP, Taper HS, Cumps J, Tulkens PM. Apoptosis in renal proximal tubules of rats treated with low doses of aminoglycosides. Antimicrob Agents Chemother 2000;44:665–675.

77. Ylikoski J, Xing-Qun L, Virkkala J, Pirvola U. Blockade of c-Jun N-terminal kinase pathway attenuates gentamicin-induced cochlear and vestibular hair cell death. Heart Res 2002;163:71–81.

78. Geleilete TJ, Melo GC, Costa RS, Volpini RA, Soares TJ, Coimbra TM. Role of myofibroblasts, macrophages, transforming growth factor-beta endothelin, angiotensin-II, and fibronectin in the progression of tubulointerstitial nephritis induced by gentamicin. J Nephrol 2002;15:633–642.

79. Takeda Y, Yoneda T, Demura M, Furukawa K, Miyamori I, Mabuchi H. Effects of high sodium intake on cardiovascular aldosterone synthesis in stroke-prone spontaneously hypertensive rats. J Hypertens 2001;19:635–639.

80. Richer C, Vacher E, Fornes P, Giudicelli JF. Antihypertensive drugs in the stroke-prone spontaneously hypertensive rat. Clin Exp Hypertens 1997;19:925–936.

81. Kodama K, Adachi H, Sonoda J. Beneficial effects of long-term enalapril treatment and low-salt intake on survival rate of Dahl salt-sensitive rats with established hypertension. J Pharmacol Exp Ther 1997;283:625–629.

82. Division of Chronic Disease Control and Community. Cardiovascular Disease Surveillance: Stroke, 1980–1989. (Atlanta, Centers for Disease Control and Prevention). 1994.

83. Patrono C. Aspirin as an antiplatelet drug. N Engl J Med 1994;330:1287–1294.

84. Fisher M. Developing therapy for acute ischemic stroke. Therapie 2002;57:564–568.

85. Xia CF, Yin H, Borlongan CV, Chao L, Chao J. Kallikrein gene transfer protects against ischemic stroke by promoting glial cell migration and inhibiting apoptosis. Hypertension 2004;42:452–459.

86. Huang ZG, Xue D, Preston E, Karbalai H, Buchan AM. Biphasic opening of the blood-brain barrier following transient focal ischemia: effects of hypothermia. Can J Neurol Sci 1999;26:298–304.

87. Patel R, McAndrew J, Sellak H, et al. Biological aspects of reactive nitrogen species. Biochim Biophys Acta 1999;141:385–400.

12 Current and Future Novel Targets of Gene Therapy for Hypertension

Michael J. Katovich, PhD, Justin L. Grobe, and Mohan K. Raizada, PhD

CONTENTS

SUMMARY

Traditional therapeutic approaches for the treatment and control of hypertension are effective in normalizing blood pressure (BP) in less than a third of patients with hypertension. These pharmacological approaches may have reached a plateau in their effectiveness and newer strategies need to be investigated to not only increase the number of patients achieving BP control, but to find ways to cure the disease instead of just manage it. Since completion of the Human Genome Project and the continuous advancement of gene delivery systems, it is now possible to investigate genetic means for the treatment and possible cure for hypertension. In this review, we discuss potential genetic targeting for treatment of hypertension. There are two generalized gene transfer approaches that have been used successfully for hypertension. One is an induction approach where genes that lower blood pressure are overexpressed. A second method is a reduction approach where products of genes that are known to increase blood pressure are decreased. There are a variety of methods that have been utilized to meet these objectives, such as "knockout" and "knock-in" animal models, and the

From: *Contemporary Cardiology: Cardiovascular Genomics*
Edited by: M. K. Raizada, et al. © Humana Press Inc., Totowa, NJ

use of sense and antisense (AS) technology. This review will focus on the sense and antisense applications, and how this technique is becoming more refined and precise through the targeting of specific tissues, the regulation and induction of components of the system, and use of other newer technologies, such as short interfering RNA (siRNA). Our lab has generally focused on the reduction approach, specifically in the genetic manipulation of components of the renin–angiotensin system (RAS). This system not only modulates BP, but has also been implicated in cardiac hypertrophy and morphology and in insulin resistance, which is highly correlated with hypertension. We will also discuss how new genes can be identified and subsequently serve as targets for the treatment of human hypertension.

Key Words: Gene therapy; viral vectors; gene delivery; animal models; hypertension; renin–angiotensin system; gene arrays.

INTRODUCTION

Hypertension is a chronic, debilitating disease that affects more than 50 million Americans (1,2). Although hypertension is defined as a condition of high blood pressure (BP) (1) (systolic BP $\geq$140 mmHg and diastolic BP $\geq$90 mmHg), it is a much more complex disorder, with a majority of hypertensive patients being insulin-resistant and/or salt sensitive (3–6). High BP is estimated to account for 6% of all deaths worldwide (7) and is the most common treatable risk factor for cardiovascular disease (CVD). A sustained elevation in BP contributes to serious health complications, such as myocardial ischemia and infarction, renal failure, stroke, and retinal damage (8–10). Vascular and cardiac remodeling occurs in hypertension, which has both hemodynamic and nonhemodynamic effects (11,12). This disorder has such a negative impact on health care that the most recent Joint National Committee on Prevention, Detection, Evaluation, and Treatment of High Blood Pressure report has suggested a new category of prehypertension in adults that have a systolic BP of 120–139 mmHg and a diastolic BP of 80–90 mmHg (13). The report states that individuals with this range of BP should be considered pre-hypertensive, and suggests health-promoting lifestyle changes to prevent CVDs.

Hypertension is an asymptomatic, chronic disease that is characterized as either primary or secondary. The latter is indicative of having a separate primary cause, whereas the primary (or essential) form of hypertension, which constitutes more than 90% of the cases, is of unknown etiology. This form of the disease is chronic, multifactoral, and multigenetic in origin, and is difficult to manage and currently not preventable or curable. Thus, the major goal of current therapies has been to control BP and prevent the complications (end-organ damage) associated with the disease, regardless of its origins. Despite the large arsenal of antihypertensive agents currently available, successful control of BP ($\leq$140/90 mmHg) is only observed in a small percentage of patients. Although only 29% of hypertensive patients in the United States have their BP controlled to the nationally recommended level of less than or equal to 140/90 mmHg with pharmacological intervention (13), the control rates are much worse in other countries around the world (14–16). Therefore proper treatment and management of hypertension is of critical importance to society and should be a matter of extreme urgency both in the United States and abroad.

ADVANTAGE OF GENE THERAPY
OVER CONVENTIONAL PHARMACOTHERAPY

Despite a large arsenal of therapeutic agents, conventional pharmacological therapy has not cured hypertension and, in fact, does not control the disease in the majority of patients. Possible reasons for poor control of BP include incorrect targets of therapy, and poor education, economics, availability of health care, follow-up care, drug availability, and compliance. Even if the "ideal drug" was available for each patient, it is more likely that compliance would be the major factor in determining patient outcome. Reasons for a lack of compliance in hypertensive patients include convenience and side effects of the drugs utilized. Convenience can refer to the drug dosing regiment, which does not always conform to a patient's everyday activities. Most pharmacological agents are short-acting ($\leq$24 h) and require multiple dosing per day. Another reason a patient may not stay on his/her medication is that symptoms related to the side effects of the drugs may be manifested in this otherwise asymptomatic disease. Patients can "feel better" when they are not on their medication, and they therefore either reduce their own dosage, or stop taking the medication altogether. Thus, we are at a stage in the treatment of hypertension where more focus must be placed on other treatment paradigms rather than further drug developments. Gene therapy offers the possibility of producing long-term effects with specificity based on the particular genetic target. Side effects may no longer be an issue, compliance would be nearly eliminated, as therapy can be directed at the source of the hypertension, and this therapy could be administered a minimal number of times over the patient's lifetime.

PHILOSOPHIES OF GENE THERAPY

Gene therapy promises to be the next frontier for treatment of and possibly a cure for complex diseases like hypertension. A variety of studies over the past few years have looked at different gene targets and gene delivery vectors as strategies. Currently, therapeutic agents are chosen by targeting the genes that are important in BP regulation. Whereas this technique should yield promising antihypertensive results, ideal gene targets would be those that have not only been implicated in hypertension, but also have been implicated in some of the target organ damage that is associated with hypertensive disease, such as the heart, kidney, vessels, etc. Over the last several years, our lab has mainly focused on the genetically manipulated renin–angiotensin system (RAS). This system has long been associated with hypertension. The RAS is essential in both the normal regulation of BP, as well as in the pathophysiology of hypertension. This system is also involved in, but not limited to, the alterations of nitric oxide metabolism (17), the impact of oxidative stress on endothelial function (18), vascular smooth muscle and cardiac hypertrophy (19,20), and insulin resistance (21,22). Additionally, there are numerous genetic link studies with components of the RAS and hypertension (23–30), as well as the successful use of both angiotensin-converting enzyme (ACE) inhibitors and angiotensin receptor blocking agents in the treatment of hypertension and some of its related complications.

There are two contrasting philosophies for gene therapy in hypertension—the reduction approach and the "induction" approach. In the "reduction" approach, genes that have been implicated in the elevation of BP are targeted, with the hope of reducing translation (in the case of a signaling molecule) or attenuating their effects by reducing their receptor's population. With the induction approach, genes that have a BP-lowering effect are introduced or upregulated with selective gene and/or promoter delivery. That is, recombinant DNA is introduced in vivo to express mRNA and increase the concentration of the targeted protein. For each of these approaches there are a variety of methodologies utilized to produce the desired effects.

There are two major contrasting paradigms that can be used to produce these genetic alterations. One is the use of transgenic animals that knock out a specific gene or overexpress a particular gene. The other approach is to alter the genetic makeup of the animal after development with induction (sense) or reduction (antisense [AS]) approaches. A potential drawback to the knockout models is that the animal may undergo some altered physiology to compensate for the removal of a particular gene. This would be especially important if the gene that is removed has a major role in the developmental process. Although knockout models have made significant contributions, any compensatory changes that the animal undergoes may reduce the power of this type of strategy. Both strategies have been successful in reducing BP or in preventing the rise in BP in experimental animals; however, we are of the opinion that the genetic alterations should occur after the developmental process to avoid any compensatory physiological adaptations that may influence the interpretation of the significance of the particular gene of interest. Therefore, this review will focus more on the postdevelopment genetic manipulations in experimental hypertension.

"Induction" Approach

Several investigators have been successful in lowering BP using the induction paradigm. Overexpressing agents that are vasodilators, such as atrial natriuretic peptide *(31–34)*, adrenomedullin *(35–38)* endothelial nitric oxide synthetase (eNOS) *(39–42)*, human tissue kallikrein *(43–55)*, superoxide dismutase *(56–58)*, and the AT2 receptor *(59)*, have been successful in reducing BP. These studies have examined different models of hypertension, and the gene transfer approach has been systemic or localized in specific tissue(s), depending on the gene target. Systemic delivery of the these transgenes in plasmid DNA or adenovirus by intravenous, intraperitoneal, or intraportal vein injections results in a reduction of BP in a variety of animal models (*see* Table 1). Innovative delivery systems have been examined by a few research groups. Chen et al. *(60)* transfected Chinese hamster ovary (CHO) cells with atrial natriuretic peptide (ANP) cDNA, and then the CHO cells were encapsulated in nonantigenic biocompatible polycaprolactone capsules, prior to their implantation into the peritoneal cavity of rats. Li et al. *(61)* used encapsulated genetically engineered fibroblasts expressing ANP. In both cases, BP was significantly reduced in hypertensive Dahl and spontaneously hypertensive rats (SHR), respectively. In most examples of the induction gene transfer approach, transgenes were administered to adult animals and BP was reduced within a week and remained below controls for 4–6 wk. The extent of the reduction in BP was dependent on the dose of DNA injected, but averaged between 20 and 40 mmHg. Some of the differences observed regarding the extent and duration of BP effects may be related to the choice of promoter directing the expression of the transgene, the route of injection, and the vehicle in which the transgene is delivered. The "induction" gene transfer approach is not restricted to systemic administration. Gene transfer of eNOS, via an adenovirus vector, into the nucleus tractus solitarii of SHR also decreased BP *(39,42)*. In all the studies undertaken, control viral injections were without effect, further demonstrating it was the transgene, and not the virus, that mediated the observed decreases in BP.

BP is not the only parameter assessed in these studies. Investigators have looked at cardiac and renal complications, which are summarized in Table 1. In addition, other parameters also have been evaluated. For instance, overexpression of human tissue kallikrien in a fructose-induced model of hypertension *(43)* not only lowered BP, but the insulin-resistant state and the number of angiotensin type I receptors (AT_1R) were also reduced. This gene transfer was without effect on control animals, which was the case in all the other gene transfer experiments described in Table 1. Other investigators (41,57) have also demonstrated that the impaired endothelial function observed in the SHR was significantly improved after gene transfer of eNOS and superoxide dismutase. The specificity of the responses to the transgene has been verified using agents that block or bind to the receptor that the upregulated protein would bind to (50,53).

Reduction Approach

Similar success in reducing BP and cardiovascular pathologies in experimental animals has been realized with the reduction gene transfer approach, which underexpresses agents that vasoconstrict vessels. The most successful agents used in this approach have targeted various components of the RAS. Table 2 summarizes the studies that have been utilized to reduce expression of various genes. These studies produce similar findings as described for the induction approach, as far as its range of effects on reducing basal BP or preventing the rise in BP in several different models of experimental hypertension. In many of these studies, administration of the AS transgene occurs during the neonatal stage and results in prevention of high BP in a variety of hypertensive models. Administration of AS to the AT_1R in 5-d-old animals completely prevented the development of hypertension in the SHR (62–65). Reverse-transcription polymerase chain reaction (RT-PCR) and receptor-binding studies confirmed a 40–60% knockdown of the endogenous AT_1R, thereby decreasing the gain of the RAS, but still leaving the system intact at a basal level (64,65). Responsiveness to angiotensin II (Ang II) is reduced in AT_1R antisense-treated rats; however, BP is only reduced in hypertensive and not in normotensive animals. This would suggest that it is an overactivity of the RAS (as opposed to altered function) that is important in hypertension. As was found with the induction gene transfer studies, not only is BP reduced but so are many of the cardiac, renal, and vascular pathophysiologies normally associated with the hypertensive state. For instance, cardiac hypertrophy, fibrosis, perivascular necrosis in cardiac tissues, and endothelial dysfunction were prevented in SHRs treated with AT_1R-AS delivered via a retroviral vector (62–65). Similar results were observed when AS to ACE was used as the transgene in a retroviral vector (66). Like the induction approach, there is also reversal of insulin-resistance in the fructose-model of hypertension with AS to the AT_1R (67). Recent reports have suggested that the RAS is important in insulin resistance (22,68,69). This implicates an association of the RAS with insulin resistance and Syndrome X. Recent clinical and experimental evidence have demonstrated that antagonism of the RAS reduces the incidence and severity of diabetes and insulin resistance (70–72), providing further rationale for the use of components of the RAS as potential transgenes in gene therapy approaches to other chronic metabolic disorders.

Generally speaking, this reduction approach appears to produce effects on BP that are more long-lasting than the induction approach; however, this may be related more to the delivery system and its resulting integration of the AS into the genome.

When retroviral vector AT_1R-AS was administered to adult SHR, we observed a transient but significant decrease in BP (73). This transient effect may be a result of the limited infection of nondividing cells by the retrovirus. Other investigators (74–78), using a viral delivery system that can infect nondividing cells, demonstrated that underexpressing genes of the RAS is effective in reducing BP in adult hypertensive rats.

Table 1
Increased Gene Expression

Transgene	Animal model	Delivery	Route	Effect on blood pressure	Comments	References
Kallikrein	Fructose-induced SD	Plasmid DNA	iv	Decreased	Decreased AT_1R, decreased endothelin, normalized insulin	43
	SHR	Adenovirus	im	No effect	Increased capillary density in ischemic muscle	44
	5/6 reduction in renal mass	Adenovirus	iv	Decreased	Left-ventricular hypertrophy attenuated, protects against renal injury and cardiac remodeling	45
	Adult and newborn SHR	Adenovirus	im	Decreased		46
	Dahl salt-sensitive	Adenovirus	iv	Decreased	Reversed cardiac hypertrophy and fibrosis and renal damage	47
	5-wk-old Goldblatt—2 Kidney/1 Clip	Adenovirus	iv	Delay of onset	Reduced left ventricular mass, protection from renal dysfunction	48
	Dahl salt-sensitive	Adenovirus	iv	Decreased	Decreased left ventricular hypertrophy, attenuated renal injury	49
	SHR	Adenovirus	iv	Delay of onset		50
	Adult and newborn SHR	Oligonucleotide	sc	Delay of onset	Gender differences	51
	SHR	Adenovirus	iv	Decreased		52
	SHR	Oligonucleotide	iv	Decreased	Decreased BP in adult but not in young SHR	53
	SHR	Plasmid DNA	im	Decreased	BP reduction attenuated with bradykinin antagonist	5
	SHR	Plasmid DNA	iv	Decreased	Hypotensive effect reversed by kallikrein inhibitor	55
Adrenomedullin	5-wk-old Goldblatt—2 Kidney/1 Clip	Adenovirus	iv	Delay of onset	Decreased left ventricular mass, decreased myocyte diameter, decreased myocardial fibrosis, decreased renal	35

(continued)

218

Gene	Model	Vector	Effect	Comments	Ref
	SHR	Plasmid DNA	iv	Decreased	2nd injection further reduced BP	38
Nitric oxide synthase	SHR	Adenovirus	icv (NTS)	Decreased	Depressor response in WKY, but greater in SHR	39
	Stroke-prone SHR	Adenovirus	iv	No effect	Improved endothelial function	40
	SHR	Plasmid DNA	iv	Decreased	2nd injection extended therapeutic time limit	41
	SHR	Adenovirus	icv (NTS)	Decreased	Decrease in HR and BP reversed by microinjection of soluble guanylate cyclase inhibitor	42
Atrial natriuretic peptide	SHR	Plasmid DNA	iv	Decreased	Increased urine volume and sodium excretion	31
	Dahl salt-sensitive	Adenovirus	iv	Decreased	Decrease in cerebral infarction, reduced thickness of arterial wall	32
	Dahl salt-sensitive	Adenovirus	iv	Decreased	Reduction in cardiac myocyte size, attenuation of glomerular sclerotic lesions	33
	4-wk-old SHR	Plasmid DNA	iv	Decreased	No effect on 12-wk-old SHR	34
Superoxide dismutase	SHR	Adenovirus	iv	Decreased	Effect greater in anesthetized compared with awake rats; improved endothelial function	56
	Stroke-prone SHR	Adenovirus	iv	No effect	Improved endothelial function	57
Heme oxygenase	5-d-old SHR	Retrovirus	ic	Delay of onset		58

SHR, spontaneously hypertensive rats; iv, intravenous; im, intramuscular; ic, intracardiac; sc, subcutaneous; icv, intracerebroventricular; WKY, Wistar–Kyoto; BP, blood pressure; SD, Sprague-Dawley rats.

Table 2
Decreased Gene Expression

Transgene	Animal model	Delivery	Route	Effect on blood pressure	Comments	References
Fibroblast growth factor	SHR	Liposome	iv	Acute decrease	Augments number of endothelial cells, ameliorated endothelial dependent response to vasoconstrictors	98
Angiotensinogen	SHR	Oligonucleotide	iv	Decrease	Plasma angiotensinogen and angiotensin II levels reduced	81
	SHR	Oligonucleotide	iv	Decrease	Angiotensinogen and angiotensin II levels reduced	82
	SHR	Oligonucleotide	icv	Decrease	Decreased AT$_1$R in PVN, decreased angiotensin II in brainstem	83
	SHR	Oligonucleotide	icv	Decrease	Decreased angiotensin II in brainstem	84
	SHR	AAV*	ic	Decrease, delay of onset	Decreased left ventricular hypertrophy, decreased angiotensinogen	96
	SHR	Asialo-glycoprotein	iv	Decrease	Reduced hepatic angiotensinogen, reduced cardiac AT$_1$R, decreased left-ventricular hypertrophy	97
	SHR	AAV	iv	Decrease	Greater effect of AAV-plasmid vector with liposome	100
	Cold-induced SD	Liposome	iv	Decrease	Decreased spontaneous drinking response	101
	Goldblatt—2 Kidney/1 Clip	Oligonucleotide	icv	Decrease	Decreased the elevated hypothalamus angiotensin II levels	105
Angiotensin converting enzyme	SHR	Retrovirus	ic	Decrease	No effect on WKY	66
AT$_1$ receptors	SHR	Retrovirus*	ic	Decrease	Decreased cardiac hypertrophy and fibrosis, similar effects seen in progeny	62
	SHR	Retrovirus*	ic	Decrease	Prevented left ventricular hypertrophy and myocardial perivascular fibrosis	63
	SHR	Retrovirus*	ic	Decrease	Decreased angiotensin II mediated responses in WKY and SHR but only decreased basal pressure in SHR	64
	SHR	Retrovirus*	ic	Decrease	Angiotensin II-induced BP and dipsogenic responses attenuated	65

Target	Model	Method	Route	Effect	Description	Ref
	Fructose-Induced SD	Retrovirus*	ic	Decrease	Prevented glucose intolerance	67
	SHR	Retrovirus	ic	Transient Decrease	Repeated daily injections for 6 d	73
	SHR	AAV*	icv (Lat. Vent)	Decrease	Intracardiac injection in 3-wk-old SHR also reduced BP	74
	SHR	Oligonucleotide	icv	Decrease		84
	L-NAME SD	Retrovirus*	ic	Decrease	Decreased left-ventricular hypertrophy, endothelial dysfunction unchanged	91
	Renin transgenic	Retrovirus*	ic	Decrease	Prevented cardiac hypertrophy	93
	Angiotensin-induced SD	Retrovirus*	ic	Decrease	Protected against angiotensin II-induced increases in BP and cardiac hypertrophy	99
	Cold-induced SD	Oligonucleotide	ic and/or icv	Decrease	Spontaneous drinking response to cold reduced	101
	Goldblatt - 2 Kidney / 1 Clip	Oligonucleotide	i.v.	Decrease		102
	SHR	Oligonucleotide	intracisternally	Decrease	Decreased cerebral infarct after middle cerebral artery occlusion	104
AT$_2$ receptors	Uni-nephrectomized SD	Oligonucleotide	interstitial pump	Increase	Increased pressor response to angiotensin II	79
	SD	Retrovirus*	ic	Increase	Increased pressor response to angiotensin II	80
Epidermal growth factor receptor	SHR	Liposome	iv	Decrease	Weekly injections for 2 mo; Decreased left-ventricular hypertrophy, but only effective in 5-wk, not 13-wk-old SHR	92
	Angiotensin-induced SD	Oligonucleotide	iv	Decrease	Normalized left-ventricular hypertrophy	108
β-adrenergic receptor	SHR	Liposome	iv	Decrease	No effect on heart rate	90
	SHR	Liposome	iv	Decrease	Decreased beta 1, but not beta 2, receptors, decreased plasma renin activity and angiotensin II	95
CPY-like kininase	DOCA salt SD	Oligonucleotide	iv	Decrease	Increased urine volume and sodium excretion	107
Tyrosine hydroxylase	SHR	Oligonucleotide	iv	Decrease	Decreased epinephrine and norepinephrine, decreased TH activity in adrenal medula	94
CYP4A1	SHR	Liposome	iv	Decrease	Decreased sensitivity to constrictor action of phenylephrine	103
Thyrotropin	SHR	Oligonucleotide	it	Decrease		106

*Injection performed at 5 d of age. SHR, spontaneously hypertensive rats; AAV, adeno-associated virus; WKY, Wistar-Kyoto; it, intrathecal; iv, intravenous; icv, intracerebroventricular; ic, intracardiac.

Further, there have been some recent studies *(79,80)* that have used gene therapy approaches to lower expression of the AT_2 receptor, which results in the increase in basal BP. Collectively, these studies indicate that both induction and reduction of components of the RAS are promising for the treatment of hypertension.

DELIVERY METHODS FOR GENE THERAPY

In hypertension, whether using an AS approach to express reduction or AS mRNA to inhibit an overexpressed protein, or using an induction or sense approach to increase the synthesis of proteins critical to the pathogenesis of the disease, one generally has to transduce somatic cells of the body. Therefore, methodologies for efficient gene transfer are paramount for successful gene therapy. Other essential components of successful gene therapy are the ability to appropriately express the gene, to have long-term survival of the transduced cell(s), and to be able to control expression of the particular gene. There have been several vehicles explored for somatic gene delivery for hypertension, such as naked DNA, liposomes, receptor-mediated delivery, and viral delivery. This last method can be further divided by the type of virus utilized: retroviral, adenoviral, adeno-associated, or lentivirus. Each system has certain advantages and disadvantages, which influence their selection. The duration of the effect of the target gene is dependent on the delivery system utilized. The following is a brief summary of some of the more common gene delivery vehicles.

Nonviral Vectors

Nonviral vectors possess some advantages over viral vectors for gene therapy, in that these vectors are usually devoid of the safety issues related to insertional mutagenesis and immunogenecity. Early attempts to modify genes to lower BP used oligodeoxynucleotides (ODN). In particular, AS-ODN was directed to the AT_1R and angiotensinogen mRNA *(81–84)*. ODN are single-stranded, short sequences of nucleotides that are made of DNA (or modified DNA) designed to interact specifically with its target mRNA by Watson–Crick basepairing. Once bound to its target mRNA, the AS-ODN inhibits protein synthesis by directly blocking translation *(85,86)*. ODNs may further work to block expression by stimulating RNase H, which sterically inhibits the mRNA from translating its message. This reduces the total number of mRNA copies and frees the AS-ODNs to hybridize again. The ODN approach has some specific disadvantages *(77,80–87)*. Its effects are long-lasting in comparison to available pharmaceutical agents, but usually the effects are still limited a week after administration. No adverse or toxic effects have been observed, they can be produced in larger quantities relatively inexpensively, and they do not cross the blood–brain barrier when given peripherally *(80)*. There have been numerous studies conducted, mostly in the SHR, with BP generally reduced anywhere from 16 to 40 mmHg for 3–7 d *(see* Tables 1 and 2). Naked AS-ODN is effective, but cationic liposomal carriers *(77,88–90)* can increase the effectiveness.

Naked DNA can be delivered directly to the cells, in a plasmid (circular, naked DNA) or with liposomes (lipid bilayers that carry the DNA into cells). These methods are relatively safe and easy. Plasmids are effective vectors, but administer relatively short transgene duration because they do not allow for integration into the genome. Human kallikrein and NOS have been manipulated using these techniques to transiently lower BP in hypertensive rats *(see* Table 1). However, these methods are not very efficient, may be cytotoxic, and only produce a transient effect *(109)*.

Modifications to nonviral vectors can increase the efficiency of gene transfer to cardiovascular tissues. Liposomes developed with cationic lipids can allow for a higher transfection efficiency of plasmid DNA. Another method to deliver DNA is a receptor-mediated method using hemagglutinating virus of Japan liposome. In this method, DNA is combined with a ligand to be internalized by a cell in a specific receptor-mediated mechanism (110). Although this method is an improvement over the basic liposomal method and is highly specific, it is more difficult to produce the modified liposomes.

Recent advances in nonviral delivery technology have infused renewed vigor into the field. These newer advances include ultrasound-mediated enhancement of gene delivery and peptide-targeted liposomal formulations to target enhancement. With regard to cardiovascular physiology, ultrasound has recently been shown to enhance transduction into vascular tissue by increasing permeability of the cell membrane. Lawrie et al. (111) has reported a 300-fold increase in gene transfer in smooth muscle cells compared with naked DNA alone using an ultrasound approach. Use of a lipid integrin DNA (LID) nonviral vector system, which is a modification of the liposomal-mediated gene delivery, consists of a standard liposomal/DNA component that is complexed with an integrin-targeting peptide. This LID vector complex can be used to attach to cell receptors on vascular tissues. This targeting has been used effectively in vitro for both vascular smooth muscles and endothelial cells (112). This technology can be a versatile one in which substitution of other peptides that can mediate selective uptake into specific cell types can be developed to enhance targeted gene delivery. If more prolonged effects are desired, the delivery of the transgene requires a viral vector. There are numerous viral vectors used for gene therapy, each having its specific advantages and disadvantages (Table 3).

Viral Vectors for Gene Therapy Approach

For hypertension, where a long-term (or permanent) control of pathophysiology is the goal, integration of the transgene into the host cell's genome is necessary. Whereas naked DNA and liposomes are incapable of this task, viruses require such actions for their life cycle. Various viral vectors have been modified and used to deliver and incorporate transgenes of interest into cells. There are four major classes of viral vectors currently being used for both in vivo and in vitro applications in hypertension (Table 3). However, the "ideal viral vector" has yet to be found. An ideal vector should be safe (have a low toxicity when delivered), should not elicit an immune response, should integrate in a predictable, safe region of the genome, must be efficiently taken up by the target tissue, and must infect the target tissue with a high enough efficiency to have a physiological effect. For practical purposes, the vector also has to be packaged with high efficiency into the viral envelope, be easily produced in high concentrations, and have enough space to accommodate the required transgene and its promoter. Each of the known viral vectors has some of these characteristics, but not all of them.

Adenovirus

Adenovirus is a double-stranded DNA virus that can infect both dividing and nondividing cells with high efficiency as it targets mammalian cells with specific membrane receptors. Viruses then enter the cells by receptor-mediated endocytosis and translocate into the nucleus. Most of the adenoviruses are episomal, and thus do not integrate into the host DNA. Because they are not integrated, the episomal DNA eventually becomes inactive or degraded, and the transgene will no longer be expressed. As the adenoviral genome

Table 3
Major Pros and Cons of Delivery Methods

Vehicle	Pros	Cons
Oligonucleotide	Easy to produce, safe to handle	Lack of target specificity, Transient expression patterns
Liposome	Easy to produce, safe to handle	Lack of target specificity, Transient expression patterns
Viruses		
Adenovirus	Infects dividing and nondividing cells	Immunogenic, transient expression, random intregration
AAV	Nonpathogenic, specific integration site (wild-type), infects nondividing cells	Very small payload
Retrovirus	Stable long-term expression, large payload	Random integration, only infects dividing cells
Lentivirus	Stable long-term expression, arge payload, infects dividing and nondividing cells	Random integration

AAV, adeno-associated virus.

expresses numerous viral proteins, the adenovirus stimulates the immune system and can cause vascular inflammation *(113,114)*. Utilization of this vector system has been shown to delay the development of hypertension in genetic and nongenetic models of hypertension for approx 1 mo (*see* Tables 1 and 2). Because of the transient expression patterns and induction of the immune response, the conventional forms of the vector have serious limitations and will likely not be used for human gene therapy for chronic diseases. With advances in virology, however, use of this vector may prove beneficial in the future.

Recent advances in engineering retroviral vectors have increased transduction of cardiovascular cells. Two methods shown to improve gene delivery into vascular beds are serotype switching and the use of antibodies. The adenovirus family is very diverse and there have been over 50 different serotypes identified. Pseudotyping technology can exploit certain serotypes to target gene delivery to specific target tissues. For CVDs, utilization of this approach has been successful in improving gene delivery. For example, serotypes 4 and 11 possess higher affinity binding and infectivity for vascular endothelial cells *(115)*. Harari et al. *(116)* reported that they were able to target activated endothelium in vitro by using an antibody-mediated adenovirus directed against e-selectin. This concept may allow for strategies to target specific vascular beds in vivo.

Adeno-Associated Virus

Adeno-associated virus (AAV) is a stable, nonpathogenic vector that can infect nondividing cells. The AAV is a parvovirus, and its replication is dependent on the presence of a helper virus. The wild-type AAV integrates in a specific region of chromosome 19. Although its site of integration is known, the recombinant AAV (rAAV) loses this property and randomly integrates. There are some limitations with this vector system because it is difficult to produce large quantities of virus and it has a limited transgene carrying capacity *(117–119)*. Although the carrying capacity is limited, this virus is amply suited for the delivery of small genes and AS cDNA, which only needs to code for a small fragment of the target gene to be effective. This virus is also fairly safe for human use. AAV is not pathogenic and is not associated with any known disease state.

To produce rAAV a helper virus (adenovirus) is required. In producing the rAAV, viral coding sequences are removed so that the source of immune reactions to viral gene expression is removed and no inflammation response is evoked in vivo. AAV infects all mammalian cells, and its expression in target tissue is long-lasting (118). With no helper virus present, AAV infection remains latent indefinitely. Upon infection of the cell with helper virus, the AAV genome is excised, replicated, packaged, and finally released by the cell.

The AAV is a good candidate for gene therapy because it is safe and has a very broad host range. AAV has been successfully used in phase 1 clinical trials for the treatment of cystic fibrosis (120). It has also been used to deliver AS to the AT_1R in hypertensive rat models. Use of rAAV containing AT_1R-AS has been administered systemically as well as centrally in the SHR (74), and resulted in a decrease in BP and a reduction in left-ventricular hypertrophy.

Retroviral Vectors

Retroviral vectors, which have a large transgene payload capacity, can be produced with high efficiency and titer. The viral genome is a single-stranded RNA that is converted to DNA in the host cell by reverse transcription mediated by viral reverse transcriptase. The DNA is then integrated into the genome and can result in long-term expression of the transgene. This virus type is highly efficient at delivering genes to dividing cells; however, this vector is not efficient at infecting nondividing cells. The other major disadvantage of retroviruses lies in their random genome integration pattern (121), which raises concerns about their safety for practical use in vivo. Despite this disadvantage, we and others have been very successful in using the retrovirus to prevent hypertension, cardiac hypertrophy, and restenosis in several experimental models (62–67,91,93,99,122).

Lentivirus

The lentiviral vectors are a subfamily of retrovirus and are the most recent addition of vectors to the rapidly developing field. The lentiviral vectors are derived from the human immunodeficiency virus type 1 (HIV-1). These highly "humanized" vectors combine the advantages of retroviral and adenoviral vectors, and they are emerging as the vectors of choice for long-term, stable in vitro and in vivo gene transfer. These vectors are attractive because they can efficiently carry large transgene cassettes (up to 18 kb in size) and they are capable of transducing both dividing and quiescent cells. Lentiviruses can allow for long-term expression of the transgene with little immune response. Lentiviruses can infect noncycling and postmitotic cells and have the potential to generate transgenic mice by infecting stem cells (123). This vector has been successfully used to transduce genes into selected tissues of adult animals with a long-term expression potential (124). However, its use in vivo has been limited by production. We have recently developed an efficient method for packaging and concentrating lentiviral vectors that consistently yields high-titer virus on a scale suitable for in vivo applications (125). We demonstrated that lentiviral vector delivered systemically can transduce several cardiovascular-relevant tissues, including the brain, and the transgene exhibited long-term (120 d, duration of experiment) expression *(126)*. Recent findings from our lab using this lentivirus to overexpress the AT_2R in SHR demonstrated that our transgene effectively transduced cardiac myocytes and significantly reduced the cardiac hypertrophy in these animals without effecting BP *(59)*. These findings provide significant information with respect to the AT_2R and cardiac hypertrophy, and suggest that the AT_2R do antagonize effects mediated by the AT_1R.

The lentivirus preparations we used were administered to 5-d-old animals. Future studies will determine the effectiveness of utilizing this vector delivery method in adults. Because the lentivirus can infect nondividing cells, it should be effective in adult animals and is most likely more applicable in a clinical setting over the retrovirus, because it could reverse the disease state in contrast to preventing the development of the disease.

CELL TYPE-SPECIFIC PROMOTERS

Numerous technological advances have afforded us the ability to underexpress (reduction approach) or overexpress (induction approach) transgenes of interest in various animal models. However, ubiquitous expression of a transgene may lead to undesirable effects. Local or targeted gene delivery has the advantage of concentrating the gene therapy in a relevant tissue, and reduces the risk of losing the vector to sites where its under- or overexpression may have deleterious consequences. One way to obviate this potential problem is to utilize tissue- or cell-selective promoters to limit transgene expression to a subset of cells or tissues. Such systems have been developed to selectively alter gene expression in the heart and vascular smooth muscle *(127,128)*. For example, tissue-specific gene expression can be enhanced by the use of specific cardiac myocytes promoters, such as mlc-v (ventricular-specific myosin light chain-2), or cardiac troponin T gene promoter *(129,130)*. Others have used a rat neuron-specific enolase promoter (Ad-NSE) to specifically target neuronal cells *(131)*. Thus, one can selectively target gene delivery to specific tissue types, provided one has utilized the appropriate tissue-specific promoter. Utilization with these specific promoters will limit expression of the transgene to specific tissue sites that are relevant for the particular disease state.

Targeting specific tissues/cells with a transgene early in development can have detrimental or even lethal effects. For example, transgenic mice with endothelially expressed genes have been reported to harbor severe developmental abnormalities *(132)*. Thus, the more optimal approach to gene therapy is the development of system(s) that allow for externally regulated control of transgene expression.

REGULATABLE PROMOTERS

Constitutive expression of a transgene may produce undesirable effects if nonphysiological levels of proteins are produced. Although gene therapy approaches have extraordinary promise, uncontrolled transgene expression may lead to deleterious consequences. Therefore, the ability to modulate transcription of a transgene or vector would be desirable for effective and safe gene therapy in humans. One way of overcoming this problem is to utilize a regulated gene expression system that uses exogenous ligands to control transgene expression. Some of these previously developed systems use inducible promoters, which are modulated by exogenous ligands, such as mifepristone *(133)*, rapamycin *(134)*, ecdysone *(135)*, or tetracycline *(136)*, to drive the expression of the transgene. These systems can allow for the activation of a transgene when needed, thereby allowing researchers and clinicians to "turn off" of the transgene expression if complications arise, or to "turn on" the transgene when it is needed. In general, these systems use an inducer or repressor that can reversibly bind the endogenous ligand, and its chimeric state then acts as a transcriptional factor for its particular promoter. Ideally, such an exogenous inducer would allow a wide therapeutic window and few, if any, side effects when compared to conventional pharmacological therapy.

Pioneering work by Bujard and Gossen *(137)* established the tetracycline transactivator system as a reliable tool for regulating transgene expression. This tetracycline *(tet)*-inducible system consists of three major components: the tetracycline-binding-transcriptional modulator protein, the corresponding tetracycline-responsive promoter element and the tetracycline-class pharmacological agent. Doxycycline (Dox) is the most commonly used tetracycline drug used with the *tet* system because it has a high affinity for the *tet* transcriptional modulator protein, has a low toxicity, and favorable pharmacokinetic properties for use in vivo *(138,139)*. This system has been used for transcriptional control of transgenes for over 10 yr, and a continuous line of modifications to the system have made it much more effective in tightly regulating gene expression *(140)*.

The original *tet* system was a "*tet*-off" version, in which application of a tetracycline caused attenuated expression of the transgene. Subsequent development of the *tet* system by Gossen et al. *(136)* resulted in the generation of a "*tet*-on" version, where application of a tetracycline causes increased transgene expression. Despite recent improvements in the *tet*-on system, including the addition of a tet-silencer protein *(141)*, this inducible system has an inherent leak in basal transgene expression and causes only mild increases in transgene expression (when compared with the range of expression of the *tet*-off system) *(142)*. Certain other problems with the *tet*-on system are currently being worked out, such as cellular toxicity, insensitivity to Dox in certain tissues, and unstable transcripts *(143,144)*. Some groups *(141,145)*, however, have suggested that differences in regulation may exist among various mouse strains.

A possible drawback with this system is that it requires two vectors, and these vectors both have to infect the same cell to achieve a properly regulated system. Despite this issue, our lab constructed dual cassette retrovirus vectors that together encoded a modified enhanced green fluorescent protein (d2EGFP) under the control *tet*-on system. Viral particles were then used to infect rat aortic vascular smooth muscle cells and pulmonary endothelial cells. Cells transduced with both vectors were examined by fluorescence microscopy for inducible expression of d2EGFP. Incubation of dual-vector infected cells with Dox caused a robust expression of d2EGFP within 48 h, whereas removal of Dox caused a disappearance of green fluorescence within 24 h, *(146)*. These results demonstrate tightly regulated gene expression using a retroviral vector system. We subsequently used this system to effectively induce AT_1R-AS, resulting in a lowering of BP in the SHR *(147)* when the animals were maintained on Dox.

However, with newer technologies, these regulatable systems will have even greater advantages. For instance, Teng et al. *(148)* have recently combined the components of the regulated system with tissue-specific properties to direct the controlled induction of an exogenous transgene to the vascular endothelium of an adult mouse by utilizing an endothelial cell-specific promoter through the *tet*-on system.

Recently some *tet*-regulated transgenic mice have been developed. This reduces the payload requirement of a gene therapy vector in these animals, because the animals already harbor half of the gene-switch system ubiquitously. Corbel and Rossi *(140)* recently summarized work on new tissue-specific tetracycline (activation and repression) transgenic mice, as well as the recent methods utilized to deliver tetracycline-regulated genes in vitro and in vivo. Ju et al. *(149)* recently generated transgenic mice with the use of an arterial smooth muscle cell (SMC)-restricted (SM22α promoter-driven), tetracycline-controlled transactivator (tTA) to effect conditional expression of a tTA-dependent transgene encoding rat vascular chymase (RVCH). The recombinant RVCH converts Ang I to Ang II in vitro. In their study, hypertension was completely reversed and the medial thickening of mesenteric arteries from $tTA^+/RVCH^+$ mice was prevented by doxycycline. Therefore, by utilizing such combined technologies, more specific and controlled targeting of selected transgenes can be employed more effectively as therapeutic tools.

More recently, use of endogenous instead of exogenous regulatable systems have been used effectively in vivo, further demonstrating the importance and versatility of effectively controlling gene expression and its application to hypertensive therapy. Kantachuvesiri et al. *(150)* have used a rat CPY1a1 enhancer/promoter sequence to control mouse Ren2 cDNA expression in rats to create an inducible model of hypertension. BP and the RAS returned to normal in the absence of the inducer. Other in vivo work has used adenovirally mediated transfer of ecdysone-inducible constructs to the heart and carotid bodies of rats *(151)*. Thus, these regulated systems offer significant advantages in utilizing gene therapy approaches to better understand disease processes and provide potential therapy for a variety of disease states.

Another example of an endogenous state-specific promoter is the hypoxia response element (HRE), which responds to hypoxic conditions within the cell. Under hypoxia, the transcription of numerous genes can be activated, including erythropoietin *(152,153)*, the β-adrenergic receptor *(154)*, glycolytic enzymes *(155,156)*, and vascular endothelial growth factor *(157,158)*, among others. Thus, this promoter could be used in various cardiovascular or metabolic disorders to regulate expression of genes that have been proven to have beneficial effects in conditions of ischemia, such as AS to the AT_1R *(159)*, the β-adrenergic receptor *(160,161)*, superoxide dismutase *(162,163)*, angiotensin-converting enzyme *(164,165)*, and vascular endothelial growth factor *(166)*.

Vigna et al. *(167)* were the first to report the generation of lentiviral vectors capable of delivering *tet*-regulated gene delivery to human hematopoietic progenitor cells ex vivo. The combination of lentiviral delivery with improved transcriptional activators of the *tet* system resulted in the regulation of an inducible gene that was maintained for over 20 wk after infection of these engineered cells. The lentivirus, with its much larger cassette site, may allow for both the tetracycline transactivator and the tetracycline response element to be housed in a single vector. We have used such a system for in vitro manipulation and are currently attempting to develop such a vector for subsequent in vivo gene therapy for hypertension in order to better control expression of our transgene of interest. Thus, these regulated systems offer significant advantages for the utilization of gene therapy approaches to better understand disease processes and to provide effective therapy for a variety of disease states.

CRE/Lox System

Another type of regulated system is an older CRE ("causes recombination")/Lox system. This technique allows for the modification of a specific gene with locus of crossover (loxP) sites flanking the specific region of interest though the use of standard gene targeting vectors in embryonic stem cells. These targeted alleles are said to be "floxed", or flanked by the loxP, and thus may not be fully functional. CRE recombinase directs recombination between loxP sites. Application of this technique in mice allows for deletion of selected material at specific times. This offers advantages over knockout models in that it can avoid the complications of not only embryonic lethality, but also the developmental compensatory changes that occur when there is a genetic knockout. Because this technology relies on homologous recombination in embryonic stem cells, its in vivo use is currently restricted to mice. Mice that are derived from these targeted embryonic stem cells are then bred to homozygosity for the targeted floxed allele and can then be crossed with other mice transgenic for CRE recombinants under the control of specific promoters to allow for a tissue-specific deletion of the floxed segment. Thus, the activity of a particular gene can be modified in a limited number of cells or tissues while the genetic content of the rest of the animal is essentially unaltered. Many tissue-specific CRE transgenic mice strains are becoming available and have provided insights into endocrine physiology in recent years. Most of these tissue-specific CRE/loxP-mediated gene deletions have been studied in endocrine or other target tissues, and have been nicely summarized by Ryding et al. *(168)*. A database cataloging these mouse models is available at http://www.mshri.on.ca/nagy/cre.htm.

Unfortunately, most CRE/loxP mouse experiments have several potential pitfalls. First, expression of CRE within a particular tissue or cell is rarely uniform, which can lead to mosaic recombination. A second potential pitfall is that of transcriptional interference by vector-derived sequences. Like strain differences observed with the *tet* system *(141,169)*, one might also anticipate that the efficiency of CRE recombination may also be strain-dependent, although there has yet to be any formal investigation of this possibility. Despite these potential drawbacks, the CRE/loxP technology is a well established genetic tool for the study of conditional deletion of genes in mice.

Vigilant Vector Approach

Recently, some groups have begun work on developing cell-state-specific promoter systems for transgenes. A popular example of this methodology is referred to as the "vigilant vector," which senses hypoxic conditions within the cell and responds by increasing transgene transcription. This approach has been used to signal dormant transgenes to become active and to protect specific tissues with high amplification of the specific transgene. In order for this system to be effective, four components are required *(170)*. The first component is stable vector that is safe and can be administered by systemic injection and in which the transgene is expressed in a particular organ or tissue. The second component is a reversible gene switch that acts as a biosensor and can detect certain physiological signals. The third component is a tissue-specific promoter, and the fourth component is an amplification system. This type of system can have broad applications. One can switch tissue-specific promoters or switch out different transgenes and/or protective genes in order to apply this vigilant approach in a variety of disease states. Tang et al. *(171)* recently characterized a hypoxic inducible double plasmid system for myocardial ischemia. This hypoxia-sensitive promoter could be used to drive transcription of hypoxia-protective genes, such as superoxide dismutase *(162)*, the β-adrenergic receptor *(160)*, and components of the RAS *(159,164)*, thus conferring some immunity to hypoxia upon these cells.

siRNA Technology

Selective downregulation (knockdown) of a specific gene can be a useful method for therapeutic intervention, provided the targeted gene is important in the pathogenesis of the disease. One way to facilitate this genetic "knockdown" is the use of AS gene technology. The major disadvantage of this method is that the transgene product (the AS mRNA) is destroyed along with the target mRNA. A recent advancement to the AS approach is a conserved posttranscriptional gene silencing (PTGS) mechanism mediated by double-stranded RNA (dsRNA). Silencing of gene expression using dsRNA, known as RNA interference (RNAi) or short interfering RNAs (siRNAs), provides a powerful tool for analyzing gene function. Although not all of the mechanisms by which this system operates are completely known, this RNAi method is more efficient than AS in that it is able to cleave the target mRNA and mark future copies of the target mRNA to be destroyed, while the interfering mRNA itself is not destroyed along with the target RNA *(172)*. It can therefore cleave and destroy multiple pieces of target RNA. An RNase III-like enzyme called a "Dicer" cuts long dsRNA, or hairpin RNAs, into double-stranded siRNAs *(173)*. These are typically 20–25 nucleotides (nt) long, and can trigger formation of an RNA silencing complex (RISC). The siRNA–RISC complex seeks out the mRNA with the targeted sequence and degrades it, effectively silencing that gene. Short dsRNAs can be synthesized in vitro and introduced into mammalian cells. Using these short siRNAs does not trigger antiviral mechanisms within the cell and can mediate gene-specific suppression in mammalian cells. As a result, a few copies of the interfering dsRNA can cause total degradation of cognate transcripts in a cell. This technology has been used successfully as a tool to analyze gene function in plants, insects, and nematodes *(174–176)*; however, use of long dsRNA in mammalian somatic cells results in activation of antiviral defense systems that can result in nonspecific degradation of RNA transcripts and a general loss of host cell protein synthesis, thus investigators soon discovered that introduction of smaller siRNA, less than 30 nt, can lead to gene specific silencing *(177)*.

Although there is significant potential for the use of this new AS technology to target specific genes associated with hypertension, important issues remain unresolved. Because there is no set pattern or rule yet discovered to determine the optimal sequence to target within a gene, investigators are encouraged to select several siRNA sequences in different locations along the gene of interest to test in order to find the most efficient site that will be important in silencing the gene of interest. A single-point mutation in certain locations of the paired region of the siRNA duplex can abolish target mRNA degradation *(177)*. siRNAs are extraordinarily effective at lowering the amounts of targeted RNA—and, by extension, proteins—frequently to undetectable levels. However, any polymorphism in the gene of interest can complicate the process. There are several web-based tools to assist in design of siRNAs (examples include those provided by Ambion [http://www.ambion.com] and Dharmacon [http://www.dharmacon.com]). Once a sequence is identified, the siRNA transgene must be chemically synthesized and transfected. Recent evidence suggests that the effectiveness of siRNAs may depend greatly on the method of transfection *(178)*. There is no uptake of siRNAs into cells, and the delivery to selected sites of therapy remains problematic *(179)*. Handling of the RNAi is laborious and complex because of ubiquitous RNAses. However, with advancing technologies, this may be a very effective means to knock down targeted disease-producing genes. Various viral vectors are being evaluated to increase infection for in vivo administration of siRNA.

Lentiviral and other retroviral systems have been shown to be effective in many settings and adenovirally based vectors are also being evaluated *(180,181)*. The ability to efficiently and stably produce and deliver sufficient amounts of siRNA to the proper target tissues still requires refinement before this new technology can be tried clinically. Xia et al. *(246)* recently described a virally mediated delivery mechanism that results in specific silencing of targeted genes through expression of siRNA. These investigators demonstrated expression of exogenous and endogenous genes in vitro and in vivo in brain and liver, and further applied this strategy to a model system of a major class of neurodegenerative disorders, finally suggesting that this virally mediated strategy could be successfully used to reduce expression of target genes to provide therapy for human diseases. Lewis et al. *(182)* recently described a method for efficient in vivo delivery of siRNAs to organs of postnatal mice. Lentivirus-based vectors may be the most promising siRNA expression system to drive gene inhibition in stem cells, because the transgenes that are expressed from the lentiviruses are not silenced during the developmental process and can thus be used to generate transgenic animals through infection of embryos *(180,183)*. Cheng et al. *(184)* recently reviewed this field, and provide an overview of its potential applications in the treatment of human disease.

MICROARRAY TECHNOLOGY AND ITS IMPLICATIONS IN GENE THERAPY

Recent advances in genomic techniques and their integration into physiology have resulted in the genesis of the "functional genomics" era. Functional genomics is a multidisciplinary approach to studying genes, their products, and interactions among them that are responsible for mediating physiological responses. Also included in functional genomics is the detection and characterization of aberrations of genetic processes that may result in diseases. Recent advances in molecular biology and technology have made it possible to monitor the expression level of numerous genes simultaneously. Cardiovascular research has focused mainly on only a small fraction of known genes; however, information gleaned from genome sequencing and the development of microarray technologies has the potential to provide for genome-wide analysis of genes that can mediate BP regulation and their potential contribution to the pathogenesis of hypertension. Protein microarrays also have been developed for protein expression analysis and interaction analysis, which may include protein–protein, ligand–receptor, enzyme–substrate, and nucleic acid–protein interactions. However, the use of high-throughput arrays (both RNA and protein) has yet to realize its full potential in cardiovascular research. Issues concerning reproducibility and preanalytic variables can make the discovery process from these methods tedious *(185,186)*.

Numerous investigators are using gene expression profiles in hypertensive models in hopes of identifying genes relevant to hypertension. Candidate genes can be identified from transcript profiling, and different strategies can be utilized to evaluate their potential relevance in the pathogenesis of hypertension. Clinical studies have demonstrated that genetic variation accounts for up to half of the phenotypic variation in BP *(187)*. Numerous studies have demonstrated links between genes of the RAS (i.e., *angiotensinogen*, *renin*, *ACE*, and AT_1R) and hypertension in various populations *(188,189)*. The use of inbred rat models of hypertension and congenic strains also has identified large chromosomal regions containing quantitative trait loci that account for genetic variation in BP

(190–193). The construction of minimal congenic strains has been used to further narrow down the particular loci involved *(194)*. However, consistent associations have been difficult to demonstrate, and little progress has been made toward identifying the specific genetic variants that contribute to a particular phenotype. Therefore, to better understand a polygenic disease such as hypertension, we need to identify which groups of genes account for the hypertensive phenotype, and how these gene clusters are regulated.

Gene expression profiling has been utilized to gain insight into disease mechanisms. Assessment of the expression of a large number of genes have been realized by the use of high-throughput gene profiling technology, such as cDNA and oligonucleotide microarrays, as well as serial analysis of gene expression (SAGE). In addition, for genomes that are not yet fully sequenced, transcript profiling of expressed sequence tags (EST) provides expression information on novel genes. The technical limitations and issues relating to analysis of microarray data have been reviewed recently *(195–198)*. Gene expression profiles most often represent complex phenotypes. Cluster analysis of expression data may distinguish particular groups of genes that are regulated in a similar manner. Profiling has been used to identify genes involved in hypertension, and usually compares differentially expressed genes in inbred genetic rat models of hypertension with their normotensive controls. Differential gene expression between these two groups, however, may not necessarily reflect causative mechanisms in hypertension. The differences may reflect a genetic difference between the strains that are unrelated to hypertension, or they may be expressed as a result of the high BP and not be related to any cause for the increase in BP. In addition, like any method, there are some technical drawbacks for the sole use of microarrays in identifying candidate genes. Some limitations and issues relating to analysis of microarray data have been reviewed recently *(196,197,199,200)*. Therefore, it is essential that other techniques, such as QTL mapping, complementation testing, or loss/gain of function experiments, be combined with the gene profiling to determine if differential gene expression reflects a causative role in hypertension *(201–203)*.

Transcript profiling of inbred genetic models of hypertension, such as the SHR, have proven useful in identifying potential genetic mechanisms of hypertension. Microarray profiling from kidneys of SHR and Wistar–Kyoto (WKY) animals has identified a number of differentially expressed genes in SHR *(203,204)*. However, even when comparing different strains of SHR, there is a large variability in genes that are differentially expressed, which underscores the genetic heterogeneity of the different strains *(203)*. These observations suggest that there can be both common and distinct genetic mechanisms in hypertension in different SHR strains.

The most appropriate tissue type for gene profiling is debatable. Most transcript profiling studies in hypertensive rats have used RNA derived from kidneys *(202,203)* to identify genes that may contribute to hypertension, as the kidney has a well-established role in long-term regulation of BP. We are currently utilizing gene expression profiling in different areas of the brain, such as the hypothalamus and brainstem, in order to identify target candidate genes that may be regulated by the brain RAS in the SHR *(205,206)*. To eliminate any genetic alteration resulting secondarily from an elevation in BP, we have also assessed gene expression profiles in primary neuronal cultures derived from the hypothalamus and brainstem areas of neonatal (prehypertensive) SHR and WKY rats *(205)*. We found that neonatal SHR neurons in culture exhibit increased AT_1R transcript expression and functional receptors as compared to WKY cultures. These results indicate that the hyperactivity of the brain RAS observed in the adult SHR is also present in the neuronal cultures *(207)*. We identified genes that are regulated by Ang II by comparing transcript profiles of neuronal cultures treated with vehicle to those treated with Ang II. Utilizing gene filtering and statistical analysis, we identified differential expression of 299 genes and 109 EST between strains *(205)*. Interestingly, SHR neurons exhibit an altered Ang II-induced pattern of gene expression as most differentially expressed genes were upregulated, whereas their expression was downregulated in WKY neurons (a complete list is available online at www.med.ufl.edu/phys/raizada/veerasingham.doc). This effort, like most of the gene expression profiling, has been of a correlational or descriptive nature. Further experiments are required to evaluate the physiological relevance of the altered gene profile of Ang II-responsive genes in SHR neurons, as well as that of genes that are differentially expressed between the two strains.

One potential therapeutic target gene in the brain that was differentially expressed in SHR compared to WKY neuronal cultures was adducin. Adducin is a ubiquitously expressed tetrameric cytoskeletal protein composed with either α/β or α/γ heterodimers, and is involved in intracellular protein trafficking, Ca^{2+} mobilization, and the phosphorylation state of certain kinases *(208)*. Genetic variations in α-adducin have been associated with primary human hypertension and the BP phenotype in Milan hypertensive rats *(25,209–211)*. Polymorphisms of the β and γ subunits may contribute to BP variation, especially when associated with α-adducin polymorphisms, consistent with the notion that biological activity of adducin is dependent on α/β or α/γ heterodimers *(25,210,211)*.

A role for adducin in BP regulation has been further supported by the demonstration of higher BP in β-adducin deficient mice than in wild-type mice *(212)*. We have identified a 22% decrease in γ-adducin *(Add3)* expression in SHR neurons compared with WKY neuronal cultures using gene expression profiling. Real-time RT-PCR confirmed the decrease in γ-adducin transcript, and Western blot analysis indicated a more dramatic decrease (approx 60%) in protein levels in SHR compared with WKY neurons in culture (206). This decrease in γ-adducin expression was maintained in the hypothalamus and brainstem of adult SHR and was also observed in mRen2 rats, suggesting that it is common to hypertensive models that exhibit an overactive brain RAS *(206)*. Furthermore, Ang II treatment of either WKY or SHR neuronal cultures resulted in a decrease of γ-adducin transcript and protein levels, indicating a regulation of expression by Ang II. These observations demonstrate a decrease in γ-adducin expression in hypothalamic and medullary areas of hypertensive rats, and support the concept that an overactive brain RAS may be responsible for the decreased expression. We also evaluated the effect of γ-adducin inhibition on the firing rate of neuronal cultures. Using intracellular delivery of γ-adducin-specific antibodies to inhibit γ-adducin resulted in an increased neuronal firing rate, which was similar to that observed with Ang II. This effect was not additive, suggesting that a common mechanism resulted in the increased firing rate *(206)*. We subsequently investigated two nongenetic models of hypertension, the chronic Ang II model and the desoxycorticosterone acetate model *(213)*. In both models, the increase in BP was associated with a 70% decrease in hypothalamic γ-adducin; however, in contrast with the genetic models of hypertension, there was no change in brainstem γ-adducin. Neuronal cultures from the WKY strain of rats, when incubated with Ang II, resulted in a 60% decrease in the neuronal γ-adducin *(213)*. Decreased γ-adducin may therefore contribute to augmented basal neuronal firing rate in cardiovascular-regulatory brain areas of hypertensive animals. Because central γ-adducin expression is decreased in SHR, we would predict that a gene therapy approach to overexpress this gene in the brain of the SHR may decrease BP and reverse hypertension, whereas deleting or reducing its expression in WKY rats would induce hypertension.

Yu et al. *(244)* demonstrated an elevation in the expression of soluble epoxide hydrolase (sEH) from the kidney of the SHR when compared with the WKY. In addition, this group showed that blocking sEH lowered the BP in the SHR. Furthermore, Sinal et al. *(214)* reported that BP is reduced in a knockout mouse model for sEH, although this change in BP was observed only in male rats. However, when the kidneys from multiple strains of SHR and WKY rats were utilized in subsequent gene profiling studies no consistent changes in this gene were observed and there was no clear correlation between expression of the gene and hypertension *(203,245)*. This led us to propose a novel hypothesis about the role of this gene in hypertension. Our hypothesis is that the expression of brain sEH may be key in the regulation of BP, and its altered expression of dysregulation could be better linked to hypertension. This hypothesis was tested and subsequently validated by demonstrating an upregulation of this enzyme in the hypothalamus and brain stem areas of the SHR by expression profiling analysis. In spite of the excellent physiological link between dysregulated expression of brain sEH and hypertension, direct gene transfer studies must be carried out to conclusively demonstrate the role of this enzyme in hypertension. It is from studies like these that gene profiling experiments that initially correlate changes in gene expression can move beyond to seek out mechanisms of functional significance.

FUTURE GENE TARGETS OF THE RAS

The RAS is classically known as a hormonal system that is involved in salt and water regulation and BP control. The RAS is one example of a system in which dysregulated expression and hyperactivity have been associated with the development and maintenance of hypertension. Both the systemic (endocrine) and tissue (paracrine/autocrine) versions of the RAS contribute to hypertension *(238,242)*. In the systemic RAS, a coordinated sequence of events involving various organs work together to generate circulating active hormone, Ang II. In this classical systemic endocrine system, angiotensinogen, which is produced in the liver, is converted to Ang I by the enzyme renin, which is secreted by the kidney. ACE is an enzyme that is found both circulating in the blood and membrane bound in numerous tissues including epithelial and endothelial cells *(215,216)*, converts ANG I to ANG II. Various areas of the brain are also rich in ACE *(217)*. Ang II produced as a result of the endocrine RAS is responsible for many short-term effects of Ang II, such as arterial vasoconstriction, aldosterone release, and sodium and water reabsorption by signaling through the AT_1R *(223,230,238)*. This classical understanding of the RAS led to the use of ACE inhibitors (ACEI) and Ang II receptor blockers (ARBs) as therapeutic agents in the treatment of hypertension. Because a hyperactive RAS is a key player in hypertension, and because 40–60% of hypertensive patients respond to ACE-inhibitors/AT_1R-antagonists, one could hypothesize that genetic manipulation of this system to inhibit signaling within the RAS may, in principle, be an ideal method to attempt a genetic cure for this disease. We and others *(62–67,73,74,84,91,93,99,101,102,104)* have used an AS technique to downregulate transcription of the ACE enzyme and/or the AT_1R to prevent the development of hypertension in both genetic and nongenetic models of experimental hypertension. However, this classical RAS is more complex, and new discoveries regarding angiotensin degradation fragments provide even more potential targets for gene therapy in hypertension.

Recently, the ACE2 enzyme has been characterized *(218,219)*. This enzyme, which initially was found in the testis, kidney, and heart, has also been identified in a wide variety of tissues and is most likely localized, much like ACE *(218–220)*. It shares 40% homology with ACE, but differs greatly in substrate specificity, and its activity is not altered by ACEI. ACE2 is one of several enzymes that catalyze the formation of degradation fragments angiotensin 1–9 (Ang 1–9) and angiotensin 1–7 (Ang 1–7) from both Ang I and Ang II, respectively *(see* Fig. 1). In mice lacking the *ACE2* gene, Allred et al. *(227)* observed a decrease in baseline BP and an enhanced pressor response during intravenous infusion of Ang II as compared with normal mice. BP was also decreased in animals that overexpressed *ACE2 (228)*. Therefore, the physiological effect of an imbalance of ACE2 over that of ACE could shift the RAS to increase vasodilator effects and reduce vasoconstrictor effects, thus resulting in a reduced BP *(see* Fig. 1). It is conceivable that the balance between ACE and ACE2 may be a pivotal mechanism in the regulation of BP and in the tissue pathophysiology (i.e., cardiac hypertrophy, renal disease) that has been associated with the tissue RAS. ACE2 also has the potential to be a better target than ACE because (1) it does not have the confounding interpretation effects that ACE does on bradykinin levels; (2) the gene has both a secreted form and a membrane-bound form that may allow us to differentiate BP effects from end-organ target pathologies; and (3) control of this unique enzyme can shift the emphasis of the entire RAS to one of vasodilation instead of vasoconstriction, and thus regulation of this enzyme may have significant therapeutic effects in the treatment of hypertension and other cardiovascular abnormalities.

Even though the actions of Ang II are best characterized, a role for other Ang peptides, such as Ang III, Ang IV, and Ang 1–7, as well as other Ang receptors, is rapidly emerging *(223–225)*. Because ACE inhibitors and ARBs are effective in treating essential hypertension, it is conceivable that some of the actions of these drugs could be mediated through these nonclassical components of the RAS. Blocking the ACE enzyme, for example, causes bradykinin levels to increase, and this leads to a lowering of BP *(226)*. Ang I levels would increase with ACE inhibition, and Ang II levels would increase with ARB treatment. In both cases, this could lead to an increase in Ang 1–7 via ACE2 and other endopeptidases. Ang 1–7 has been suggested to antagonize Ang II action directly at the AT_1R as well as indirectly via other pathways (such as antagonizing ACE) and its concentrations are increased during ACE inhibition *(221,222)*. Although Ang 1–7 is catabolized by ACE, it is also considered a competitive inhibitor of ACE *(219)*. This new knowledge of the RAS suggests several potential genetic targets. Overexpression of ACE2, or increased production of Ang 1–7, are two future possible targets for gene therapy in the treatment of hypertension.

Most studies of the RAS have focused on the AT_1R subtype. This subtype is one that is responsible for most of the known actions of Ang II, such as vasoconstriction, enhancement of noradrenergic neurotransmission, and release of hormones from the adrenal gland *(229,230)*. There is an additional receptor subtype that can be activated by Ang II, the AT_2R *(229,230)*. This receptor, like the AT_1R, is a G protein-coupled receptor with seven transmembrane regions *(229–233)*. Although similar in size (363 amino acids for AT_2R and 359 amino acids for AT_1R), there is only 34% homology between the two receptor subtypes. The AT_2R is more widely distributed in fetal tissues, and it has been suggested that this receptor is involved in developmental processes *(229–233)*. Generally, the actions of AT_2Rs oppose those of the AT_1R *(229–233)*. AT_2R knockout models

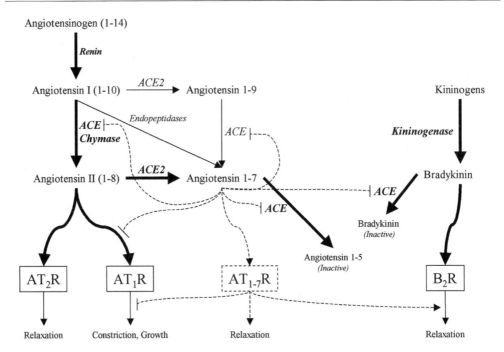

Fig. 1 The renin–angiotensin system. ACE, angiotensin-coverting enzyme; AT_1R, angiotensin type I receptors; AT_2R, angiotension type II receptors; B_2R, bradykinin type II receptors.

exhibit increases in basal BP and/or show enhanced pressor responses to Ang II *(234,235)*. Further, we have shown recently that overexpression of the AT_2R inhibits cardiac hypertrophy in the SHR *(59)* and that underexpression of the AT_2R can elevate BP in Sprague-Dawley animals *(80)*. The recent finding that the AT_2R can act in a constitutive manner *(236)* is also intriguing, and may suggest some clinical significance. Its use as a genetic target will continue to be examined.

In contrast to the classical systemic (endocrine) RAS, there is the local-tissue (paracrine/autocrine) RAS. Components of the classical, systemic RAS are found in numerous tissues *(237–240)*. Ang II and its other active degradation fragments can be produced within given tissues, and thus have their physiological effects locally at that (or neighboring) tissues. This paracrine/autocrine system appears to play a major role in long-term cardiovascular regulation, especially in regulating cardiac hypertrophy and remodeling of the arteriole vasculature in other tissues *(241–243)*. We have demonstrated that overexpression of the AT_2R *(59)* or underexpression of the AT_1R *(62–64,91,93,99)* is effective in preventing cardiac hypertrophy in genetic and nongenetic models of experimental hypertension. Targeting specific tissues with gene therapy approaches may be able to reverse and/or prevent the pathophysiological alterations that occur in hypertensive and other cardiovascular diseases. Figure 1 identifies most of the well-characterized components of the RAS, and thus identifies some current and future targets for gene therapy.

SUMMARY AND PERSPECTIVES

Hypertension is a prevalent disease in which current intervention with pharmaceutical agents is effective in only about one-third of patients. Additionally, the current pharmacological approach aims to control BP, and will not lead to prevention or cure of the disease. Gene therapy has the potential to prevent and/or cure hypertension, as clinical findings strongly support the notion that hypertension is genetically based. Many of these clinical findings involve components of the RAS, although there are many other candidate genes. Although there are numerous technologies available to use for discovery and examination of candidate genes, and for the delivery and manipulation of gene therapies, each has its own strengths and weaknesses. Current knowledge of the pathways that can lead to hypertension can suggest some of these potential genes, but this method will not reveal novel pathways or mechanisms to study and target. Microarray expression profiling studies can be used to identify a number of differentially expressed genes, but the challenge remains to determine the physiological relevance of these findings, and to identify which of these genes are linked to the development and/or maintenance of hypertension. The combination of gene expression profiling and the phenotypic characterization of in vitro and in vivo loss- or gain-of-function experiments has the potential to identify genes involved in the pathogenesis of hypertension, and thereby presents novel targets for therapy. Our primary research task then, still remains, to identify significant candidate genes.

REFERENCES

1. Deshmukh R, Smith A, Lilly LS. Hypertension. In: Pathophysiology of heart disease. (Lilly LS, ed.). 1998; Williams & Wilkins, Baltimore, MD: 267–288.
2. American Heart Association Heart Disease and Stroke Statistics, 2004. Update Dallas, TX; American Heart Association, 2003. www.americanheart.org/statistics/index.html
3. Sowers, JR. Is hypertension an insulin-resistant state? Metabolic changes associated with hypertension and antihypertensive therapy. Am Heart J 1991;122:932–935.
4. Ferrannini E, Natali A. Essential hypertension, metabolic disorders, and insulin resistance. Am Heart J 1991;4:1274–1282.
5. Reaven GL. Insulin resistance, hyperinsulinemia, and hypertriglyceridemia in the etiology and clinical course of hypertension. Am J Med 1991;90(suppl 2A):7S–12S.
6. Cusi D, Barlassina C, Taglietti MV. Genetics of human arterial hypertension. J Nephrol 2003;16:609–615.
7. Murray CJ, Lopez AD. Global mortality, disability, and the contribution of risk factors: Global Burden of Disease Study. Lancet 1997;349:1436–1442.
8. Stamler J, Stamler R, Neaton JD. Blood pressure, systolic and diastolic, and cardiovascular risks. Arch Intern Med 1993;153:598–615.
9. Whelton PK. Epidemiology of hypertension. Lancet 1994;334:101–106.
10. Devereux RB, Pickering TG, Harshfield GA, et al. Left ventricular hypertrophy in patients with hypertension: importance of blood pressure response to regularly recurring stress. Circulation 1983;68:470–476.
11. Wang X, Ren B, Liu S, Sentex E, Tappia PS, Dhalla NS. Characterization of cardiac hypertrophy and heart failure due to volume overload in the rat. J Appl Physiol 2003;94:752–763.
12. de Simone G, Pasanisi F, Contaldo F. Link of nonhemodynamic factors to hemodynamic determinants of left ventricular hypertrophy. Hypertension 2001;38:13–18.
13. Chobanian AV, Bakris GL, Black HR, et al., and the national high blood pressure educational program coordinating committee. Seventh report of the Joint National Committee on Prevention, Detection, Evaluation and Treatment of High Blood Pressure. Hypertension 2003;42:1206–1252.
14. Joint National Committee on Prevention, Detection, Evaluation and Treatment of High Blood Pressure: The sixth report of the Joint National Committee on Prevention, Detection, Evaluation and Treatment of High Blood Pressure. Arch Intern Med 1997;157:2413–2446.
15. Joffres MR, Ghadirian P, Fodor JG, Petrasovits A, Cockalingam A, Hamet P. Awareness, treatment, and control of hypertension in Canada. Am J Hypertens 1997;10:1097–1102.
16. Wolf-Maier K, Cooper RS, Kramer H, et al. Hypertension treatment and control in five European countries, Canada, and the United States. Hypertension 2004;43:10–17.

17. Liu R, Persson AE. Angiotensin II stimulates calcium and nitric oxide release from Macula densa cells through AT1 receptors. Hypertension 2004;43:649–653.
18. Zhou MS, Jaimes EA, Raij L. Inhibition of oxidative stress and improvement of endothelial function by amlodipine in angiotensin II-infused rats. Am J Hypertens 2004;17:167–171.
19. Higashi M, Shimokawa H, Hattori T, et al. Long-term inhibition of Rho-kinase suppresses angiotensin II-induced cardiovascular hypertrophy in rats in vivo: effect on endothelial NAD(P)H oxidase system. Circ Res 2003;93:767–775.
20. Yamakawa T, Tanaka S, Kamei J, Kadonosono K, Okuda K. Phosphatidylinositol 3-kinase in angiotensin II-induced hypertrophy of vascular smooth muscle cells. Eur J Pharmacol 2003;478:39–46.
21. Yavuz D, Koc M, Toprak A, et al. Effects of ACE inhibition and AT1-receptor antagonism on endothelial function and insulin sensitivity in essential hypertensive patients. J Renin Angiotensin Aldosterone Syst 2003;4:197–203.
22. Henriksen EJ, Jacob S. Angiotensin converting enzyme inhibitors and modulation of skeletal muscle insulin resistance. Diabetes Obes Metab 2003;5:214–222.
23. Levesque S, Moutquin JM, Lindsay C, Roy M-C, Rousseau. Implications of an AGT halotype in multigene association study with pregnancy hypertension. Hypertension 2004;43:71–78.
24. Sethi AA, Nordestgaard BG, Agerholm-Larsen B, Frandsen E, Jensen G, Tybjaerg-Hansen A. Angiotensinogen polymorphisms and elevated blood pressure in the general population. Hypertension 2001;37:875–881.
25. Clark CJ, Davies E, Anderson NH, et al. α-adducin and angiotensin I-converting enzyme polymorphisms in essential hypertension. Hypertension 2000;36:990–994.
26. Tsai C-T, Fallin D, Chiang F-T, et al. Angiotensinogen gene haloytpe and hypertension. Interactions with ACE gene I Allele. Hypertension 2003;41:9–15.
27. Ueda S, Elliot HL, Morton JJ, Connell JMC. Enhanced pressor response to angiotensin I in normotensive men with the deletion genotype (DD) for angiotensin converting enzyme. Hypertension 1995;25:1266–1269.
28. Jeunemaitre X, Soubrier F, Kotelevtsev YV, et al. Molecular basis of human hypertension: role of angiotensinogen. Cell 1992;71:169–180.
29. Zee RY, Lou YK, Griffiths LR, Morris BJ. Association of a polymorphism of the angiotensin 1-converting enzyme gene with essential hypertension. Biochem Biophys Res Commun 1992;184:9–15.
30. Bonnardeaux A, Davies E, Jeunemaitre X, et al. Angiotensin II type 1 receptor gene polymorphisms in human essential hypertension. Hypertension 1994;24:63–69.
31. Qin YJ, Zhang JF, Wei YJ, Ding JF, Chen KH, Tang J. Gene suture—a novel method for intramuscular gene transfer and its application in hypertension therapy. Life Sci 1999;65:2193–203.
32. Lin KF, Chao J, Chao L. Atrial natriuretic peptide gene delivery reduces stroke-induced mortality rate in Dahl salt-sensitive rats. Hypertension 1999;33(1 Pt 2):219–224.
33. Lin KF, Chao J, Chao L. Atrial natriuretic peptide gene delivery attenuates hypertension, cardiac hypertrophy, and renal injury in salt-sensitive rats. Hum Gene Ther 1998;9:1429–1438.
34. Lin KF, Chao J, Chao L. Human atrial natriuretic peptide gene delivery reduces blood pressure in hypertensive rats. Hypertension 1995;26(6 Pt 1):847–853.
35. Wang C, Dobrzynski E, Chao J, Chao L. Adrenomedullin gene delivery attenuates renal damage and cardiac hypertrophy in Goldblatt hypertensive rats. Am J Physiol Renal Physiol 2001;280:F964–F971.
36. Zhang JJ, Yoshida H, Chao L, Chao J. Human adrenomedullin gene delivery protects against cardiac hypertrophy, fibrosis, and renal damage in hypertensive Dahl salt-sensitive rats. Hum Gene Ther 2000;11:1817–1827.
37. Dobrzynski E, Wang C, Chao J, Chao L. Adrenomedullin gene delivery attenuates hypertension, cardiac remodeling, and renal injury in deoxycorticosterone acetate-salt hypertensive rats. Hypertension 2000;36:995–1001.
38. Chao J, Jin L, Lin KF, Chao L. Adrenomedullin gene delivery reduces blood pressure in spontaneously hypertensive rats. Hypertens Res 1997;20:269–277.
39. Hirooka Y, Sakai K, Kishi T, Ito K, Shimokawa H, Takeshita A. Enhanced depressor response to endothelial nitric oxide synthase gene transfer into the nucleus tractus solitarii of spontaneously hypertensive rats. Hypertens Res 2003;26:325–331.
40. Alexander MY, Brosnan MJ, Hamilton CA, et al. Gene transfer of endothelial nitric oxide synthase but not Cu/Zn superoxide dismutase restores nitric oxide availability in the SHRSP. Cardiovascular Res 2000;47:609–617.
41. Lin KF, Chao L, Chao J. Prolonged reduction of high blood pressure with human nitric oxide synthase gene delivery. Hypertension 1997;30(3 Pt 1):307–313.

42. Tai MH, Hsiao M, Chan JY, et al. Gene delivery of endothelial nitric oxide synthase into nucleus tractus solitarii induces biphasic response in cardiovascular functions of hypertensive rats. Am J Hypertens 2004;17:63–70.

43. Zhao C, Wang P, Xiao X, et al. Gene therapy with human tissue kallikrein reduces hypertension and hyperinsulinemia in fructose-induced hypertensive rats. Hypertension 2003;42:1026–1033.

44. Emanueli C, Salis MB, Stacca T, et al. Rescue of impaired angiogenesis in spontaneously hypertensive rats by intramuscular human tissue kallikrein gene transfer. Hypertension 2001;38:136–141.

45. Wolf WC, Yoshida H, Agata J, Chao L, Chao J. Human tissue kallikrein gene delivery attenuates hypertension, renal injury, and cardiac remodeling in chronic renal failure. Kidney Int 2000;58:730–739.

46. Zhang JJ, Wang C, Lin KF, Chao L, Chao J. Human tissue kallikrein attenuates hypertension and secretes into circulation and urine after intramuscular gene delivery in hypertensive rats. Clin Exp Hypertens 1999;21:1145–1160.

47. Chao J, Zhang JJ, Lin KF, Chao L. Adenovirus-mediated kallikrein gene delivery reverses salt-induced renal injury in Dahl salt-sensitive rats. Kidney Int 1998;54:1250–1260.

48. Yayama K, Wang C, Chao L, Chao J. Kallikrein gene delivery attenuates hypertension and cardiac hypertrophy and enhances renal function in Goldblatt hypertensive rats. Hypertension 1998;31:1104–1110.

49. Chao J, Zhang JJ, Lin KF, Chao L. Human kallikrein gene delivery attenuates hypertension, cardiac hypertrophy, and renal injury in Dahl salt-sensitive rats. Hum Gene Ther 1998;9:21–31.

50. Jin L, Zhang JJ, Chao L, Chao J. Gene therapy in hypertension: adenovirus-mediated kallikrein gene delivery in hypertensive rats. Hum Gene Ther 1997;8:1753–1761.

51. Chao J, Yang Z, Jin L, Lin KF, Chao L. Kallikrein gene therapy in newborn and adult hypertensive rats. Can J Physiol Pharmacol 1997;75:750–756.

52. Chen LM, Chao L, Chao J. Adenovirus-mediated delivery of human kallistatin gene reduces blood pressure of spontaneously hypertensive rats. Hum Gene Ther 1997;8:341–347.

53. Chao J, Jin L, Chen LM, Chen VC, Chao L. Systemic and portal vein delivery of human kallikrein gene reduces blood pressure in hypertensive rats. Hum Gene Ther 1996;7:901–911.

54. Xiong W, Chao J, Chao L. Muscle delivery of human kallikrein gene reduced blood pressure in hypertensive rats. Hypertension 1995;25(4 Pt 2):715–719.

55. Wang C, Chao L, Chao J. Muscle delivery of human kallikrein gene reduces blood pressure in hypertensive rats. Hypertension 1995;25(4 Pt 2):715–719.

56. Chu Y, Iida S, Lund DD, et al. Gene transfer of extracellular superoxide dismutase reduces arterial pressure in spontaneously hypertensive rats: role of heparin-binding domain. Circ Res 2003;92:461–468.

57. Fennell JP, Brosnan MJ, Frater AJ, et al. Adenovirus-mediated overexpression of extracellular superoxide dismutase improves endothelial dysfunction in a rat model of hypertension. Gene Ther 2002;9:110–117.

58. Sabaawy HE, Zhang F, Nguyen X, et al. Human heme oxygenase-1 gene transfer lowers blood pressure and promotes growth in spontaneously hypertensive rats. Hypertens 2001;38:210–215.

59. Metcalfe BL, Huentelman MJ, Parilak LD, et al. Prevention of cardiac hypertrophy by angiotensin II type 2 receptor gene transfer. Hypertension 2004;43:1233–1238.

60. Chen LG, Qu Y, Peng WZ, Wang YQ, Xiao J, Wang ZR. Encapsulated ANP cDNA transfection cells attenuate hypertension in hypertensive rats. Space Med Eng (Beijing) 2003;16:77–78.

61. Li T, Liang H, Lu G, Shi R, Lu S. Hypotensive effect of encapsulated genetically engineered fibroblasts expressing mutant atrial natriuretic peptide in hypertensive rats. Zhonghua Yi Xue Za Zhi 2002;82:1086–1089.

62. Reaves PY, Gelband CH, Wang H, et al. Permanent cardiovascular protection from hypertension by the AT(1) receptor antisense gene therapy in hypertensive rat offspring. Circ Res 1999;85:e44–e50.

63. Martens JR, Reaves PY, Lu D, et al. Prevention of renovascular and cardiac pathophysiological changes in hypertension by angiotensin II type 1 receptor antisense gene therapy. Proc Natl Acad Sci USA 1998;3;95:2664–2669.

64. Lu D, Raizada MK, Iyer S, Reaves P, Yang H, Katovich MJ. Losartan versus gene therapy: chronic control of high blood pressure in spontaneously hypertensive rats. Hypertension 1997;30(3 Pt 1):363–370.

65. Iyer SN, Lu D, Katovich MJ, Raizada MK. Chronic control of high blood pressure in the spontaneously hypertensive rat by delivery of angiotensin type 1 receptor antisense. Proc Natl Acad Sci USA 1996;93:9960–9965.

66. Wang H, Katovich MJ, Gelband CH, Reaves PY, Phillips MI, Raizada MK. Sustained inhibition of angiotensin I-converting enzyme (ACE) expression and long-term antihypertensive action by virally mediated delivery of ACE antisense cDNA. Circ Res 1999;85:614–622.

67. Katovich MJ, Reaves PY, Francis SC, Pachori AS, Wang HW, Raizada MK. Gene therapy attenuates the elevated blood pressure and glucose intolerance in an insulin-resistant model of hypertension. J Hypertens 2001;19:1553–1558.

68. Henriksen EJ, Jacob S. Angiotensin converting enzyme inhibitors and modulation of skeletal muscle insulin resistance. Diabetes Obes Metab 2003;5:214–222.

69. Katovich MJ, Pachori A. Effects of inhibition of the renin-angiotensin system on the cardiovascular actions of insulin. Diabetes Obes Metab 2000;2:3–14.

70. Dahlof B, Devereux RB, Kjeldsen SE, et al., LIFE Study Group. Cardiovascular morbidity and mortality in the Losartan Intervention For Endpoint reduction in hypertension study (LIFE): a randomised trial against atenolol. Lancet 2002;359:995–1003.

71. Lindholm LH, Ibsen H, Dahlof B, et al., LIFE Study Group. Cardiovascular morbidity and mortality in patients with diabetes in the Losartan Intervention For Endpoint reduction in hypertension study (LIFE): a randomised trial against atenolol. Lancet 2002;359:1004–1010.

72. Lindholm LH, Ibsen H, Borch-Johnsen K, et al., for the LIFE study group. Risk of new onset diabetes in the Losartan Intervention For Endpoint reduction in hypertension study. J Hypertens 2002;20:1879–1886.

73. Katovich MJ, Gelband CH, Reaves P, Wang HW, Raizada MK. Reversal of hypertension by angiotensin II type 1 receptor antisense gene therapy in the adult SHR. Am J Physiol 1999;277(3 Pt 2):H1260–H1264.

74. Phillips MI, Mohuczy-Dominiak D, Coffey M, et al. Prolonged reduction of high blood pressure with an in vivo, nonpathogenic, adeno-associated viral vector delivery of AT1-R mRNA antisense. Hypertension 1997;29(1 Pt 2):374–380.

75. Phillips MI. Antisense inhibition and adeno-associated viral vector delivery for reducing hypertension. Hypertension 1997;29(1 Pt 2):177–187.

76. Phillips MI. Gene therapy for hypertension: sense and antisense strategies. Expert Opin Biol Ther 2001;1:655–662.

78. Phillips MI. Gene therapy for hypertension: the preclinical data. Hypertension 2001;38(3 Pt 2):543–548.

79. Moore AF, Heiderstadt NT, Huang E, et al. Selective inhibition of the renal angiotensin type 2 receptor increases blood pressure in conscious rats. Hypertension 2001;37:1285–1281.

80. Wang H-W, Gallinat S, Li H-W, Sumners C, Raizada MK, Katovich MJ. Elevated blood pressure in normotensive rats produced by "knockdown" of the angiotensin type 2 receptor. Exp Physiol 2004;89:313–322.

81. Tomita N, Morishita R, Higaki J, et al. Transient decrease in high blood pressure by in vivo transfer of antisense oligodeoxynucleotides against rat angiotensinogen. Hypertension 1995;26:131–136.

82. Wielbo D, Simon A, Phillips MI, Toffolo S. Inhibition of hypertension by peripheral administration of antisense oligodeoxynucleotides. Hypertension 1996;28:147–151.

83. Phillips MI, Wielbo D, Gyurko R. Antisense inhibition of hypertension: a new strategy for renin-angiotensin candidate genes. Kid Int 1994;46:1554–1556.

84. Gurko R, Wielbo D, Phillips MI. Antisense inhibition of AT1 receptor mRNA and angiotensinogen mRNA in the brain of spontaneously hypertensive rats reduces hypertension of neurogenic origin. Regul Pept 1993;49:167–174.

85. Galderisi U, Cascino A, Giordano A. Antisense oligonucleotides as therapeutic agents. J Cell Physiol 1999;181:251–257

85a. Lavrovshy Y, Chen S, Roy AK. Therapeutic potential and mechanism of action of oligonucleotides and ribozymes. Biochem Mol Med 1997;62:11–22.

86. Neckers L, Whitesell L, Rosolen A, Geselowitz DA. Antisense inhibition of oncogene expression. Crit Rev Oncogen 1992;3:175–231.

87. Kagiyama S, Kagiyama T, Phillips MI. Antisense oligonucleotides strategy in the treatment of hypertension. Curr Opin Mol Ther 2001;3:258–264.

88. Phillips MI, Galli SM, Mehta JL. The potential role of antisense oligodeoxynucleotide therapy for cardiovascular disease. Drugs 2000;60:239–248.

89. Phillips MI. Somatic gene therapy for hypertension. Braz J Med Biol Res 2000;33:715–721.

90. Zhang YC, Bui JD, Shen L, Phillips MI. Antisense inhibition of beta(1)-adrenergic receptor mRNA in a single dose produces a profound and prolonged reduction in high blood pressure in spontaneously hypertensive rats. Circulation 2000;15;101:682–688.

91. Reaves PY, Beck CR, Wang HW, Raizada MK, Katovich MJ. Endothelial-independent prevention of high blood pressure in L-NAME-treated rats by angiotensin II type I receptor antisense gene therapy. Exp Physiol 2003;88:467–473.

92. Kagiyama S, Qian K, Kagiyama T, Phillips MI. Antisense to epidermal growth factor receptor prevents the development of left ventricular hypertrophy. Hypertension 2003;41(3 Pt 2):824–829.

93. Pachori AS, Numan MT, Ferrario CM, Diz DM, Raizada MK, Katovich MJ. Blood pressure-independent attenuation of cardiac hypertrophy by AT(1)R-AS gene therapy. Hypertension 2002;39:969–975.

94. Kumai T, Tateishi T, Tanaka M, Watanabe M, Shimizu H, Kobayashi S. Tyrosine hydroxylase antisense gene therapy causes hypotensive effects in the spontaneously hypertensive rats. J Hypertens 2001;19:1769–1773.

95. Clare Zhang Y, Kimura B, Shen L, Phillips MI. New beta-blocker: prolonged reduction in high blood pressure with beta(1) antisense oligodeoxynucleotides. Hypertension 2000;35(1 Pt 2):219–224.

96. Kimura B, Mohuczy D, Tang X, Phillips MI. Attenuation of hypertension and heart hypertrophy by adeno-associated virus delivering angiotensinogen antisense. Hypertension 2001;37(2 Part 2):376–380.

97. Makino N, Sugano M, Ohtsuka S, Sawada S, Hata T. Chronic antisense therapy for angiotensinogen on cardiac hypertrophy in spontaneously hypertensive rats. Cardiovasc Res 1999;44:543–548.

98. Cuevas P, Garcia-Calvo M, Carceller F, et al. Correction of hypertension by normalization of endothelial levels of fibroblast growth factor and nitric oxide synthase in spontaneously hypertensive rats. Proc Natl Acad Sci USA 1996;93:11,996–12,001.

99. Pachori AS, Wang H, Gelband CH, Ferrario CM, Katovich MJ, Raizada MK. Inability to induce hypertension in normotensive rat expressing AT(1) receptor antisense. Circ Res. 2000;86:1167–1172.

100. Tang X, Mohuczy D, Zhang YC, Kimura B, Galli SM, Phillips MI. Intravenous angiotensinogen antisense in AAV-based vector decreases hypertension. Am J Physiol. 1999;277(6 Pt 2):H2392–H2399.

101. Peng JF, Kimura B, Fregly MJ, Phillips MI. Reduction of cold-induced hypertension by antisense oligodeoxynucleotides to angiotensinogen mRNA and AT1 receptor mRNA in brain and blood. Hypertension 1998;31:1317–1323.

102. Galli SM, Phillips MI. Angiotensin II AT(1A) receptor antisense lowers blood pressure in acute 2-kidney, 1-clip hypertension. Hypertension 2001;38:674–678.

103. Wang MH, Zhang F, Marji J, Zand BA, Nasjletti A, Laniado-Schwartzman M. CYP4A1 antisense oligonucleotide reduces mesenteric vascular reactivity and blood pressure in SHR. Am J Physiol Regul Integr Comp Physiol 2001;280:R255–R261.

104. Yamakawa H, Phillips MI, Saavedra JM. Intracisternal administration of angiotensin II AT1 receptor antisense oligodeoxynucleotides protects against cerebral ischemia in spontaneously hypertensive rats. Regul Pept 2003;111:117–122.

105. Kagiyama S, Varela A, Phillips MI, Galli SM. Antisense inhibition of brain renin angiotensin system decreases blood pressure in chronic 2-kidney, 1-clip hypertensive rats. Hypertension 2001;37:371–375.

106. Suzuki S, Pilowsky P, Minson J, et al J. Antisense to thyrotropin releasing hormone receptor reduces arterial blood pressure in spontaneously hypertensive rats. Circ Res 1995;77:679–683.

107. Hayashi I, Majima M, Fujita T, et al. In vivo transfer of antisense oligonucleotide against urinary kininase blunts deoxycorticosterone acetate-salt hypertension in rats. Br J Pharmacol 2000;131:820–806.

108. Kagiyama S, Eguchi S, Frank GD, Inagami T, Zhang YC, Phillips MI. Angiotensin II-induced cardiac hypertrophy and hypertension are attenuated by epidermal growth factor receptor antisense. Circulation 2002;106:909–912.

109. Wivel NA, Wilson JM. Methods of gene delivery. Hematol Oncol Clin North Am 1998;12:483–501

110. Mann MJ, Morishita R, Gibbons GH, vonderLeyen HE, Dzau VJ. DNA transfer into vascular smooth muscle using fusigenic Sendai virus (HJV) liposomes. Mol Cell Biochem 1997;172:2–12.

111. Lawrie A, Brisken AF, Francis SE, et al. Ultrasound enhances reporter gene expression after transfection of vascular cells in vitro. Circulation 1999;99:2617–2620.

112. Parkes R, Meng QH, Siapati KE, McEwan JR, Hart SL. High efficiency transfection of porcine vascular cells in vitro with a synthetic vector system. J Gene Med 2002;4:292–299.

113. Kovesdi I, Brough DE, Bruder JT, Wickham TJ. Adenoviral vectors for gene transfer. Curr Opin Biotechnol 1997;8:583–589.

114. Lu D, Yang H, Raizada, MK. Attenuation of ANG II actions by adenovirus delivery of AT1 receptor antisense in neurons and SMC. Am J Physiol 1998;274:H719–H727.

115. Zhang LQ, Mei YF, Wadell G. Human adenovirus serotypes 4 and 11 show higher binding affinity and infectivity for endothelial and carcinoma cell lines than serotype 5. J Gen Virol 2003;84(Pt 3):687–695.

116. Harari OA, Wickham TJ, Stocker CJ, et al. Targeting an adenoviral gene vector to cytokine-activated vascular endothelium via E-selectin. Gene Ther 1999;6:801–807.

117. Flotte TR, Carter BJ. Adeno-associated virus vectors for gene therapy. Gene Ther 1995;2:357–362.

118. Hallek, M. Wendtner CM. Recombinant adeno-associated virus (rAAV) vectors for somatic gene therapy: recent advances and potential clinical applications. Cytokines Mol. Ther. 1996;2:69–79.

119. Langer JC, Klotman ME, Hanss B, et al. Adeno-associated virus gene transfer into renal cells: potential for in vivo gene delivery. Exp Nephrol 1998;6:189–194.
120. Flotte T, Carter B, Conrad C, et al. Phase I study of an adeno-associated virus-CFTR gene vector in adult CF patients with mild lung disease. Hum Gene Ther 1996;10;7:1145–1159.
121. Guntaka RV, Swamynathan SK. Retroviral vectors for gene therapy. Indian J Exp Biol 1998;36:359–345.
122. Gardon M, Raizada MK, Katovich MJ, Berecek KH, Gelband CH. Gene therapy for hypertension and restenosis. J Renin Angiotensin Aldosterone Syst 2000;1:211–216.
123. Rubinson DA, Dillon CP, Kwiatkowski AV, et al. A lentivirus-based system to functionally silence genes in primary mammalian cells, stem cells and transgenic mice by RNA interference. Nat Genet 2003;33:401–406.
124. Naldini L, Blomer U, Gage FH, Trono D, Verma IM. Efficient transfer, integration, and sustained long-term expression of the transgene in adult rat brains injected with a lentiviral vector. Proc Natl Acad Sci USA 1996;93:11,382–11,388.
125. Huentelman MJ, Reaves PY, Katovich MJ, Raizada MK. Large-scale production of retroviral vectors for systemic gene delivery. Methods Enzymol 2002;346:562–573.
126. Coleman JE, Huentelman MJ, Kasparov S, et al. Efficient large-scale production and concentration of HIV-1-based lentiviral vectors for use in vivo. Physiol Genomics 2002;12:221–228.
127. Ribault S, Neuville P, Mechine-Neuville A, et al. Chimeric smooth muscle-specific enhancer/promoters: valuable tools for adenovirus-mediated cardiovascular gene therapy. Circ Res 2001;88:468–475.
128. Hoggatt AM, Simon GM, Herring BP. Cell-specific regulatory modules control expression of genes in vascular and visceral smooth muscle tissues. Circ Res 2002;91:1151–1159.
129. Franz WM, Rothmann T, Frey N, Katus HA. Analysis of tissue-specific gene delivery by recombinant adenoviruses containing cardiac-specific promoters. Cardiovasc Res 1997;35:560–566.
130. Wang Q, Sigmund CD, Lin JJ. Identification of cis elements in the cardiac troponin T gene conferring specific expression in cardiac muscle of transgenic mice. Circ Res 2000;86:478–484.
131. Navarro V, Millecamps S, Geoffroy MC, et al. Efficient gene transfer and long-term expression in neurons using a recombinant adenovirus with a neuron-specific promoter. Gene Ther 1999;6:1884–1892.
132. Carmeliet P, Lampugnani MG, Moons L, et al. Targeted deficiency or cytosolic truncation of the VE-cadherin gene in mice impairs VEGF-mediated endothelial survival and angiogenesis. Cell 1999;98:147–157.
133. Wang Y, O'Malley BW Jr, Tsai SY, O'Malley BW. A regulatory system for use in gene transfer. Proc Natl Acad Sci USA 1994;91:8180–8184.
134. Pollock R, Issner R, Zoller K, Natesan S, Rivera VM, Clackson T. Delivery of a stringent dimerizer-regulated gene expression system in a single retroviral vector. Proc Natl Acad Sci USA 2000;97:13,221–13,226.
135. No D, Yao TP, Evans RM. Ecdysone-inducible gene expression in mammalian cells and transgenic mice. Proc Natl Acad Sci USA 1996;16;93:3346–3351.
136. Gossen M, Freundlieb S, Bender G, Muller G, Hillen W, Bujard H. Transcriptional activation by tetracyclines in mammalian cells. Science 1995;268:1766–1769.
137. Gossen M, Bujard H. Tight control of gene expression in mammalian cells by tetracycline-responsive promoters. Proc Natl Acad Sci USA 1992;89:5547–5551.
138. Gossen M, Bujard H. Anhydrotetracycline, a novel effector for tetracycline controlled gene expression systems in eukaryotic cells. Nucleic Acids Res 1993;21:4411–4412.
139. Efrat S, Fusco-DeMane D, Lemberg H, Emran OL, Wang X. Conditional transformation of a pancreatic β-cell line derived from transgenic mice expressing a tetracycline-regulated oncogene. PNAS 1995;92:3576–3580.
140. Corbel SY, Rossi FMV. Latest developments and in vivo use of the Tet system: ex vivo and in vivo delivery of tetracycline-regulated genes. Curr Opin Biotechnol 2002;13:448–452.
141. Zhu Z. Ma B, Homer RJ, Zheng T, Elias JA. Use of the tetracycline controlled transcriptional silencer (tTS) to eliminate transgene leak in inducible overexpression transgenic mice. J Biol Chem 2001;276:25,222–25,229.
142. Imhof MO, Chatellard P, Mermod N. A regulatory network for the efficient control of transgene expression. J Genetic Med 2000;2:107–116.
143. Baron U, Gossen M, Bujard H. Tetracycline-controlled transcription in eukaryotes: novel transactivators with graded transactivation potential Nucleic Acids Res 1997;25:2723–2729.
144. Urlinger S, Baron U, Thellmann M, Hasan MT, Bujard H, Hillen W. Exploring the sequence space for tetracycline-dependent transcriptional activators: novel mutations yield expanded range and sensitivity. PNAS 2000;97:7963–7968.

145. Robertson A, Perea J, Tolmachova T, Thomas PK, Huxley C. Effects of mouse strain, position of integration and tetracycline analogue on the tetracycline conditional system in transgenic mice. Gene 2002;282:65–74.

146. Raizada MK, Francis SC, Wang H, Gelband CH, Reaves PY, Katovich MJ. Targeting of the renin-angiotensin system by antisense gene therapy: a possible strategy for the long-term control of hypertension. J Hypertens 2000;18:353–362.

147. Pachori AS, Huentelman MJ, Francis SC, Gelband GH, Katovich MJ, Raizada MK. The future of hypertension therapy: sense, antisense or nonsense? Hypertension 2001;37:357–364.

148. Teng PI, Dichiara MR, Komuves LG, Abe K, Quertermous T, Topper, JN. Inducible and selective transgene expression in murine vascular endothelium. Physiol. Genomics 2002;11:99–107.

149. Ju H, Gros R, You X, Tsang S, Husain M, Rabinovitch M. Conditional and targeted overexpression of vascular chymase causes hypertension in transgenic mice. Proc Natl Acad Sci USA 2001;98:7469–7474.

150. Kantachuvesiri S, Fleming S, Peters J, et al. Controlled hypertension: a transgenic toggle switch reveals differential mechanisms underlying vascular disease. J Biol Chem 2001;276:36,727–36,733.

151. Hoppe UC, Marban E, Johns DC, Adenovirus-mediated inducible gene expression *in vivo* by a hybrid ecdysone receptor. Mol Ther 2000;1:159–164.

152. Madan A, Curtin PT. A 24-base-pair sequence 3' to the human erythropoietin gene contains a hypoxia-responsive transcriptional enhancer. Proc Natl Acad Sci USA 1993;90:3928–3932.

153. Beck I, Ramirez S, Weinmann R, Caro J. Enhancer element at the 3'-flanking region controls transcriptional response to hypoxia in the human erythropoietin gene. J Biol Chem. 1991;266:15,563–15,566.

154. Eckhart AD, Yang N, Xin X, Faber JE. Characterization of the alpha1B-adrenergic receptor gene promoter region and hypoxia regulatory elements in vascular smooth muscle. Proc Natl Acad Sci USA 1997;94:9487–9492.

155. Webster KA, Gunning P, Hardeman E, Wallace DC, Kedes L. Coordinate reciprocal trends in glycolytic and mitochondrial transcript accumulations during the in vitro differentiation of human myoblasts. J Cell Physiol. 1990;142:566–573.

156. Semenza GL, Jiang BH, Leung SW, et al. Hypoxia response elements in the aldolase A, enolase 1, and lactate dehydrogenase A gene promoters contain essential binding sites for hypoxia-inducible factor 1. J Biol Chem 1996;271:32,529–32,537.

157. Forsythe JA, Jiang BH, Iyer NV, et al. Activation of vascular endothelial growth factor gene transcription by hypoxia-inducible factor 1. Mol Cell Biol 1996;16:4604–4613.

158. Minchenko A, Salceda S, Bauer T, Caro J. Hypoxia regulatory elements of the human vascular endothelial growth factor gene. Cell Mol Biol Res 1994;40:35–39.

159. Yang BC, Phillips MI, Zhang YC, et al. Critical role of AT1 receptor expression after ischemia/reperfusion in isolated rat hearts: beneficial effect of antisense oligodeoxynucleotides directed at AT1 receptor mRNA. Circ Res 1998;83:552–559.

160. Chen H, Zhang YC, Li D, et al. Protection against myocardial dysfunction induced by global ischemia-reperfusion by antisense-oligodeoxynucleotides directed at beta(1)-adrenoceptor mRNA. J Pharmacol Exp Ther 2000;294:722–727.

161. Chen EP, Bittner HB, Akhter SA, Koch WJ, Davis RD. Myocardial recovery after ischemia and reperfusion injury is significantly impaired in hearts with transgenic overexpression of beta-adrenergic receptor kinase. Circulation 1998;98(19 Suppl):II249–II253.

162. Chen EP, Bittner HB, Davis RD, Folz RJ, Van Trigt P. Extracellular superoxide dismutase transgene overexpression preserves post ischemic myocardial function in isolated murine hearts. Cir 1996;94(9 Suppl):II412–II417.

163. Wang P, Chen H, Qin H, et al. Overexpression of human copper, zinc-superoxide dismutase (SOD1) prevents post ischemic injury. Proc Natl Acad Sci USA 1998;95:4556–4560.

164. Chen H, Mohuczy D, Li D, et al. Protection against ischemia/reperfusion injury and myocardial dysfunction by antisense-oligodeoxynucleotide directed at angiotensin-converting enzyme mRNA. Gene Ther 2001;8:804–810.

165. Divisova J, Vavrinkova H, Tutterova M, Kazdova L, Meschisvili E. Effect of ACE inhibitor captopril and L-arginine on the metabolism and on ischemia-reperfusion injury of the isolated rat heart. Physiol Res 2001;50:143–152.

166. Minchenko A, Salceda S, Bauer T, Caro J. Hypoxia regulatory elements of the human vascular endothelial growth factor gene. Cell Mol Biol Res 1994;40:35–39.

167. Vigna et al. (Vigina E, Cavalieri S, Ailles L, Geuna M, Loew R, Bujard H, Naldini L. Robust and efficient regulation of transgene expression in vivo by improved tetracycline-dependent lentiviral vectors. Mol Ther 2002;5:252–261.

168. Ryding ADS, Sharp MGF, Mullins JJ. Conditional transgenic technologies. J Endocrinol 2001;171:1–14.

169. Robertson A, Perea J, Tolmachova T, Thomas PK, Huxley C. Effects of mouse strain, position of integration and tetracycline analogue on the tetracycline conditional system in transgenic mice. Gene 2002;282:65–74.

170. Tang Y, Schmitt-Ott K, Qian K, Kagiyama S, Phillips MI. Vigilant vectors: adeno-associated virus with a biosensor to switch on amplified therapeutic genes in specific tissues in life-threatening diseases. Methods 2002;28:259–266.

171. Tang Y, Jackson M, Qian K, Phillips MI. Hypoxia inducible double plasmid system for myocardial ischemia gene therapy. Hypertension 2002;39(2 Pt 2):695–698.

172. Gibson, SA, Shillitoe EJ. Ribozymes. Their functions and strategies for their use. Mol Biotechnol 1997;7:125–137.

173. Shuey DJ, McCallus DE, Giordano T. RNAi: gene-silencing in therapeutic intervention. Drug Discov Today 2002;7:1040–1046.

174. Guru T. A silence that speaks volumes. Nature 2000;404:804–808.

175. Ingelbrecht I, Van Houdt H, English J, Que Q, Napoli CA. Chalcone synthase co suppression phenotypes in petunia flowers: comparison of sense and antisense constructs and single-copy vs. complex T-DNA sequences. Plant Mol Biol 1994;31:957–973.

176. Fire A, Xu S, Montgomery MK, Kostas SA, Driver SE, Mello CC. Potent and specific genetic interference by double stranded RNA in *Caenorhabditis elegans*. Nature 1998;391:806–811.

177. Elbashir SM, Harborth J, Lendeckel W, Yalcin A, Weber K, Tuschl T. Duplexes of 21-nucleotide RNAs mediate RNA interference in cultured mammalian cells. Nature 2001;411:494–498.

178. Walters DK, Jelinek DF. The effectiveness of double stranded short inhibitory RNAs (siRNAs) may depend on the method of transfection. Antisense Nucleic Acid Drug Dev 2002;12:411–418.

179. Tuschl T, Borkhardt A. Small Interfering RNAs: a revolutionary tool for the analysis of gene function and gene therapy. Mol Intervent 2002;2:158–167.

180. Pfeifer A, Ikawa M, Dayn Y, Verma IM. Transgenes by lentiviral vectors: lack of gene silencing in mammalian embryonic stem cells and preimplantation embryos. Proc Natl Acad Sci USA 2002;99:2140–2145.

181. Shen C, Buck AK, Liu X, Winkler M, Reske SN. Gene silencing by adenovirus-delivered siRNA. FEBS Lett 2003;539:111–114.

182. Lewis DL, Hagstrom JE, Loomis AG, Wolff JA, Herweijer H. Efficient delivery of siRNA for inhibition of gene expression in postnatal mice. Nat Genet 2002;32:107–108.

183. Lois C, Hong EJ, Pease S, Brown EJ, Baltimore D. Germline transmission and tissue specific expression of transgenes derived from lentiviral vectors. Science 2002;295:868–872.

184. Cheng JC, Moore TB, Sakamoto KM. RNA interference and human disease. Mol Genet Metabol 2003;80:121–128.

185. Boguski MS, McIntosh MW. Biomedical informatics for proteomics. Nature 2003;422:233–237.

186. Templin MF, Stoll D, Schrenk M, Traub PC, Vohringer CF, Joos TO. Protein microarray technology. Drug Discov Today 2002;7:815–822.

187. Ward R. Familial aggregation and genetic epidemiology of blood pressure. In: Hypertension: pathophysiology, diagnosis and management. (Laragh JH, Brenner BM, eds). Raven, New York: 1990;81–100.

188. Luft FC. Hypertension as a complex genetic trait. Semin Nephrol 2002;22:115–126.

189. Zhu X, Cooper RS. Linkage disequilibrium analysis of the renin-angiotensin system genes. Curr Hypertens Rep 2003;5:40–46. .

190. Hamet P, Pausova Z, Adarichev V, Adaricheva K, Tremblay J. Hypertension: genes and environment. J Hypertens 1998;16:397–418.

191. Pravenec, M., Krenova D, Kren V, et al. Congenic strains for genetic analysis of hypertension and dyslipidemia in the spontaneously hypertensive rat. Transplant Proc 1999;31:1555–1556.

192. Rapp JP. Genetic analysis of inherited hypertension in the rat. Physiol Rev 2000;80:135–172.

193. Stoll M, Kwitek-Black AE, Cowley AW Jr, et al. New target regions for human hypertension via comparative genomics. Genome Res 2000;10:473–482.

194. Cicila GT, Garrett MR, Lee SJ, Liu J, Dene H, Rapp, JP. High-resolution mapping of the blood pressure QTL on chromosome 7 using Dahl rat congenic strains. Genomics 2001;72:51–60.

195. Cook SA, Rosenzweig A. DNA microarrays: implications for cardiovascular medicine. Circ Res 2002;91:559–564.

196. Patino WD, Mian OY, Hwang P M. Serial analysis of gene expression: technical considerations and applications to cardiovascular biology. Circ Res 2002;91:565–569.

197. Nadon R, Shoemaker J. Statistical issues with microarrays: processing and analysis. Trends Genet 2002;18:265–271.
198. Quackenbush J. Computational analysis of microarray data. Nat Rev Genet 2001;2:418–427.
199. Pravenec M, Wallace C, Aitman, TJ, Kurtz, TW. Gene Expression profiling in hypertensive research. A critical perspective. Hypertension 2003;41:3–8.
200. Cook SA, Rosenzweig A. DNA microarrays: implications for cardiovascular medicine. Circ Res 2002;91:559–564.
201. Aitman TJ, Glazier AM, Wallace CA, et al. Identification of Cd36 (Fat) as an insulin-resistance gene causing defective fatty acid and glucose metabolism in hypertensive rats. Nat Genet 1999;21:76–83.
202. McBride MW, Carr FJ, Graham D, et al. Microarray analysis of rat chromosome 2 congenic strains. Hypertension 2003;41:847–853.
203. Okuda T, Sumiya T, Iwai N, Miyata T. Difference of gene expression profiles in spontaneous hypertensive rats and Wistar-Kyoto rats from two sources. Biochem Biophys Res Commun 2002;296:537–543.
204. Okuda T, Sumiya T, Mizutani K, et al. Analyses of differential gene expression in genetic hypertensive rats by microarray. Hypertens Res 2002;25:249–255.
205. Veerasingham SJ, Sellers KW, Raizada MK. Functional genomics as an emerging strategy for the investigation of central mechanisms in experimental hypertension. Prog Biophys Mol Biol 2004;84:107–123.
206. Yang H, Francis SC, Sellers K, et al. Hypertension-linked decrease in the expression of brain gamma-adducin. Circ Res 2002;91:633–639.
207. Raizada MK, Lu D, Tang W, Kurian P, Sumners C. Increased angiotensin II type-1 receptor gene expression in neuronal cultures from spontaneously hypertensive rats. Endocrinology 1993;132:1715–1722.
208. Matsuoka Y, Li X, Bennett V. Adducin: structure, function and regulation. Cell Mol Life Sci 2000;57:884–895.
209. Bianchi G, Tripodi G, Casari G, et al. Two point mutations within the adducin genes are involved in blood pressure variation. Proc Natl Acad Sci USA 1994;91;3999–4003.
210. Wang J G, Staessen JA, Barlassina C, et al. Association between hypertension and variation in the alpha- and beta- adducin genes in a white population. Kidney Int 2002;62:2152–2159.
211. Zagato L, Modica R, Florio M, et al Genetic mapping of blood pressure quantitative trait loci in Milan hypertensive rats. Hypertension 2000;36:734–739.
212. Marro ML, Scremin OU, Jordan MC, et al. Hypertension in beta-adducin-deficient mice. Hypertension 2000;36,449–453.
213. Yang H, Reaves PY, Katovich MJ, Raizada MK. Decreases in hypothalamic gamma adducin in rat models of hypertension. Hypertension 2004;43:324–328.
214. Sinal CJ, Miyata M, Tohkin M, Nagata K, Bend JR, Gonzalez FJ. Targeted disruption of soluble epoxide hydrolase reveals a role in blood pressure regulation. J Biol Chem. 2000;275:40,504–40,510.
215. Baudin B, Berard M, Carrier JL, Legrand Y, Drouet L. Vascular origin determines angiotensin I-converting enzyme expression in endothelial cells. Endothelium 1997;5:73–84.
216. Schulz WW, Hagler HK, Buja LM, Erdos EG. Ultrastructural localization of angiotensin I-converting enzyme (EC 3.4.15.1) and neutral metalloendopeptidase (EC 3.4.24.11) in the proximal tubule of the human kidney. Lab Invest 1988;59:789–797.
217. McKinley MJ, Albiston AL, Allen AM, et al. The brain renin-angiotensin system: location and physiological roles. Int J Biochem Cell Biol 2003;35:901–918.
218. Tipnis SR, Hooper NM, Hyde R, Karran E, Christie, G. A human homolog of angiotensin-converting enzyme. J Biol Chem 2000;275;33,238–33,243.
219. Donoghue M, Hsieh F, Baronas E, et al. A novel angiotensin-converting enzyme-related carboxypeptidase (ACE2) converts angiotensin I to angtiotensin 1–9. Circ Res 2000;87:1–9.
220. Harmer D, Gilbert M, Borman R, Clark KL. Quantitative mRNA expression profiling of ACE2, a novel homologue of Angiotensin converting enzyme. FEBS Lett 2002;532:107–110.
221. Stegbauer J, Vonend O, Oberhauser V, Rump, LC. Effects of Angiotensin-(1–7) and other bioactive components of the renin-angiotensin system on vascular resistance and noradrenaline release in rat kidney. J Hypertens 2003;21:1391–1399.
222. Zhu Z, Zhong J, Zhu S, Liu D, van der Giet M, Tepel M. Angiotensin 1-7 inhibits angiotensin II inducted signal transduction. J Cardiovasc Pharmacol 2002;40:693–700.
223. Cesari M, Rossi GP, Pessina AC. Biological properties of the Angiotensin peptides other than Angiotensin II: implications for hypertension and other cardiovascular diseases. J Hypertens 2002;20:793–799.
224. Reaux A, Fournie-Zaluski MC, Lloren-Cortes C. Angiotensin III: a central regulator of vasopressin release and blood pressure. Trends Endocrinol Metab 2001;12:157–162.

225. Roks AJM, Henning RH. Angiotensin peptides: ready to re(de)fine the Angiotensin system? J Hypertens 2003;21:1269–1271.
226. Tom B, Dendorfer A, Danser AHJ. Bradykinin, angiotensin 1-7 and ACE inhibitors: how do they interact. Int. J Biochem Cell Biol 2003;35:792–801.
227. Allred AJ, Donoghue M, Acton S, Coffman TM. Regulation of blood pressure by the Angiotensin converting enzyme homologue ACE2. 35th annual meeting of the American Soc Nephrol Nov 1–4, 2002.
228. Donoghue M, Wakimoto H, Maguire CT, et al. Heart block, ventricular tachycardia, and sudden death in ACE2 transgenic mice with downregulated connexins. J Mol Cell Cardiol 2003;35:1043–1053.
229. Chung O, Stoll M, Unger T. Physiological and pharmacological implications of AT1 versus AT2 receptors. Blood Press Suppl 1996;2:47–52.
230. Matsukawa T, Ichikawa I. Biological function of angiotensin and its receptors. Ann Rev Physiol 1997;59:395–412.
231. Gallinat S, Busche S, Raizada MK, Sumners C. The angiotensin II type 2 receptor: an enigma with multiple variations. Am J Physiol Endocrinol Metab 2000;278:E357–E374.
232. DeGasparo M, Catt K, Inagami J, Wright JW, Unger T. International Union of Pharmacology. XVIII. The Angiotensin II receptors. Pharmacol Rev 2000;52:415–472.
233. Unger T, The angiotensin type 2 receptor. Variations on an enigmatic theme. J Hypertens 1999;17:1775–1786.
234. Hein L, Barsh GS, Pratt RE, Dzau VJ, Kobilka BK. Behavioral and cardiovascular effects of disrupting the angiotensin II type 2 receptor gene in mice. Nature 1995;377:744–747.
235. Ichiki T, Labosky PA, Shiota C, et al. Effects on blood pressure and exploratory behaviour of mice lacking angiotensin II type-2 receptor. Nature 1995;377:748–750.
236. Miura S, Karnik SS. Ligand-independent signals from angiotensin II type 2 receptor induce apoptosis. Embro J 2000;19:4026–4035.
237. Dzau, V.J. Tissue renin-angiotensin system in myocardial hypertrophy and failure. Arch Intern Med 1993;153:937–942.
238. Dzau, V.J. Circulating versus local renin-angiotensin system in cardiovascular homeostasis. Circulation 1988;77:(6 Pt 2):I4–I13.
239. Crockcroft JR, O'Kane KPJ, Webb DJ. Tissue angiotensin generation and regulation of vascular tone. Pharmacol Ther 1995;65:193–213.
240. Bader M, Peters J, Baltatu O, Muller DN, Luft FC, Ganten D. Tissue renin-angiotensin systems: new insights from experimental animal models in hypertension research. J Mol Med 2001;79:76–102.
241. Crockcroft JR, O'Kane KPJ, Webb DJ. Tissue angiotensin generation and regulation of vascular tone. Pharmacol Ther 1995;65:193–213.
242. Bader M, Peters J, Baltatu O, Muller DN, Luft FC, Ganten D. Tissue renin-angiotensin systems: new insights from experimental animal models in hypertension research. J Mol Med 2001;79:76–102.
243. Blaufarb IS, Sonnenblick EH. The renin angiotensin system in left ventricular remodeling. Am J Cardiol 1996;77:8C–16C.
244. Yu Z, Xu F, Huse LM, et al. Soluble epoxide hydrolase regulates hydrolysis of vasoactive epoxyeicosatrienoic acids. Circ Res. 2000;87:992–998.
245. Fornage M, Hinojos CA, Nurowska BW, et al. Polymorphism in soluble epoxide hydrolase and blood pressure in spontaneously hypertensive rats. Hypertension 2000;40:485–490.
246. Xia H, Mao Q, Paulson HL, Davidson BL. siRNA-mediated gene silencing in vitro and in vivo. Nat Biotechnol 2002;20:1006–1010.

13 Application of Viral Gene Transfer in Studies of Neurogenic Hypertension

Sergey Kasparov, MD, PhD,
A. G. Teschemacher, PhD,
and Julian F. R. Paton, PhD

CONTENTS

INTRODUCTION
VIRAL VEHICLES FOR GENE DELIVERY INTO CENTRAL NEURONES
APPLICATIONS OF SOMATIC GENE TRANSFER IN STUDIES OF CENTRAL
    MECHANISMS OF BLOOD PRESSURE CONTROL
CONCLUSIONS
REFERENCES

SUMMARY

This chapter reviews the use of viral gene transfer to disentangle the complexities of neurogenic hypertension. Viral gene manipulation allows lasting and controllable genetic manipulation in selected areas of the brain in different species and strains, including experiments in the spontaneously hypertensive rat, an established model of hypertension. Recent evidence indicates that, in contrast to pharmacological tools that may act on any cellular target within a given area of the brain, viral vectors deliver transgene in a nonuniform manner, and its concentration in different types of cells may vary greatly. This occurs as a result of both transductional tropism of a viral vector system and the transcriptional activity of the promoter in different cellular types which are present in any brain nucleus. Properties of adenoviral and lentiviral vectors are compared and contrasted. Application of viral vectors for overexpression of biologically active molecules, expression of dominant negative proteins, pathway tracking, and other experiments to study central mechanisms of cardiovascular control are discussed. In summary, virally mediated gene delivery to the brain is a powerful research tool that can be used to address a wide range of questions related to mechanisms of human essential hypertension.

Key Words: Hypertension; viral vectors; adenovirus; gene expression; gene targeting.

From: *Contemporary Cardiology: Cardiovascular Genomics*
Edited by: M. K. Raizada, et al. © Humana Press Inc., Totowa, NJ

INTRODUCTION

In spite of recent advances in the treatment of hypertension, many patients fail to respond to standard therapies targeted mainly at regulating blood volume, electrolyte balance, and the peripheral renin-angiotensin system. In a recent review, S. J. Mann writes: "One such form of hypertension is the often overlooked entity of neurogenic hypertension. These implications *underscore the need for further clinical and basic research attention concerning neurogenically mediated hypertension" (1)*. The purpose of this chapter is to renew attention to this overlooked entity by considering novel molecular strategies to disentangle the complexities of neurogenic hypertension.

The lack of understanding of the mechanisms of neurogenic hypertension to which S. J. Mann alludes justifies interest in new methods of analysis of this disease, which would allow us to study these mechanisms with a new level of precision. Many such methods have evolved during the last decade or so, and currently converge under the umbrella of physiological genomics. Availability of fully sequenced genomes and the vast numbers of readily accessible clones greatly facilitates the use of genetic manipulations in order to reveal the roles of individual genes and their families under normal, as well as pathological, conditions.

We have chosen to employ viral vectors to manipulate genes within the central nervous system structures regulating blood pressure. Virally mediated gene delivery to the brain is a powerful research tool, which can be used to address a wide range of questions including those concerning central cardiovascular control mechanisms. So, what are the advantages of the viral approach?

Why Viral Vectors?

First, viral vectors allow evaluation of the long-term outcomes of various experimental manipulations on blood pressure control. It is not a secret that many conclusions about central mechanisms of blood pressure control have originated from acute experiments in anesthetized animals. Meanwhile, human hypertension is a chronic condition and, thus, it becomes imperative to also look at long-term manipulations within specific brain structures for a more complete understanding of this condition. In addition, acute experimentation usually occurs under anesthesia which has very profound effects on nearly every transmitter system relevant to blood pressure control (reviewed in ref. 2). Nowadays, chronic recording of arterial blood pressure using radiotelemetry in rats or mice has negated these problems. However, one problem that remains is the chronic central delivery of pharmacological agents directly into specific brain nuclei. Here, viral gene manipulation is of great advantage because, following a single microinjection, it enables chronic alteration of brain signalling in a chosen structure that can last for many days or even weeks *(3–8)*. Moreover, in experiments of this kind it is possible to obtain an intraexperimental control (e.g., monitor blood pressure before and after the genetic manipulation in the same animal). This is important, because it greatly facilitates interpretation of the results *(see* section titled "Application of Somatic Gene Transfer in Studies of Central Mechanism of Blood Pressure"). In addition, pharmacological approaches are, in many cases, impossible because of the lack of suitable drugs, especially for recently discovered targets and for those awaiting discovery.

Second, viral gene manipulation is a flexible approach, because the same vectors can be used in many species. There is little doubt, for a variety of reasons, that the rat will remain the species of choice for neuroscience studies including those concerned with hypertension. In the context of this chapter, it is a great advantage that this approach can be applied to the spontaneously hypertensive rat (SHR) and the outcome compared directly with its normotensive progenitor strain, the Wistar–Kyoto rat (WKY), or any other control strain (3,9). Whereas germline transgenesis in the rat is extremely technically challenging and time-consuming, viral gene delivery does allow effective manipulation of central signaling pathways (10). Although the SHR is not an ideal model of essential hypertension in humans, it has nevertheless served for many years as a valuable model of this disease and, with its normotensive progenitor control WKY, remains an important resource. Moreover, in addition to SHR, there are many other models of hypertension in the rat.

Third, viral gene transfer enables both site-specific and, in some cases, cell-type-specific genetic manipulation. Viral vectors can be delivered stereotaxically into any area of the brain and, if needed, retrograde transduction performed with some types of vectors (11–13) (Fig. 1). However, all brain nuclei are heterogeneous in terms of their histochemistry and connectivity. Many nuclei harbor excitatory glutamatergic and inhibitory γ-aminobutyric acid (GABA)-ergic neurons, and changes in both of these transmitter systems have been implemented in pathological hypertension (14–18). Additionally, catecholaminergic cell groups (e.g., A2 in the nucleus tractus solitarius [NTS], A6 in the Locus Coeruleus, C1 in the rostral ventro-lateral medulla) have all been implicated in pathological hypertension (19–23). Moreover, each group of neurones is embedded in a network of glia and blood vessels containing endothelial and vascular smooth muscle cells. Thus, it now becomes necessary to selectively target a cell type with a specific phenotype within a heterogeneous population using modified viral delivery vectors with cell-specific promoters and analyze their exact roles in pathological hypertension.

Finally, we should not forget that a large volume of information about the biochemical changes in central signaling mechanisms in hypertension has been obtained in highly reductionistic models, such as cell lines. For example, the PC12 line has been derived from pheochromocytoma and used as a model of central catecholaminergic neurones. Cell lines such as these are convenient in particular because DNA can be easily introduced using well-established methods, such as calcium phosphate transfection or liposome-based carriers. However, central neurones are very different from these simple models and to make a definitive conclusion about the function of brain circuits, genetic manipulation must also be made in vivo. Central neurones are generally very resistant to chemical methods of gene delivery, and here viruses again offer a powerful alternative. For example, if a hypothesis links hypertension to a change in a signaling cascade in catecholaminergic neurones of a particular cell group within the brainstem, viral vectors make it possible to perform a variety of experiments specifically on this cell type.

Nonuniform Transductional and Transcriptional Efficacy of Viral Vectors

We would like to draw the reader's attention to one very important feature of viral gene transfer experiments: the nonuniformity of transgene expression. Pharmacological analytical tools injected into the central nervous system affect all cells that have the appropriate binding site or receptor. In contrast, virally delivered transgenes may or may not be effective in some cells depending on the efficiency of the virus at both entering the cell and inducing expression of the transgene once it has reached the nucleus. The ability of the virus to enter the cell and the subsequent transcriptional activity of its expression cassette are two critical rate-limiting steps. Indeed, this gave rise to the concept of targeted

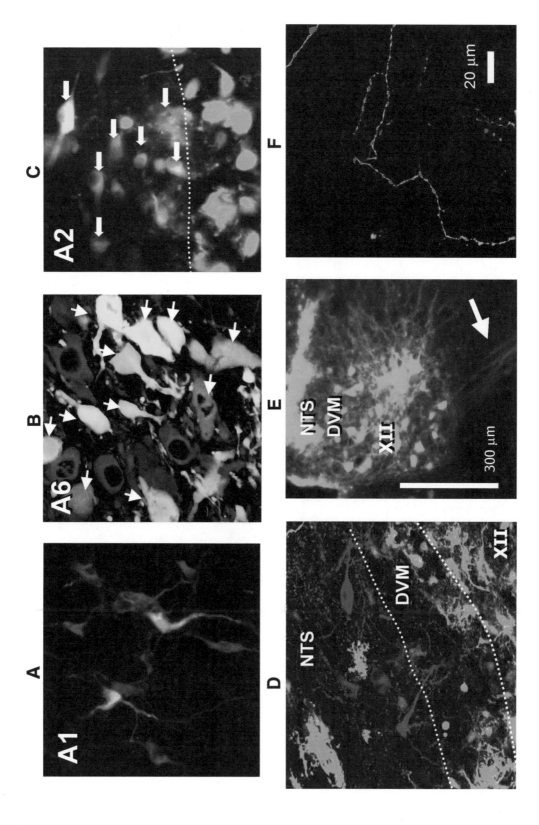

viral gene delivery, which can occur at either a transductional (i.e., at the stage of viral entry) or transcriptional level. Detailed analysis of viral targeting is outside of the scope of this chapter, and more information can be found in recent reviews *(24–27)*. It is essential, however, to realize that as a result of the natural tropism of viral capsids (and/or the protcin coat of enveloped viruses), and the striking variability of promoter activity in different neuronal populations (reviewed in more detail in ref. *27*), the transgene probably is *never* expressed at the same level in all cells in the brain area in which the viral vector was injected. Indeed, a "false negative outcome" can occur if the transgene is expressed at very low, physiologically insufficient levels. On the other hand, expression of a biologically active molecule in cells that normally do not express this molecule may alter their function in an unpredictable manner. These considerations are important for interpretation of viral gene transfer experiments and have led us to perform a more thorough characterisation of the expression profile of a number of viral vectors in cardiovascular areas of both the brainstem and diencephalon *(27,28)*.

In this chapter we will give an overview of currently available viral gene delivery systems and illustrate how they can be used to advance our understanding of the central mechanisms of hypertension.

Fig. 1. (A) Retrogradely transfected noradrenergic neurones in the A1 brainstem area. Adenoviral vector (AVV) PRSx8-enhanced green fluorescent protein (EGFP) (1 μL of 2.2*10^8 PFU) was injected in the paraventricular area of the hypothalamus. Five days later, sections were prepared and immunostained for dopamine β-hydroxylase (DBH; red fluorescence of the CY3 conjugated secondary antibody). This image in an overlay of the EGFP and CY3 channels obtained separately using spectral confocal microscope. Note that both EGFP-expressing neurones are also DBH-positive, and therefore appear yellow. (Reproduced from Kasparov et al. *[27]*, with permission). **(B,C)** AVV PRSx8-EGFP was injected into either Locus Coeruleus (A6) or dorsal vagal complex (including the A2 group). Six days later, the tissue was fixed and processed for DBH. The images are overlays of EGFP (green) and DBH (red) channels of confocal images. Note that in the A6, all transduced neurones appear yellow (arrows) owing to co-localization with the DBH stain. In contrast, in the dorsal vagal complex, whereas the EGFP-expressing cells in nucleus tractus solitarii (NTS) were DBH-positive A2 cells (yellow color, thick arrows), the underlying neurones of the dorsal vagal motor nucleus (below the dotted line) also expressed high levels of EGFP (green color, DBH-negative). Data contributed by D. Lonergan (University of Bristol). **(D,E)** AVV HCMV-EGFP expression profile in the dorsal vagal complex. Two injections of 0.5μL of 2.7*10^8 PFU of the vector were made at 300 and 400 μm from the dorsal surface of the medulla. The tissue was then processed for DBH. The NTS is devoid of EGFP-expressing neurons; no EGFP-expressing cells in NTS area were DBH-positive. Some glial cells can be seen. In contrast, there are numerous EGFP-expressing cells (both glia and neurones) in the deeper cholinergic motor nuclei. In particular, many of the neurones of the motor nucleus of the hypoglossal nerve expressed EGFP. These cells could be easily identified on low-power images (right panel) by their long axons projecting toward the ventral edge of the medulla. **(F)** AVV PRSx8-EGFP was used to visualize catecholaminergic neurones and their beaded axons in organotypic slice cultures of the rat brainstem. Vectors were applied to plating media and fluorescent neurones visualized after more than 3 d using conventional and confocal fluorescent microscopy. (Further details in ref. *27*.)

VIRAL VEHICLES FOR GENE DELIVERY
INTO CENTRAL NEURONES

Vectors for gene delivery into the brain have been derived from a number of viral genomes, such as adenoviruses, adeno-associated viruses (AAVs), retroviruses and related lentiviruses, herpes simplex virus, and some others. So far, studies of central mechanisms of cardiovascular control have mainly employed adenoviral vectors (AVV) and retroviral vectors, including lentiviral vectors (LVV) *(3,5,10–12,29–33)*. These viruses can infect various cell types present in the brain (i.e., neurones, glia, endothelial, and vascular muscle cells) and result in long-lasting gene expression without noticeable adverse effects. Vectors derived from the AAV have been successfully used for gene delivery to peripheral targets *(34,35)*, but they are also well-equipped for gene delivery into central neurones *(36)*. Finally, a replicating pseudorabies virus has been used to retrogradely transfect vagal cardioinhibitory neurones *(13)*.

General Properties of AVV and LVV

AVV and LVV are very different in respect to their genomic organization, structure, and life cycle. Whereas AVV vectors are descendants of the widespread pathogens associated with mild human infections of the respiratory tract and eyes, LVV vectors have been derived from either a deadly human immunodeficiency virus (HIV) or a feline immunodeficiency virus (FIV). From the practical point of view, the most important features of any viral gene delivery system include its safety in use (i.e., nonvirulent), cellular tropism in the brain, transgene carrying capacity, rapidity, longevity and stability of gene expression, the degree of an immune response induced, the ability for retrograde transduction, and the speed and cost of production.

In contrast to AVV, LVV are able to stably insert the transgene into the host genome, whereas the transgenes delivered by AVV remain episomal. Thus, AVV-delivered transgenes may be relatively rapidly eliminated (2–3 wk), especially in dividing cells, such as endothelial cells, whereas LVV induce expression for months. In central neurones, this difference might be less evident because the longevity of expression seems to be largely dependent on the promoter used. Some AVV constructs have been reported to drive expression for at least 9 mo *(37)*. In terms of capacity, currently the majority of laboratories use AVV with deletions in the E1 region (with additional deletions in the E2 and/or E3 and E4 regions). With these deletions, which render the virus replication deficient, AVV can accommodate approx 7 kb of a transgene. This is enough for one or even two expression cassettes. Various versions of AVV have been made, some of which express two different proteins from two separate promoters *(38)*. In addition, high-capacity AVV lacking most of their genome have been generated *(39)*, but production of these vectors remains too complicated for them to replace the currently used E1-E2/E3 deleted AVV. In contrast, HIV-derived self-inactivating LVV, such as those developed by Iwakuma et al. *(40)* and further modified by Coleman et al. *(41)*, have most of the viral genome deleted and, in principle, can accommodate approx 11–12 kb. Size limitations within the viral backbone are important, particularly when large transgenes are inserted or when cell-specific expression is desirable. To achieve cell specificity in transgenic animals, researchers commonly use long promoter sequences (several kb) upstream of a particular gene to drive the expression *(42)* or even bacterial artificial chromosomes (tens of kb; *[43]*). Clearly, viral vectors have restrictions imposed by the size of viral particles, but it proves possible to target expression to at least some subsets of cells relevant to central cardiovascular control (see section titled "Future Potential of Viral Gene Transfer," and Fig. 4). Parenthetically, in contrast to AVV and LVV, AAV have even smaller capacity. Even the most advanced versions of these vectors accommodate inserts no larger than approx 4 kb, which limits their use for expression of large cassettes (44).

TRANSDUCTIONAL TROPISM OF THE AVV AND LVV

AVV particles are very different from LVV in that they are nonenveloped and their ability to invade cells is dependent entirely on the proteins present in their fibers and capsid. It has been demonstrated that the serotype affects the neuronal tropism of the AVV, and apparently fibers of the Ad17 serotype might be best suitable for targeting neurones (45). Nevertheless, most of the AVV vectors currently used have been derived from serotype 5. Adenovirus fiber protein interacts with a range of protein receptors present on the membranes of many cells, such as the Major Histocompatibility Complex class I molecule and the "Coxsackie–adenovirus" receptor (CAR). Modifications of the AVV fiber protein may change its tropism and alter its ability to infect certain cell types (for review, see ref. 26). Recently, using this approach, Omori et al. (46) have redirected AVV to microglia which lack CAR. This was achieved by incorporating the Arg-Gly-Asp motif containing peptide into the HI loop of the fiber knob. This motif enables interaction with αV integrins, ubiquitously expressed on the surface of mammalian cells. Similarly, Baker and his colleagues were able to modify the HI loop to detarget AVV from CAR and, instead, direct it to endothelial cells (47,48). Thus, modifications of adenoviral capsid can lead to the development of vectors with an even better ability to preferentially target different cell types present in brain, such as glia, endothelium, or, perhaps, neuronal subsets. Thus, alteration of vector tropism may be achieved by modification of the capsid proteins.

AXONAL TRANSPORT AND TARGETING REMOTE SITES IN THE BRAIN

The ability of a viral vector to transduce remote neurones via retrograde transport may have major implications for its use in experimental neuroscience. This feature is heavily dependent on the properties of the viral particle, but could also be influenced by the phenotype of the targeted neurones. There has been some controversy regarding the ability of the conventional AVV (serotype 5) to transduce neurones retrogradely, but this issue has been recently resolved by a number of studies. For example, through the use of AVV with the Rous sarcoma virus long terminal repeat as the promoter, retrograde transduction was obtained after microinjections into the caudate putamen (49). Transfected cells (predominantly dopaminergic) were found in substantia nigra compacta that was 2 mm from the site of injection, ruling out viral diffusion as the method of transfection. Nashimura et al. (50) achieved retrograde transfection through intrahippocampal AVV injections using a modified chicken β-actin promoter (51) rather than human cytomegalovirus (HCMV). Neurones retrogradely transduced in these experiments were located in the cerebral cortex and were likely to be glutamatergic. Irnaten et al. (12) used AVV with an HCMV-driven construct to retrogradely transduce, from the pericardial sac, cholinergic neurones in nucleus ambiguus located in the ventrolateral medulla. Sinnayah (11) found retrogradely transfected neurones in the subfornical organ after injection of AVV with the HCMV promoter into the supraoptical nucleus (the exact transmitter phenotype of these cells is not known). Collectively, these data indicate that AVV are able to retrogradely invade various types of neurones that have different neurochemical profiles. Finally, we have also observed retrograde transduction of noradrenergic and adrenergic cells using AVV with the PRSx8 promoter, which is highly active in these cell types. For example, after injection of AVV PRSx8-enhanced green fluorescent protein (EGFP), into the paraventricular area of hypothalamus in the rat, noradrenergic neurones expressing EGFP were found in cardiovascular regions of the NTS and in the A1 area of the ventrolateral medulla (Fig. 1A). Moreover, injection of the same construct into the dorsal horn of the spinal cord resulted in EGFP-expressing noradrenergic neurones in locus coeruleus and some ventral brainstem noradrenergic groups. Therefore, we believe that transgene expression in remote sites after AVV microinjections may occur within the central nervous system, provided that the promoter used is active in these projection neurones.

In contrast with AVV, LVV have an additional protein coat or envelope wrapped around the capsid. The coat is associated with the capsid but consists of a separate protein encoded by separate genes. Because this coat is involved in the binding of the viral particle to the cellular membrane, modifications of the coat can alter the transductional properties of the vector, just as we described above for AVV. Most vectors used currently, irrespectively of the virus they have been derived from (i.e., HIV or FIV), are pseudotyped in that they employ a foreign protein coat, such as the vesicular stomatitis virus glycoprotein G (VSVG) (11,40,41). The VSVG coat enables LVV to deliver transgenes to a wide range of cells including neurones and glia (41). Pseudotyping with other protein coats generates new properties. The VSVG-pseudotyped vectors seem to have negligible ability for retrograde transduction. In contrast with an AVV, for example, VSVG-pseudotyped FIV did not retrogradely transduce neurones in the subfornical organ when injected into the supraoptical nucleus (11). This feature of VSVG-pseudotyped LVV may be important for functional studies when gene manipulation needs to be restricted to the injected brain area. Additionally, when an elongation factor 1α(EF1α)-EGFP LVV with the VSVG envelope was injected into the hypothalamus of the rat, no GFP-expressing neurones in remote areas, such as the brainstem, could be found (Kasparov, Paton, Huentelman, and Raizada, unpublished observation). Other coat proteins, such as the rabies-G envelope protein, however, alter this property permitting retrograde axonal transfection as demonstrated with the equine infectious anemia virus-bearing HCMV-βGal expression cassette (52). A good example of how the type of coat protein may change the cellular tropism of the LVV in the brain is that of the Ross River virus glycoproteins changing targeting by the FIV from neurones (characteristic of VSVG coat) to glia (53).

AAV VECTORS FOR GENE DELIVERY IN THE BRAIN

AAV used currently have been derived from the serotype 2 AAV. These viruses have a small, nonenveloped capsid and are efficient in transducing central neurones (54–57). Their tropism to other potentially interesting cell types, such as endothelial vascular cells, is lower than that of the AVV but can be increased by a capsid modification (57). Recently, it has been demonstrated that as with the AVV, AAV can also transduce neurones retrogradely: for example, expression occurred in the entorinal cortex after injection into the hippocampus (58). AAV lack almost their entire native genome and therefore do not cause expression of their capsid proteins in transduced cells. Because capsid proteins can trigger an immune response, these vectors are advantaged by this property, making them particularly suitable for systemic use in tissues outside of the brain–blood barrier. For some time, it had been thought that AAV integrate their transgenes into the host chromosome, similar to the wild-type AAV, but this does not seem to apply to vectors derived from it. Thus, AAV-delivered transgenes remain largely episomal. Nevertheless, the expression following AAV transduction usually lasts for months which, together with an absence of any immune response, makes these vectors one of the favorite prototypes for gene therapy research. For further information on AAV vectors, see recently published reviews *(27,56,59,60)*.

APPLICATIONS OF SOMATIC GENE TRANSFER IN STUDIES OF CENTRAL MECHANISMS OF BLOOD PRESSURE CONTROL

In the following, we describe the types of experiments that can be performed using viral vectors that are capable of efficient gene delivery into central structures regulating cardiovascular homeostasis.

Overexpression Experiments

A common experiment is to overexpress a certain protein in a brain structure of interest in order to increase the activity of this protein and monitor the outcome chronically. This approach has been used in a number of studies by Hirooka and colleagues *(5,61–65)*. For example, in *(1)* an AVV with HCMV promoter was used to overexpress the endothelial isoform of nitric oxide synthase (eNOS) in the rostral ventrolateral medulla (RVLM), a major region providing descending sympato-excitatory drive. The experiments were carried out in two strains of rats—the stroke-prone SHR and its progenitor strain, the WKY rat. Arterial pressure was chronically monitored using radiotelemetry. Seven days after gene transfer, mean arterial pressure and heart rate decreased in both groups but these falls were significantly larger in the SHR. In addition, baroreceptor reflex input–output function was increased in both rat groups. A control for the nonspecific effects of the viral transduction was made using an AVV expressing β-galactosidase, which caused no change in the parameters measured. The authors argued that an increase in nitric oxide (NO) production in RVLM improves the impaired baroreceptor reflex control in SHR. In a previous study from the same group *(65)*, eNOS was overexpressed in the NTS. The increased production of NO was demonstrated using microdialysis. In eNOS-transfected animals, blood pressure and heart rate were significantly decreased 5–10 d after gene transfer.

In these studies, the cellular targets to which the transgene was delivered was not established: it is not known whether the bulk of the eNOS-expressing cells were neurones, glia, or vascular cells (smooth muscle or endothelium). NO is thought to freely diffuse through cellular membranes and may reach targets in cells located some distance away from the source of release. But how far it travels under physiological conditions is not entirely clear *(66)*. In the experiments described above, eNOS activity will appear in the cells determined by both the transductional tropism of the AVV and the transcriptional activity of HCMV promoter. This is very likely to be a different subset of cells from the ones producing eNOS endogenously. In the NTS, AVV with the HCMV promoter largely targets glial cells, and transgene expression in local endothelial cells has also been documented *(see* ref. *27)*. Because NO can easily cross cellular membranes, its overproduction in these experiments means that it could still reach its receptor (soluble guanylate cyclase) located in cells adjacent to the transfected cells. However, if the overexpressed molecule had to act on the target within the same cell, any mismatch between the expression profile of the viral vector and the distribution of the target molecule could lead to a false negative or otherwise unpredictable outcome. Moreover, the action of high local concentrations of NO on the targets *within* the cells in which the AVV causes eNOS overexpression might result in nonphysiological responses.

In summary, overexpression of eNOS will produce large quantities of NO comparable to a chronic infusion of an NO donor into the structure. This provides a good method of chronic delivery of a substance without the need of repeated injections into a single brain locus, which is technically unachievable in many brain structures. However, both overexpression of eNOS and delivery of a pharmacological agent are unlikely to accurately mimic the physiological scenario in terms of providing a site- or cell-specific source of NO at a physiologically relevant concentration.

AVV with the HCMV promoter was also used to overexpress mitochondrial or cytoplasmatic superoxide dismutase isoforms to demonstrate involvement of reactive oxygen species (ROS) in the pressor, and dipsogenic responses induced by intracerebroventricular (icv) administration of angiotensin II (Ang II) in mice *(8)*. ROS have been implicated in the pathogenesis of neurodegenerative disease but, in addition, are currently thought to act as second messengers in some signaling systems. In the Zimmerman et al. study *(8)*, AVV were administered in the lateral ventricle of the mouse brain and the outcome evaluated 3 d later. Arterial pressure and heart rate were monitored before and after intraventricular administration of Ang II. Overexpression of both mitochondrial and cytoplasmatic isoforms strongly antagonized responses to icv injections of Ang II. The dipsogenic action of Ang II was also significantly antagonized. These studies have established a role for ROS in an AT_1 receptor-mediated signaling pathway regulating the cardiovascular system. The transgene in these studies was found predominantly in the brain tissue surrounding the ventricles and the subfornical organ, a circumventricular organ with a high density of AT_1 receptors known to be involved in blood-to-brain communication. Thus, AT_1 receptors in the subfornical organ may trigger hypertension via signaling cascade involving ROS. More recently, the same group has found that overexpression of Cu/Zn superoxide dismutase in subfornical organ and organum vasculosum of the lamina terminalis (this was achieved using icv injection of AVV) reduced sympathetic tone in mice with cardiac failure triggered by myocardial infarction *(67)*. Interestingly, ROS scavenging did not affect the sympathetic tone in control animals without cardiac failure, suggesting that ROS signaling becomes activated only under these pathological conditions. The authors conclude that in heart failure, ROS within the circumventricular organs may mediate central sympathoactivation by circulating molecules such as Ang II and aldosterone *(67)*.

We used a similar strategy to address the role for ROS in the AT1-receptor mediated signaling in the NTS, except that we overexpressed catalase instead of superoxide dismutase. We also used an AVV with HCMV promoter, but in our case this approach failed to prevent the depressant action of Ang II on baroreceptor reflex-mediated bradycardia in spite of the significantly elevated catalase activity in the area of transfection *(10)*. Clearly, this reflects differences in the signalling mechanisms employed by the same receptor in the two different brain areas. However, the methodology of viral gene transfer leaves room for alternative interpretations that have to be considered. First, is it possible that in the NTS, AVV with the HCMV promoter did not lead to sufficient catalase expression in the cells that mediate the AT1 receptor-mediated baroreceptor reflex attenuation? The precise nature of these cells is still unclear, but our current evidence suggests that they could be the eNOS-bearing endothelial cells. From our experiments, in which eNOS dominant negative protein, expressed using an AVV with HCMV promoter, was able to antagonize AT_1 receptor-mediated effects in NTS *(see* Figs. 2 and 3), we reckon that this is unlikely to be the case. Second, it is not impossible that the catalase expressed was inefficient in inactivating the ROS generated by AT_1 receptor activation in the NTS. This argument is more difficult to dismiss, but we could argue that the lack of the effect of the catalase overexpression was consistent with the inability of a number of pharmacological blockers to antagonize various steps in the cascade signaling pathway downstream of ROS generation *(10)*.

In summary, these studies illustrate some of the potential experimental applications of virally mediated transgenesis for overexpression of a protein in different central nervous structures to evoke chronic alterations in cardiovascular function.

Expression of Antisense Oligonucleotides and siRNA-Mediated Gene Suppression

Viral vectors have also been used in "loss-of-function" experiments in order to chronically decrease expression of a certain gene. There is more than one way to achieve this. Lu and Raizada *(68)* successfully used a retroviral vector to express an antisense sequence to the 5'end of the AT_{1B} receptor gene. The vectors were applied to primary cultures from brainstem to down-regulate AT_1 receptor expression. This experiment resulted in downregulation of all measured responses to Ang II, including c-fos and noradrenaline transporter expression.

Although the antisense approach has been used successfully by some groups *(35,68,69)*, the more recent reports about small interfering RNAs (siRNA) being able to selectively target specific mRNA species into the degradation pathway have evoked huge interest from the scientific community *(70,71)*. Most published studies to date have employed synthetic double-stranded RNA oligonucleotides *(72–74)*. However, it is also possible to use viral vectors to express siRNA to the same effect *(75–78)*. These vectors are designed in such a way that transcription results in generation of hairpin-like RNA, which acts similarly to the conventional siRNA. Viral vectors for expression of siRNA have been made on the basis of polymerase II promoters, such as HCMV *(78)*, and polymerase III promoters such as U6 *(75)* and H1 *(79)*. Polymerase III promoters are currently thought to be optimal for siRNA hairpin expression because they provide a high rate of transcription of small RNA molecules in a wide range of cells. Moreover, the mechanisms of the initiation and termination of transcription by polymerase III allow production of precise lengths of transcripts that do not undergo mRNA-specific posttranscriptional modifications, which interfere with siRNA function. Some systems of that kind are available commercially. Viral vectors with polymerase III-derived inducible siRNA expression systems have also been developed *(79)*. At this point, this technology has not been applied in studies of central cardiovascular control, but this is just a matter of time.

Expression of Dominant-Negative Proteins

It is possible to suppress the function of certain proteins by expression of dominant negative proteins. This principle usually employs protein–protein interaction, for example, between the dominant negative protein and a catalytic subunit of an enzyme. We were interested in the role of NO in baroreceptor reflex control at the level of the NTS. A number of pharmacological tools were used *(32)* to demonstrate that various blockers of NO production prevented a well-documented inhibitory action of Ang II on this reflex in the NTS (80,81). Viral gene transfer of a dominant negative form of eNOS was then employed for two reasons. First, we believed that it would be more selective for the "endothelial" NOS isoform (as opposed to the "neuronal" or nNOS isoform) than the available pharmacological antagonists. Second, it was important to evaluate the role of NO in NTS chronically, and long-term pharmacological blockade of eNOS in NTS is technically not achievable. To suppress endogenous eNOS in the NTS, an AVV was used to express a truncated form of eNOS (TeNOS) under the control of the HCMV promoter (82). Although TeNOS lacks catalytic activity, it is correctly localized to the membrane. TeNOS acts as a dominant negative inhibitor of wild-type eNOS activity through heterodimerization with the native protein (83). We demonstrated that in animals that had received three bilateral injections in the NTS of the TeNOS AVV 5–6 d prior to the test, Ang II, which normally strongly suppresses baroreceptor reflex when administered into the NTS, was ineffective (Fig. 2) (32). Similarly, the NO precursor L-arginine, which also inhibited the baroreceptor reflex when injected into the NTS of naïve rats, failed to modulate the baroreceptor reflex in TeNOS-transfected animals. There appeared to be no evidence of any aberrant effects of the AVV because: (1) the baseline baroreceptor reflex sensitivity was not altered by TeNOS expression; and, (2) an EGFP-expressing AVV did not cause any detectable alterations in baroreceptor reflex function and multiple other physiological variables measured.

More recently, the same construct was used chronically in normotensive conscious freely-moving rats instrumented with radio transmitters to record their blood pressure and heart rate. This approach gives a continuous definitive measure of arterial pressure. After the implantation of transmitters, the basal level of blood pressure, heart rate, and spontaneous baroreceptor reflex gain were determined by a time–series method. Subsequently, the animals were then reanesthetized and the AVV-TeNOS microinjected into the NTS. TeNOS expression evoked a gradual increase in baroreceptor reflex gain between d 7 and 21 after gene transfer, peaking at d 21 (1.68 ± 0.20 ms/mmHg). This value was significantly higher compared to that before gene transfer (1.13 ± 0.09 ms/mmHg). It was also significantly elevated compared with two groups of control animals: those that received an NTS microinjection of an AVV expressing EGFP, which acted as a viral control, and those that received a microinjection of saline. In addition, heart rate decreased 14–21 d after TeNOS gene transfer. However, blood pressure was not affected. These results indicate that eNOS is constitutively active within the NTS, and acts to regulate baroreceptor reflex gain and heart rate but not resting blood pressure in normotensive WKY rats (3). In addition, these data suggest that baroreflex gain (at least the cardiac component) is controlled independently from arterial pressure by the NTS. This prompted the question as to whether eNOS activity in NTS of the SHR was important for the known depressed baroreceptor reflex gain in this animal model. Our preliminary data indicate that when TeNOS was expressed in 10- to 11-wk-old SHR, baroreceptor reflex sensitivity increased, whereas systolic blood pressure decreased (84). These results suggest that in this model of pathological hypertension, endogenous eNOS activity in the NTS is elevated compared with normotensive rats and plays a major role in determining levels of both arterial pressure and baroreceptor reflex gain. For reasons which will become apparent later, it is worth mentioning that in all of these vectors, transgene expression was driven by the HCMV promoter.

We have also used AVV expressing dominant negative proteins to dissect out the intracellular signaling pathway utilized by Ang II to suppress the baroreceptor reflex

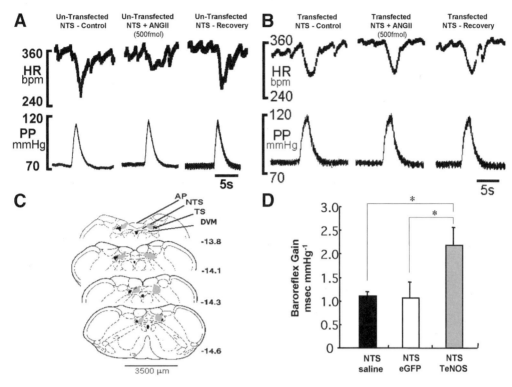

Fig. 2. Examples of the usefulness of adenoviral vector (AVV)-mediated expression of a dominant negative protein in the nucleus tractus solitarii (NTS) for cardiovascular control. Angiotensin II (Ang II) injections into the NTS attenuate the reflex bradycardia to baroreceptor stimulation (A). This was shown to be dependent on endothelial nitric oxide synthase (eNOS) because adenoviral transfection with a dominant negative "TeNOS" (a truncated form of eNOS) prevented the effect of Ang II (B). Transfection sites (indicated by grey shading) were localized within the NTS as revealed by expression of enhanced green fluorescent protein (EGFP) using a second adenovirus (C). Chronic expression of TeNOS in rats fitted with telemetry devices to record arterial pressure revealed a significant elevation in baroreceptor reflex sensitivity in normotensive rats (D). Note that neither saline injections into NTS or expression of EGFP in this nucleus altered baroreceptor reflex gain. AP, area postrema; DVM, dorsal vagal motor nucleus; HR, heart rate in beats per min (bpm); PP, perfusion pressure; TS, solitary tract. (Data taken from refs. *3* and *32*.)

within the NTS *(10)*. In contrast, HCMV-EGFP-injected animals were no different from naïve rats in terms of Ang II action on the baroreceptor reflex in NTS. However, expression of a dominant negative Gq protein driven by the human elongation factor (EF1α) promoter in NTS strongly antagonized the depressant action of Ang II on the baroreceptor reflex (Fig. 3). This was an important finding because Gq is one of the established intracellular links between G protein-coupled receptors, such as the AT_1 receptor, and intracellular Ca^{2+} stores. These data were consolidated using conventional pharmacological approaches to block intracellular signalling pathways *(10)*. In the same study, some AVV with HCMV-driven constructs were also used. One of them expressed a dominant form of Akt (or protein kinase B). However, this intervention was without effect on Ang II inhibition of the baroreceptor reflex, which was consistent with the outcome of pharmacological experiments *(85)*. In summary, AVV expressing various dominant-negative proteins helped us to unravel the functional significance of eNOS in

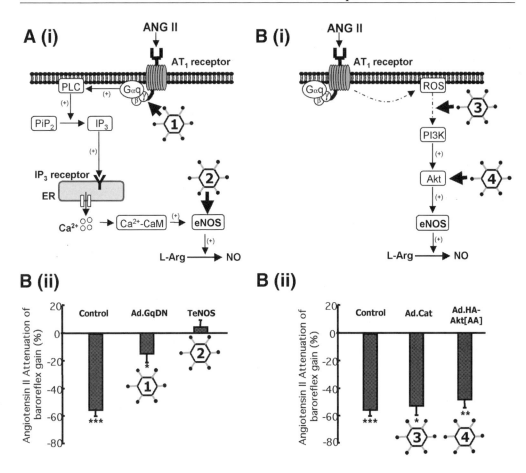

Fig. 3. Determining the intracellular signaling pathway activated by angiotensin II (Ang II) to inhibit the baroreceptor reflex. Two possible pathways were tested **(A,B)**. Using adenoviral gene transfer (and pharmacological antagonists—*see* ref. *10*) to disrupt pathway A prevented the Ang II-induced attenuation of the baroreceptor reflex. Two adenoviruses were used to express dominant negative proteins to block Gq (AVV 1) and endothelial nitric oxide synthase (eNOS) (AVV 2). In contrast, reducing reactive oxygen species (ROS) by overexpressing catalase (AVV 3) or expressing a dominant-negative to block protein kinase B activity (Akt; AVV 4) were unable to prevent the baroreceptor reflex attenuation by Ang II. It has been hypothesized that pathway A is responsible for the Ang II-induced activation of eNOS. (Data taken from refs. *10* and *32*.)

the NTS for long-term control of baroreceptor reflex sensitivity and arterial pressure in conscious normotensive and hypertensive animals, as well as the intracellular signaling pathway that links AT_1 receptor to baroreflex inhibition.

Three Methodological Aspects of Using Dominant-Negative Proteins

First, expression of the dominant-negative protein might give a more accurate portrait of the function of endogenous molecules than their overexpression, provided that the dominant-negative protein is specific and potent. Indeed, if a biologically active transgene appears in different cellular phenotypes that normally do not express it (as is the case with most overexpression experiments), this may give the wrong idea about the function of this transgene. In contrast, a dominant-negative protein is not supposed to have any functional consequence in cells other than to block the activity of the native protein, if it is present. Theoretically at least, it could be argued that the use of dominant-negative proteins should be somewhat more selective, and any effect more reliably interpreted than the responses that occur following overexpression of proteins in the "gain-of-function" experiments.

Second, as mentioned previously, we have used largely AVV with the HCMV promoter, with one exception being the EF1α-driven construct. We want to draw attention to this issue because this is an example of a case where viral transgenesis differs radically from the use of a pharmacological blocker: expression of a transgene might result in its inadvertent targeting of a subset of cells with a specific phenotype. As mentioned previously, we have recently found that HCMV-driven expression is not as ubiquitous in the brain as is sometimes thought (27). A striking result was obtained in experiments in organotypic brainstem slice cultures co-transfected with two AVV at the same time: the first AVV contained an HCMV-DsRed expression cassette (DSRed is a far-red shifted fluorescent protein from coral), whereas in the second AVV expression of EGFP was controlled by the PRSx8 artificial promoter, which is highly active in noradrenergic, adrenergic, and some vagal preganglionic neurons. In several brainstem noradrenergic cell groups, no colocalization of DsRed and EGFP could be detected in numerous (>50) cells using spectral confocal microscopy (for details, see 86). In contrast, co-infection with HCMV-DsRed AVV and HCMV-EGFP AVV resulted in more than 90% of double-labeled cells (many of which had the characteristic glial morphology; unpublished observation). These results were consistent with the outcome of in vivo experiments where noradrenergic neurones in the locus coeruleus did express EGFP, but did not express DsRed after injection of a mixture of PRSx8-EGFP and HCMV-DsRed AVV, although red fluorescent cells were visible outside this nucleus (27). Interestingly, HCMV-EGFP AVV caused robust expression in brainstem cholinergic motor nuclei of the hypoglossal nerve (Fig. 1D,E). The ability of AVV with the HCMV promoter to efficiently target glia has also been documented before both in vivo (87) and in acute brain slices (88). In addition, AVV with HCMV-EGFP can transduce local vascular endothelium after brainstem microinjections in vivo (89). Therefore, it is possible, and even likely, that HCMV-controlled vectors discriminate against some cellular phenotypes in favor of others and the physiological outcome of these experiments may be the result of expression in nonneuronal cellular compartments, such as the local vascular cells or glia.

A dominant-negative approach has also been employed to analyze the role of Rho/Rho kinase pathway in the NTS (6). Rho is a small GTPase, present in many cells, that can be activated by a number of extracellular signals. In the GTP-bound state, Rho binds to numerous intracellular targets to activate them. One such target is Rho kinase. The dominant-negative Rho kinase bears mutations in its adenosine triphosphate-binding domain and effectively inhibits the Rho-mediated phosphorylation of its numerous down-stream targets. AVV with HCMV promoter to drive expression of this dominant negative protein were injected into the NTS of both WKY and SHR, from which blood pressure was measured using radiotelemetry. In both strains a transient drop in heart rate and blood pressure was observed between d 4 and d 7, but this was more dramatic in the SHR. The authors also found that in the SHR, Rho redistributes to the plasma membrane from the cytosol, and that phosphorylation of one of the downstream targets of Rho kinase in SHR is enhanced. In addition, a small but statistically significant decrease in both eNOS and nNOS protein was found after Rho-kinase dominant-negative protein expression in the NTS. In this study, an AVV with the HCMV promoter was used (6). Thus, based on our evidence *(27)*, it can be predicted that only a small minority of targets transduced by this vector in the NTS could be neurones. What then could be the cellular target of the Rho-kinase dominant-negative expression in the NTS described by Ito et al. *(6)*? Clearly, in contrast with the previously discussed eNOS overexpression experiments, the Rho-kinase dominant-negative could only act on Rho signaling within the same cells expressing the transgene. Given that the effect was very transient (3 d only), it is possible that the local endothelial cells were responsible for it; these cells can express transgenes by injection of AVV with HCMV promoter in the brain *(89)*. They are exposed to the immune system and are likely to be rapidly eliminated as a result the residual expression of the adenoviral proteins. A change in eNOS expression reported in that study could be consistent with this suggestion *(6)*.

In conclusion, the examples presented illustrate the usefulness of expressing dominant-negative proteins in unraveling neuronal mechanisms in central regulation of cardiovascular function. These have allowed identification of ligand-mediated intracellular cascades *and* the simultaneous physiological consequences of perturbing such pathways on blood pressure regulation. There is no doubt that viral gene transfer coupled with radiotelemetry provides a powerful tool for the cardiovascular neuroscientist. However, further refinement of viral constructs is required. As exemplified by the AVV with HCMV-driven trangenes, caution is required when interpreting data and ascribing functional effects to a specific cell type within the brain.

Tracking Cardioascular Circuits Using Retrograde Viral Transfection

Certain types of viruses (e.g., the pseudorabies virus) can be used to track neuronal pathways as a result of their retrograde transport and ability to express transgenes, such as EGFP, in connected central neurones, which presumably form a neuroanatomical circuit. Irnaten et al. *(13)* used the Bartha strain of swine pathogenic presudorabies virus in a study on cardiorespiratory networks. Pseudorabies virus is an attenuated replicating pathogen, and is therefore different from all other vectors mentioned in this chapter because it is *not* replication-deficient. It enters neurones via their peripheral axonal terminals and invades the soma by retrograde transport. Once in a neuronal soma, the virus replicates within a few hours, becomes highly concentrated in dendritic processes, and then leaves its host at sites of synaptic contact. It is thought that glial processes limit the lateral spread of virions to unrelated nerve cells and contribute to a predominantly transsynaptic pattern of viral spread *(see* refs. *90,91)*. Irnaten et al. *(13)* engineered a Bartha virus mutant to express EGFP using an endogenous gG promoter present in that virus. Two days after the injection of the virus into the pericardial sac of rat pups, EGFP fluorescent cardiovagal neurones could be identified in the nucleus ambiguus. However, an adjacent population of motoneurones with their axons in the superior laryngeal did not express EGFP. Electrophysiological analysis revealed that the EGFP-expressing neurones could generate action potentials and had currents similar to those in nearby nontransfected neurones. If pups were sacrificed 3 d after pericardial injections, EGFP labeling was also found in the periambigual area and NTS. However, in vivo analysis of transfected pups revealed that viral infection caused a clear shift in the baroreceptor reflex input–output curve measured at d 3, suggesting a change in the functional state of the reflex pathway *(13)*. In conclusion, this viral approach allows clear identification of cardiac vagal motoneurones, and in this regard is similar to that achieved using conventional fluorescent retrograde tracers, such as rhodamine beads. It appears, however, that interneurones antecedent to the motoneurones are much more difficult to study. It is highly unlikely that the infected neurones retain normal neurophysiological characteristics for any length of time because of the detrimental effects of rapidly replicating virus.

AVV can also be used for retrograde tracing, but they do not pass transsynaptically. Moreover, as AVV do not cause any deleterious effects in the neurones they infect, they can also be used to coexpress a functional protein along with a fluorescent reporter. For example, cardiac parasympathetic preganglionic neurones in nucleus ambiguus were retrogradely transfected with AVV after injection of this virus into the pericardial sac of P4–P10 rat pups *(12)*. The AVV contained two transgenes in a head-to-head orientation, both under control of the HCMV promoter. One of these cassettes expressed EGFP, and the other—the ϵ-subunit of $GABA_A$ receptor. Two to four days after viral injection medullary slices were prepared. Retrogradely transduced fluorescent neurones could be identified and their electrophysiological characteristics studied using the patch clamp technique. It was found that expression of the ϵ-subunit in cardiac vagal motoneurones blocked the pentobarbitone-induced potentiation of GABAergic currents.

Finally, and as mentioned previously, we have developed a method for selective retrograde transduction of subsets of brainstem noradrenergic neurones which may be used to analyze their function *(27)*.

Future Potential Applications of Viral Gene Transfer

There may be several other applications of viral gene transfer in studies of central cardiovascular control; we wish to describe two. First, our laboratory recently demonstrated direct recording of transmitter release from individual visualized varicosities of brainstem noradrenaline-containing neurones. An AVV was constructed to express EGFP under control of the PRSx8 promoter, which is highly active in noradrenergic neurones *(see* previous section). In slice cultures, catecholaminergic neurones displayed characteristic beaded axons that were readily identifiable using either conventional fluorescent or confocal microscopy (Fig. 1F). Moreover, these axons could be traced for hundreds of microns. Using fine carbon electrodes, microamperometric recordings of noradrenaline release from these varicosities can be made (Fig. 4). Thus, this novel approach will allow for the first time a study of the modulation of noradrenaline release from characterized central neurones of normotensive and hypertensive rat strains. Second, the "vigilant vector" introduced by Phillips and colleagues *(92)* has a number of unique characteristics. It has both a cardiac myocyte-specific promoter (a truncated version of MLC2v) and an enhancer, with the hypoxia response element operating within a single AAV. This construct drives expression of antisense RNA to the AT_1 receptor in the heart in hypoxia-inducible manner. The motivation for such a construct was based on the problem of myocardial ischemia, which initially is a progressive asymptomatic condition. Following a hypoxic episode in the heart, AT_1 receptor antisense expression could help alleviate consequences of ischemia, because this receptor contributes to this condition. Such vigilant vectors have not yet been applied to the central nervous system, but it is conceivable that expressing transgenes to depress AT_1 receptors in specific cell types could be most beneficial in neurogenic hypertension. Cascades which link neuronal activity to c-fos gene expression could possibly be exploited to achieve inducibility as described in ref. *93.*

CONCLUSIONS

There is no question that genetic manipulation to address biological questions has recently become a universal research tool in all areas of physiology. As illustrated herein,

A   **B**

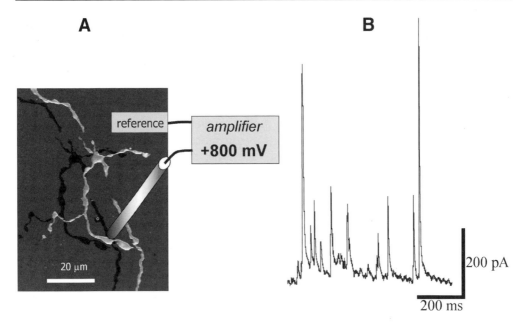

Fig. 4. Detection of noradrenaline release from visualized varicosities of A1 neurones. **(A)** Schematic to illustrate the principle of microamperometric catecholamine detection. Oxidation of the catecholamine at the preset electrode potential generates current, as shown in panel B. In these experiments, a 5-μm carbon fiber electrode was positioned directly on the visualized enhanced green flurorescent protein (EGFP)-fluorescent axonal varicosities. **(B)** A current trace illustrates bursts of vesicular noradrenaline release from a single varicosity.

viral vectors offer an efficient method of gene transfer, and can be used to perform a variety of experiments in order to address mechanisms of central cardiovascular control. So far, mainly AVV and LVV have been used in these studies, but AAV also has very attractive features. All available viral vectors target (albeit sometimes inadvertently) the transgene to one or more cell types in the brain (glia, different components of blood vessels, various neuronal phenotypes). This occurs at both the transductional (e.g., at the stage of viral entry into the cells) and transcriptional levels (e.g., via the mechanisms which control gene expression), and needs to be taken into account when interpreting the functional outcome of such experiments. It is expected that in the near future, viral vector production will become faster and cheaper, and that viruses will be completely nonimmunogenic, with targeted cellular tropism in which expression is controllable and suitable for both in vivo and in vitro applications. It may also become important to further refine protocols for production of large quantities of vectors, such as LVV, for systemic applications. Finally, further research should focus on developing short and powerful promoters suitable for directing virally mediated expression to selected populations of cells. Viral gene manipulation in the brainstem has already been successfully used to identify mechanisms relating to cardiovascular control, as well as the alterations that occur and that may contribute to hypertension. In this type of research, viral gene transfer is particularly valuable because it is fully compatible with other established conventional experimental strategies, such as hypertensive rat models and long-term telemetric monitoring of blood pressure.

ACKNOWLEDGMENTS

We wish to thank Professor D. Murphy (Henry Wellcome Laboratories for Integrative Neuroscience & Endocrinology, University of Bristol, UK) for his generous assistance in our initial developments of viral vectors. We are grateful to Drs. D. Lonergan and H. Waki, who contributed to some of the data described in this chapter. PRSx8 was provided by Drs. K.-S. Kim and D.-Y Hwang, Harvard University. We gratefully acknowledge the financial support of the British Heart Foundation, the Wellcome Trust, and the Royal Society.

REFERENCES

1. Mann SJ. Neurogenic essential hypertension revisited: the case for increased clinical and research attention. Am J Hypertens 2003;16:881–888.
2. KeetonTK, Campbell WB. The pharmacologic alteration of renin release. Pharmacol Rev 1980;31:81–227.
3. Waki H, Kasparov S, Wong L-F, Murphy D, Shimizu T, Paton JFR. Chronic inhibition of eNOS activity in NTS enhances baroreceptor reflex in conscious rats. J Physiol 2003;546:233–242.
4. Paton JF, Waki H, Kasparov S. In vivo gene transfer to dissect neuronal mechanisms regulating cardio-respiratory function. Can J Physiol Pharmacol 2003;81:311–316.
5. Kishi T, Hirooka Y, Kimura Y, et al. Overexpression of eNOS in RVLM improves impaired baroreflex control of heart rate in SHRSP. Rostral ventrolateral medulla. Stroke-prone spontaneously hypertensive rats, Hypertension 2003;41:255–260.
6. Ito K, Hirooka Y, Sakai K, et al. Rho/Rho-kinase pathway in brain stem contributes to blood pressure regulation via sympathetic nervous system: possible involvement in neural mechanisms of hypertension. Circulation Res 2003;92:1337–1343.
7. Kishi T, Hirooka Y, Sakai K, Shigematsu H, Shimokawa H, Takeshita A. Overexpression of eNOS in the RVLM causes hypotension and bradycardia via GABA release. Hypertension 2001;38:896–901.
8. Zimmerman MC, Lazartigues E, Lang JA, Sinnayah P, Ahmad IM, Spitz DR, Davisson RL. Superoxide mediates the actions of angiotensin II in the central nervous system., Circulation Res 2002;91:1038–1045.
9. Waki H, Kasparov S, Katahira K, Shimizu T, Murphy D, Paton JF. Dynamic exercise attenuates spontaneous baroreceptor reflex sensitivity in conscious rats. Exper Physiol 2003;88:517–526.
10. Wong LF, Polson JW, Murphy D, Paton JF, Kasparov S. Genetic and pharmacological dissection of pathways involved in the angiotensin II-mediated depression of baroreflex function. FASEB J Online 2002;16:1595–1601.
11. Sinnayah P, Lindley TE, Staber PD, Cassell MD, Davidson BL, Davisson RL. Selective gene transfer to key cardiovascular regions of the brain: comparison of two viral vector systems. Hypertension 2002;39:603–608.
12. Irnaten M, Walwyn WM, Wang J, et al. Pentobarbital enhances GABAergic neurotransmission to cardiac parasympathetic neurons, which is prevented by expression of $GABA_A$ e subuni. Anesthesiology 2002;97:717–724.
13. Irnaten M, Neff RA, Wang J, Loewy AD, Mettenleiter TC, Mendelowitz D. Activity of cardiorespiratory networks revealed by transsynaptic virus expressing GFP. J Neurophysiol 2001;85:435–438.
14. Chalmers J. Brain, blood pressure and stroke. J Hypertens 1998;16:1849–1858.
15. de Wardener HE. The hypothalamus and hypertension. Physiol Rev 2001;81:1599–1658.
16. Haywood JR, Mifflin SW, Craig T, et al. γ-Aminobutyric acid (GABA)A function and binding in the paraventricular nucleus of the hypothalamus in chronic renal-wrap hypertension. Hypertension 2001;37:614–618.
17. Arnolda L, Minson J, Kapoor V, Pilowsky P, Llewellyn-Smith I, Chalmers J, Amino acid neurotransmitters in hypertension. Kidney Int Suppl 1992;37:S2–S7.
18. Yamada K, Moriguchi A, Mikami H, Okuda N, Higaki J, Ogihara T. The effect of central amino acid neurotransmitters on the antihypertensive response to angiotensin blockade in spontaneous hypertension. J Hypertens 1995;13:1624–1630.
19. Dampney RAL, Goodchild AK, Tan E. Identification of cardiovascular cell groups in the brain stem. Clin Exper Hypertens 1984;6:205–220.

20. Dampney RAL. Functional organization of central pathways regulating the cardiovascular system. Physiol Rev 1994;74:323–364.
21. Lu D, Yu K, Paddy MR, Rowland NE, Raizada MK. Regulation of norepinephrine transport system by angiotensin II in neuronal cultures of normotensive and spontaneously hypertensive rat brains. Endocrinology 1996;137:763–772.
22. MacLean MR, Raizada MK, Sumners C. The influence of angiotensin II on catecholamine synthesis in neuronal cultures from rat brain. Biochem Biophys Res Comm 1990;167:492–497.
23. MacLean MR, Phillips MI, Summers C, Raizada MK. α1-Adrenergic receptors in the nucleus tractus solitarii region of rats with experimental and genetic hypertension. Brain Res 1990;519:261–265.
24. Baker AH. Adenoviral vectors for gene therapy. Mol Biotechnol 2003;25:101–102.
25. Nicklin SA, Dishart KL, Buening H, et al. Transductional and transcriptional targeting of cancer cells using genetically engineered viral vectors. Cancer Lett 2003;201:165–173.
26. Wickham TJ. Targeting adenovirus. Gene Ther 2000;7:110–114.
27. Kasparov S, Teschemacher AG, Hwang D-Y, Kim K-S, Lonergan T, Paton JFR. Viral Vectors as Tools for Studies of Central Cardiovascular Control. Prog Biophys Mol Biol 2004;84:251–277.
28. Lonergan T, Teschemacher AG, Paton JFR, Kasparov S. Expression profile of adenoviral vectors incorporating hCMV, synapsin-1 and PRSx8 promoters in brainstem centres of cardiovascular control. J Physiol 2004;http://www.physoc.org/publications/proceedings/archive/index.asp.
29. Katovich MJ, Reaves PY, Francis SC, Pachori AS, Wang HW, Raizada MK. Gene therapy attenuates the elevated blood pressure and glucose intolerance in an insulin-resistant model of hypertension. J Hypertens 2001;19:1553–1558.
30. Wang H, Lu D, Reaves PY, Katovich MJ, Raizada MK. Retrovirally mediated delivery of angiotensin II type 1 receptor antisense in vitro and in vivo. Methods Enzymol 1999;314:581–590.
31. Stec DE, Davisson RL, Haskell HE, Davidson BL, Sigmund CD. Efficient liver-specific deletion of a floxed human angiotensinogen transgene by adenoviral delivery of Cre recombinase in vivo. J Biol Chem 1999;274:21,285–21,290.
32. Paton JFR, Deuchars J, Ahmad Z, Wong L-F, Murphy D, Kasparov S. Adenoviral vector demonstrates that angiotensin II-induced depression of the cardiac baroreflex is mediated by endothelial nitric oxide synthase in the nucleus tractus solitarii of the rat. J Physiol 2001;531:445–458.
33. Hirooka Y, Sakai K, Kishi T, Takeshita A. Adenovirus-mediated gene transfer into the NTS in conscious rats. A new approach to examining the central control of cardiovascular regulation. Ann NY Acad Sci 2001;940:197–205.
34. Phillips MI. Gene therapy for hypertension: the preclinical data. Hypertension 2001;38:543–548.
35. Phillips MI. Gene therapy for hypertension: sense and antisense strategies. Exp Opin Biol Ther 2001;1:655–662.
36. Kugler S, Kilic E, Bahr M. Human synapsin 1 gene promoter confers highly neuron-specific long-term transgene expression from an adenoviral vector in the adult rat brain depending on the transduced area. Gene Ther 2003;10:337–347.
37. Glover CP, Bienemann AS, Hopton M, Harding TC, Kew JN, Uney JB. Long-term transgene expression can be mediated in the brain by adenoviral vectors when powerful neuron-specific promoters are used. J Gene Med 2003;5:554–559.
38. Hwang D-Y, Carlezon WA Jr, Isacson O, Kim K-S. A high-efficiency synthetic promoter that drives transgene expression selectively in noradrenergic neurons. Hum Gene Ther 2001;12:1731–1740.
39. Thomas CE, Schiedner G, Kochanek S, Castro MG, Lowenstein PR. Peripheral infection with adenovirus causes unexpected long-term brain inflammation in animals injected intracranially with first-generation, but not with high-capacity, adenovirus vectors: Toward realistic long-term neurological gene therapy for chronic diseases. Proc Natl Acad Sci USA 2000;97:7482–7487.
40. Iwakuma T, Cui Y, Chang L-J. Self-Inactivating lentiviral vectors with U3 and U5 modifications. Virology 1999;261:120–132.
41. Coleman JE, Huentelman MJ, Kasparov S, et al. Efficient Large-Scale Production and Concentration of HIV-1-Based Lentiviral Vectors For Use In vivo. Physiol Genom 2003;12:221–228.
42. Jin X, Mathers PH, Szabo G, Katarova Z, Agmon A. Vertical bias in dendritic trees of non-pyramidal neocortical neurons expressing GAD67-GFP in vitro. Cerebral Cortex 2001;11:666–678.
43. Gong S, Zheng C, Doughty ML, et al. A gene expression atlas of the central nervous system based on bacterial artificial chromosomes. Nature 2003;425:917–925.
44. Kugler S, Kilic E, Bahr M. Human synapsin 1 gene promoter confers highly neuron-specific long-term transgene expression from an adenoviral vector in the adult rat brain depending on the transduced area. Gene Ther 2003;10:337–347.

45. Chillon M, Bosch A, Zabner J, et al. Group D adenoviruses infect primary central nervous system cells more efficiently than those from group C. J Virol 1999;73:2537–2540.

46. Omori,N., Mizuguchi,H., Ohsawa,K., et al. Modification of a fiber protein in an adenovirus vector improves in vitro gene transfer efficiency to the mouse microglial cell line. Neurosci Lett 2002;324:145–148.

47. Nicklin SA, Von Seggern DJ, Work LM, et al. Ablating adenovirus type 5 fiber-CAR binding and HI loop insertion of the SIGYPLP peptide generate an endothelial cell-selective adenovirus. Mol Ther 2001;4:534–542.

48. White SJ, Nicklin SA, Sawamura T, Baker AH. Identification of peptides that target the endothelial cell-specific LOX-1 receptor. Hypertension 2001;37:449–455.

49. Bilang-Bleuel,A., Revah,F., Colin,P., et al. Intrastriatal injection of an adenoviral vector expressing glial-cell- line-derived neurotrophic factor prevents dopaminergic neuron degeneration and behavioral impairment in a rat model of Parkinson disease. Proc Natl Acad Sci USA 1997;94:8818–8823.

50. Nishimura I, Uetsuki T, Dani SU, et al. Degeneration in vivo of rat hippocampal neurons by wild-type Alzheimer amyloid precursor protein overexpressed by adenovirus-mediated gene transfer. J Neurosci 1998;18:2387–2398.

51. Niwa H, Yamamura K, Miyazaki J. Efficient selection for high-expression transfectants with a novel eukaryotic vector. Gene 1991;108:193–199.

52. Mazarakis ND, Azzouz M, Rohll JB, et al. Rabies virus glycoprotein pseudotyping of lentiviral vectors enables retrograde axonal transport and access to the nervous system after peripheral delivery. Hum Mol Genet 2001;10:2109–2121.

53. Kang Y, Stein CS, Heth JA, et al. In vivo gene transfer using a nonprimate lentiviral vector pseudotyped with Ross River Virus glycoproteins. J Virol 2002;76:9378–9388.

54. Davidson BL, Chiorini JA. Recombinant adeno-associated viral vector types 4 and 5. Preparation and application for CNS gene transfer. Methods Mol Med 2003;76:269–285.

55. Okada T, Nomoto T, Shimazaki K, et al. Adeno-associated virus vectors for gene transfer to the brain. Methods 2002;28:237–247.

56. Paterna JC, Büeler H. Recombinant adeno-associated virus vector design and gene expression in the mammalian brain. Methods 2002;28:208–218.

57. Nicklin SA, Buening H, Dishart KL, et al. Efficient and selective AAV2-mediated gene transfer directed to human vascular endothelial cells. Mol Ther 2001;4:174–181.

58. Kaspar BK, Erickson D, Schaffer D, Hinh L, Gage FH, Peterson DA. Targeted retrograde gene delivery for neuronal protection. Mol Ther 2002;5:50–56.

59. Büning H, Nicklin SA, Perabo L, Hallek M, Baker AH. AAV-based gene transfer. Curr Opin Mol Ther 2003;5:367–375.

60. Davidson BL, Breakefield XO. Viral vectors for gene delivery to the nervous system. Nat Rev Neurosci 2003;4:353–364.

61. Hirooka Y, Sakai K, Kishi T, Ito K, Shimokawa H, Takeshita A. Enhanced depressor response to endothelial nitric oxide synthase gene transfer into the nucleus tractus solitarii of spontaneously hypertensive rats. Hypertens Res 2003;26:325–331.

62. Hirooka Y, Kishi T, Sakai K, Shimokawa H, Takeshita A. Effect of overproduction of nitric oxide in the brain stem on the cardiovascular response in conscious rats. J Cardiovasc Pharmacol 2003;41(Suppl 1):S119–S126.

63. Kishi T, Hirooka Y, Ito K, Sakai K, Shimokawa H, Takeshita A. Cardiovascular effects of overexpression of endothelial nitric oxide synthase in the rostral ventrolateral medulla in stroke-prone spontaneously hypertensive rats. Hypertension 2002;39:264–268.

64. Matsuo I, Hirooka Y, Hironaga K, et al. Glutamate release via NO production evoked by NMDA in the NTS enhances hypotension and bradycardia in vivo. Am J Physiol Reg Integr Comp Physiol 2001;280:R1285–R1291.

65. Sakai K, Hirooka Y, Matsuo I, Eshima K, Shigematsu H, Shimokawa H, Takeshita A. Overexpression of eNOS in NTS causes hypotension and bradycardia in vivo. Hypertension 2000;36:1023–1028.

66. Paton JFR, Kasparov S, Paterson DJ. Nitric oxide and autonomic control of heart rate: a question of specificity. Trends Neurosci 2002;25:626–631.

67. Lindley TE, Doobay MF, Sharma RV, Davisson RL. Superoxide is involved in the central nervous system activation and sympathoexcitation of myocardial infarction-induced heart failure. Circulation Res 2004;94:402–409.

68. Lu D, Raizada MK. Delivery of angiotensin II type 1 receptor antisense inhibits angiotensin action in neurons from hypertensive rat brain. Proc Natl Acad Sci USA 1995;92:2914–2918.

69. Kagiyama S, Qian K, Kagiyama T, Phillips MI. Antisense to epidermal growth factor receptor prevents the development of left ventricular hypertrophy. Hypertension 2003;41:824–829.

70. Shi Y. Mammalian RNAi for the masses. Trends Genet 2003;19:9–12.

71. Couzin J. Breakthrough of the year. Small RNAs make big splash. Science 2002;298:2296–2297.

72. Czauderna F, Fechtner M, Aygun H, et al. Functional studies of the PI(3)-kinase signalling pathway employing synthetic and expressed siRNA, Nucleic Acids Res 2003;31:670–682.

73. Higuchi H, Yamashita T, Yoshikawa H, Tohyama M. Functional inhibition of the p75 receptor using a small interfering RNA. Biochem Biophys Res Comm 2003;301:804–809.

74. Sorensen DR, Leirdal M, Sioud M. Gene silencing by systemic delivery of synthetic siRNAs in adult mice. J Mol Biol 2003;327:761–766.

75. Miller VM, Xia H, Marrs GL, et al. Allele-specific silencing of dominant disease genes. Proc Natl Acad Sci USA 2003;100:7195–7200.

76. Rubinson DA, Dillon CP, Kwiatkowski AV, et al. A lentivirus-based system to functionally silence genes in primary mammalian cells, stem cells and transgenic mice by RNA interference. Nat Genet 2003;33:401–406.

77. Barton GM, Medzhitov R. Retroviral delivery of small interfering RNA into primary cells. Proc Natl Acad Sci USA 2002;99:14,943–14,945.

78. Xia H, Mao Q, Paulson HL, Davidson BL. siRNA-mediated gene silencing in vitro and in vivo. Nat Biotechnol 2002;20:1006–1010.

79. Wiznerowicz M, Trono D. Conditional suppression of cellular genes: lentivirus vector-mediated drug-inducible RNA interference. J Virol 2003;77:8957–8961.

80. Casto R, Phillips MI. Angiotensin II attenuates baroreflexes at nucleus tractus solitarius of rats. Am J Physiol Regul Integr Comp Physiol 1986;250:R193–R198.

81. Casto R, Phillips MI. Baroreflex resetting by infusions of angiotensin II into the nucleus tractus solitarius. Federation Proceedings 1985;44:3645.

82. Kantor DB, Lanzrein M, Stary SJ, et al. A role for endothelial NO synthase in LTP revealed by adenovirus-mediated inhibition and rescue. Science 1996;274:1744–1748.

83. Lee CM, Robinson LJ, Michel T. Oligomerization of endothelial nitric oxide synthase. Evidence for a dominant negative effect of truncation mutants. J Biol Chem 1995;270:27,403–27,406.

84. Kasparov S, Waki H, Okwuadigbo E, Murphy D, Paton JFR. Endothelial nitric oxide synthase in the nucleus tractus solitarii (NTS) attenuates baroreflex and increases blood pressure in spontaneously hypertensive rat (SHR): evidence from in vivo gene transfer. Soc Neurosci Abst 2002;28:861.1.

85. Wong L-F, Kasparov S, Murphy D, Paton JFR. Angiotensin II-mediated signal transduction mechanisms in the nucleus of the solitary tract (NTS) that depress the baroreflex. Soc Neuroci Abst 2001;27:837.4.

86. Kasparov S, Teschemacher A, Paton JFR. Dynamic confocal imaging in acute brain slices and organotypic slice cultures using a spectral confocal microscope with single photon excitation. Exper Physiol 2002;87:715–724.

87. Kugler S, Kilic E, Bahr M. Human synapsin 1 gene promoter confers highly neuron-specific long-term transgene expression from an adenoviral vector in the adult rat brain depending on the transduced area. Gene Ther. 2003;10:337–347.

88. Stokes CEL, Murphy D, Paton JFR, KasparovS. Dynamics of a transgene expression in acute rat brain slices transfected with adenoviral vectors. Exper Physiol 2003;88:459–466.

89. Kasparov S, Paton JFR. Somatic gene transfer: implications for cardiovascular control. Exper Physiol 2000;85:747–755.

90. Aston-Jones G, Card JP. Use of pseudorabies virus to delineate multisynaptic circuits in brain: opportunities and limitations. J Neurosci Method 2000;103:51–61.

91. Loewy AD. Viruses as transneuronal tracers for defining neural circuits. Neurosci Biobehav Rev 1998;22:679–684.

92. Phillips MI, Tang Y, Schmidt-Ott K, Qian K, Kagiyama S. Vigilant vector: heart-specific promoter in an adeno-associated virus vector for cardioprotection. Hypertension 2002;39:651–655.

93. Stokes CEL, Teschemacher A, Murphy D, Paton JFR, Kasparov S. Visualisation of c-fos activation in living neurones of the paraventricular nucleus of hypothalamus using adenoviral gene transfer. FASEB J 2003;17:abstract# 564.4.

14 Vigilant Vectors

Intelligent Gene Vectors for Cardioprotection in Myocardial Ischemia

M. Ian Phillips, PhD, DSc and Yi Tang, PhD

SUMMARY

The study describes the development of a vigilant vector for protection against myocardial ischemia. The concept is a vector that can be systemically injected that waits in the heart for an ischemic attack. The vector then switches on cardioprotective genes specifically in the heart to save the cells from apoptosis and maintain cardiac performance. Using the adeno-associated virus (AAV), we have developed a double vector system (a sensor and an effector vector), that has a gene switch responsive to hypoxia, and a myosin light chain 2 ventricular (MLC-2v) promoter so that expression only occurs in the heart. The gene switch causes expression of therapeutic genes, such as heme oxygenase 1 (HO-1) and super oxide dismutase (SOD), to provide cardioprotective effects. The sensor AAV contains an oxygen-dependent domain (ODD) of hypoxia-inducible factor-1 (HIF-1α). The vector is switched on by low oxygen (<1%) and switched off by normoxia. To amplify the cardioprotective effect, an amplification system is added to the gene switch. This system consists of the yeast gene, GAL4, together with the NFκβ protein P_{65}. The MLC-2v promoter drives the expression of a fusion protein of GAL4/p65 exponentially with low oxygen. This fusion protein binds to the effector component of the amplification system in a second AAV or plasmid. The effector

From: *Contemporary Cardiology: Cardiovascular Genomics*
Edited by: M. K. Raizada, et al. © Humana Press Inc., Totowa, NJ

AAV has a GAL4 upstream sequence-binding site. Binding to this site by the fusion protein causes the expression of cardioprotective genes at a rate that increases exponentially as oxygen levels are reduced. This has been successfully tested in vitro in myocardial cells, including both embryonic prenatal and adult rat cardiomyocytes; and in vivo in mouse myocardial ischemic hearts.

Key Words: Vigilant vector; myocardial ischemia; gene switch; AAV vector; cardioprotection MLC-2v promoter.

INTRODUCTION

Vigilant vectors are intelligent in that they are designed to switch on or off *(1)*. This is an advance over current gene therapies where a gene is used to replace a mutated gene but is secreted constitutively. Many life-threatening and chronic diseases create physiological signals that could be used to switch on therapeutic genes. We are developing a gene therapy approach in which a systemically injected vigilant vector waits for these signals and switches genes on to protect specific tissues with high amplification. The concept of a vigilant vector requires four components (Fig. 1). The first component is a safe and stable vector that can be administered by systemic injection and can express transgenes in a particular organ or tissue. The adeno-associated virus (AAV) vector is safe and stable for this purpose. The second component is a reversible gene switch which acts as a biosensor that can detect certain physiological signals. We are developing a hypoxia switch, based on the oxygen-dependent degradation (ODD) domain of hypoxia-inducible factor (HIF-1α). The third component is a tissue-specific promoter, and we have used the myosin light chain-2 ventricular (MLC-2v) promoter for specific expression in the heart. The fourth component is an amplification system. For this we have developed a double-plasmid/vector system based on the yeast GAL4, and human transcriptional activator p65 to produce a transactivating fusion protein that binds to a GAL4 activation sequence in an activating plasmid that then expresses high levels of cardioprotective genes. Repeated bouts of hypoxia in coronary artery disease lead to silent or overt myocardial tissue damage *(2)*. In diabetes, the signal is high glucose; in cancer, the signals are tumor markers.

We have found that the design is not obvious. A single vector containing the gene switch promoter and transgene does not, by itself, produce enough protective genes when the gene switch is on. This may be because of interference between the switch sequences and the promoter sequences. Therefore, we have developed a double-plasmid (or vector) system to greatly amplify the transgene expression to provide the maximum protection.

To demonstrate how these components come together in an adeno-associated viral vector to make a vigilant vector, we have focused on designing the vector for use in protecting the heart during ischemia *(2,3)*. Therefore, the gene switch senses hypoxia and the promoter is specific in the heart.

VECTOR

For the vector, the recombinant adeno-associated virus (rAAV) is proving to be a stable, nonpathological vector *(4,5)*. Our data and data from other studies show that a single injection of rAAV (serotype 2) expresses transgenes in tissue for at least 6–18 mo *(5)*.

Single Vector Model

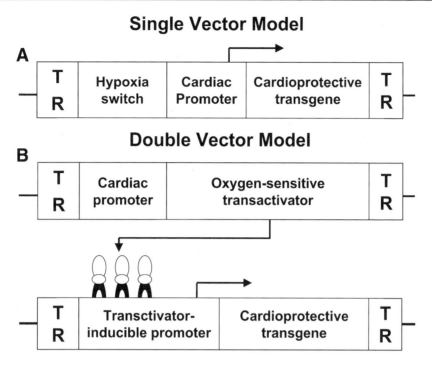

Fig. 1. Two models for the vigilant vector. (**A**) Single-vector model. Hypoxia switch, cardiac promoter, and cardioprotective transgene are adapted between the inverted terminal repeats (TR) of adeno-associated virus (AAV). (**B**) Double-vector model. In a single AAV, the cardiac promoter controls an oxygen-sensitive transactivator. The transactivator produces a fusion protein which binds to the inducible promoter and activates transcription of cardioprotective transgene in the second AAV.

GENE SWITCH

For ischemia, the gene switch for the vector has to sense hypoxia. Hypoxia triggers a multifaceted adaptive response in mammalian cells, which is primarily mediated by a family of transcription factor termed HIF-1α and its cognate DNA recognition site, known as hypoxia response element (HRE) *(6,7)*. By utilizing HIF-1α or HRE, we have studied three models of hypoxic switch (Fig. 2).

To test the ability of HRE to induce transcription under hypoxia in cardiomyocytes, we tethered HRE to the SV40 promoter or MLC-2v *(8)* promoter and put them upstream of a luciferase reporter gene (Fig. 2A).

Under normal oxygen condition, the HIF-1α is undetectable *(7)* as a result of its rapid destruction by the ubiquitin–proteosome system *(9–13)*. But during hypoxia, HIF-1α is no longer degraded, and accumulates exponentially as cellular O_2 decreases *(12)*. Within the HIF-1α, there is an ODD domain (amino acids [aa] 401–603) *(11,13,14)*. It independently controls ubiquitin–proteosome-mediated degradation of HIF-1α. The deletion of this entire region stabilized the HIF-1α. Conversely, the ODD domain alone confers oxygen-dependent instability when fused to a stable protein, Gal4. Thus, the vigilant vector contains an oxygen-sensitive chimeric transactivator (GAL4/ODD/p65), which

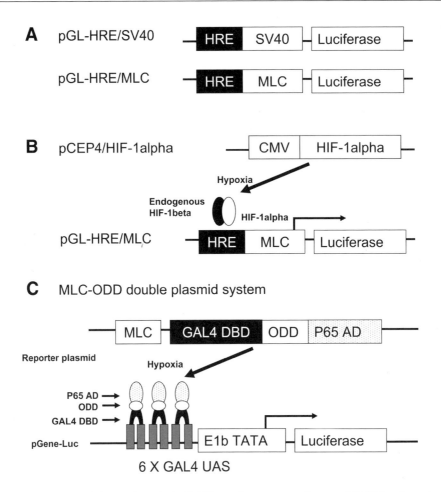

Fig. 2. Three models of a hypoxia switch. (**A**) Hypoxia-response element (HRE) has been inserted upstream of either the SV40 or the myosin light chain 2 ventricular (MLC-2v) promoter to switch on luciferase expression in response to hypoxia. (**B**) Coexpression of hypoxia-inducible factor (HIF)-1α-containing plasmid with the HRE/MLC-2v promoter. Under hypoxia, the HIF-1α subunit is stable and activated to dimerize the HIF-1β subunit. This binds to the HRE, stimulating transcription from the HRE/MLC-2v promoter. (**C**) Oxygen-sensitive chimeric transactivator (GAL4/ODD/p65), which is expressed by the transactivator plasmid under the control of the MLC-2v promoter. It can accumulate under hypoxia and activate the inducible promoter containing the GAL4 upstream activation sequence in the reporter plasmid.

was constructed by inserting ODD between the yeast GAL4 DNA-binding domain and p65 activation domain.

TISSUE SPECIFICITY

The method of using vigilant vector is to inject them systemically. Therefore, they will be ubiquitously distributed. However, by adding a tissue-specific promoter, the vector is designed to be expressed in only one tissue. To specifically express transgenes in the heart, we have used the MLC-2v promoter, which is is highly specific for the heart, during both embryonic and postnatal development (8) The MLC-2v promoter is 3.0 kb, but the proximal 250-basepair (bp) sequences, which contain the TATA box and several conserved *cis* regulatory heart factor (HF) sequences, HF-1 (HF-1a and HF-1b) *(15–17)*, HF-2 *(17,18)*, and HF-3, are sufficient to confer not only cardiac muscle specificity, but also ventricularly restricted expression *(18–22)*.

What is not obvious is that we could reduce the length of the MLC-2v to 280 bp and still produce heart specificity. We tested the specificity of a 1700-kb MLC-2v promoter in rAAV in vivo and a 280-bp MLC-2v promoter in vitro.

CARDIOPROTECTIVE GENES

There are several genes that could be considered for protection of the heart during ischemia. In previous studies, we showed that antisenses to angiotensin II type-1 receptor *(23,24)*, antisense to adrenergic β_1-receptor *(25)*, or antisense to angiotensin-converting enzyme *(26)* protect rat hearts from ischemia–reperfusion injury. Recent use has shown that heme oxygenase-1 (HO-1) is cardioprotective when delivered in a vigilant vector *(27)*. HO-1 degrades the prooxidant heme and generates carbon monoxide and antioxidant bilirubin *(28)*. Alternatively, superoxide dismutase (SOD) protects the heart against superoxide radicals generated during ischemia–reperfusion *(28,29)*. Thus, these genes are good choices for cardioprotective transgenes in the vector.

TRANSGENE AMPLIFICATION

It may seem obvious to use a single plasmid or vector containing the required elements. But, when testing a single vector with the gene switch for hypoxia and an MLC-2v promoter, we found that there was not the expected increase in transgene expression at 1% O_2. Therefore, we developed an amplification system using two plasmids (double-plasmid system) (Fig. 3)—one plasmid or vector is the sensor, the second is the effector. The sensor contains a transcriptional activator (GAL4/p65) which consists of yeast GAL4 DNA-binding domain and p65 activation domain *(30)*. When activated, the gene products form a fusion that binds to a GAL4 upstream activating sequence (UAS) inserted in the effector plasmid, and powerfully activates transgene transcription. We tested the amplification effect of this system on MLC-2v, SV40, and cytomegalovirus (CMV) promoters. In addition to amplification, this double-plasmid system provides a convenient platform for the regulation of gene expression in response to hypoxia by replacing the GAL4/p65 with a chimera containing the oxygen-sensitive gene switch ODD (Fig. 2C) or using HRE/SV40 enhancer/promoter to control GAL4/p65.

METHODS

Construction of AAV-Based Plasmids

We inserted a rat 1.7-kb MLC-2v promoter and the coding sequence of GFP between the inverted terminal repeats of AAV vector to construct pMLC-2v–GFP *(2)*.

The plasmid, gene luciferase (pGL) with HRE and simian virus (SV) 40 promoter (pGL-HRE/SV40 *[31]*), was derived from pGL-SV40 (pGL2-Promoter, Promega, Madison, WI) by insertion of a 68-bp human enolase (ENO) 1 HRE sequence (–416 to –349, GenBank accession no. X16287) into the 5′ flank of the SV40 promoter. The HRE sequence was also inserted into the 5′ flank of the MLC-2v promoter in the pGL-MLC to generate pGL-HRE/MLC *(2)*.

pCEP4 (a specific plasma mold from Invitrogen, Carlsbad, CA)/HIF-1α *(32)*, which contains human HIF-1α cDNA sequence downstream of a CMV promoter.

A   **Single Plasmid System:**

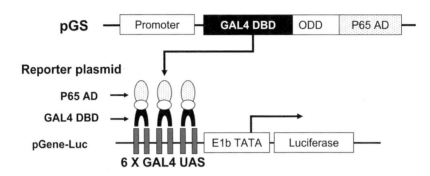

B   **Double Plasmid System:**

Fig. 3. The amplification system. **(A)** A single-plasmid system is the traditional way to express transgene, in which a promoter drives transgene (luciferase) expression directly in one plasmid. However, this does not produce enough transgene. **(B)** A double-plasmid system can amplify the power of promoter based on the strong transcription activity of GAL4/p65 fusion protein. The promoters in the transactivator plasmid gene sensor (pGS) tested included SV40, HRE/SV40, cytomegalovirus (CMV), and myosin light chain 2 ventricular (MLC-2v) promoter. The reporter plasmid contains GAL4 upstream activation sequence (UAS) in front of an adenovirus E1b TATA box and the firefly luciferase reporter gene. The fusion protein binds to the GAL4 UAS and promotes an amplified transgene expression.

We have developed the use of the ODD domain as a gene switch for hypoxia. ODD (aa 394–603) *(13)* was amplified by polymerase chain reaction (PCR) from pCEP4/HIF-1α *(31)* and inserted in-frame between the coding sequence of GAL4 DNA-binding domain and p65 activation domain (GAL4/ODD/p65) in plasmid gene sensor (pGS)-MLC to generate pGS-MLC-ODD. The key to the invention, which is not obvious, is the insertion of ODD between GAL4 and p65, which confers a powerful O_2 switch action when linked to a promoter.

Transgene Amplification Plasmids

SINGLE-PLASMID SYSTEM

The single-plasmid system is shown in Fig. 3A. Three promoters have been inserted in front of the transgene, which in this case is a luciferase reporter gene. pGL-SV40 (Promega, CA) contains SV40 promoter. Plasmid myosin light chain promoter-luciferase harbors a 281-bp (–264 to 17, GenBank accession no. U26708) fragment of MLC-2v promoter. Plasmid cytomegalovirus promoter-luciferase has CMV enhancer and promoter.

DOUBLE-PLASMID SYSTEM

To activate a highly amplified transgene expression, the double-plasmid system (Fig. 3B) is used. For the transactivator plasmid, pGS-CMV expresses a chimeric transcription factor consisting of the yeast GAL4 DNA-binding domain (aa 1–93) *(33)* and the human p65 activation domain (aa 283–551) *(34)* from nuclear factor (NF)-κB under the control of a CMV enhancer/promoter. The CMV promoter has been replaced with an SV40 promoter, HRE/SV40 enhancer/promoter, or 281-bp MLC-2v promoter to generate pGS-SV40, pGS- HRE/SV40, and pGS-MLC, respectively. For the reporter plasmid, pGene-Luc encodes luciferase driven by six copies of a 17-bp GAL4 UAS *(35)* and an adenovirus-derived E1b TATA box *(36)*. It was derived from pGene/V5-His/*lacZ* (Invitrogen, Carlsbad, CA) by replacing the *lacZ* coding sequence with a luciferase cDNA. The identity of clones was confirmed by nucleotide sequence analysis.

Testing the Plasmids In Vitro

A rat embryonic cardiac myoblast cell line, H9c2 (CRL1446; ATCC, Manassas, VA), was maintained in Dulbecco's modified Eagle's medium supplemented with sodium pyruvate and 10% fetal bovine serum. Cells were cultured under normoxic conditions (5% CO_2, 20% O_2, 75% N_2, v/v) in a humidified incubator at 37°C. For hypoxic treatment, cells were put into hypoxia chambers. The chambers were connected to a tank with premixed gas (1% O_2, 5% CO_2, and 94% N_2) at one end and to a vacuum at the other end. Hypoxia condition was achieved by evacuating and gassing the chambers for six times. Then the tightly sealed chambers were incubated at 37°C. The oxygen level in the chamber and medium is around 7.6 mmHg, which was monitored by an OxyLite probe (Oxford Optronix, Oxford, UK).

Cells were transfected at a confluence of 50–60%. Transfection was performed with LipofectAMINE (Invitrogen) according to manufacturer's protocol. pRL-CMV (Promega) or pRL-TK (Promega) coding *Renilla* luciferase was used to control transfection efficiency. Luciferase assays were performed with dual luciferase assay system (Promega). Results were quantified with a Monolight 3010 luminometer (Pharmingen, San Diego, CA) and expressed as a ratio of firefly luciferase activity over *Renilla* luciferase activity.

Intracardiac Injection

For intracardiac injection, the animal is lightly anesthetized with an inhalant, such as metofan or isoflurene, and placed on its back. The needle of the syringe is injected under the xiaphoid process, angled slightly left to enter the left-ventricular chamber. The syringe is drawn back until blood is seen and then the injectate is deposited directly into blood. The advantage of this method is that it utilizes direct injections that are rapidly distributed through the body. In our experience with this method of injection *(37)*, we have not seen any toxic response or infection.

RESULTS

Cardiac Specificity

In vivo, the pGL-MLC was specifically expressed in cardiomyocytes. After transient transfection, the luciferase expression in cardiomyocytes (H9c2) is 29.38 ± 13.11-fold higher than that in rat glioma cells (C6) *(2)* and 20.07 ± 1.71-fold higher than that in pulmonary vein endothelial cells. The transfection efficiency in three cell lines was normalized by the expression of an internal control plasmid containing ubiquitous viral promoter (CMV or thymidine kinase promoter).

In vivo, 4 wk after a systemic injection into adult mice or 5-d-old rats, the transduction of rAAV-MLC-2v-GFP was shown by PCR of DNA in many tissues, such as spleen, liver, lung, kidney, and heart. The tissue-specific expression of GFP mRNA under MLC-2v promoter was examined by reverse transcription (RT)-PCR and was detected only in heart (2). The presence of GFP protein was further examined by immunofluorescence staining, which was apparent in the heart of the treated animal and absent in the control animal (injected with saline). GFP was undetectable in the kidney and liver of the same treated animals and controls (2).

Hypoxia-Inducible Gene Switches

H9c2 cells were transfected with pGL-HRE/SV40 alone, pGL-HRE/MLC alone, or both HIF-1α and pGL-HRE/MLC and then subjected to 1% O_2 for 24 h (Fig. 4). The luciferase expression of HRE/SV40 (Fig. 4A) construct increased by 7.12 ± 1.52-fold in cells incubated under hypoxia relative to cells incubated under 20% O_2. However, pGL-HRE/MLC did not show significant hypoxic induction. In the presence of overexpressed HIF-1α, HRE/MLC showed three- to fourfold increases under hypoxia (Fig. 4B).

The MLC-ODD double-plasmid system was tested under 1% O_2 for 24 h (Fig. 5). In H9c2 cells, this system showed 5.75 ± 1.38-fold increase of expression. This system worked even better in the primary culture of adult rat cardiomyocyte, with the hypoxia induction ratio at 17.89 ± 4.85. Without ODD, GAL4/p65 fusion protein did not increase reporter expression. Therefore, the ODD was acting as a biosensor for low oxygen.

The Amplification Effect

For a strong promoter, such as CMV, the double-plasmid system could increase the power of CMV promoter up to 3.52 ± 0.33-fold over that of the single-plasmid (Fig. 5). For a relatively weak promoter, such as SV40, there was a 410.56 ± 84.42-fold increase (3). For a tissue-specific promoter, such as MLC-2v, the increase was 346.08 ± 22.50-fold without compromising cardiac specificity expression. Although by adding a higher dose of transactivator plasmid we could further increase the expression level of the MLC double-plasmid system, the tissue specificity was decreased. The double-plasmid system also effectively increased the level of HRE/SV40 promoter up to 412.79 ± 185.27-fold at 1% O_2 and 205.35 ± 65.44-fold at 20% O_2 and still maintained its hypoxic induction ability (3). The HRE/SV40 double-plasmid system started increasing expression at 4 h; this increase is reversible (Fig. 6).

Time of Onset

Although we do not know the time of onset of gene activity in vivo, we have tested time-of-onset in vitro. Careful measurements of O_2 levels in the cultures have revealed that it takes 2.6–3.8 h after O_2 has been reduced from 20 to 1% in a closed chamber to reach 1% in the culture medium. The reporter gene in vector in this cell culture system was significantly higher at 4–6 h. Therefore, subtracting the time to reach 1% in the media, the activation of the system is about 0.2–1.4 h. This indicates that using Western blotting of transgenes such as HO-1, we can detect expression within 10–30 min after ligation of the left anterior descending coronary artery in mice (27). The time for therapeutic genes to act is within this time frame, except in absolute anoxia.

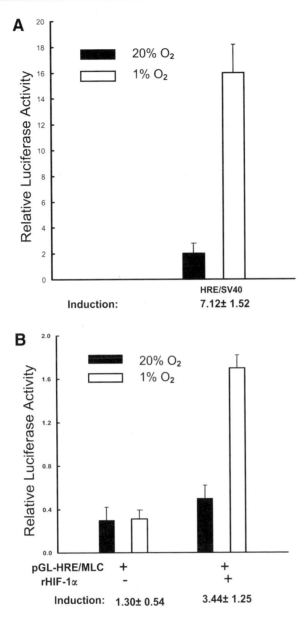

Fig. 4. The hypoxia-inducible ability of hypoxia-response element (HRE) containing gene switch. (**A**) HRE can switch SV40 promoter on in response to 1% O_2; 2 μg/well pGL-HRE/SV40 was transfected into H9c2 cells along with 100 ng/well pRL-TK control plasmid in 60-mm dishes. Duplicate plates were incubated in either 20 or 1% O_2 for 24 h before preparation of cell lysates. Results are expressed as a ratio of firefly luciferase activity over *Renilla* luciferase (relative luciferase activity). The ratio of relative luciferase activity in cells at 1% O_2 compared to 20% O_2 was also calculated to determine induction by hypoxia (mean ± standard deviation (SD) $n = 3$ independent experiments). (**B**) HRE/myosin light chain 2 ventricular (MLC-2v) enhancer/promoter alone could not augment luciferase expression under hypoxia. However, in the presence of rHIF-1α, HRE/MLC-2v could increase luciferase expression by three to fourfold in response to hypoxia. H9c2 cells were cotransfected with 2 μg/well pGL-HRE/MLC and 100 ng/well pRL-TK, in the absence or the presence of recombinant hypoxia-inducible factor (rHIF)-1α. The cells were exposed to 1 or 20% O_2 for 24 h (mean ± SD; $n = 4$ independent samples).

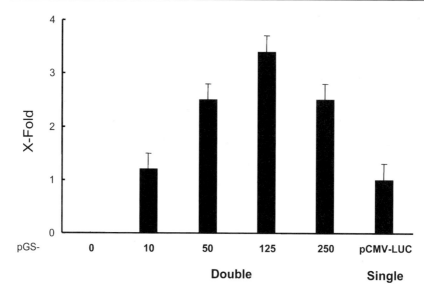

Fig. 5. The double-plasmid system amplified the power of the cytomegalovirus (CMV) promoter. For double-plasmid system transfection, H9c2 cells seeded in six-well plates received 125 ng/well control pRL-TK, 250 ng/well reporter plasmid (pGene-Luc), 0–250 ng/well transactivator plasmid (pGS-CMV), and various amounts of empty vector such that all cells received a total of 625 ng plasmid per well. The transfection of 250 ng/well pCMV-Luc served as the single plasmid system. The relative luciferase activity from double-plasmid transfection was normalized to that obtained from the single-plasmid system (X-Fold) (mean ± SD; $n = 3$ independent samples).

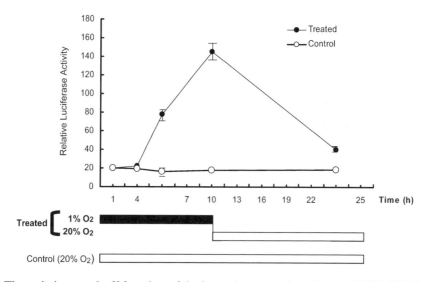

Fig. 6. The switch on-and-off function of the hypoxia-responsive element (HRE)/SV40 double-plasmid system. H9c2 cells were transfected with 10 ng/well pGS-HRE/SV40 and 2 µg/well pGene-Luc. The cells in the treated group were first exposed at 1% O_2 for 10 h and then returned to 20% O_2 for another 14 h. Thus, the luciferase expression was first increased during the hypoxic period, then dropped down after reoxygenation. The cells in the control group were continuously incubated at 20% O_2 (mean ± SD; $n = 3$–6 independent samples).

DISCUSSION

Current gene therapy strategies insert genes, but the expression of transgenes is constitutive. This produces an unphysiological expression pattern of protein production, including inappropriate downregulation of effector systems, cellular toxicity, and pathophysiology *(38,39)*. Therefore, being able to switch a vector on or off is a highly desirable aspect for gene therapy. Several inducible gene expression systems have been proposed. These systems are usually composed of two or three co-expressed vectors. One vector (in some cases there are two) expresses a chimeric transcription factor, which functions as a gene switch. This switch is regulated by the administration of a small molecule. The other vector contains reporter gene downstream of the switch-controllable promoter. The systems are as follows. (1) The *tet* on–off system, a tetracycline *(tet)*-regulated system, is either a *tet*-repressible or a tet-activating system. In the presence of the antibiotic tetracycline—a *tet*-repressor containing transactivator (tTA) does not bind to a tTA-dependent promoter, and prevents transcription. By withdrawing *tet*, the system is turned on *(40)*. In the *tet*-activating system, the transactivator contains a mutant *tet* repressor that requires doxycycline, a *tet* derivative, for specific DNA binding. Thus, the system is turned on in the presence of doxycycline and turned off without doxycycline *(41)*. (2) The ecdysone-inducible system *(42)* uses three plasmids. Two plasmids express retinoid X receptor and ecdysone receptor/VP16 fusion protein. Ecdysone binds to and activates the ecdysone receptor/VP16. The activated fusion protein and retinoid X receptor will heterodimerize and bind to ecdysone response element in the presence of muristerone A, which is a synthetic analog of ecdysone, to transactivate transcription. (3) The antiprogestin-regulated gene switch is a transactivator consisting of the truncated human progesterone receptor ligand-binding domain in the middle of the VP16 transactivation domain and the yeast GAL4 DNA-binding domain. This fusion protein activates GAL4 binding site-contained promoter in response to progesterone antagonists *(43)*, such as RU486/mifeprostone *(46)*. (4) The dimerization-based gene switch system co-expresses two fusion proteins, one consisting of FKBP and DNA-binding domain, and the other containing FRAP and the transactivation domains *(45)*. These two fusion proteins are associated by rapamycin through FKBP and FRAP. The heterodimeric protein complex activates transcription from an inducible promoter.

The weakness of all of these regulatable systems is that they need exogenous drugs as inducers. Not only does this produce unwanted side effects, but it also defeats the purpose of gene therapy, which is to be highly specific and nontoxic. For example, tetracycline deposits in bone and stains teeth *(46)*. Long-term administration may lead to bacteria resistance. RU486/mifeprostone is a progesterone antagonist *(43)*. Rapamycin has growth-inhibitory and immunosuppressive effects.

Therefore, the vigilant vector is designed to respond directly to endogenous pathophysiological signals, such as hypoxia, and to switch off when normotoxia returns without any drug being given. HRE alone as a hypoxic gene switch, fused to either a similar virus (SV40) promoter *(31,47)* or a CMV promoter *(48)*, has been reported to successfully increase the gene expression in response to hypoxia. We have obtained similar positive results when we tested HRE/SV40 promoter in cardiomyocytes *(3)*. However, under hypoxia, HRE alone was not able to upregulate transcription from a tissue-specific promoter, MLC-2v promoter *(2)*, in cardiomyocyte cultures. Overexpressed HIF-1α could help HRE to regulate the MLC-2v promoter, but the expression level was quite low. We designed the oxygen-sensitive (ODD) transactivator and put it under the control of the MLC-2v promoter. This has proven effective in both sensitivity to O_2 and heart under hypoxic conditions, such as myocardial ischemia (27).

According to the results of other groups (49) and ours, tissue-specific promoters are relatively weak compared to nonspecific promoters, such as CMV. The challenge is to increase the promoter strength without losing specificity. Several methods have been employed in the attempt to circumvent the power limitation of the MLC-2v promoter. An SV40 enhancer can increase the activity of MLC-2v promoter by at least 10-fold, but it decreases its cardiac specificity (50). Although three copies of the HF-1, HF-2, and HF-3 elements did not compromise the specificity of the MLC-2v promoter (2), there was only a threefold increase in activity. Overexpression of HF-1β leads to just a two- to threefold increase in the activity of the MLC-2v promoter (2). The double-plasmid method dramatically increased the power of the MLC-2v promoter by more than 300-fold and still maintained its specificity. This method could be applied to other tissue-specific promoters.

Our strategy needs two plasmids to cooperate, and in the context of rAAV, it will be a double-virus system. This raises the question of whether two viruses can enter the same cell. Several methods using two rAAVs to overcome its size limitation provide supporting evidence for our strategy. Relying on the intrinsic property of rAAV to undergo intermolecular concatamerization (51,52), one approach (53) has used a vector encoding multiple enhancer sequences to increase the transgene expression in a second, co-infected transgene-containing vector. The other option (54) is to split a large gene into two parts and separately package them into two individual rAAV vectors. After being co-infected into target cells, these two rAAV vectors form head-to-tail heterodimers and restore the coding sequence of the transgene after RNA splicing. Therefore, there are solutions for two rAAVs to enter the same cell and work together, should the simple empirical test of injecting two vectors at the same time prove inadequate.

The cardioprotective genes listed in the introduction protect ischemic heart through different mechanisms. We have used HO-1 for ischemia (27) but, to provide full protection, cotransfer of multiple protective genes may be necessary. For example, a rat model of Parkinson's disease coexpression of the L-dopa synthesizing enzyme, tyrosine hydroxylase, and its cofactor synthetic enzyme, GTP-cyclohydrolase-1, by rAAV provided substantial functional improvement (55). However, the effects after delivery of the tyrosine hydroxylase gene alone have been disappointing. Thus, the double virus system could be expanded to a triple (or more) virus system, with one transactivator virus expressing a strong oxygen-sensitive regulator, and several other viruses carrying different protective genes under the inducible promoter.

The concept of a vigilant vector has broad applicability. By switching the tissue-specific promoters, gene switches, and protective genes, this concept can be developed and applied generally to a number of other disease states. Among these are diabetes type 1, in which glucose would switch on preproinsulin genes, cancer where tumor markers could switch on antigrowth and antiangiogenic genes; and stroke in which hypoxia could switch on tPA. One could further imagine that a vigilant vector could lie in wait to protect against the cellular effects of biological warfare attacks, inhibiting, for example, the uptake of anthrax toxin.

REFERENCES

1. Phillips MI, Tang Y, Schmidt-Ott K, Qian K, Kagiyama S. Vigilant vector: heart-specific promoter in an adeno-associated virus vector for cardioprotection. Hypertension. 2002;39(2 Pt 2):651–655.

2. Bleske BE, Shea MJ. Current concepts of silent myocardial ischemia. Clin Pharm 1990;9:339–357.
3. Tang Y, Jackson M, Qian K, Phillips MI. Hypoxia inducible double plasmid system for myocardial ischemia gene therapy. Hypertension. 2002;39(2 Pt 2):695–698.
4. Song S, Embury J, Laipis PJ, Berns KI, Crawford JM, Flotte TR. Stable therapeutic serum levels of human alpha-1 antitrypsin (AAT) after portal vein injection of recombinant adeno-associated virus (rAAV) vectors. Gene Ther 2001;8:1299–1306.
5. Phillips MI, Mohuczy-Dominiak D, Coffey M, et al. Prolonged reduction of high blood pressure with an in vivo, nonpathogenic, adeno-associated viral vector delivery of AT1-R mRNA antisense. Hypertension 1997;29(1 Pt 2):374–380.
6. Wang GL, Semenza GL. General involvement of hypoxia-inducible factor 1 in transcriptional response to hypoxia. Proc Natl Acad Sci USA 1993;90:4304–4308.
7. Wang GL, Jiang BH, Rue EA, Semenza GL. Hypoxia-inducible factor 1 is a basic-helix-loop-helix-PAS heterodimer regulated by cellular O2 tension. Proc Natl Acad Sci USA 1995;92:5510–5514.
8. Franz WM, Breves D, Klingel K, Brem G, Hofschneider PH, Kandolf R. Heart-specific targeting of firefly luciferase by the myosin light chain-2 promoter and developmental regulation in transgenic mice. Circ Res 1993;73:629–638.
9. Kallio PJ, Wilson WJ, O'Brien S, Makino Y, Poellinger L. Regulation of the hypoxia-inducible transcription factor 1alpha by the ubiquitin-proteasome pathway. J Biol Chem 1999;274:6519–6525.
10. Salceda S, Caro J. Hypoxia-inducible factor 1alpha (HIF-1alpha) protein is rapidly degraded by the ubiquitin-proteasome system under normoxic conditions. Its stabilization by hypoxia depends on redox-induced changes. J Biol Chem 1997;272:22,642–22,647.
11. Huang LE, Gu J, Schau M, Bunn HF. Regulation of hypoxia-inducible factor 1alpha is mediated by an O2-dependent degradation domain via the ubiquitin-proteasome pathway. Proc Natl Acad Sci USA 1998;95:7987–7992.
12. Jiang BH, Semenza GL, Bauer C, Marti HH. Hypoxia-inducible factor 1 levels vary exponentially over a physiologically relevant range of O2 tension. Am J Physiol 1996;271(4 Pt 1):C1172–C1180.
13. Jaakkola P, Mole DR, Tian YM, et al. Targeting of HIF-alpha to the von Hippel-Lindau ubiquitylation complex by O2-regulated prolyl hydroxylation. Science 2001;292:468–472.
14. Ivan M, Kondo K, Yang H, et al. HIFalpha targeted for VHL-mediated destruction by proline hydroxylation: implications for O2 sensing. Science 2001;292:464–468.
15. Zhu H, Nguyen VT, Brown AB, et al. A novel, tissue-restricted zinc finger protein (HF-1b) binds to the cardiac regulatory element (HF-1b/MEF-2) in the rat myosin light-chain 2 gene. Mol Cell Biol 1993;13:4432–4444.
16. Navankasattusas S, Zhu H, Garcia AV, Evans SM, Chien KR. A ubiquitous factor (HF-1a) and a distinct muscle factor (HF-1b/MEF-2) form an E-box-independent pathway for cardiac muscle gene expression. Mol Cell Biol 1992;12:1469–1479.
17. Zhu H, Garcia AV, Ross RS, Evans SM, Chien KR. A conserved 28-base-pair element (HF-1) in the rat cardiac myosin light-chain-2 gene confers cardiac-specific and alpha-adrenergic-inducible expression in cultured neonatal rat myocardial cells. Mol Cell Biol 1991;11:2273–2281.
18. Lee KJ, Ross RS, Rockman HA, et al. Myosin light chain-2 luciferase transgenic mice reveal distinct regulatory programs for cardiac and skeletal muscle-specific expression of a single contractile protein gene. J Biol Chem 1992;267:15,875–15,885.
19. Lee KJ, Hickey R, Zhu H, Chien KR. Positive regulatory elements (HF-1a and HF-1b) and a novel negative regulatory element (HF-3) mediate ventricular muscle-specific expression of myosin light-chain 2-luciferase fusion genes in transgenic mice. Mol Cell Biol 1994;14:1220–1229.
20. Henderson SA, Spencer M, Sen A, Kumar C, Siddiqui MA, Chien KR. Structure, organization, and expression of the rat cardiac myosin light chain-2 gene. Identification of a 250-base pair fragment which confers cardiac-specific expression. J Biol Chem 1989;264:18,142–18,148.
21. Griscelli F, Gilardi-Hebenstreit P, Hanania N, et al. Heart-specific targeting of beta-galactosidase by the ventricle-specific cardiac myosin light chain 2 promoter using adenovirus vectors. Hum Gene Ther 1998;9:1919–1928.
22. Franz WM, Rothmann T, Frey N, Katus HA. Analysis of tissue-specific gene delivery by recombinant adenoviruses containing cardiac-specific promoters. Cardiovasc Res 1997;35:560–566.
23. Yang BC, Phillips MI, Ambuehl PE, Shen LP, Mehta P, Mehta JL. Increase in angiotensin II type 1 receptor expression immediately after ischemia-reperfusion in isolated rat hearts. Circulation 1997;96:922–926.
24. Yang BC, Phillips MI, Zhang YC, et al. Critical role of AT1 receptor expression after ischemia/ reperfusion in isolated rat hearts: beneficial effect of antisense oligodeoxynucleotides directed at AT1 receptor mRNA. Circ Res 1998;83:552–559.

25. Chen H, Zhang YC, Li D, et al. Protection against myocardial dysfunction induced by global ischemia-reperfusion by antisense-oligodeoxynucleotides directed at beta(1)-adrenoceptor mRNA. J Pharmacol Exp Ther 2000;294:722–727.

26. Chen H, Mohuczy D, Li D, et al. Protection against ischemia/reperfusion injury and myocardial dysfunction by antisense-oligodeoxynucleotide directed at angiotensin-converting enzyme mRNA. Gene Ther 2001;8:804–810.

27. Tang YL, Tang Y, Zhang YC, Qian K, Shen L, Phillips MI. Protection from ischemic heart injury by a vigilant heme oxygenase-1 plasmid system. Hypertension 2004;43:1–6.

28. Melo LG, Agrawal R, Zhang L, et al. Gene therapy strategy for long-term myocardial protection using adeno-associated virus-mediated delivery of heme oxygenase gene. Circulation 2002;105:602–607.

29. Chen EP, Bittner HB, Davis RD, Folz RJ, Van Trigt P. Extracellular superoxide dismutase transgene overexpression preserves postischemic myocardial function in isolated murine hearts. Circulation 1996;94(9 Suppl):II412–II417.

30. Wang Y, O'Malley BW Jr, Tsai SY, O'Malley BW. A regulatory system for use in gene transfer. Proc Natl Acad Sci USA 1994;91:8180–8184.

31. Semenza GL, Jiang BH, Leung SW, et al. Hypoxia response elements in the aldolase A, enolase 1, and lactate dehydrogenase A gene promoters contain essential binding sites for hypoxia-inducible factor 1. J Biol Chem 1996;271:32,529–32,537.

32. Jiang BH, Rue E, Wang GL, Roe R, Semenza GL. Dimerization, DNA binding, and transactivation properties of hypoxia-inducible factor 1. J Biol Chem 1996;271:17,771–17,778.

33. Keegan L, Gill G, Ptashne M. Separation of DNA binding from the transcription-activating function of a eukaryotic regulatory protein. Science 1986;231:699–704.

34. Schmitz ML, Baeuerle PA. The p65 subunit is responsible for the strong transcription activating potential of NF-kappa B. EMBO J 1991;10:3805–3817.

35. Giniger E, Varnum SM, Ptashne M. Specific DNA binding of GAL4, a positive regulatory protein of yeast. Cell 1985;40:767–774.

36. Lillie JW, Green MR. Transcription activation by the adenovirus E1a protein. Nature 1989;338:39–44.

37. Kimura B, Mohuczy D, Tang X, Phillips MI. Attenuation of hypertension and heart hypertrophy by adeno-associated virus delivering angiotensinogen antisense. Hypertension 2001;37(2 Part 2):376–380.

38. Isgaard J, Carlsson L, Isaksson OG, Jansson JO. Pulsatile intravenous growth hormone (GH) infusion to hypophysectomized rats increases insulin-like growth factor I messenger ribonucleic acid in skeletal tissues more effectively than continuous GH infusion. Endocrinology 1988;123:2605–2610.

39. Wolf E, Kahnt E, Ehrlein J, Hermanns W, Brem G, Wanke R. Effects of long-term elevated serum levels of growth hormone on life expectancy of mice: lessons from transgenic animal models. Mech Ageing Dev 1993;68:71–87.

40. Gossen M, Bujard H. Tight control of gene expression in mammalian cells by tetracycline-responsive promoters. Proc Natl Acad Sci USA 1992;89:5547–5551.

41. Gossen M, Freundlieb S, Bender G, Muller G, Hillen W, Bujard H. Transcriptional activation by tetracyclines in mammalian cells. Science 1995;268:1766–1769.

42. No D, Yao TP, Evans RM. Ecdysone-inducible gene expression in mammalian cells and transgenic mice. Proc Natl Acad Sci USA 1996;93:3346–3351.

43. Vegeto E, Allan GF, Schrader WT, Tsai MJ, McDonnell DP, O'Malley BW. The mechanism of RU486 antagonism is dependent on the conformation of the carboxy-terminal tail of the human progesterone receptor. Cell 1992;69:703–713.

44. Wang Y, DeMayo FJ, Tsai SY, O'Malley BW. Ligand-inducible and liver-specific target gene expression in transgenic mice. Nat Biotechnol 1997;15:239–243.

45. Rivera VM, Clackson T, Natesan S, et al. A humanized system for pharmacologic control of gene expression. Nat Med 1996;2:1028–1032.

46. Cohlan SQ. Tetracycline staining of teeth. Teratology 1977;15:127–129.

47. Boast K, Binley K, Iqball S, et al. Characterization of physiologically regulated vectors for the treatment of ischemic disease. Hum Gene Ther 1999;10:2197–21208.

48. Shibata T, Giaccia AJ, Brown JM. Development of a hypoxia-responsive vector for tumor-specific gene therapy. Gene Ther 2000;7:493–498.

49. Buttrick PM, Kass A, Kitsis RN, Kaplan ML, Leinwand LA. Behavior of genes directly injected into the rat heart in vivo. Circ Res 1992;70:193–198.

50. Jin Y, Pasumarthi KB, Bock ME, Chen Y, Kardami E, Cattini PA. Effect of "enhancer" sequences on ventricular myosin light chain-2 promoter activity in heart muscle and nonmuscle cells. Biochem Biophys Res Commun 1995;210:260–266.

51. Duan D, Sharma P, Yang J, et al. Circular intermediates of recombinant adeno-associated virus have defined structural characteristics responsible for long-term episomal persistence in muscle tissue. J Virol. 1998;72:8568–8577. Erratum in: J Virol 1999;73:861.
52. Yang J, Zhou W, Zhang Y, Zidon T, Ritchie T, Engelhardt JF. Concatamerization of adeno-associated virus circular genomes occurs through intermolecular recombination. J Virol 1999;73:9468–9477.
53. Duan D, Yue Y, Yan Z, Engelhardt JF. A new dual-vector approach to enhance recombinant adeno-associated virus-mediated gene expression through intermolecular cis activation. Nat Med 2000;6:595–598.
54. Sun L, Li J, Xiao X. Overcoming adeno-associated virus vector size limitation through viral DNA heterodimerization. Nat Med 2000;6:599–602.
55. Kirik D, Georgievska B, Burger C, et al. Reversal of motor impairments in parkinsonian rats by continuous intrastriatal delivery of L-dopa using rAAV-mediated gene transfer. Proc Natl Acad Sci USA 2002;99:4708–4713.

15 Gene Therapy for Cerebral Arterial Diseases

Yoshimasa Watanabe, MD
and Donald D. Heistad, MD

CONTENTS

INTRODUCTION
MINIMUM REQUIREMENTS FOR CEREBROVASCULAR GENE THERAPY
ESSENTIAL TOOLS FOR ALTERATION OF GENE EXPRESSION
ACCESS TO CEREBRAL ARTERIES
TARGETS OF CEREBROVASCULAR GENE THERAPY
SAFETY AND FUTURE DIRECTIONS OF CLINICAL APPLICATIONS
CONCLUSION
REFERENCES

SUMMARY

Although there has been steady progress towards cardiovascular gene therapy in humans, gene therapy for cerebrovascular disorders is still in its infancy. Several major steps, including gene transfer to cerebral arteries and alteration of gene expression, have been taken. There are several promising targets for cerebrovascular gene therapy, such as prevention of cerebral vasospasm after subarachnoid hemorrhage, stimulation of formation of collateral vessels to ischemic brain, and treatment of atherosclerotic lesions in carotid arteries. Some major obstacles, however, must be overcome before cerebrovascular gene therapy can be clinically used in humans. A key to cerebrovascular gene therapy is the development of safe and effective vectors for gene/nucleotide delivery. In addition, advances in understanding the biology of diseases and vectors will be of great value.

Key Words: Gene therapy; adenoviruses; cerebral arteries; carotid arteries; cerebral vasospasm; collateral circulation; carotid stenosis.

INTRODUCTION

Since the first successful experiments of in vivo gene transfer to blood vessels were reported in 1990 *(1)*, many investigators have explored gene therapy for cardiovascular diseases. Results have been reported in several clinical trials of gene therapy for cardio-

From: *Contemporary Cardiology: Cardiovascular Genomics*
Edited by: M. K. Raizada, et al. © Humana Press Inc., Totowa, NJ

vascular diseases, including coronary artery disease and limb ischemia (2–4). In relation to cerebrovascular disorders, however, no clinical trials for gene therapy have been reported yet.

Previously, we discussed the possibility of cerebrovascular gene therapy (5), and suggested several therapeutic targets including (1) prevention of cerebral vasospasm after subarachnoid hemorrhage (SAH), (2) stimulation of collateral blood flow to ischemic regions of the brain by angiogenesis, and (3) treatment of atherosclerotic lesions of extracranial cerebral arteries by inhibition of thrombosis or proliferation of lesions, stabilizing plaques, and prevention of restenosis after angioplasty. Recent studies using animal models demonstrate the feasibility of gene therapy for some of these targets. Some major obstacles, however, must be overcome before clinically applied to humans.

Here, we summarize the current status of studies aimed at cerebrovascular gene therapy, and discuss future directions and application in humans. Two different targets for cerebrovascular gene therapy are cerebral vasculatures and parenchymal cells of the brain. In this review, we focus on gene therapy targeted to cerebral arterial diseases.

MINIMUM REQUIREMENTS
FOR CEREBROVASCULAR GENE THERAPY

The essence of gene therapy is the correction of pathological molecular mechanisms of diseases by alteration of gene expression in a target organ or cells. Although there have been setbacks in establishing gene therapy in patients (6,7), potential advantages, such as specific and prolonged effects provided by the manipulation of specific genes, and utilization of gene expression mechanisms of the host, would make gene therapy an attractive alternative to pharmacological therapy.

For establishment of cerebrovascular gene therapy, there are several minimal requirements: first, efficient means for alteration of gene expression must be readily available. Second, access to cerebral arteries must be provided by devices or procedures that are applicable to patients. Third, alteration of gene expression must produce therapeutic effects with minimal effect on normal functions of cells and organs. Fourth, appropriate targets of treatment must be selected in terms of mechanisms and temporal characteristics of pathological process. In other words, mechanisms of the pathogenesis of target diseases must be known at the molecular level, and the time course of the effects of gene therapy must fit within the "therapeutic time window" of target diseases. Lastly, safety and ethical issues must be resolved before its clinical use in humans (8).

ESSENTIAL TOOLS FOR ALTERATION OF GENE EXPRESSION

Basic strategies for gene therapy consist of (1) expression of deficient genes or "reconstitution," (2) overexpression of therapeutic genes, and (3) downregulation of pathogenic gene expression. These "therapeutic" alterations of gene expression are achieved by delivery of genes or nucleotides with therapeutic potency into an organ or cells.

Vectors have generally been used for the delivery of genes or nucleotides into blood vessels (9), because uptake of "naked" DNA into the vascular wall is very limited. Replication-deficient recombinant adenoviruses are widely used for delivery of genes, both in experimental gene transfer to cerebral blood vessels and in some clinical trials of cardiovascular gene therapy (9,10). In contrast with retroviral vectors, both dividing and nondividing cells are efficiently transfected with adenoviral vectors, which is a major advantage of the vectors in transfecting quiescent vascular cells *(11)*. Adenoviral vectors, however, readily provoke the host's inflammatory and immune responses, with damage to the vascular wall and early loss of transgene expression *(12–14)*. To reduce immune responses in vascular tissue, modified second- and third-generation adenoviral vectors have been produced, but they still have substantial immunogenicity *(15,16)*.

Several studies have used adeno-associated viruses (AAVs) as an alternative for adenoviral vectors *(17,18)*. AAV vectors are characterized by low toxicity and incorporation of delivered DNA into the host's genomic DNA, resulting in longer-term expression of transgene production. The small size of transgene capacity and difficulties in large-scale production and purification, however, are limitations for use of the vectors in gene therapy *(19)*.

In terms of the safety of vectors, nonviral, cationic liposomal vectors are advantageous over viral vectors, because liposomes facilitate cellular DNA uptake with no substantial toxicity *(20,21)*. In addition, liposomal vectors are capable of carrying large-sized DNA. Liposome-mediated gene transfer has been used in vascular tissue in vivo *(9)*, although efficiency of transfection to vascular tissue is low in comparison with virally mediated gene transfer *(22,23)*.

As an alternative to gene transfer of therapeutic molecules, administration of oligodeoxyribonucleotide (ODN) has been used for downregulation of target genes in the cardiovascular system *(24)*. This method includes techniques utilizing inactivation of mRNA with antisense or ribozyme ODNs, and inhibition of mRNA expression with "decoy" ODNs that interact with transcription factors. This strategy is attractive because it can potentially alter the initial steps in the chain of pathological changes. There also may be problems, however, with low transfection efficiencies, short half-lives, and toxicity of ODNs *(24,25)*.

At present, adenovirus-mediated gene transfer appears to be the most promising method of gene therapy for cerebral arterial diseases. Development of alternative approaches may be extremely useful for safe and more effective gene therapy.

ACCESS TO CEREBRAL ARTERIES

For gene therapy, the most important characteristics of cerebral arteries that must be addressed are that the arteries supply a tissue that is very susceptible to ischemia, and that the function of specific regions within the brain is unique. Thus, it is essential to avoid ischemia, even in small regions of the brain. The first successful in vivo gene transfer to blood vessels was achieved in segments of the iliofemoral artery of pigs by intraluminal administration of a retroviral vector or liposomes containing a reporter gene, with interruption of blood flow for 30 min using a double-balloon catheter *(1)*. Even in the carotid artery of certain animals, in vivo gene transfer can be achieved by the same approach, which usually requires interruption of blood flow for 10–30 min (for examples, *see* refs. *13,23,26*). This method, however, may produce ischemic damage to the brain in humans, especially in patients who are at risk for cerebral ischemia.

Vectors or ODNs can be administered from the outside of vessels in order to circumvent the requirement for interruption of blood flow, which is usually needed for the intraluminal approach. For the intracranial circulation, transfection of vascular and perivascular cells can be achieved by injection of vectors or ODNs into cerebrospinal fluid (CSF). For example the injection of an adenoviral vector containing a reporter gene into the cisterna magna of rats effectively transfected cells in adventitia and perivascular

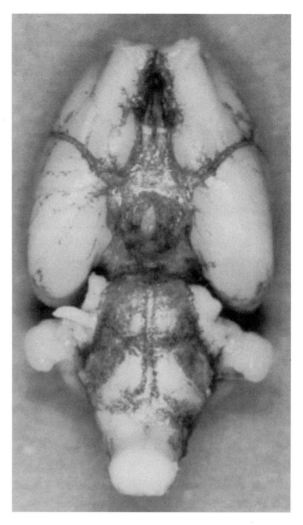

Fig. 1. Adenovirus-mediated gene transfer of bacterial β-galactosidase (βGal) to cerebral arteries. Rat brain was examined histochemically after intracisternal injection of adenovirus encoding βGal. Expression of βGal (dark staining) was seen on the ventral surface of the brain, especially along major cerebral arteries. (Reprinted with permission from ref. *27*.)

tissue surrounding cerebral arteries on the surface of the brain *(27)* (Fig. 1). Selective gene transfer to specific arteries is difficult by this method, but widespread transfection may be advantageous for treatment of some types of cerebrovascular disorders, such as cerebral vasospasm after SAH (*see* Subheading entitled "Cerebral Vasospasm After SAH"). The same technique has been applied to adenovirus-mediated gene transfer in other species including primates *(28–31)*. In several studies, ODNs were also administered via the cisterna magna, and found to be distributed in all layers of intracranial cerebral arteries *(25,32)*.

For the extracranial carotid artery, injection of vectors into the periarterial sheath can be used for perivascular gene delivery *(33)*. In addition to avoiding interruption of cerebral blood flow, there appears to be less inflammatory response in the vascular wall than with the intravascular approach *(34)*. Perivascular gene/nucleotide delivery to the carotid artery has also been demonstrated by use of the "paintbrush" technique for adenoviral vectors *(35)* or by placement of slow-releasing polymers containing ODNs or plasmid cDNAs *(36,37)*.

In addition to the perivascular approach, recent development of a new method utilizing a contrast-enhanced ultrasound technique provides intraluminal delivery of ODNs or plasmids to extracranial carotid arteries without interrupting blood flow *(38–40)*. Transfer of genes or ODNs into the vascular wall is localized within the area of insonation by this method, although the approach may produce systemic dissemination of ODNs or plasmids.

With the development of methods for gene/nucleotide delivery to cerebral arteries, functional efficacy of the methods has been tested in normal animals before being applied to disease models. For example, delivery of endothelial nitric oxide synthase (eNOS) gene into the vessel wall has been studied *(26,30,41)*. Overexpression of eNOS, in endothelium or even in adventitia, enhances agonist-induced, nitric oxide (NO)-mediated vasorelaxation.

Currently, genes or nucleotides can be delivered only to some accessible segments of cerebral arteries, as discussed earlier. Further improvements in methods for delivery to cerebral arteries that are currently not accessible will provide more effective and selective targeting of gene/nucleotide delivery. In addition, cells in different layers of the vessel wall are transfected heterogeneously. For example, medial smooth muscle cells usually are not transfected, whereas endothelium and adventitia are the primary sites of gene delivery and expression after adenovirus-mediated gene transfer *(27,33,42)*. Therapeutic effects in the medial layer of the vessel wall, however, may be obtained indirectly by alteration of production of biomolecules that are released form endothelial cells or adventitial cells.

TARGETS OF CEREBROVASCULAR GENE THERAPY

In general, difficulty in maintaining long-term effects is one of the major limitations of current gene therapy techniques, especially for the treatment of chronic diseases. Nevertheless, a transient therapeutic effect may be suitable for treatment of several cardiovascular disorders, such as prevention of restenosis after angioplasty, and therapeutic angiogenesis for ischemic tissue, as suggested previously *(10)*. In this context, chronic cerebral ischemia with poor collateral circulation and acute brain diseases or insults accompanied by functional disorders of cerebral arteries, such as cerebral vasospasm, are potential targets of gene therapy. So far, prevention of cerebral vasospasm after SAH has been a major focus of research, and therapeutic angiogenesis in the brain has recently become an additional target. Prevention of neointimal formation after endothelial injury has also been studied extensively in carotid arteries.

Cerebral Vasospasm After SAH

Cerebral vasospasm, which is a delayed and sustained constriction of cerebral arteries after SAH, is refractory to prevention by conventional methods, and may cause severe ischemic damage to the brain *(43,44)*. It is a good target for gene therapy because of the unique characteristics of the syndrome: delayed onset of vasospasm allows a period of time for transgene expression or downregulation of expression of a specific gene, and the transiency of the risk of the syndrome will not require prolonged alteration of gene expression. In addition, the perivascular approach via CSF for gene/nucleotide delivery allows alteration of gene expression in arteries over a wide area at the base of the brain, which are exposed to subarachnoid blood. This approach has been used in reported gene therapy experiments for cerebral vasospasm. For adenovirus-mediated gene transfer, the presence of subarachnoid blood does not attenuate transgene expression in cerebral vessels *(45,46)*.

Although mechanisms that lead to cerebral vasospasm are not fully understood, recent evidence suggests involvement of multiple mechanisms *(47,48)*. Several strategies of gene therapy for vasospasm, including enhancement of vasodilator mechanisms, downregulation of vasoconstrictor signaling, and modification of stress-induced cellular responses, have been tested as summarized in Table 1.

Effects of adenovirus-mediated gene transfer of eNOS have been examined in animal models of SAH. The rationale for this approach is that there is evidence for impairment of endothelium-dependent, NO-induced vasorelaxation after SAH *(49)*. In these studies, however, overexpression of eNOS in cerebral arteries generally failed to prevent vasospasm *(50,51)*, although agonist-induced, NO-mediated vasorelaxation was improved in ex vivo organ bath studies *(51)*. Because NOS activity and NO production were elevated after eNOS gene transfer *(50)*, failure to prevent vasospasm may be due to inactivation of NO by oxyhemoglobin *(47,52)* or decreased cellular levels of cyclic guanosine monophosphate (cGMP) *(53,54)*.

In contrast to the attempts to enhance NO-mediated vasorelaxation after SAH, gene transfer of calcitonin gene-related peptide (CGRP), a vasodilator neuropeptide, prevented vasospasm after SAH *(55,56)* (Fig. 2A). Gene transfer of CGRP increases the level of cAMP in the basilar artery *(28)*, and this is thought to result in activation of K^+ channels, such as adenosine triphosphate (ATP)-sensitive K^+ channels (K_{ATP} channels), producing hyperpolarization of smooth muscle membrane and relaxation of cerebral arteries *(57,58)*. This strategy has a good rationale, because the smooth muscle cell membrane is depolarized, and relaxation in response to activators of K_{ATP} channels is preserved or enhanced in cerebral arteries after experimental SAH *(59–61)*.

Several other studies have examined the effects of the downregulation of genes related to smooth muscle contraction. The potent vasoconstrictor endothelin-1 (ET-1) and mitogen-activated protein kinase (MAPK), a key intracellular signaling molecule that regulates contraction of smooth muscle in some vessels, have been implicated in the pathophysiology of cerebral vasospasm after SAH *(47,62–64)*. In order to downregulate the expression of these molecules, an antisense ODN against preproET-1 or MAPK was injected into CSF of animals with experimental SAH *(25,65,66)*. Although this approach was reported to be effective in small animals, little effect was found in larger animals, perhaps because a physical barrier of subarachnoid clot prevented ODNs from entering into cerebral arteries *(65)*.

Modification of stress-induced cellular responses by inhibition of nuclear factor (NF)κB, a key transcription factor in vascular inflammatory responses, or by overexpression of heme oxygenase-1 (HO-1), an inducible isoform of key enzymes for catabolism of heme, has been tested after SAH. The rationale is that inflammatory responses in cerebral arteries are implicated in the pathogenesis of cerebral vasospasm *(67–69)*, and induction of HO-1 is thought to be a protective mechanism in cerebral arteries after SAH *(70–72)*. Both strategies, with the administration of "decoy" ODN for NFκB into CSF or by adenoviral gene transfer of HO-1 to cerebral arteries, were effective in reducing vasospasm after experimental SAH *(32,73)*.

Table 1
Gene Therapy for Prevention of Vasospasm After Experimental Subarachnoid Hemorrhage (SAH)

Target molecules	Strategy	Gene/nucleotide delivery	Treatment protocol	Reduction of vasospasm	Animals	Refs
eNOS	Gene transfer	Adenovirus	At the time of SAH	No	Dog	50
			24 h before SAH	Yes	Dog	51
preproCGRP	Gene transfer	Adenovirus	30 min after SAH	Yes	Rabbit	55
					Dog	56
preproET-1	Antisense	ODN	30 min after SAH	Yes[a]	Dog	65
			24 h before HI	Yes[b]	Rat	25
MAPK	Antisense	ODN	At the time of SAH	Yes	Rat	66
NF-κB	Decoy	ODN	At the time of SAH	Yes	Rabbit	32
HO-1	Gene transfer	Adenovirus	At the time of SAH	Yes	Rat	73
ecSOD	Gene transfer	Adenovirus	30 min after SAH	Yes	Rabbit	78

eNOS, endothelial nitric oxide synthase; CGRP, calcitonin gene-related peptide; ET-1, endothelin-1; MAPK, mitogen-activated protein kinase; NF-κB, nuclear factor-κB; HO-1, hemeoxygenase-1; ecSOD, extracellular superoxide dismutase; ODN, oligodeoxynucleotide; HI, hemolysate injection.
[a]In combination with recombinant tissue plasminogen activator.
[b]Hemolysate-induced spasm.

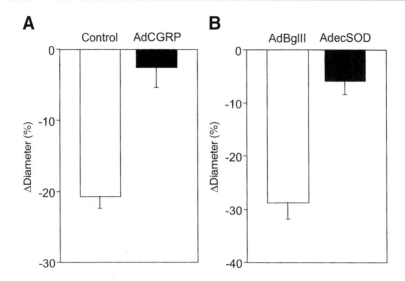

Fig. 2. Reduction of vasospasm following subarachnoid hemorrhage (SAH) after gene transfer of calcitonin gene-related peptide (CGRP) or extracellular superoxide dismutase (ecSOD) in rabbits. Adenovirus encoding preproCGRP (AdCGRP) or ecSOD (AdecSOD) was injected into the cisterna magna 30 min after intracisternal injection of autologous blood. The percentage changes in the diameter (Δdiameter) of the basilar artery were evaluated by vertebral arteriography performed before and two days after SAH. **(A)** Effects of AdCGRP. Control, animals injected with artificial cerebrospinal fluid or adenovirus encoding βGal. **(B)** Effects of AdecSOD. AdBglII, animals injected with adenovirus containing no transgene. Values are mean ± SEM.

As a means for enhancement of cellular protection, gene transfer of superoxide dismutase (SOD) has also been tested. Elevated superoxide levels in the subarachnoid space may contribute to cerebral vasospasm *(74–76)*. Superoxide impairs NO-mediated relaxation of cerebral arteries by inactivation of NO, and may trigger oxidative cell damage by production of peroxynitrite and other reactive oxygen species, such as hydroxyl radical. Gene transfer of extracellular SOD (ecSOD), an isoform of SOD that binds to extracellular matrix of vascular tissue, reduced vasospasm *(77,78)* (Fig. 2B).

Several positive results suggest that prevention of vasospasm after SAH is a promising target for clinical use of the gene therapy technique. Most studies, however, have been performed in SAH models of small animals, in which severity and temporal profile of vasospasm are different from those in humans. Thus, preclinical experiments are needed in larger animals. In addition, mechanisms of development, maintenance, and resolution of cerebral vasospasm are not fully understood yet, so there is no clear target for treatment of vasospasm at present. Further research addressing pathogenesis of vasospasm will greatly benefit the development of effective gene therapy for vasospasm after SAH.

Collateral Circulation in the Brain

Development of collateral circulation in ischemic tissue is an alternative strategy to recanalization of an occluded artery. This strategy, also referred to as "therapeutic angiogenesis," has been applied in clinical trials on the treatment of myocardial or limb ischemia by gene transfer of angiogenic growth factors, such as vascular endothelial growth factor (VEGF), hepatocyte growth factor (HGF), and basic fibroblast growth factor (bFGF) (*see* ref. *79* for review). In recent studies using a cerebral hypoperfusion model in rats, delivery of the genes for HGF or VEGF into CSF stimulated angiogenesis in the brain and increased cerebral blood flow *(80)*. Gene transfer of bFGF is also effective in inducing neovascularization in the brain of normal rats *(81)*.

Thus, therapeutic angiogenesis may be applicable to treatment of chronic cerebral ischemia/hypoperfusion produced by disease of extracranial arteries. It is not yet clear, however, whether gene therapy for angiogenesis will be useful for treatment of focal brain ischemia. Neovascularization in the ischemic limb of mice is effectively achieved by intravenous administration of bone marrow-derived endothelial progenitor cells (EPCs) transfected ex vivo with the VEGF gene *(82)*. EPC-mediated gene therapy may be applicable to focal cerebral ischemia, because EPCs contribute to neovascularization in the ischemic area of the brain after occlusion of the middle cerebral artery in mice *(83)*.

After accumulation of experience from clinical trials in peripheral circulation, several issues have been raised regarding safety of gene transfer technique for therapeutic angiogenesis *(10)*. For cerebral circulation, it is possible that vascular malformations may develop at the site of angiogenesis, and predispose to brain hemorrhage. In addition, brain edema is a possible complication after gene transfer of VEGF, which increases vascular permeability and produces edema in limbs after gene transfer. Angiogenesis induced by gene transfer of HGF, however, may not produce brain edema *(84)*.

Stenotic Lesions of the Carotid Artery

Restenosis of arteries, which is a major problem after coronary angioplasty and stenting, is a potential target for gene therapy *(85)*. For treatment of stenotic lesions of carotid arteries, carotid endarterectomy and angioplasty with stenting are now widely used. Restenosis of the carotid artery after those procedures may be an appropriate target for gene therapy, although the incidence of restenosis in the carotid artery may not be as high as in coronary and iliofemoral arteries *(86–88)*. Neointima formation after endothelial injury in the carotid arteries of small animals is widely used as an experimental model for restenosis after angioplasty, and gene therapies have been tested for inhibition of neointima formation using this model (Table 2).

The most common approach in early studies for the prevention of neointima formation was direct inhibition of smooth muscle proliferation by inducing cell-cycle arrest. Several strategies, including antisense ODN-based gene targeting of essential components or positive regulators of the cell cycle *(89–93)*, inhibition of the key transcription factor E2F by decoy ODN administration *(94)*, and gene transfer of negative regulators of the cell cycle *(95–100)* were found to be effective in reducing neointima formation of carotid arteries. Some of those approaches have been applied to patients with coronary artery disease in clinical trials *(3,101)*.

Other studies have demonstrated a reduction of neointima formation by inhibition of smooth muscle proliferation and/or migration in injured carotid arteries through several approaches, such as downregulation of expression of growth factors or a growth factor receptor by antisense strategies *(102–104)*, gene transfer of dominant negative mutants of mitogenic signaling molecules *(37,105,106)*, and applications of decoy ODNs for key transcription factors in smooth muscle proliferation *(107,108)*. Recent studies have suggested efficacy of other approaches, including facilitation of apoptosis of neointimal smooth muscle cells by changing expression of apoptotic or antiapoptotic factors *(109,110)* and inhibition of migration of medial smooth muscle cells by gene transfer of tissue inhibitors of metalloproteinase *(111,112)*.

Table 2
Gene Therapy for Carotid Stenosis After Arterial Injury

Category	Target gene/molecules	Strategy	Gene/nucleotide delivery	Refs
Cell cycle	cdc2 kinase, cdk2 kinase, PCNA, cyclin B1, c-*myb*, c-*myc*	Antisense	HVJ-L, ODN	89–93
	E2F	Decoy	HVJ-L	94
	p21CIP1, p27KIP1, GAX, GATA-6, p53, Rb protein	Gene transfer	Adenovirus	95–100
Growth factor	bFGF, TGF-β1	Antisense	Adenovirus, plasmid	102,104
Mitogenic signal	PDGFR β-chain	Antisense	ODN	103
	H-ras, MAPKK, STAT3 (dominant-negative mutants)	Gene transfer	Plasmid, adenovirus	37,105,106
	AP-1, Egr-1	Decoy	ODN	107,108
Apoptotic signal	Fas-ligand	Gene transfer	Adenovirus	109
	bcl-x$_L$	Antisense	ODN	110
Metalloproteinase inhibitor	TIMP-1, TIMP-2	Gene transfer	Adenovirus	111,112
NO-cGMP system	NOS isoforms, PKG catalytic domain	Gene transfer	HVJ-L, adenovirus	115–117,120
PGI$_2$	PGI$_2$ synthase	Gene transfer	Plasmid, HVJ-L	118,119
Antithrombotic	Hirudin, TFPI	Gene transfer	Adenovirus	121,122

PCNA, proliferative cell nuclear antigen; Rb, retinoblastoma; MAPKK, mitogen-activated protein kinase kinase; STAT, signal transducer and activator of transcription; PDGFR, platelet-derived growth factor receptor; AP-1, activator protein-1; Egr-1, early growth response factor-1; bFGF, basic fibroblast growth factor; TGF, transforming growth factor; TIMP, tissue inhibitor of matrix metalloproteinase; NOS, nitric oxide synthase; PKG, protein kinase G; PGI$_2$, prostaglandin I$_2$; TFPI, tissue factor pathway inhibitor; ODN, oligodeoxynucleotide; HVJ-L, hemagglutinating virus of Japan-liposome complex.

Facilitation of re-endothelialization is an attractive concept for treatment of injured arteries. In rabbit femoral artery, gene transfer of VEGF reduced formation of neointima and the frequency of thrombotic occlusion by accelerating re-endothelialization after endothelial injury *(113)*. Gene transfer of VEGF has been tested for prevention of coronary restenosis in patients undergoing angioplasty *(114)*. Reconstitution of production of endothelium-derived mediators with antiproliferative and antithrombotic properties, such as NO and prostaglandin I_2 (PGI_2), in the injured vessel wall is an alternative strategy to facilitation of re-endothelialization. Gene transfer of NOS isoforms *(115–117)* or PGI_2 synthase *(118)* has been reported to be effective for reducing neointima formation in injured carotid arteries. Overexpression of PGI_2 synthase also has been reported to accelerate endothelial regeneration after balloon injury *(119)*. In accordance with these studies, neointima formation was reduced by gene transfer of the catalytic domain of protein kinase G *(120)*, or antithrombotic molecules, such as hirudin or tissue factor pathway inhibitor *(121,122)*.

Thus, there are many possible choices for gene therapy for carotid restenosis. Results of most studies, however, may not be directly relevant to clinical settings, because of the challenges of intraluminal gene/nucleotide delivery with interruption of carotid blood flow. Several studies, however, suggest feasibility of the perivascular approach (for examples, *see* refs. *37,92,103*). A solution for the problem of the intraluminal approach may be provided by recent developments in catheter- or stent-based gene/nucleotide delivery systems, which may enable safe and effective intraluminal approaches for the carotid artery *(123–125)*. Again, experimental models in most studies involve small animals, and long-term outcome of the treatments is unclear because the follow-up period in most studies is only a few weeks. Preclinical studies with an experimental design that is more relevant to the clinical setting are needed.

Prevention of thrombotic events, including both acute occlusion at the lesion site and thromboembolism to distal arterial branches, is also important for patients with carotid atherosclerotic lesions, even if the lesions do not produce hemodynamically significant stenosis. For this purpose, regression or stabilization of plaques is an appropriate target for gene therapy. Several studies have demonstrated feasibility of gene therapy for atherosclerotic lesions in the aorta of mice *(126–128)*.

SAFETY AND FUTURE DIRECTIONS OF CLINICAL APPLICATIONS

After reasonably successful and promising initial steps toward the establishment of cerebrovascular gene therapy, concerns about safety have emerged as the major obstacle and urgent problem. Concerns about systemic adenoviral toxicity and insertional mutagenesis induced by a retroviral vector have been reinforced after serious adverse effects were reported in patients from clinical trials *(6,7)*. In relation to cerebrovascular gene therapy, systemic toxicity after adenovirus-mediated gene transfer is unlikely because administration of adenoviruses is local. Similarly, because adenoviruses currently are used predominantly, insertional mutagenesis is not an issue. Inflammatory and immune responses caused by adenoviral vectors, however, are problematic even after local administration. For example, inflammatory changes in cerebral arteries after adenoviral gene transfer may exacerbate vasospasm because inflammation is an important characteristic in cerebral vessels after SAH *(67–69)*.

Intense efforts are underway to minimize adverse effects of adenoviral vectors, because adenoviral vectors are a very promising choice of vectors. A simple method is concomitant use of cationic polymer/lipids or calcium phosphate, which enhances transgene expression in cerebral arteries, and thereby allows use of lower titers of adenoviral vectors *(129,130)*. A technology for constructing a new generation of adenoviral vectors also may help to reduce adverse effects *(19)*. Helper-dependent, or "gutless" or "gutted," adenoviral vectors, which do not contain most genes encoding viral proteins, allow efficient transfection but produce less inflammatory and immune responses than other adenoviral vectors. A recent study demonstrated long-term transgene expression after systemic gene transfer with this vector in mice *(127)*, although dose-dependent acute toxicity has been reported in nonhuman primates *(131)*. A relatively minor challenge is purification, with contamination by the helper virus, which is required for production of the helper-dependent adenovirus. A great challenge, however, is large-scale production of the vector. Improvements in production of the vector may address concerns about large-scale production *(132,133)*.

Tissue-selective targeting of vectors and/or transgene expression is useful for reducing adverse effect and increasing therapeutic effect *(134,135)*. For example, over-expression of VEGF gene can be regulated by a hypoxia-inducible enhancer *(136)*. This method may enable selective angiogenesis in ischemic tissue and prevent unwanted, excessive angiogenesis in normal tissue.

For the safe use of vectors, data regarding the pharmacokinetics of vectors in animals, and ultimately in humans, will be required *(137)*. In addition, even when a beneficial effect is anticipated, adverse effects of specific genes or nucleotides must be clarified. Because cerebrovascular gene therapy targets vascular tissue in close proximity to neurons, evaluation of changes in brain function, including the neuropsychological effects, induced by transgene products or nucleotides will be important.

CONCLUSION

Cerebrovascular gene therapy is still in its infancy, and many basic studies have yet to be performed in order to fulfill minimum requirements for its clinical use. Some aspects of the fundamental technology for gene therapy have been developed but, in working toward cerebrovascular gene therapy trials, further improvements are needed for production of safe and effective vectors. In addition, continued advances in understanding the biology of diseases and vectors will be useful *(8)*.

It is unlikely that cerebrovascular gene therapy will be used widely in patients in the near future, but we are optimistic that improvement of methods for gene therapy will ultimately result in its clinical use.

ACKNOWLEDGMENTS

Original studies by authors were supported by funds from the Veterans Administrations, NIH Grants HL16066, HL62984, NS24621, DK54759, a Carver Research Program of Excellence, the Wendy Hamilton Trust, and an award from the American Heart Association (0120641Z).

REFERENCES

1. Nabel EG, Plautz G, Nabel GJ. Site-specific gene expression in vivo by direct gene transfer into the arterial wall. Science 1990;249:1285–1288.
2. Grines CL, Watkins MW, Helmer G, et al. Angiogenic Gene Therapy (AGENT) trial in patients with stable angina pectoris. Circulation 2002;105:1291–1297.

3. Kutryk MJB, Foley DP, van den Brand M, et al. Local intracoronary administration of antisense oligo-nucleotide against c-myc for the prevention of in-stent restenosis. J Am Coll Cardiol 2002;39:281–287.

4. Rajagopalan S, Mohler ER III, Lederman RJ, et al. Regional angiogenesis with vascular endothelial growth factor in peripheral arterial disease: a phase II randomized, double-blind, controlled study of adenoviral delivery of vascular endothelial growth factor 121 in patients with disabling intermittent claudication. Circulation 2003;108:1933–1938.

5. Heistad DD, Faraci FM. Gene therapy for cerebral vascular disease. Stroke 1996;27:1688–1693.

6. Lehrman S. Virus treatment questioned after gene therapy death. Nature 1999;401:517–518.

7. Marshall E. Second child in French trial is found to have leukemia. Science 2003;299:320.

8. Khurana VG, Meyer FB. Translational paradigms in cerebrovascular gene transfer. J Cereb Blood Flow Metab 2003;23:1251–1262.

9. Smith RC, Walsh K. Local gene delivery to the vessel wall. Acta Physiol Scand 2001;173:93–102.

10. Isner JM, Vale PR, Symes JF, Losordo DW. Assessment of risks associated with cardiovascular gene therapy in human subjects. Circ Res 2001;89:389–400.

11. Chu Y, Heistad DD. Gene transfer to blood vessels using adenoviral vectors. Methods Enzymol 2002;346:263–276.

12. Newman KD, Dunn PF, Owens JW, et al. Adenovirus-mediated gene transfer into normal rabbit arteries results in prolonged vascular cell activation, inflammation, and neointimal hyperplasia. J Clin Invest 1995;96:2955–2965.

13. Vassalli G, Agah R, Qiao R, Aguilar C, Dichek DA. A mouse model of arterial gene transfer: antigen-specific immunity is a minor determinant of the early loss of adenovirus-mediated transgene expression. Circ Res 1999;85:25e–32e.

14. Channon KM, Qian H, Youngblood SA, et al. Acute host-mediated endothelial injury after adenoviral gene transfer in normal rabbit arteries: impact on transgene expression and endothelial function. Circ Res 1998;82:1253–1262.

15. Wen S, Schneider DB, Driscoll RM, Vassalli G, Sassani AB, Dichek DA. Second-generation adenoviral vectors do not prevent rapid loss of transgene expression and vector DNA from the arterial wall. Arterioscler Thromb Vasc Biol 2000;20:1452–1458.

16. Qian HS, Channon K, Neplioueva V, W et al. Improved adenoviral vector for vascular gene therapy: beneficial effects on vascular function and inflammation. Circ Res 2001;88:911–917.

17. Rolling F, Nong Z, Pisvin S, Collen D. Adeno-associated virus-mediated gene transfer into rat carotid arteries. Gene Ther 1997;4:757–761.

18. Richter M, Iwata A, Nyhuis J, et al. Adeno-associated virus vector transduction of vascular smooth muscle cells in vivo. Physiol Genomics 2000;2:117–127.

19. Kay MA, Glorioso JC, Naldini L. Viral vectors for gene therapy: the art of turning infectious agents into vehicles of therapeutics. Nat Med 2001;7:33–40.

20. Nabel GJ, Nabel EG, Yang Z, et al. Direct gene transfer with DNA-liposome complexes in mela-noma: expression, biologic activity, and lack of toxicity in humans. Proc Natl Acad Sci USA 1993;90:11,307–11,311.

21. Templeton NS, Lasic DD. New directions in liposome gene delivery. Mol Biotechnol 1999;11:175–180.

22. Laitinen M, Pakkanen T, Donetti E, et al. Gene transfer into the carotid artery using an adventitial collar: comparison of the effectiveness of the plasmid-liposome complexes, retroviruses, pseudotyped retroviruses, and adenoviruses. Hum Gene Ther 1997;8:1645–1650.

23. Lee SW, Trapnell BC, Rade JJ, Virmani R, Dichek DA. In vivo adenoviral vector-mediated gene transfer into balloon-injured rat carotid arteries. Circ Res 1993;73:797–807.

24. Morishita R, Aoki M, Kaneda Y, Ogihara T. Gene therapy in vascular medicine: recent advances and future perspectives. Pharmacol Ther 2001;91:105–114.

25. Onoda K, Ono S, Ogihara K, et al. Inhibition of vascular contraction by intracisternal administration of preproendothelin-1 mRNA antisense oligoDNA in a rat experimental vasospasm model. J Neurosurg 1996;85:846–852.

26. Channon KM, Qian H, Neplioueva V, et al. In vivo gene transfer of nitric oxide synthase enhances vasomotor function in carotid arteries from normal and cholesterol-fed rabbits. Circulation 1998;98:1905–1911.

27. Ooboshi H, Welsh MJ, Rios CD, Davidson BL, Heistad DD. Adenovirus-mediated gene transfer in vivo to cerebral blood vessels and perivascular tissue. Circ Res 1995;77:7–13.

28. Toyoda K, Faraci FM, Russo AF, Davidson BL, Heistad DD. Gene transfer of calcitonin gene-related peptide to cerebral arteries. Am J Physiol 2000;278:H586–H594.

29. Christenson SD, Lake KD, Ooboshi H, Faraci FM, Davidson BL, Heistad DD. Adenovirus-mediated gene transfer in vivo to cerebral blood vessels and perivascular tissue in mice. Stroke 1998;29:1411–1416.

30. Chen AFY, Jiang S, Crotty TB, et al. Effects of in vivo adventitial expression of recombinant endothelial nitric oxide synthase gene in cerebral arteries. Proc Natl Acad Sci USA 1997;94:12,568–12,573.

31. Driesse MJ, Kros JM, Avezaat CJJ, et al. Distribution of recombinant adenovirus in the cerebrospinal fluid of nonhuman primates. Hum Gene Ther 1999;10:2347–2354.

32. Ono S, Date I, Onoda K, et al. Decoy administration of NF-κB into the subarachnoid space for cerebral angiopathy. Hum Gene Ther 1998;9:1003–1011.

33. Ríos CD, Ooboshi H, Piegors D, Davidson BL, Heistad DD. Adenovirus-mediated gene transfer to normal and atherosclerotic arteries: a novel approach. Arterioscler Thromb Vasc Biol 1995;15:2241–2245.

34. Schneider DB, Sassani AB, Vassalli G, Driscoll RM, Dichek DA. Adventitial delivery minimizes the proinflammatory effects of adenoviral vectors. J Vasc Surg 1999:543–550.

35. Khurana VG, Weiler DA, Witt TA, et al. A direct mechanical method for accurate and efficient adenoviral vector delivery to tissues. Gene Ther 2003;10:443–452.

36. Edelman ER, Simons M, Sirois MG, Rosenberg RD. *c-myc* in vasculoproliferative disease. Nature 1995;359:67–70.

37. Indolfi C, Avvedimento EV, Rapacciuolo A, et al. Inhibition of cellular *ras* prevents smooth muscle cell proliferation after vascular injury in vivo. Nat Med 1995:541–545.

38. Porter TR, Hiser WL, Kricsfeld D, et al. Inhibition of carotid artery neointimal formation with intravenous microbubbles. Ultrasound Med Biol 2001;27:259–265.

39. Taniyama Y, Tachibana K, Hiraoka K, et al. Local delivery of plasmid DNA into carotid artery using ultrasound. Circulation 2002;105:1233–1239.

40. Huber PE, Mann MJ, Melo LG, et al. Focused ultrasound (HIFU) induces localized enhancement of reporter gene expression in rabbit carotid artery. Gene Ther 2003;10:1600–1607.

41. Kullo IJ, Mozes G, Schwartz RS, et al. Adventitial gene transfer of recombinant endothelial nitric oxide synthase to rabbit carotid arteries alters vascular reactivity. Circulation 1997;96:2254–2261.

42. Schulick AH, Dong G, Newman KD, Virmani R, Dichek DA. Endothelium-specific in vivo gene transfer. Circ Res 1995;77:475–485.

43. Dorsch NWC. Cerebral arterial spasm—a clinical review. Br J Neurosurg 1995;9:403–412.

44. Treggiari-Venzi MM, Suter PM, Romand J. Review of medical prevention of vasospasm after aneurysmal subarachnoid hemorrhage: a problem of neurointensive care. Neurosurgery 2001;48:249–262.

45. Onoue H, Tsutsui M, Smith L, Stelter A, O'Brien T, Katusic ZS. Expression and function of recombinant endothelial nitric oxide synthase gene in canine basilar artery after experimental subarachnoid hemorrhage. Stroke 1998;29:1959–1966.

46. Muhonen MG, Ooboshi H, Welsh MJ, Davidson BL, Heistad DD. Gene transfer to cerebral blood vessels after subarachnoid hemorrhage. Stroke 1997;28:822–829.

47. Sobey CG, Faraci FM. Subarachnoid haemorrhage. What happens to the cerebral arteries? Clin Exp Pharmacol Physiol 1998;25:867–876.

48. Dietrich HH, Dacey RG Jr. Molecular keys to the problems of cerebral vasospasm. Neurosurgery 2000;46:517–530.

49. Faraci FM, Heistad DD. Regulation of the cerebral circulation: role of endothelium and potassium channels. Physiol Rev 1998;78:53–97.

50. Stoodley M, Weihl CC, Zhang Z, et al. Effect of adenovirus-mediated nitric oxide synthase gene transfer on vasospasm after experimental subarachnoid hemorrhage. Neurosurgery 2000;46:1193–1203.

51. Khurana VG, Smith LA, Baker TA, Eguchi D, O'Brien T, Katusic ZS. Protective vasomotor effects of in vivo recombinant endothelial nitric oxide synthase gene expression in a canine model of cerebral vasospasm. Stroke 2002;33:782–789.

52. Macdonald RL, Weir BKA. A review of hemoglobin and the pathogenesis of cerebral vasospasm. Stroke 1991;22:971–982.

53. Sobey CG, Heistad DD, Faraci FM. Effect of subarachnoid hemorrhage on dilatation of rat basilar artery in vivo. Am J Physiol 1996;271:H126–H132.

54. Sobey CG, Quan L. Impaired cerebral vasodilator responses to NO and PDE V inhibition after subarachnoid hemorrhage. Am J Physiol 1999;277:H1718–H1724.

55. Toyoda K, Faraci FM, Watanabe Y, et al. Gene transfer of calcitonin gene-related peptide prevents vasoconstriction after subarachnoid hemorrhage. Circ Res 2000;87:818–824.

56. Satoh M, Perkins E, Kimura H, Tang J, Chu Y, Heistad DD, Zhang JH. Posttreatment with adenovirus-mediated gene transfer of *calcitonin* gene-related peptide to reverse cerebral vasospasm in dogs. J Neurosurg 2002;97:136–142.

57. Nelson MT, Huang Y, Brayden JE, Hescheler J, Standen NB. Arterial dilations in response to calcitonin gene-related peptide involve activation of K^+ channels. Nature 1990;344:770–773.

58. Kitazono T, Heistad DD, Faraci FM. Role of ATP-sensitive K^+ channels in CGRP-induced dilatation of basilar artery in vivo. Am J Physiol 1993;265:H581–H585.

59. Harder DR, Dernbach P, Waters A. Possible cellular mechanism for cerebral vasospasm after experimental subarachnoid hemorrhage in the dog. J Clin Invest 1987;80:875–880.

60. Sobey CG, Heistad DD, Faraci FM. Effect of subarachnoid hemorrhage on cerebral vasodilatation in response to activation of ATP-sensitive K^+ channels in chronically hypertensive rats. Stroke 1997:392–397.

61. Zuccarello M, Bonasso CL, Lewis AI, Sperelakis N, Rapoport RM. Relaxation of subarachnoid hemorrhage-induced spasm of rabbit basilar artery by the K^+ channel activator cromakalim. Stroke 1996;27:311–316.

62. Zimmermann M, Seifert V. Endothelin and subarachnoid hemorrhage: an overview. Neurosurgery 1998;43:863–876.

63. Laher I, Zhang JH. Protein kinase C and cerebral vasospasm. J Cereb Blood Flow Metab 2001;21:887–906.

64. Fujikawa H, Tani E, Yamaura I, et al. Activation of protein kinases in canine basilar artery in vasospasm. J Cereb Blood Flow Metab 1999;19:44–52.

65. Ohkuma H, Parney I, Megyesi J, Ghahary A, Findlay JM. Antisense preproendothelin-oligoDNA therapy for vasospasm in a canine model of subarachnoid hemorrhage. J Neurosurg 1999;90:1105–1114.

66. Satoh M, Parent AD, Zhang JH. Inhibitory effect with antisense mitogen-activated protein kinase oligodeoxynucleotide against cerebral vasospasm in rats. Stroke 2002;33:775–781.

67. Peterson JW, Kwun B, Hackett JD, Zervas NT. The role of inflammation in experimental cerebral vasospasm. J Neurosurg 1990;72:767–774.

68. Bavbek M, Polin R, Kwan A, Arthur AS, Kassell NF, Lee KS. Monoclonal antibodies against ICAM-1 and CD18 attenuate Cerebral vasospasm after experimental subarachnoid hemorrhage in rabbits. Stroke 1998;29:1930–1936.

69. Handa Y, Kabuto M, Kobayashi H, Kawano H, Takeuchi H, Hayashi M. The correlation between immunological reaction in the arterial wall and the time course of the development of cerebral vasospasm in a primate model. Neurosurgery 1991;28:542–549.

70. Suzuki H, Kanamaru K, Tsunoda H, et al. Heme oxygenase-1 gene induction as an intrinsic regulation against delayed cerebral vasospasm in rats. J Clin Invest 1999;104:59–66.

71. Ono S, Zhang Z-D, Marton LS, et al. Heme oxygenase-1 and ferritin are increased in cerebral arteries after subarachnoid hemorrhage in monkeys. J Cereb Blood Flow Metab 2000;20:1066–1076.

72. Suzuki H, Muramatsu M, Kojima T, Taki W. Intracranial heme metabolism and cerebral vasospasm after aneurismal subarachnoid hemorrhage. Stroke 2003;34:2796–2800.

73. Ono S, Komuro T, Macdonald RL. Heme oxygenase-1 gene therapy for prevention of vasospasm in rats. J Neurosurg 2002;96:1094–1102.

74. Mori T, Nagata K, Town T, Tan J, Matsui T, Asano T. Intracisternal increase of superoxide anion production in a canine subarachnoid hemorrhage model. Stroke 2001;32:636–642.

75. Shishido T, Suzuki R, Qian L, Hirakawa K. The role of superoxide anions in the pathogenesis of cerebral vasospasm. Stroke 1994;25:864–868.

76. McGirt MJ, Parra A, Sheng H, et al. Attenuation of cerebral vasospasm after subarachnoid hemorrhage in mice overexpressing extracellular superoxide dismutase. Stroke 2002;33:2317–2323.

77. Nakane H, Chu Y, Faraci FM, Oberley LW, Heistad DD. Gene transfer of extracellular superoxide dismutase increases superoxide dismutase activity in cerebrospinal fluid. Stroke 2001;32:184–189.

78. Watanabe Y, Chu Y, Andresen JJ, Nakane H, Faraci FM, Heistad DD. Gene transfer of extracellular superoxide dismutase reduces cerebral vasospasm following subarachnoid hemorrhage. Stroke 2003;34:434–440.

79. Ylä-Herttuala S, Alitalo K. Gene transfer as a tool to induce therapeutic vascular growth. Nat Med 2003;9:694–701.

80. Yoshimura S, Morishita R, Hayashi K, et al. Gene transfer of hepatocyte growth factor to subarachnoid space in cerebral hypoperfusion model. Hypertension 2002;39:1028–1034.

81. Yukawa H, Takahashi JC, Miyatake S, et al. Adenoviral gene transfer of basic fibroblast growth factor promotes angiogenesis in rat brain. Gene Ther 2000;7:942–949.

82. Iwaguro H, Yamaguchi J, Kalka C, et al. Endothelial progenitor cell vascular endothelial growth factor gene transfer for vascular regeneration. Circulation 2002;105:732–738.

83. Hess DC, Hill WD, Martin-Studdard A, Carroll J, Brailer J, Carothers J. Bone marrow as a source of endothelial cells and NeuN-expressing cells after stroke. Stroke 2002;33:1362–1368.

84. Shimamura M, Sato N, Oshima K, et al. Novel therapeutic strategy to treat brain ischemia: overexpression of hepatocyte growth factor gene reduced ischemic injury without cerebral edema in rat model. Circulation 2004;109:424–431.

85. Kibbe MR, Billiar TR, Tzeng E. Gene therapy for restenosis. Circ Res 2000;86:829–833.

86. Strandness DE Jr. Screening for carotid disease and surveillance for carotid restenosis. Semin Vasc Surg 2001;14:200–205.

87. Chakhtoura EY, Hobson RW II, Goldstein J, et al. In-stent restenosis after carotid angioplasty-stenting: incidence and management. J Vasc Surg 2001;33:220–226.

88. Ecker RD, Pichelmann MA, Meissner I, Meyer FB. Durability of carotid endarterectomy. Stroke 2003;34:2941–2944.

89. Morishita R, Gibbons GH, Ellison KE, et al. Single intraluminal delivery of antisense cdc2 kinase and proliferating-cell nuclear antigen oligonucleotides results in chronic inhibition of neointimal hyperplasia. Proc Natl Acad Sci USA 1993;90:8474–8478.

90. Abe J, Zhou W, Taguchi J, et al. Suppression of neointimal smooth muscle cell accumulation *in vivo* by antisense cdc2 and cdk2 oligonucleotides in rat carotid artery. Biochem Biophys Res Commun 1994;198:16–24.

91. Morishita R, Gibbons GH, Kaneda Y, Ogihara T, Dzau VJ. Pharmacokinetics of antisense oligodeoxyribonucleotides (cyclin B1 and cdc 2 kinase) in the vessel wall in vivo: enhanced therapeutic utility for restenosis by HVJ-liposome delivery. Gene 1994;149:13–19.

92. Simons M, Edelman ER, DeKeyser J, Langer R, Rosenberg RD. Antisense *c-myb* oligonucleotides inhibit intimal arterial smooth muscle cell accumulation *in vivo*. Nature 1992;359:67–70.

93. Bennet MR, Anglin S, McEwan JR, Jagoe R, Newby AC, Evan GI. Inhibition of vascular smooth muscle cell proliferation in vitro and in vivo by c-myc antisense oligodeoxynucleotides. J Clin Invest 1994;93:820–828.

94. Morishita R, Gibbons GH, Horiuchi M, et al. A gene therapy strategy using a transcription factor decoy of the E2F binding site inhibits smooth muscle proliferation in vivo. Proc Natl Acad Sci USA 1995;92:5855–5859.

95. Chang MW, Barr E, Lu MM, Barton K, Leiden MJ. Adenovirus-mediated over-expression of the cyclin/cyclin-dependent kinase inhibitor, p21 inhibits vascular smooth muscle cell proliferation and neointima formation in the rat carotid artery model of balloon angioplasty. J Clin Invest 1995;96:2260–2268.

96. Chen D, Krasinski K, Chen D, et al. Down regulation of cyclin-dependent kinase 2 activity and cyclin A promoter activity in vascular smooth muscle cells by p27^{KIP1}, an inhibitor of neointima formation in the rat carotid artery. J Clin Invest 1997;99:2334–2341.

97. Yonemitsu Y, Kaneda Y, Tanaka S, et al. Transfer of wild-type p53 gene effectively inhibits vascular smooth muscle cell proliferation in vitro and in vivo. Circ Res 1998;82:147–156.

98. Smith RC, Branellec D, Gorski DH, et al. p21^{CIP1}-mediated inhibition of cell proliferation by overexpression of the gax homeodomain gene. Gene Dev 1997;11:1674–1689.

99. Mano T, Luo Z, Malendowicz SL, Evans T, Walsh K. Reversal of GATA-6 downregulation promotes smooth muscle differentiation and inhibits intimal hyperplasia in balloon-injured rat carotid artery. Circ Res 1999;84:647–654.

100. Chang MW, Eliav B, Seltzer J, et al. Cytostatic gene therapy for vascular proliferative disorders with a constitutively active form of the retinoblastoma gene product. Science 1995;267:518–522.

101. Mann MJ, Whittemore AD, Donaldson MC, et al. Ex-vivo gene therapy of human vascular bypass grafts with E2F decoy: the PREVENT single-centre, randomized, controlled trial. Lancet 1999;354:1493–1498.

102. Hanna AK, Fox JC, Neschis DG, Safford SD, Swain JL, Golden MA. Antisense basic fibroblast growth factor gene transfer reduces neointimal thickening after arterial injury. J Vasc Surg 1997;25:320–325.

103. Sirois MG, Simons M, Edelman ER. Antisense oligonucleotide inhibition of PDGFR-β receptor subunit expression directs suppression of intimal thickening. Circulation 1997;95:669–676.

104. Merrilees M, Beaumont B, Scott L, Hermanutz V, Fennessy P. Effect of TGF-β1 antisense S-oligonucleotide on synthesis and accumulation of matrix proteoglycans in balloon catheter-injured neointima of rabbit carotid arteries. J Vasc Res 2000;37:50–60.

105. Indolfi C, Avvedimento EV, Rapacciuolo A, et al. In vivo gene transfer: prevention of neointima formation by inhibition of mitogen-activated protein kinase kinase. Bas Res Cardiol 1997;92:378–384.

106. Shibata R, Kai H, Seki Y, et al. Inhibition of STAT3 prevents neointima formation by inhibiting proliferation and promoting apoptosis of neointimal smooth muscle cells. Hum Gene Ther 2003;14:601–610.

107. Kume M, Komori K, Matsumoto T, et al. Administration of a decoy against the activator protein-1 binding site suppresses neointimal thickening in rabbit balloon-injured arteries. Circulation 2002;105:1226–1232.

108. Ohtani K, Egashira K, Usui M, et al. Inhibition of neointimal hyperplasia after balloon injury by cis-element 'decoy' of early growth response gene-1 in hypercholesterolemic rabbits. Gene Ther 2004;11:126–132.

109. Sata M, Perlman H, Muruve DA, et al. Fas ligand gene transfer to the vessel wall inhibits neointima formation and overrides the adenovirus-mediated T cell response. Proc Natl Acad Sci USA 1998;95:1213–1217.

110. Pollman MJ, Hall JL, Mann MJ, Zhang L, Gibbons GH. Inhibition of neointimal cell bcl-x expression induces apoptosis and regression of vascular disease. Nat Med 1998;4:222–227.

111. Cheng L, Mantile G, Pauly R, et al. Adenovirus-mediated gene transfer of the human tissue inhibitor of metalloproteinase-2 blocks vascular smooth muscle cell invasiveness in vitro and modulates neointimal development in vivo. Circulation 1998;98:2195–2201.

112. Dollery CM, Humphries SE, McClelland A, Latchman DS, McEwan JR. Expression of tissue inhibitor of matrix metalloproteinases 1 by use of an adenoviral vector inhibits smooth muscle cell migration and reduces neointimal hyperplasia in the rat model of vascular balloon injury. Circulation 1999;99:3199–3205.

113. Asahara T, Chen D, Tsurumi Y, et al. Accelerated restitution of endothelial integrity and endothelium-dependent function after phVEGF$_{165}$ gene transfer. Circulation 1996;94:3291–3302.

114. Laitinen M, Hartikainen J, Hiltunen MO, et al. Catheter-mediated vascular endothelial growth factor gene transfer to human coronary arteries after angioplasty. Hum Gene Ther 2000;11:263–270.

115. von der Leyen HE, Gibbons GH, Morishita R, et al. Gene therapy inhibiting neointimal vascular lesion: in vivo transfer of endothelial cell nitric oxide synthase gene. Proc Natl Acad Sci USA 1995;92:1137–1141.

116. Qian H, Neplioueva V, Shetty GA, Channon KM, George SE. Nitric oxide synthase gene therapy rapidly reduces adhesion molecule expression and inflammatory cell infiltration in carotid arteries of cholesterol-fed rabbits. Circulation 1999;99:2979–2982.

117. Shears LL II, Kibbe MR, Murdock AD, et al. Efficient inhibition of intimal hyperplasia by adenovirus-mediated inducible nitric oxide synthase gene transfer to rats and pigs in vivo. J Am Coll Surg 1998;187:295–306.

118. Todaka T, Yokoyama C, Yanamoto H, et al. Gene transfer of human prostacyclin synthase prevents neointimal formation after carotid balloon injury in rats. Stroke 1999;30:419–426.

119. Numaguchi Y, Naruse K, Harada M, et al. Prostacyclin synthase gene transfer accelerates reendothelialization and inhibits neointimal formation in rat carotid arteries after balloon injury. Arterioscler Thromb Vasc Biol 1999;19:727–733.

120. Sinnaeve P, Chiche J, Gillijns H, et al. Overexpression of a constitutively active protein kinase G mutant reduces neointima formation and in-stent restenosis. Circulation 2002;105:2911–2916.

121. Rade JJ, Schulick AH, Virmani R, Dichek DA. Local adenoviral-mediated expression of recombinant hirudin reduces neointima formation after arterial injury. Nat Med 1996;2:293–298.

122. Atsuchi N, Nishida T, Marutsuka K, et al. Combination of a brief irrigation with tissue factor pathway inhibitor (TFPI) and adenovirus-mediated local TFPI gene transfer additively reduces neointima formation in balloon-injured rabbit carotid arteries. Circulation 2001;103:570–575.

123. Marshall DJ, Palasis M, Lepore JJ, Leiden JM. Biocompatibility of cardiovascular gene delivery catheters with adenovirus vectors: an important determinant of the efficiency of cardiovascular gene transfer. Mol Ther 2000;1:423–429.

124. Perlstein I, Connolly JM, Cui X, et al. DNA delivery from an intravascular stent with a denatured collagen-polylactic-polyglycolic acid-controlled release coating: mechanisms of enhanced transfection. Gene Ther 2003;10:1420–1428.

125. Takahashi A, Palmer-Opolski K, Smith RC, Walsh K. Transgene delivery of plasmid DNA to smooth muscle cells and macrophages from a biostable polymer-coated stent. Gene Ther 2003;10:1471–1478.

126. Inoue S, Egashira K, Ni W, et al. Anti-monocyte chemoattractant protein-1 gene therapy limits progression and destabilization of established atherosclerosis in apolipoprotein E-knockout mice. Circulation 2002;106:2700–2706.

127. Belalcazar LM, Merched A, Carr B, et al. Long-term stable expression of human apolipoprotein A-I mediated by helper-dependent adenovirus gene transfer inhibits atherosclerosis progression and remodels atherosclerotic plaques in a mouse model of familial hypercholesterolemia. Circulation 2003;107:2726–2732.

128. Jalkanen J, Leppänen P, Pajusola K, et al. Adeno-associated virus-mediated gene transfer of a secreted decoy human macrophage scavenger receptor reduces atherosclerotic lesion formation in LDL receptor knockout mice. Mol Ther 2003;8:903–910.

129. Toyoda K, Nakane H, Heistad DD. Cationic polymer and lipids augment adenovirus-mediated gene transfer to cerebral arteries in vivo. J Cereb Blood Flow Metab 2001;21:1125–1131.

130. Toyoda K, Andresen JJ, Zabner J, Faraci FM, Heistad DD. Calcium phosphate precipitates augment adenovirus-mediated gene transfer to blood vessels in vitro and in vivo. Gene Ther 2000;7:1284–1291.

131. Brunetti-Pierri N, Palmer DJ, Beaudet AL, Carey KD, Finegold M, Ng P. Acute toxicity after high-dose systemic injection of helper-dependent adenoviral vectors into nonhuman primates. Hum Gene Ther 2004;15:35–46.

132. Sakhuja K, Reddy PS, Ganesh S, et al. Optimization of the generation and propagation of gutless adenoviral vectors. Hum Gene Ther 2003;14:243–254.

133. Palmer D, Ng P. Improved system for helper-dependent adenoviral vector production. Mol Ther 2003;8:846–852.

134. Peng K, Russell SJ. Viral vector targeting. Curr Opin Biotechnol 1999;10:454–457.

135. Wickham TJ. Targeting adenovirus. Gene Ther 2000;7:110–114.

136. Lee M, Rentz J, Bikram M, Han S, Bull DA, Kim SW. Hypoxia-inducible VEGF gene delivery to ischemic myocardium using water-soluble lipopolymer. Gene Ther 2003;10:1535–1542.

137. Pislaru S, Janssens SP, Gersh BJ, Simari RD. Defining gene transfer before expecting gene therapy: putting the horse before the cart. Circulation 2002;106:631–636.

III | REGENERATIVE TISSUES FOR THE DISEASED CARDIOVASCULAR SYSTEM

16   Therapeutic Angiogenesis
and Vasculogenesis
for Tissue Regeneration

Paolo Madeddu, MD, FAHA

CONTENTS

INTRODUCTION
DIFFERENT MODELS OF VASCULAR GROWTH
DISEASE-RELATED IMPAIRMENT OF ANGIOGENESIS
    AND VASCULOGENESIS
THERAPEUTIC ANGIOGENESIS/VASCULOGENESIS:
    PROMISES AND LIMITATIONS
CONCLUSIONS
REFERENCES

SUMMARY

Therapeutic angiogenesis/vasculogenesis represents a new approach to treating patients with ischemic disease not curable with conventional treatment. Manipulation of the angiogenesis program and transplantation of progenitor cells is hoped to overcome endogenous liabilities that impede appropriate healing in atherosclerotic or diabetic patients. Viral vectors represent the usual means for delivering curative genes, but new nonviral methods are gaining importance for their safer profile. The number of angiogenic substances suitable for therapeutic purposes is rapidly growing, and combinatory strategies offer distinctive advantages. Combating endothelial death or interfering with vascular destabilization may prevent organ failure. Ex vivo engineered endothelial progenitor cells have been proposed for the treatment of peripheral and myocardial ischemia. The approach eliminates the drawback of immune response against viral vectors and makes repeating the therapeutic procedure in case of injury recurrence feasible. Genetic manipulation of stem cells opens new avenues for regenerative medicine.

Key Words: Angiogenesis; vasculogenesis; viral vectors; gene therapy; endothelial.

From: *Contemporary Cardiology: Cardiovascular Genomics*
Edited by: M. K. Raizada, et al. © Humana Press Inc., Totowa, NJ

INTRODUCTION

Gene therapy consists of the transfer of nucleic acid sequences to somatic cells for therapeutic purposes. The gene can be directly transferred to the host, or first delivered to cells in culture to make them capable of synthesizing transgene product. Transfected cells can then be introduced into the recipient organism, where they start releasing the therapeutic agent. One of the most promising applications of gene therapy is the promotion of vascular growth. Angiogenesis gene therapy and somatic progenitor cell transplantation have opened new therapeutic possibilities for patients with ischemic disease not curable with conventional treatment. Optimization of the two approaches is now required to increase efficacy and minimize possible side effects. In the near future, it is expected that gene therapy and stem cell transplantation will be used in combination because of the significant technical overlap and reciprocal advantages of the two strategies *(1)*.

DIFFERENT MODELS OF VASCULAR GROWTH

Angiogenesis

Postnatal neovascularization was originally considered to consist of angiogenesis, i.e., activation of preexisting endothelial cells (ECs) which proliferate, migrate, and sprout *in situ*. Angiogenic sprouting is essential for the development of several physiological and pathological settings, such as endometrial proliferation, postischemic recovery, wound healing, and cancer growth *(2)*. Angiogenesis occurs in stages: (1) vasodilatation and extravasation of plasma proteins that provide the provisional scaffold for migrating ECs; (2) interruption of EC mutual contact and detachment from basement membrane with contribution of extracellular matrix proteinases; (3) EC migration and tube formation; (4) stabilization and remodeling of newly formed vessels into three-dimensional networks; and (5) destabilization and regression of unnecessary microvessels.

Growth factors (GFs) that guide EC proliferation and migration are named direct angiogenic factors. In addition, indirect angiogenic GFs modulate the release of direct factors from cells recruited into sites of angiogenesis. Factors with potential for therapeutic angiogenesis have been classified as belonging to GF families, chemokines, transcription factors, and substances with pleiotropic activity (Table 1).

Under conditions of anemia, hypoxia-inducible transcription factor triggers a coordinated response by inducing expression of endothelial GFs *(3)*. Angiogenesis is also induced by metabolic stimuli, including hypoglycemia and acidosis.

THE VEGF FAMILY

Vascular endothelial growth factor (VEGF) represents the prototypical angiogenic factor (Fig. 1). By interacting with endothelial tyrosine kinase VEGF receptors VEGFR-1 (flt-1) and VEGFR-2 (flk-1/KDR), VEGF-A regulates the progression phase of angiogenesis and induces ECs to proliferate, migrate, and survive *(4)*. VEGF-B exists as two protein isoforms, VEGF-B$_{167}$ and VEGF-B$_{186}$, resulting from alternatively spliced mRNA. VEGF-B specifically binds to VEGFR-1. However, it also forms heterodymers with VEGF-A, a property that influences receptor specificity and final biologic effects. Recent studies indicate that VEGF-B promotes angiogenesis in association with an activation of Akt and eNOS-related pathways *(5)*. VEGF-C, with related receptors VEGFR-2 and VEGFR-3 (flt-4), represents an apparently redundant pathway for postnatal angiogenesis. VEGF-C was shown to stimulate nitric oxide (NO) release from ECs and

Table 1
Factors With Angiogenic Properties

Growth factors	Chemokines	Transcription factors	Pleiotropic substances
VEGF Family	MCP-1	HIF	Tissue kallikrein
FGF Family		EGR	PAR-activators
Angiopoietins		Prox	Thrombin
HGF, PDGF-BB		Cyr61	
IGF-1, IGF-2			Secreted frizzled-related protein
NGF			Nitric oxide

VEGF, vascular endothelial growth factor; FGF, fibroblast growth factor; HGF, hepatocyte growth factor; PDGF, platelet-derived growth factor; IGF, insuline-like growth factor; NGF, nerve growth factor; MCP-1, monocyte chemoattractant protein-1; HIF, hypoxia-inducible factor; EGR, early growth response gene; PAK, protease-activated receptor.

to induce neovascularization in a rabbit model of hind limb ischemia (6). Evidence also indicates a role for VEGF-C in pathological angiogenesis and lympho-angiogenesis (7).

THE ANGIOPOIETINS FAMILY

Angiopoietin-1 (Ang-1), which acts through the Tie-2 receptor, is essential for normal embryonic development, whereas in the adults, it decreases vascular permeability and stabilizes networks initiated by VEGF, presumably by stimulating an interaction between ECs and pericytes (Fig. 1) (8,9). Ang-2 is highly expressed at sites of normal and pathological vascular remodeling. It contributes to stabilizing the shape of native vessels, rendering a quiescent capillary responsive to VEGF-A. However, in the absence of the appropriate stimulus for vessel growth, expression of Ang-2 in endothelium is associated with vessel regression (10).

THE FGF FAMILY

Members of fibroblast growth factor (FGF) family promote the recruitment of mesenchymal cells to vessel walls, an essential mechanism for muscolarization of nascent capillaries (11,12). FGF-2 activates the extracellular signal-regulated kinase 1 and 2 (ERK 1/2) through its specific receptors. It has been implicated in protective pathways that increase cell survival, promote neovascularization, and elicit cardioprotection. However, FGFs also contribute to cancer angiogenesis.

PLEIOTROPIC AGENTS

The number of newly discovered angiogenic substances is rapidly increasing. Recently, a role for the kallikrein–kinin system in angiogenesis has been proposed by our group (Fig. 2) (13,14). Knockouts for kallikrein and kinin receptors are viable, thus suggesting that the system is not essential to embryo vasculogenesis. In adulthood, kinin B_1 receptor and tissue kallikrein gene expression is upregulated under conditions of myocardial or limb ischemia (13,15). The functional importance of these expressional changes is documented by the fact that native angiogenic response to ischemia is blunted by chronic B_1 receptor antagonism or genetic deletion of the same receptor (16). Furthermore, disruption of B_2 receptor gene results in myocardial capillary rarefaction and ischemia with aging (17).

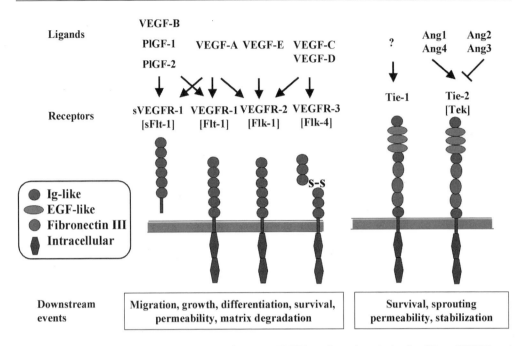

Fig. 1. The vascular endothelial growth factor (VEGF) and angiopoietin families. VEGF and angiopietins cooperate in the generation of new vessels and their rearrangement. VEGF interacts with endothelial tyrosine kinase VEGF receptors VEGFR-1 (flt-1) and VEGFR-2 (flk-1/KDR); VEGF-A regulates the progression phase of angiogenesis and induces endothelial cells to proliferate, migrate, and survive. Other isoforms of VEGF are displayed together with their receptors. A soluble form of VEGFR-1 (s-flt-1) is present in circulation and may form complexes with VEGFs, thus inhibiting their biological functions. Angiopoietins activate Tie receptors and interact with VEGF for vascular stabilization. Placental growth factor (PIGF) belongs to VEGF family and exerts its function through bimoling of VEGF-1.

Neurotrophic Control of Angiogenesis

The neurotrophin nerve growth factor (NGF), known to regulate neuronal survival and differentiation, acts as a stimulator of angiogenesis and arteriogenesis *(18)*. Thus, chemical signals derived from nerves may drive vascular growth. In addition, NGF high-affinity tyrosine kinase receptor (trkA) and low-affinity p75 receptor are present on ECs and vascular smooth muscle cells (VSMC), suggesting the existence of paracrine/autocrine loops of the polypeptide on these cells. NGF exerts direct mitogenic and prosurvival effects on ECs via trkA phosphorylation and subsequent activation of ERK1/2 and VEGF/phosphatidyl-3' kinase (PI3K)/Akt-B/NO pathways *(18)*. Instead the functions of p75 remain undefined, although recent studies support a dual role for p75 acting as co-receptor modulating NGF-mediated trkA activity, as well as promoter of signaling cascades that result in the induction of apoptosis. Thus, relative expression of NGF subtype receptors on cellular surface can provide a bifunctional switch for survival or death decisions *(19)*.

Semaphorins' Guidance of Neoangiogenesis

The motility and morphogenesis of ECs is controlled by spatio-temporally regulated activation of integrin adhesion receptors, and integrin activation is stimulated by major

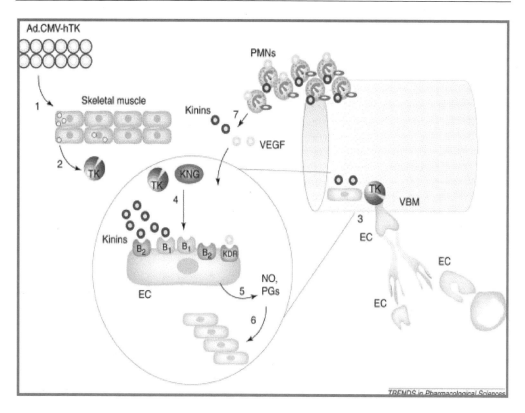

Fig. 2. Mechanisms mediating kallikrein-induced angiogenesis. Tissue kallikrein gene was delivered to skeletal muscle via a viral vector. Transduced protein is released from myocytes and generate kinins. Binding of kinins with receptors on endothelial cells stimulates nitric oxide and prostacyclin release. Kinins also stimulate the recruitment of inflammatory cells that are rich of growth factors. In addition, kallikrein induces the activation of matrix proteinases. Recent studies indicate that kallikrein acts through the intracellular kinase Akt, by a mechanism independent of vascular endothelial growth factor. PMNs, polymorphonuclear leukocytes; VEGF, vascular endothelial growth factor; KNG, kininogen; EC, endothelial cell; VBM, vinblastine, methotrexate, and bleomycin; NO, nitric oxide; PGs, prostaglandins (Adapted from ref. *19a.*)

determinants of vascular remodeling. During vascular development and experimental angiogenesis, ECs generate autocrine chemorepulsive signals of class 3 semaphorins (SEMA3 proteins) that localize at nascent adhesive sites in spreading endothelial cells. Disrupting endogenous SEMA3 function in ECs stimulates integrin-mediated adhesion and migration to extracellular matrices, whereas exogenous SEMA3 proteins antagonize integrin activation. Expression of dominant negative SEMA3 receptors in chick embryo ECs locks integrins in an active conformation, and severely impairs vascular remodeling. *Sema3a*-null mice show vascular defects as well. Thus, during angiogenesis, endothelial SEMA3 proteins endow the vascular system with the plasticity required for its reshaping by controlling integrin function *(20)*.

Vasculogenesis

It was principal merit of Asahara and Isner having documented that vasculogenesis, which is *de novo* vessel formation by bone marrow (BM)-derived endothelial progenitor cells (EPC), plays an important role in postnatal neovascularization triggered by ischemia, wounding, or cancer.

EPCs have been identified not only in bone marrow but also in peripheral blood *(21,22)*. These cells are rapidly mobilized from BM into the circulation from where they colonize ischemic areas and differentiate into mature ECs. Similarly, EPCs are mobilized in areas of vascular trauma or acute myocardial infarction *(23,24)*. The increase in circulating EPCs was positively correlated to increased plasma VEGF levels in these patients *(24)*.

MODULATORS OF VASCULOGENESIS

The molecular events regulating vasculogenesis are largely unknown. Mobilization and recruitment of such elements by VEGF is supported by several findings. VEGFR-1 and VEGFR-2 are expressed on EPCs *(25)*. Furthermore, EPCs isolated from circulation are capable of secreting VEGF in liquid culture *(26)*. After VEGF administration in mice, EPCs increase in the circulation- and display-enhanced proliferative and migratory activity *(27)*. Likewise, patients given *VEGF* gene transfer for the treatment of peripheral ischemia show a significant increase in circulating EPCs, thus suggesting that VEGF overexpression can mobilize EPCs. In addition to the direct effects on EPC mobilization, VEGF can also induce the release of hematopoietic GFs, such as granulocyte-macrophage colony-stimulating factor *(28,29)*. Modulation of EPC kinetics has been similarly observed in response to granulocyte colony-stimulating factor and stem cell factor (SCF, sKitL) *(29)*. Matrix metalloproteinase-9 appears to play an essential role for EPC recruitment from the BM, an effect that involves SCF release *(30)*.

The same factors responsible for mobilization may also be implicated in EPC migration and incorporation. For instance, increased statement of VEGF is paralleled by EPC recruitment into sites of vascular injury or exogenous VEGF delivery. In accordance, EPC homing is guided by VEGF and stromal cell-derived factor-1 (SDF-1) *(31)*. The latter binds to the chemokine receptor CXCR-4, which is highly expressed on EPCs *(32)*.

Arteriogenesis

Arteries provide the bulk flow to tissue; thus, interconnection of the arterial system is necessary to give relief to ischemic organs. The mechanisms of angiogenesis and arteriogenesis differ significantly. Arteriogenesis is driven by shear stress which stimulates EC to send chemoattractant signals to monocytes *(33)*. These cells produce GFs and proteinases, which promote VSMC proliferation. Members of FGF family and platelet-derived growth factor (PDGF)-BB are involved in arteriogenesis, whereas VEGF seems to stimulate capillary growth more efficiently. The identification of substances regulating collateralization has great relevance from a therapeutic viewpoint. Substantial differences exist regarding the rate and characteristics of microvascular growth among species. For instance, reparative angiogenesis is very fast in rats compared with mice. In the rabbit, arteriogenesis is more efficient than in mice and rats. All these differences should be taken into account when attempting to extrapolate therapeutic efficacy of an angiogenic substance from preclinical models to clinical trials.

Vascular Regression

Vessel destabilization is a natural process that intervenes to finish the angiogenic process once perfusion matches the metabolic request. In general, there is a perfect balance between the number of capillaries and cells. In skeletal and myocardial muscle this ratio is equal to 1. In addition, there is an optimal distance for oxygen and nutrient diffusion from capillary to cells. When too many vessels are generated, compensatory mechanisms intervene to switch off the angiogenic program. There are, however, different ways by which the angiogenic process is terminated. In healthy animals, neoangiogenesis generally results in a well-organized and persistent vascular network. In contrast, under conditions like diabetes, proliferating ECs are committed to premature death by apoptosis. This generates a vicious cycle that leads to persistent hypoxia, cellular death, and eventually organ failure (34,35).

Thrombospondins inhibit angiogenesis through direct effects on ECs and indirect effects on GF mobilization or activation. Ang-2 acts as a destabilizer at low levels of VEGF expression. Inhibitory PAS domain protein, C-reactive protein, chemokines binding CXCR3, VEGF soluble receptors Flt-1 and Tie-2, and proteinase products (such as fragments of kininogen and angiotensinogen) inhibit angiogenesis and contribute to vessel regression (36).

DISEASE-RELATED IMPAIRMENT OF ANGIOGENESIS AND VASCULOGENESIS

Under disease conditions, impaired neovascularization results in part from diminished vascular GF production. However, endogenous expression of cytokines is not the only factor responsible for the deficit. In fact, primary dysfunction of ECs may configure a picture that we have defined as endotheliopathy (Fig. 3) (36). For instance, diabetic or hypercholesterolemic animals—like patients affected by similar diseases—exhibit alterations in EC proliferation and viability (37,38). Excessive apoptotic endothelial and muscular cell loss progressively occurs in the hind limb of diabetic animals, and rapid acceleration intervenes at occasion of arterial obstruction (35). Although the cellular dysfunction does not necessarily preclude a favorable response to cytokine replacement therapy, the extent of hemodynamic recovery does not match that of control healthy animals; thus suggesting a limitation imposed by a diminished responsiveness of EPCs/ECs.

Aging, another condition associated to impaired neovascularization, might also lead to dysfunctional EPCs and defective vasculogenesis (39,40). Consistently, EPCs from older patients with clinical ischemia have significantly less therapeutic efficiency in rescuing ischemic hind limb of mice compared with those from younger ischemic patients (41).

Recently, Vasa et al. have evaluated EPC kinetics and their relationship to clinical disorders. They showed that the number and migratory activity of circulating EPCs inversely correlates with risk factors for coronary artery disease, such as smoking, family history, and hypertension (42). Hill et al. reached the conclusion that circulating EPCs may represent a surrogate biological marker for assessing cardiovascular risk (43). In addition, EPC and monocyte kinetics might provide indications on the therapeutic efficacy of transplantation approach (44).

THERAPEUTIC ANGIOGENESIS/VASCULOGENESIS: PROMISES AND LIMITATIONS

This novel therapeutic approach is intended to overcome the limits in GF production and endothelial cell dysfunction inherent to aging and degenerative disease.

Delivery Techniques

For angiogenesis gene therapy to be successful, a curative gene must be delivered to the right target without endangering distant tissues where angiogenesis could be delete-

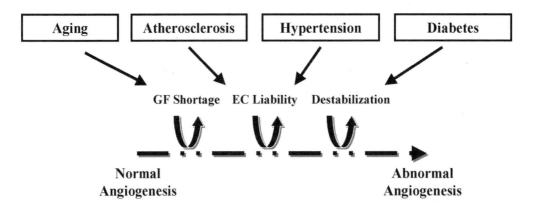

Fig. 3. Aging, atherosclerosis, hypertension, and diabetes alter the function of endothelial cells and hamper the action of growth factors. Excessive activation of apoptosis leads to progressive microvascular rarefaction in diabetic muscle and myocardium.

rious. Delivery systems are mainly based on viral and nonviral vectors. There are various barriers that impede an easy entering of exogenous genetic material into cells (Fig. 4). Genetic material has to be taken up using receptor-mediated mechanisms or endocytosis, followed by endosomal release and nuclear import. Integration into host genoma is required for persistent transgene expression.

Plasmids

Naked plasmid DNA is taken up by cells with low efficiency. However, muscle tissue represents an exception, because relatively high expression levels have been reported after plasmid injection. Carrier molecules were used to increase plasmid-based gene transfer efficiency, including liposomes or polymer complexes. Plasmids are expressed for short periods, but have the advantage of easier manufacturing and safer profile compared with viral vectors.

Adenoviral Vectors

Recombinant viruses are widely used for gene delivery. Viruses have developed efficient mechanisms to overcome the endosomal barrier. Viral protein often contains membrane-active domains mediating the delivery of viral genome to the cytoplasm after activation in the endosome.

Adenoviral vectors (AV) have been widely used for gene therapy as a result of their ability to transduce nondividing cells very efficiently. They are made replication deficient by producing point mutations, deletions, insertions, and combinations directed toward a specific AV gene or genes, such as the El gene. AV vectors can be amplified and produced in high titres (10^{11}–10^{13} virus particle/mL^{-1}) and accommodate transgene cassette up to 10 kb. Further, they allow relatively transient gene expression, a positive prerogative in reparative angiogenesis. AV are also utilized to achieve transient genetic engineering of stem cells.

Most currently used AV are based on serotype 2 and serotype 5. A high prevalence of antibodies against these serotypes is observed in humans, whereas the prevalence of antibodies against serotype 35 is low. The capsid protein is the major target for neutralizing antibodies. Immunogenicity precludes repetition of gene transfer in case of disease recurrence. Therefore, strong efforts have been made to overcome immune reactions.

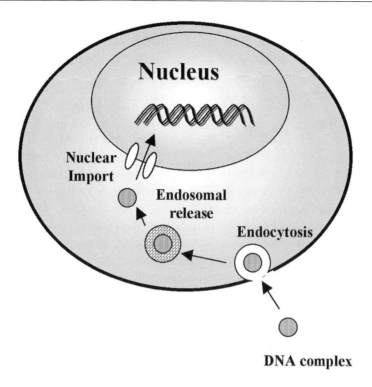

DNA complex

Fig. 4. Genetic material has to pass several obstacles before being incorporated into cells. Generally, exogenous DNA cannot enter the cell, but viruses exploit endocytosis for incorporation.

Construction of chimeric adenovirus vectors may offer definite advantages with respect to immunogenity, thereby allowing more durable transgene expression. Chimeric adenoviral vectors, Ad5/H3, generated by replacing the *Ad5* hexon gene with the hexon gene of Ad3, were not neutralized by antibodies in mice previously injected with Ad5 adenoviral vectors *(45)*.

ADENO-ASSOCIATED VIRAL VECTORS

Adeno-associated virus (AAV) is a small single-strand DNA parvovirus that is defective, nonpathogenic, and largely diffused in the general population. More than 90% of the parental viral genome is deleted in AAV-based vectors. Consequently, no viral protein is expressed from AAV vectors in transduced cells. Recent advances enhanced the production capability of high-titer stocks of AAV. Accordingly, vectors that express different genes can be mixed before transduction in order to obtain the simultaneous statement of two or more different proteins in the same tissue. AAV has been shown to infect primate hematopoietic progenitor cells with reasonable efficiency; but its use involves coinfection with a helper virus, such as adenovirus or herpes simplex virus. Use of recombinant AAV will require the development of optimized cotransfection and helper plasmid strategies for productive infection. Finally, AAV has a broad host range, but displays an exquisite tropism for nervous and muscular tissue. The efficiency of AAV transduction in skeletal and cardiac muscle cells, as well as in smooth muscle cells, is very high, and transgene statement persists for long periods of time. It is possible to insert regulatory motifs in coding sequence so as to switch off transgene expression whenever necessary. All these properties make AAV vectors valuable tools for delivery of single factors or of their combination in therapeutic angiogenesis and vasculogenesis.

RETROVIRAL VECTORS

Retroviral vectors (RV), such as the murine leukemia virus, can accept up to 8 kb of exogenous DNA, and require cell division in order to integrate in their genome. Therefore, most ex vivo retroviral gene transfer protocols include the addition of a variety of stimulatory cytokines to induce cell cycling before sequential addition of vector-containing supernatants. Vectors derived from lentivirus (LV) offer major advantages over other RV, because they do not depend on the proliferation of target cells for 'stable' transduction and induce very little immune response. These two features, together with the relative ease of production, make LV vectors an ideal tool for the design of experimental models involving gene transfer into progenitor populations. Recently, LV vectors have been used for stable expression of marker genes in hematopoietic progenitors, thus opening new perspectives to stem cell gene transfer studies. For instance, ECPs harvested from peripheral blood can be engineered to secrete proangiogenic substances and then reintroduced into the organism. However, concerns have been raised that LV-mediated transgene integration into the host genoma may induce gene mutations or unregulated transgene expression leading to generation of vascular tumours in the implantation site. Furthermore, the development of leukemia in two children several months after retroviral gene transfer for severe combined immunodeficiency and the demonstration of the causal role of insertional oncogenesis in this process has shed serious doubts on the safety of randomly integrating vectors *(46)*.

Two strategies may avoid insertional oncogenesis: (1) the development of vectors with site-specific integration; and (2) the development of episomal replicative vectors. Most currently used episomal replicative systems are based on the Epstein–Barr virus origin of replication. However, these systems require the use of a viral transactivator (Epstein–Barr nuclear antigen-1). Because the Epstein–Barr virus-based system may be associated with oncogenesis, episomal replicative systems functioning independent of a viral transactivator must be considered in the future.

NONVIRAL VECTORS

The negative side effects of viral vectors might be prevented by delivery of transgene via synthetic molecules. Cationic lipids and polycationic molecules bind to DNA by electrostatic interactions, leading to hydrophobic collapse with formation of nano-particles, which are resistant to DNase. Masking positive charges to reduce interactions with blood components and proteins can be accomplished with hydrophilic polymers, such as polyethylene glycol. Transferrin has been used for targeting specific receptors which are expressed by plasma membranes. Fab-antibodies for cell surface markers also enabled efficient gene delivery. Synthetic viral proteins have been successfully incorporated in nonviral vectors to enhance intracellular delivery of transferred DNA, including influenza-derived peptides. Nonviral vectors are nonefficient in passing nuclear membrane. Incorporation of peptides containing nuclear localization signals can help overcome this bottleneck

TRANSCRIPTION FACTORS

Engineered transcription factors present an advantage over conventional gene transfer, which relies on expression of an exogenous cDNA. Engineered factors can activate or repress endogenous genes in the appropriate dosage. Rebar et al. documented that zinc-finger transcription factor induces expression of native VEGF isoforms, apparently leading to the formation of a well organized neovascularization instrumental to wound healing (47).

Dosage Effects

At variance with traditional drugs, the effective dosage of gene therapy is hard to predict because it depends on infectivity of the viral vector, the half-life of the angiogenic molecule and its ability to diffuse to adjacent tissue, a peculiarity of those transgenes carrying a secretory signal sequence. In relation to the last assumption, it should be noted however that even angiogenic GF lacking a signal sequence might be released as a result of lysis of infected cells or by a nonclassic pathway.·

The localization of transgene product can be monitored in preclinical models of angiogenesis by different techniques, including immunohistochemistry (Fig. 5A). More problematic is tracing transgene expression in patients. In addition, a few studies have addressed the relation between infecting dosage and biological effects (Fig. 5B). We found that low-dosage gene therapy can be successfully applied to stimulate angiogenesis, thus improving the therapeutic/risk index of the strategy. In addition, incremental increases of recombinant angiogenic protein did not necessarily produce additional effects, possibly as a result of the saturation of downstream mechanisms or activation of contraregulatory factors (Fig. 6).

Biological effects of angiogenesis gene therapy are highly dependent on the modality and volume of injection. Inverse transfection efficiency relative to body weight was evidenced by cumulative observations in different species. Mice displayed 60-fold, and rats 50-fold, increased capacity to be infected as compared with pigs or humans. This is because of greater tissue diffusion of gene transfer vectors and smaller volume of rodent skeletal and myocardial muscle. Tissue damage occurs more easily during manipulation of small animals, which may further facilitate transduction efficiency.

Gene Targeting to Specific Vascular Sites

The endothelium once was considered an homogeneous inert population of elements separating circulation from surrounding tissue. Established evidence indicates instead that functional and structural diversity of ECs is the result of molecular differences among EC populations. Recently, organ-specific endothelial antigens have been characterized using in vivo phage display, a technique in which peptide libraries, expressed on the surface of bacteriophages, bind to EC surface molecules. In vivo phage display creates a map of addresses that can be used for targeting therapeutic agents to tissues affected by vascular disease or cancer. This strategy might be applied to enhance the specificity of therapeutic angiogenesis.

Angiogenesis Gene Therapy

This approach is based on the concept that supplementation with GFs would overcome the endogenous deficit of cytokines and result in more robust angiogenic response (48). Potentiation of microcirculation by therapeutic angiogenesis has been applied in models of myocardial and peripheral ischemia and subsequently exploited for the treatment of wound-healing and peripheral neuropathy. Following successful application in animal models, these concepts have been transferred from the bench to the bedside. However, the results of first controlled clinical trials using $VEGF_{165}$ or FGF-2 in patients with ischemic heart disease did not result in the level of efficacy for which researchers had hoped. A list of phase 2 and 3 clinical trials is provided in Table 2.

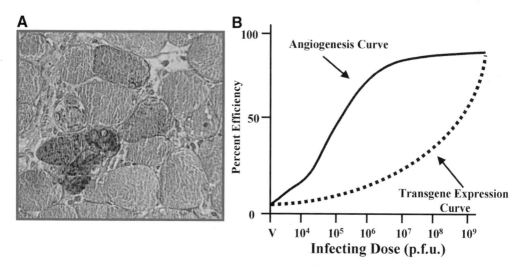

Fig. 5. Immunohistochemical localization of transgenic kallikrein in skeletal myofibers after gene delivery into mouse adductor muscle (**A**). Dosage-related effect of gene transfer on recombinant protein expression and number of newly formed vessels (**B**). The curves are markedly different, with recombinant protein increasing exponentially with infecting dosage, whereas vessel growth reaches a plateau at relatively moderate infecting dosage.

The reasons for this partial success are matter of discussion. Preclinical gene therapy protocols are generally performed in otherwise healthy animals, which hardly reflects the condition seen under pathologic conditions in humans. Furthermore, animal studies are carried out without consensus statements on surgical methods to determine ischemia. For limb ischemia, the femoral artery is dissected free from its proximal origin to the bifurcation into the saphenous and popliteal arteries, closed by electro-coagulation or silk ligatures, and excised. More drastic lesions, including femoral vein and nerve, or milder interventions have been reported. For instance, electro-coagulation of the upper part of femoral artery is recommended to avoid excessive sufferance in nonimmuno-competent or otherwise non-healing animals. It is obvious that none of these methods reflects the natural event that, in humans, leads to thrombosis and ischemia. Advanced atherosclerotic lesions can growth sufficiently large to occlude the lumen of a vessel. However, the majority of clinical syndromes, including ischemic stroke and myocardial infarction, predominantly arise from rupture or erosion of a preexisting atherosclerotic plaque and consequent thrombus formation. Furthermore, no animal model really mimics the transient ischemia that occurs in patients with angina or recurrent claudication.

In the majority of clinical trials, one angiogenic substance has been administered. Given the complexity of the angiogenesis program, it appears rather naïve thinking that administration of a single angiogenic molecule would be sufficient to generate a well-tempered and durable neovascularization. Furthermore, unregulated vascular GF overexpression leads to functionally inefficient neovascularization. To overcome the above limitations, combinatory approaches and expression-regulated gene transfer have been proposed. However, because relatively few titration studies have been performed so far, little is known regarding the appropriate dosage, the duration of treatment, and the schedule of combinations. An empirical approach ignoring these aspects is likely to produce a series of hazardous side effects in critical patients, thus raising public hostility and halting research in vascular medicine.

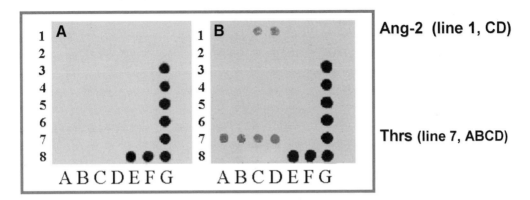

Fig. 6. Microarray of angiogenesis gene expression in muscles injected with kallikrein (**B**) or reporter gene luciferase (**A**). Angiogenesis inducer kallikrein stimulates the induction of thrombospondins which are regarded as angiogenesis terminators.

Another unsolved problem regards the phenotypic variability of different vascular beds in terms of responsiveness to angiogenic and antiapoptotic stimuli and the impact of disease states on this variability. This would imply the use of different therapeutic factors to stimulate collateral growth depending on the specific tissue (for instance, heart vs limb) and disease (for instance, atherosclerosis vs diabetic microangiopathy).

Therapeutic Vasculogenesis

Recent evidence suggests that EPCs may provide an opportunity for therapeutic interventions of regenerative medicine. Indeed, transplantation of exogenous EPCs, isolated from adult peripheral blood, cord blood, or bone marrow, has shown great promise as a potential means to combat cardiovascular disease *(49–52)*. In animal models of ischemia, transplanted EPCs augmented reparative neovascularization either through differentiation into mature ECs, or indirectly through paracrine stimulation of resident EC proliferation. Furthermore, EPCs interfere with ischemia-induced cardiomyocyte apoptosis, thus preventing inappropriate cardiac remodeling and failure *(53)*.

Preliminary evidence suggests that the strategy may have therapeutic utility for the treatment of ischemic disease in humans *(54)*. However, many issues must be settled before the EPC transplantation can be extensively and safely applied to patients, including establishing the source, optimal dosage, and cell subfraction most suitable for therapeutic purpose.

EPCs are generally enriched from circulating mononuclear cells based on adherence on fibronectin and labeling with acetylated low-density lipoprotein (LDL) and ulexlectin *(55)*. This definition is now questioned because cells that coexpress specific endothelial and stem/progenitor markers, such as CD34, VEGFR-2/KDR, AC133, and VE-cadherin, are extremely rare in peripheral blood. Accordingly, the term EPCs should be more appropriately attributed to a purified precursor cell population. Because 10% of ECs in the neovascularization are estimated to derive from differentiation of circulating EPC *(56)*, angioblasts might be more abundant in the blood than previously thought *(57)*. Accordingly, angioblast-like properties have been attributed to CD34– CD14+ cells, showing the capacity to differentiate into macrophages, dendritic cells, or ECs depending on environmental cues *(57)*. Alternatively, a small subset of circulating stem cells,

Table 2
Phase II and Phase III Angiogenesis Trials

Trial	Therapeutic agent	Disease target	Endpoint	n	Results
VIVA	Rec. VEGF prot.	CHD	ETT	178	Negative
FIRST	Rec. FGF-2 prot.	CHD	ETT	337	Negative
TRAFFIC	Rec. FGF-2 prot	PAOD	ETT	190	Positive
GM-CSF	Rec. GM-CSF prot.	CHD	Coll Flow	21	Positive
AGENT	Ad.-FGF-4	CHD	ETT	79	Positive
VEGF PVDT	Ad.-VEGF$_{165}$	PAOD	Angiogr	54	Positive
KAT	Ad.-VEGF$_{165}$	CHD	ST-segm Perfusion	103	Positive for plasmid/liposome
REVASC	Ad.-VEGF$_{121}$	CHD		67	
RAVE	Ad.-VEGF$_{121}$	PAOD			Negative

CHD, coronary heart disease; PAOD, peripheral artery occlusive disease; ETT, exercise tolerance test; GM-CSF, granulocyte-macrophage colony-stimulating factor; n, number of patients.

318

endowed of self-renewal capacity and regenerative potential, could be responsible for the high incorporation and differentiation rate.

However, shortage of EPCs in peripheral circulation, together with disease-related dysfunction, still limits extensive application of primary EPC transplant *(58)*. Another problem regards the substantial loss of functional EPCs in the first few hours after transplantation. The therapeutic implications of this phenomenon probably have been underestimated, and relevance of apoptosis in jeopardizing vasculogenesis still awaits experimental and clinical documentation.

Certain technical improvements could help to overcome the problems delineated above. They include (1) local instead of systemic delivery of EPCs, (2) chemokine supplementation to promote BM-derived EPC mobilization, (3) enrichment procedures or culture-expansion of EPCs, (4) enhancement of EPC function by gene transduction, i.e., gene-modified EPC therapy, and (5) use of selected subpopulation of EPC endowed with capacity of stimulating vasculogenesis and myogenesis *(59)*.

Gene-Modified EPC Therapy

Advances in our ability to genetically manipulate cells ex vivo has provided the technological platform to implement EPC biology and circumvent the potential hazard of direct gene transfer. Furthermore, the approach eliminates the drawback of immune response against viral vectors and makes feasible repeating the therapeutic procedure in case of injury recurrence. Another advantage is represented by the possibility of using EPCs as delivery system for curative substances to target organs. Figure 7 shows the major features of ex vivo gene therapy.

THERAPEUTIC APPLICATIONS OF TRANSDUCED EPCs

Transduction of holoclone-generating epidermal cells with RV has led to the first clinical trial of gene therapy for the genetically-determined skin disease epidermolysis bullosa *(60)*. Genetic modification of EPCs to overexpress angiogenic GFs, to enhance signaling pathways implicated in the angiogenic response, and to potentiate biological activity and viability of EPCs is still in its beginning phase, but some therapeutic results have been already reported.

Iwaguro et al. have recently shown that gene-modified EPCs can rescue impaired neovascularization in an animal model of limb ischemia *(58)*. Transplantation of heterologous EPCs transduced with adenovirus-encoding human $VEGF_{165}$ not only improved neovascularization and hemodynamic recovery, but also resulted in better clinical outcome; i.e., limb amputation was reduced by 64% as compared with controls. Notably, the approach allowed a reduction of the dose of EPCs needed to achieve limb salvage by 30 times. Thus, combining EPC cell therapy with *VEGF* gene therapy may be one option by which the limitations imposed by paucity and dysfunctional activity of EPCs may be overcome. Several important questions, however, remain unsettled. It is not clear if transplanted EPCs enhance angiogenesis, vasculogenesis, or both. In addition, Iwaguro et al. failed to define the fate and possible side effects of systemic EPC delivery, including pathological angiogenesis in tissues distant from ischemic limb. A side-by-side comparison of VEGF-transduced EPCs vs direct *VEGF* gene transfer should help to understand the relative value of the new combinatory strategy.

Loss of telomerase activity has been suggested to activate the molecular mechanisms that lead to cellular senescence. Recently, Murosawa et al. demonstrated that EPC

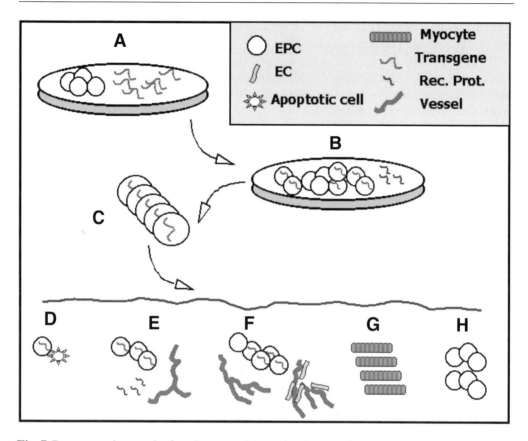

Fig. 7. Representative graph of ex vivo gene therapy for therapeutic angiogenesis/vasculogenesis. **(A)** In vitro endothelial progenitor cells (EPCs) are cultured, expanded, and infected with adenovirus or other vectors encoding angiogenic genes (red). **(B)** Infected EPCs are further expanded and tested for their ability to release recombinant protein (violet). **(C)** Transfected EPC are injected into target tissue. **(D)** Some EPCs are destroyed after transplantation. **(E)** Surviving EPCs release angiogenic recombinant protein that in turn stimulates vessel growth (angiogenesis) from resident endothelial cells (ECs). **(F)** EPCs differentiate into mature ECs and form new vessels (vasculogenesis). **(G)** EPCs differentiate in myocytes or other mesenchimal cells under the influence of environmental stimuli. **(H)** EPCs holoclones can colonize targeted tissue, thus constituting a permanent reservoir of regenerative value in case of injury recurrence.

telomerase activity can be enhanced by transfection with human telomerase reverse transcriptase *(hTERT)* gene transfer *(61)*. This resulted in improved migratory and mitogenic activity, better resistance to starvation-induced apoptosis, and augmented reparative neovascularization. The authors concluded that enhanced regenerative activity of EPCs by *hTERT* transfer may provide novel therapeutic strategy for postnatal neovascularization in severe ischemic disease patients.

Similar approaches could be used with chemokines and GFs. One possible target is the serine/threonine protein kinase Akt (also known as PKB), a key mediator of intracellular signal transduction processes. Overexpression of constitutively activated Akt mutants in many cell types promotes cellular transformation by two distinct mechanisms: (1) stimulation of proliferation under conditions in which cells should normally be growth-arrested; and (2) inhibition of apoptosis. Another interesting possibility is to use SDF-1 to augment EPC-mediated vasculogenesis. In vitro, expression of CXCR4, the receptor of

SDF-1, was reportedly detected in $66 \pm 3\%$ of EPCs after 7-d culture *(32)*. Furthermore, SDF-1 attenuates EPC apoptosis by 75%. In vivo, locally injected SDF-1 into athymic ischemic hind limb muscle of nude mice combined with human EPC transplantation increased local accumulation of fluorescence-labelled EPCs in ischemic muscle and increased capillarization and tissue perfusion recovery. It would be of paramount importance to see if SDF-1 transfection can trigger autocrine activation of EPCs and improve their viability.

Improvement of EPC engraftment could be obtained by silencing their apoptotic signaling. Techniques available to this aim include the use of antisense RNA, RNA interference and hammerhead, and hairpin RNAses.

CONCLUSIONS

Therapeutic angiogenesis/vasculogenesis represents a new approach to treat patients with ischemic disease not curable with conventional treatment. Advances in our ability to genetically manipulate cells ex vivo has provided the technological platform to implement stem cell biology and circumvent the potential hazards of direct gene transfer. Ex vivo engineered endothelial progenitor cells have shown promising therapeutic profile for treatment of ischemia and for delivery of curative substances to target organs. Thus, genetic manipulation of stem cells represent a novel option for tissue regeneration.

ACKNOWLEDGMENT

These studies were supported in part by a grant from Ministero Italiano della Salute Ricerca Finalizzata: *"Trattamento dell'ischemia miocardia e della cardiopatia ischemica mediante autotrapianto di cellule staminali toti-potenti"* (2003–2004) and a grant from Ministero Italiano della Ricerca Scientifica e dell'Università (MIUR)-FIRB Project (2003–2005).

REFERENCES

1. Nabel E. Stem cells combined with gene transfer for therapeutic vasculogenesis. Magic bullets? Circulation 2001;105:672–674.
2. Risau W. Mechanism of angiogenesis. Nature 1997;386:671–674.
3. Semenza GL. Hypoxia inducible factor 1: master regulator of O_2 homeostasis. Curr Opin Genet Dev 1999;8:588–594.
4. Ferrara N, T Devis-Smyth. The biology of vascular endothelial growth factor. Endocr Rev 1997;18:4–25.
5. Silvestre JS, Tamarat R, Ebrahimian TG, et al. Vascular endothelial growth factor-B promotes in vivo angiogenesis. Circ Res 2003;93:114–123.
6. Witzenbichler B, Asahara T, Murohara T, et al. Vascular endothelial growth factor-C (VEGF-C/VEGF-2) promotes angiogenesis in the setting of tissue ischemia. Am J Pathol 1998;153:381–394.
7. Ferrara N, Alitalo K. Clinical applications of angiogenic growth factors and their inhibitors. Nat Med 1999;5:1359–1364.
8. Suri C, McClain J, thurston G, et al. Increased vascularization in mice overexpressing angiopoietin-1. Science 1998;282:468–471.
9. Chae JK, Ki, I, Lim ST, et al. Coadministration of angiopoietin-1 and vascular endothelial growth factor enhances collateral vascularization. Arterioscler Thromb Vasc Biol 2000;20:2573–2578.
10. Maisonpierre PC, Suri C, Jones PF, et al. Angiopoietin-2, a natural antagonist for Tie2 that disrupts in vivo angiogenesis. Science 1997;277:55–60.
11. Bussolino F, Mantovani, A, Persico, G, et al. Molecular mechanisms of blood vessel formation. Trends Biochem Sci 1997;22:251–256.

12. Hanahan D. Signaling vascular morphogenesis and maintenance. Science 1997;277:48–50.
13. Emanueli C, Salis, MB, Chao, J, et al. Adenovirus-mediated human tissue kallikrein gene delivery induces angiogenesis in normoperfused skeletal muscle. Arterioscler Thromb Vasc Biol 2000;20:2379–2385.
14. Emanueli C, Minasi, A, Zacheo, A, et al. Local delivery of human tissue kallikrein gene accelerates spontaneous angiogenesis in mouse model of hindlimb ischemia. Circulation 2001;103:125-132.
15. Tschope C, Heringer-Walther, S, Koch M, et al. Upregulation of bradykinin B1-receptor expression after myocardial infarction. Br J Pharmacol 2000;129:1537–1538.
16. Emanueli C, Salis MB, Stacca, T, et al. Targeting kinin B1 receptor for therapeutic neovascularization. Circulation 2002;105:360–366.
17. Maestri R, Milia, AF, Salis, MB, et al. Cardiac hypertrophy and microvascular deficit in kinin B2 receptor knockout mice. Hypertension 2003;41:1151–1155.
18. Emanueli C, Salis, MB, Pinna, A, et al. Nerve growth factor promotes angiogenesis and arteriogenesis in ischemic hindlimbs. Circulation 2002;106:2257–2262.
19. Chao M, Casaccia-Bonnefil, P, Carter, B, et al. Neurotrophin receptors: mediators of life and death. Brain Res Rev 1998;26:295–301.
19a. Emanueli C, Madeddu P. Targeting kinin receptors for the treatment of tissue ischaemia. Trends Pharmacol Sci 2001;22:478–484.
20. Serini G, Valdembri, D, Zanivan, S, et al. Class 3 semaphorins control vascular morphogenesis by inhibiting integrin function. Nature 2003;424:391–397.
21. Asahara T, Murohara T, Sullivan, A, et al. Isolation of putative progenitor endothelial cells for angiogenesis. Science 1997;275:965–967.
22. Asahara T, Masuda, H, Takahashi, T, et al. Bone marrow origin of endothelial progenitor cells responsible for post-natal vasculogenesis in physiological and pathological neovascularization. Circ Res 1999;85:221–228.
23. Gill M, Dias, S, Hattori, K, et al. Vascular trauma induces rapid but transient mobilization of VEGFR2+AC133+ endothelial precursor cells. Circ Res 2001;88:167–174.
24. Shintani S, Murohara, T, Ikeda, H. et al. Mobilization of endothelial progenitor cells in patients with acute myocardial infarction. Circulation 2001;103:2776–2779.
25. Rafii S, Heissig, B, Hattori, K, et al. Efficient mobilization and recruitment of marrow-derived endothelial and hematopoietic stem cells by adenoviral vectors expressing angiogenic factors. Gene Ther 2002;9:631–641.
26. Pelosi E, Valtieri, M, Coppola, S, et al. Identification of the hemangioblast in postnatal life. Blood 2002;100:3203–3208.
27. Asahara T, Takahashi, T, Masuda, H, et al. VEGF contributes to postnatal neovascularization by mobilizing bone marrow-derived endothelial progenitor cells. EMBO J 1999;18:3964–3972.
28. Bautz F, Raffi, S, Kanz, L, et al. Expression and secretion of vascular endothelial growth factor-A by cytokine-stimulated hematopoietic progenitor cells: possible role in the hematopoietic microenvironment. Exp Hematol 2000;28:700–706.
29. Takahashi T, Kalka, C, Masuda, H, et al. Ischemia- and cytokine-induced mobilization of bone marrow-derived endothelial progenitor cells for neovascularization. Nat Med 1999;5:434–438.
30. Heissig B, Hattori, K, Dias, S, et al. Recruitment of stem and progenitor cells from the bone marrow niche requires MMP-9 mediated release of kit-ligand. Cell 2002;109:625–637.
31. Yamaguchi J, Kusano, KF, Masuo, O, et al. Stromal cell-derived factor-1 effects on ex vivo expanded endothelial progenitor cell recruitment for ischemic neovascularization. Circulation 2003;107: 1322–1325.
32. Mohle R, Bautz, F, Rafii, S, et al. The chemokine receptor CXCR-4 is expressed on CD34+ hematopoietic progenitors and leukemic cells and mediates transendothelial migration induced by stromal cell-derived factor-1. Blood 1998;91:4523–4530.
33. Shaper W, Scholz D. Factors regulating arteriogenesis. Arterioscler Thromb Vasc Biol 2003;23:1143–1151.
34. Emanueli C, Salis, MB, Pinna, A, et al. Prevention of diabetes-induced microangiopathy by human tissue kallikrein gene transfer. Circulation 2002;106:993–999.
35. Emanueli C, Graiani, G, Salis, MB, et al. Prophylactic gene therapy with human tissue kallikrein ameliorates limb ischemia recovery in IDDM mice. Diabetes 2004;53:1096–1103.
36. Emanueli C, Madeddu P. Angiogenesis gene therapy to rescue ischemic tissues: achievements and future directions. Br J Pharmacol 2001;133:951–958.
37. Rivard A, Silver, M, Chen, D, et al. Rescue of diabetes-related impairment of angiogenesis by intramuscular gene therapy with adeno-VEGF. Am J Pathol 1999;154:355–363.

38. Van Belle E, Rivard, A, Chen, D, et al. Hypercholesterolemia attenuates angiogenesis but does not preclude augmentation by angiogenic cytokines. Circulation 1997;96:2667–2674.
39. Rivard A, et al. Age-dependent impairment of angiogenesis. Circulation 1999;99:111–120.
40. Shimadu T, Takeshita, Y, Murohara, T, et al. Angiogenesis and vasculogenesis are impaired in the precocious-aging klotho mouse. Circulation 2004 110:1148–1155.
41. Masuda H, Asahara T. Post-natal endothelial progenitor cells for neovascularization in tissue regeneration. Cardiovasc Res 2003;93:162–169.
42. Vasa M, Fichtischerer, S, Aicher, A, et al. Number and migratory activity of circulating endothelial progenitor cells inversely correlate with risk factors for coronary artery disease. Circ Res 2001;89:E1–E7.
43. Hill JM, Zalos, G, Halcox, JP, et al. Circulating endothelial progenitor cells, vascular function, and cardiovascular risk. N Engl J Med 2003;348:593–600.
44. Urbich C, Heeschen, C, Aicher, A, et al. Relevance of monocytic features for neovascularization capacity of circulating endothelial progenitor cells. Circulation 2003;108:2511–2516.
45. Wu H, Dmitriev, I, Kashentseva, E, et al. Construction and characterization of adenovirus serotype 5 packaged by serotype 3 hexon. J Virol 2002;76:12,775–12,782.
46. Kaiser J. Gene therapy. RAC's advice: proceed with caution. Science 2002;298:2113–2115.
47. Rebar EJ, Huang, Y, Hickey, R, et al. Induction of angiogenesis in a mouse model using engineered transcription factors. Nature Med 2002;8:1427–1432.
48. Henry TD, Abraham JA. Review of preclinical and clinical results with vascular endothelial growth factors for therapeutic angiogenesis. Curr Interv Cardiol Rep 2000;2:228–241.
49. Orlic D, Kajstura, J, Chimenti, S, et al. Bone marrow cells regenerate infarcted myocardium. Nature 2001;410:701–705.
50. Murohara T, Ikeda, H, Duan, J, et al. Transplanted cord blood-derived endothelial precursor cells augment postnatal neovascularization. J Clin Invest 2000;105:1527–1536.
51. Kawamoto A, Gwon, HC, Iwaguro, H, et al. Therapeutic potential of ex vivo expanded endothelial progenitor cells for myocardial ischemia. Circulation 2001;103:634–637.
52. Kalka C, Masuda, H, Takahashi, T, et al. Transplantation of ex vivo expanded endothelial progenitor cells for therapeutic neovascularization. Proc Natl Acad Sci USA 2000;97:3422–3427.
53. Kocher AA, Schuster, MD, Szaboles, MJ, et al. Neovascularization of ischemic myocardium by human bone-marrow-derived angioblasts prevents cardiomyocyte apoptosis, reduces remodeling and improves cardiac function. Nat Med 2001;7:430–436.
54. Assmus B, Schachinger, V, Teupe, C, et al. Transplantation of progenitor cells and regeneration enhancement in acute myocardial infarction (TOPCARE-AMI). Circulation 2002;106:3009–3017.
55. Rehman J, Li, J, Orschell, CM, et al. Peripheral blood "endothelial progenitor cells" are derived from monocyte/macrophages and secrete angiogenic growth factors. Circulation 2003;107:1164–1169.
56. Crosby JR, Kaminski, WE, Schatterman, G, et al. Endothelial cells of hematopoietic origin make a significant contribution to adult blood vessel formation. Circ Res 2000;87:728–730.
57. Harraz M, Jiao, C, Hanlon, HD, et al. CD34- blood-derived human endothelial cell progenitors. Stem Cells 2001;19:301–312.
58. Iwaguro H, Yamaguchi, J, Kalka, et al. Endothelial progenitor cell vascular endothelial growth factor gene transfer for vascular regeneration. Circulation 2001;105:732–738.
59. Madeddu P. Emanueli C, Polosi E, et al. Transplanation of low dose CD24+Kdr+ cells promotes vascular and muscular regeneration in ischemic limbs. FASEB J. 2004 Sep 2 [Epub ahead of print].
60. Dellambra E, et al. Corrective transduction of human epidermal stem cells in laminin 5-dependent junctional epidermolysis bullosa. Hum Gene Ther 1998;9:1359–1370.
61. Murasawa S, Llevadot, J, Silver, M, et al. Constitutive human telomerase reverse transcriptase expression enhances regenerative properties of endothelial progenitor cells. Circulation 2002;106:1133–1139.

17 Cell Transplantation

The New Frontier

Shafie Fazel, MD, MSc,
Paul W. M. Fedak, MD, MSc,
Richard D. Weisel, MD,
Denis Angoulvant, MD, MSc,
Terrence M. Yau, MD, MSc,
and Ren-Ke Li, MD, PhD

CONTENTS

SUMMARY

Cell transplantation of noncontractile cells into ischemic or dilated cardiomyopathic hearts prevents progressive failure and improves cardiac function by incompletely understood mechanisms. Significant angiogenesis and extracellular matrix remodeling occur after cell transplantation, but these effects do not fully explain the improvement in systolic function of the heart. Recent provocative results suggest that cell transplantation may be able to induce neocardiomyogenesis, and may enhance regional systolic function by recruiting stem cells that differentiate into functioning cardiomyocytes. Enhancing these effects using a combined modality that includes transplantation of genetically modified cells may hold the key to future cardiac regeneration.

Key Words: Cardiomyopathy; cell transplantation; genetic modification; angiogenesis; stem cells; extracellular matrix.

From: *Contemporary Cardiology: Cardiovascular Genomics*
Edited by: M. K. Raizada, et al. © Humana Press Inc., Totowa, NJ

INTRODUCTION

The discussion of cardiac cell transplantation within the context of a book dedicated to cardiovascular genomics is precarious but timely. Gene therapy evolved out of the central concept that providing one gene may reverse or prevent the progression of disease caused by the deficiency or altered function of a single gene. Intense investigation into the application of gene therapy has not only provided us with the opportunity to improve genetic techniques, genetic engineering, and gene delivery, but has taught us about the biology of single-gene disease processes, as outlined in the other chapters of this book. The process, however, has also highlighted the limitations of single-gene therapy. Even in diseases where the disease process is solely attributed to a single-gene defect, such as cystic fibrosis, gene-therapy strategies have yet to prove their clinical efficacy. Furthermore, the majority of the disease burden in the developed world is not caused by single-gene deficiencies but by degenerative disease processes that are largely multifactorial and polygenic. For instance, ischemic cardiomyopathy and heart failure are predicated on ongoing micro- and macrovascular atherosclerosis, micro- and macromyocardial infarctions and cell necrosis, ongoing myocardial ischemia and cell apoptosis, extracellular matrix remodeling with progressive left-ventricular dilatation, production of an inflammatory cytokine milieu, and distant effects, such as neurohormonal activation. Although gene therapy has been used to target a specific pathway in a complex degenerative process, such as angiogenesis in ischemic cardiomyopathy, the overexpression of a single gene late in the process will not be sufficient to halt it.

In a parallel to gene therapy, it was initially thought that if the principal insult that precipitates heart failure is myocyte death, then replacement of cardiomyocytes should reverse the heart failure phenotype. This original concept has now been significantly altered and revised. We and others have been unable to transplant cells that eventually beat in synchrony with the heart. In spite of this apparent major limitation, cell transplantation works (1). Various labs working with different animal models of heart failure, using a variety of cells have all, more or less, shown improvement in systolic function, prevention of ventricular dilatation, and prevention of heart failure. Albeit poorly understood, cell transplantation has begun to be enthusiastically investigated in human trials (2–6). The central question becomes: why should myocardial transplantation of noncontracting muscle cells or bone marrow cells prevent heart failure? We propose that unlike gene therapy, cell therapy invokes multiple endogenous processes that are capable of halting degenerative myocardial failure, such as angiogenesis, extracellular matrix remodeling, and perhaps cardiomyogenesis by stem cell recruitment. If living tissue heals, cell transplantation may work by cellularizing a largely acellular scar and converting it to living tissue, thus permitting and potentiating the mobilization of endogenous repair mechanisms. Here, the field of cell transplantation into postmitotic organs, such as the heart, directly encroaches on the fields of stem cells and stem cell plasticity. Our attention will, therefore, be focused mostly on these new frontiers of myocardial regeneration.

CELL TRANSPLANTATION PREPARES THE HEART FOR REPAIR

Angiogenesis

When the field of myocardial cell transplantation was in its infancy, investigators did not evaluate the extent of neovascularization caused by cell transplantation because they did not expect it. Now it is well-known that a major effect of cell engraftment is the induction of angiogenesis (Table 1), perhaps by the release of cytokines and growth factors, the participation of the cells in new vessel formation, and the recruitment of endothelial and smooth muscle cell precursors, progenitors, and/or stem cells. Compared with gene or protein angiogenic therapies, cell transplantation not only provides the signals for new vessels to grow into the ischemic region, but the donor cells provide the necessary cellular building blocks for new vessel formation in a region where cells are likely scarce. Angiogenesis in the absence of myogenesis may not influence overall heart function, but improving perfusion to the infarct region may itself modify the remodeling of both the injured region and the remaining myocardium. Increasing perfusion may salvage hibernating native cardiomyocytes and/or restore damaged cells. Increased perfusion may also aid in the restoration of injured matrix that in turn may facilitate donor cell incorporation, donor-to-host cell communications, and increased structural support and stability. This section highlights some of the advances that have occurred in investigating the effects of differentiated, progenitor, and stem cell transplantation on angiogenesis (capillary formation) and vasculogenesis (muscular vessel formation).

Considering the cell-type dependency of this process, the data suggests that cell transplantation-induced vasculogenesis is independent of the process of inflammation. We now know that vasculogenesis involves endothelial cell budding, endothelial progenitor cell (EPC) homing and differentiation, and bone marrow mesenchymal stem cell (MSC) mobilization and differentiation to smooth muscle cells to form the muscular media of the new vessels. The reviewed literature should be read, with the following serving as an underlying central question: why should cell transplantation cause vasculogenesis?

TRANSPLANTATION OF DIFFERENTIATED CELLS

Smooth muscle cell transplantation causes neovascularization in injured myocardium. Smooth muscle cells, under pathologic conditions, can de-differentiate, migrate, proliferate, and secrete extracellular matrix to heal vascular injuries. They also secrete factors, such as nitric oxide, basic fibroblast growth factor (bFGF) and vascular endothelial growth factor (VEGF) involved in the angiogenic process (7–9). Li et al. (10) successfully transplanted smooth muscle cells into the cryo-necrosed left ventricle of adult rats and observed a four- to fivefold increase in blood vessel formation, and significant improvement in contractile function. In a pig model of myocardial infarction followed by transplantation of uterine smooth muscle cells, we recently showed extensive formation of de novo muscular blood vessels (unpublished observation). Transplantation of vascular smooth muscle cells in the same model did not induce a similar degree of arteriolar and venular blood vessel formation. The uterine smooth muscle cells improved myocardial function more than the vascular smooth muscle cells, suggesting that part of the benefit of cell transplantation arose from its effects on vasculogenesis.

Likewise, albeit to a more limited degree, transplantation of skeletal myoblasts is also able to induce angiogenesis. Skeletal myoblasts are skeletal muscle precursor cells that have the capacity for self renewal and differentiation. Since the first experiment reported by Chiu et al. (11) of the successful engraftment of skeletal myoblasts, several studies have assessed the ability of these cells to improve postinfarction cardiac function (12–14). Initial studies did not demonstrate significant increase in angiogenesis caused by myoblast transplantation (15). However, in a study evaluating VEGF-transfected skeletal myoblasts, Suzuki et al. (16) showed that implantation of nontransfected skeletal myoblasts still resulted in significantly increased capillary number.

Table 1
Cell Transplantation and Neovascularization

Cells	Strategy	Results	Ref.
Fetal rat stomach SMC	IM, 4 wk after cryo injury, rats	4 wk: increased capillary density	*10*
Skeletal myoblasts + VEGF	IM, 1 h after MI, rats	4 wk: increased capillary density in VEGF transfected > nontransfected > medium	*102*
EPCs	IM, 4 wk after MI, pigs	4 wk: increased capillary density. Improvement of myocardial function	*31*
EPCs	IC, 5 d after MI, humans	4 mo: improvement of coronary flow reserve	*3*
BMD-MC	IM, 4 wk after MI, pigs	4 wk: increased endothelial cell number and myocardial perfusion	*32*
BMD-MC	TCS, 2 wk after MI, pigs	2 wk: increased angiogenesis	*33*
BMD-MC	IM, after creation of a coronary stenosis, rats	2 mo: increased capillary density, blood flow, angiopoietin 1 and VEGF expression	*34*
BMD-MC	IM, 60 min after MI, pigs	3 wk: increased capillary density, blood flow, and angiographic collateral vessels	*37*
BMD-MC	IC, 5–9 d after MI, humans	3 mo: improvement of myocardial perfusion	*5*

(continued)

328

Cell type	Method/model	Results	Ref.
BMD-MC	IM, ICM, humans	3 mo: improvement of myocardial perfusion	103
BMD-MC	IM, ICM, humans	2 mo: improvement of myocardial perfusion	104
HSC	IM, 5 h after MI, mice	9 d: donor-derived endothelial cells and SMCs in *de novo* capillaries and arterioles. Donor-derived cardiomyocytes	42
MSC	Intraaortic, 2 wk after MI, rats	4 wk: donor-derived endothelial cells, cardiomyocytes and fibroblasts	46
MSCs treated with 5-aza	IM, 3 wk after cryo injury, rats	8 wk: increased capillary density	105
MSCs treated with 5-aza	IM injection 4 wk after MI, pigs	4 wk: increased capillary density	106
MSCs treated with 5-aza	IM injection of noninjured heart, mice	1, 4, 8, and 12 wk: increased capillary density. Donor-derived endothelial cells	50

SMC, smooth muscle cells; EPC, endothelial progenitor cells; BMD-MC, bone marrow-derived mononuclear cells; HSC, hematopoietic stem cells; MSC, mesenchymal stem cells; 5-aza, 5-azacytidine; IM, intramyocardial; IC, intracoronary; TCS, transcoronary sinus; MI, myocardial infarction; ICM, ischemic cardiomyopathy.

Recently, we investigated the enhancement of cell transplantation-mediated angiogenesis/vasculogenesis by transfecting the implanted cells with VEGF *(17)*. We had hypothesized that over-expression of VEGF would enhance the beneficial effects of cell transplantation. Surprisingly, in our initial experiments, the greater degree of angiogenesis did not correlate with improvement in myocardial function *(17)*. These observations are akin to our observations that endothelial cell transplantation caused significant angiogenesis but did not improve function *(18)*. As such, increased angiogenesis does not necessarily imply greater functional benefit, whereas the process of vasculogenesis (as seen in our uterine smooth muscle cell experiments) appears to be directly correlated with functional improvement. Interestingly, our most recent results suggest that VEGF-enhanced cell transplantation causes significant upregulation of Flk-1 and Flt-1, VEGF receptors, in the infarct border zone (manuscript in preparation). That is, the VEGF transgene, which should only be highly expressed in the middle of the infarcted scar where the cells were transplanted, caused an upregulation of its receptors in the nontransplanted host cells located in the infarct border zone. This observation demonstrates for the first time that cell transplantation can affect host cells through both a paracrine, and perhaps a matrix-mediated, mechanism, and that cross-talk between the host and transplanted cells occurs.

TRANSPLANTATION OF PROGENITOR AND STEM CELLS

EPCs are bone marrow-derived progenitor cells that are implicated in the maintenance of endothelium through their ability to mature into endothelial cells and to support the process of angiogenesis *(19)*. They have a common precursor with hematopoietic stem cells (HSCs) *(20)* and can be isolated from bone marrow or peripheral blood mononuclear cells *(21–23)*. These cells express both the endothelial cell marker VEGF-receptor-2, and progenitor cell markers CD34 and/or CD133 *(24,25)*. The number of circulating EPCs in the peripheral blood of humans is low under normal conditions, but can be significantly increased by bone marrow mobilization with granulocyte-colony stimulating factor (G-CSF) and VEGF *(26,27)*.

Recently, Kaushal et al. *(28)* showed that in vitro expanded EPCs were able to recreate functional small vessels or cause angiogenesis. Human EPCs, when infused into athymic nude rats after myocardial infarction, induced significant angiogenesis, reduced host cardiomyocyte apoptosis, and prevented adverse remodeling *(29,30)*. Kawamoto et al. *(31)* recently reported a significant increase in capillary density, angiographic collateral development, and left-ventricular ejection fraction 4 wk after transplantation of autologous EPCs in a swine model of myocardial infarction. Similarly, Kocher et al. *(30)* also showed that infusion of human EPCs in rats after myocardial infarction resulted in vasculogenesis. A recent clinical trial conducted by Assmus et al. *(3)* reported the feasibility and safety of intracoronary infusion of autologous EPCs after myocardial infarction in humans. Their preliminary evidence also suggests an increase in the perfusion of the implanted area.

The above studies clearly implicate EPCs in neovascularization. The possibility that differentiated cell transplantation also causes mobilization and homing of EPCs to the transplanted site requires investigation.

It appears that induction of angiogenesis is not limited to circulating EPCs because unselected bone marrow resident cells can also induce significant angiogenesis *(32–34)*. Bone marrow contains many cell types that include MSCs and hematopoietic stem cells

(HSCs). Bone marrow-derived progenitors have the capacity to home to different tissue, proliferate, and acquire the phenotypes of the host organ *(35,36)*. Kamihata et al. *(37)* reported that 16% of the bone marrow-derived mononuclear cells (BMD-MCs) that they implanted in a swine model of myocardial infarction expressed bFGF, VEGF, and angiopoietin 1, suggesting that the cells are precursors or progenitors of endothelial-like cells. Orlic et al. *(35)* reported that bone marrow cells mobilized by stem cell factor (SCF) and G-CSF also participated in angiogenesis. In the TOPCARE-AMI trial, Assmus et al. *(3)* observed a similar beneficial effect of unselected BMD-MCs and EPCs on normal-ization of coronary flow reserve. These results suggest either that the bone marrow cell preparations are "contaminated" with significant number of EPCs, or that other bone marrow-derived cells are also able to participate in the process of angiogenesis.

Evidence suggests that HSCs may participate in angiogenesis. HSCs have been shown to transdifferentiate to multiple lineages *(38)* (reviewed later). HSC participation in neovascularization is somewhat anticipated because they are mobilized by angiogenic factors such as VEGF and angiopoietin-1 *(39,40)*, and have a common precursor with the EPCs, the hemangioblast *(41)*. Indeed, Orlic et al. *(42)* observed a significant degree of neovascularization after transplantation of HSCs into the infarct border zone in a murine model. Jackson et al. *(43)* similarly reported that 3% of endothelial cells in ischemic myocardium expressed the marker of donor cells after bone marrow transplantation in lethally irradiated mice.

The other stem cell population that resides in the bone marrow, the MSC, also has been shown to significantly increase neovascularization after engraftment into injured myocardium *(44–46)*. MSCs are a self-renewing clonal precursor of nonhematopoietic tissues that provide the microenvironment for hematopoiesis. They can be induced to differentiate into cells of mesenchymal lineage including fibroblasts, fat, cartilage, bone, skeletal, and cardiac muscle *(47–49)*. Human MSCs do not express markers of EPCs and are not reported to transdifferentiate into endothelial cells *(48,49)*. However, Gojo et al. *(50)* recently reported that immortalized murine MSCs treated in vitro with 5-azacytidine were able to transdifferentiate into endothelial cells, pericytes, and smooth muscle cells. Dr. C. Verfaillie's laboratory *(51)* showed that the culture-adherent por-tion of bone marrow contains a subset of cells—multipotent adult progenitor cells—that capably participated in the generation of all adult mouse tissues when injected into the blastocyst. These cells express the VEGF receptors Flk1 and other phenotypic markers of endothelial lineage after VEGF stimulation. The contribution of MSCs, which are traditionally selected as the culture-dish adherent cells of the bone marrow, to neovascularization may be accounted for by the presence of the multipotent adult progenitor cells in the preparations.

Thus, several subsets of bone marrow cells, circulating progenitor cells, and differen-tiated cells are capable of inducing significant angiogenesis. These observations argue that a common mechanism must exist by which the various cell types induce angiogenesis and/or vasculogenesis. It appears that this mechanism is not cell-type-specific, but the extent of it depends on the cell type. Vasculogenesis requires the expression of various angiogenic cytokines and growth factors in addition to the recruitment of other cells, such as the EPCs and MSCs. It is unlikely that transplanted stomach smooth muscle cells, for instance, possess the machinery to independently induce significant angiogenesis. The cross-talk between the transplanted cells and the host cells is likely to be an important mediator. The challenge in the future will involve enhancing this cross-talk to induce the endogenous repair mechanisms that allow more efficient neovascularization.

Extracellular Matrix Remodeling

Another beneficial effect of cell engraftment is the prevention of adverse matrix remodeling. The extracellular matrix provides the structural framework for coordinated cardiomyocyte contraction, and sequesters growth factors and cytokines. The myocardial matrix thus assembles a dynamic microenvironment in which molecular cues converge to maintain tissue architecture by regulating cell orientation, shape, growth, and survival *(52–55)*. Maladaptive remodeling of the cardiac matrix impairs structural support for cardiomyocytes and leads to ventricular dilatation and both systolic and diastolic dysfunction *(56,57)*. The engraftment of transplanted cells likely reorganizes the degraded matrix of the host myocardium and secretes new matrix elements, and may thereby regenerate normal myocardial tissue architecture. This process may also improve the structural support for native heart cells and, by tethering transplanted cells to actively contracting host tissue, may improve myocardial function. We are currently in the process of measuring the impact of cell transplantation on the extracellular matrix, both in the infarct zone as well as in the remote myocardium.

Myogenesis

Considering that the transplanted cells significantly induce angiogenesis and may induce beneficial matrix remodeling, one wonders what other repair mechanisms are mobilized by the process of transplantation. Recent evidence suggests that injured or stressed myocardium is able to recruit cardiac-derived c-Kit[+] stem cells or bone marrow-derived c-Kit[+] hematopoietic stem cells (reviewed later). Therefore, mechanisms exist in the body to allow mobilization and homing of appropriate stem cells to the injured heart to give rise to an unknown degree of neocardiomyogenesis and neovascularization. It is possible that cell transplantation enhances the mobilization of such mechanisms that are obviously inadequate to prevent progressive heart failure in patients after a myocardial infarction. The aforementioned mechanisms may only be in place to replace the low level cell loss that occurs with physiologic apoptosis of cardiomyocytes, and are overwhelmed by massive cardiomyocyte loss. Cell duress may be responsible for mobilizing stem cells, and the massive amount of noncardiomyocyte cell duress that occurs with cell transplantation may significantly potentiate these endogenous repair mechanisms. The beneficial effects of matrix remodeling and vasculogenesis may act as adjunct mechanisms that allow, enhance, or aid these processes. We propose that cell transplantation amplifies not only the signals that promote stem cell mobilization and proliferation, but also their effects on extracellular matrix and angiogenesis. That is, the transplanted cells may pave the way for the successful engraftment of recruited cardiac and bone marrow stem cells.

BONE MARROW STEM CELLS AND STEM CELL PLASTICITY

Traditionally, hematopoietic stem cells reside in the c-Kit[+], Sca-1[+], Thy[lo], and Lin[neg/low] fraction of the bone marrow *(58,59)*. Until recently, these cells were thought to only give rise to hematopoietic cells. Mice that bear a partial mutation in c-Kit-receptor tyrosine kinase activity are partially deficient in hematopoietic stem cells and readily accept bone marrow transplantation without prior lethal irradiation. Complete mutation of this transmembrane protein results in an embryonic lethal phenotype. The c-Kit receptor is a membrane-bound signaling tyrosine kinase expressed on HSCs, neural-crest-derived stem cells, and primordial germ cells, but not on mature hematopoietic cells *(60)*. The c-Kit ligand,

(SCF), upon c-Kit binding, dimerizes the receptor with subsequent autophosphorylation and activation of intracellular signaling, leading to stem cell survival, proliferation, and mobilization (61,62).

Work from Dr. M. Goodell's laboratory at the Baylor College of Mcdicine has identified an alternate method of stem cell purification that has had an impact on identifying other tissue-resident stem cells. In a series of experiments, Goodell and colleagues were able to show that the Hoechst dye-excluding fraction of the bone marrow, the side population or SP cells, were able to stably reconstitute the bone marrow of irradiated recipients in long-term reconstitution experiments (63). Further work from the same lab suggested that the bone marrow SP cells have the potential to differentiate into cardiomyocytes in ischemic myocardium (60). These observations, coupled with a myriad of investigations reporting that adult stem cells from the bone marrow can differentiate into non-lymphohematopoietic tissues, such as myocytes (64), hepatocytes (65), microglia and macroglia (66), and neuronal tissue (67,68), have given rise to the burgeoning field of "stem cell plasticity."

SP cells have also been isolated from muscle tissue. In fact, when these muscle SP cells from wild-type donors where transplanted into *mdx* mice, a mouse model of muscular dystrophy, new muscle cells were noted to express the dystrophin gene (69). These muscle cells must have been derived from the transplanted muscle SP cells. Furthermore, the muscle SP cells reconstituted the bone marrow of lethally irradiated hosts (70). Subsequent work demonstrated that muscle-resident SP cells were likely hematopoietic in origin (71). But why would hematopoietic stem cells reside in the muscle? Are they contaminating cells with no function, or do they exist in other tissues for tissue repair? And more interesting, why would muscle-resident hematopoietic stem cells be able to correct the genetic deficiency in muscle tissue? Last, if stem cells exist in skeletal muscle tissue, do stem cells exist within the fabric of cardiac muscle tissue?

Perhaps the most intriguing observation comes from investigation of neural stem cells. When grown in culture, these cells form spheroids and are capable of generating oligodendrocytes, neurons, and astrocytes. When transplanted into irradiated hosts, they too were capable of reconstituting the bone marrow (72). Work of other investigators suggests that the bone marrow cells are also capable of giving rise to neurons (68). Whether this process occurs by transdifferentiation, dedifferentiation followed by redifferentiation to another fate, or fusion of bone marrow cells with existing neurons is unclear, and is the subject of intense investigation.

The series of observations demonstrating that single cells from one tissue can give rise to cells of another tissue across germline boundaries prompted Dr. H. Blau (73) from Stanford University to publish an editorial in the journal *Cell* in which she argued that perhaps stemness is a cell function, and that stem cells are cells that perform that function. Central to her argument is the concept that most cells have the capability, under the appropriate condition, to be stem-like; that is, they have the capability of dedifferentiating, proliferating, and redifferentiating. These are tantalizing suggestions that beg the question: why would cells retain such activity, or is there a physiological role for stem cell plasticity? The theme that seems to be emerging is that stem cells are critical mediators of tissue response to injury.

BONE MARROW STEM CELLS AND MYOCARDIAL INJURY

Whereas the heart was previously viewed as a postmitotic organ, recent evidence suggests that the myocardium has some replicative potential, and it may have the potential for self-repair or self-regeneration *(74)*. Examination of cell division in both normal and pathological human myocardium revealed myocyte proliferation rates of 14 to 140 per million myocytes *(75)*. In the infarct border zone, estimates of cardiomyocyte proliferation approached 4–5% of the total cardiomyocyte number *(76)*.

Mobilization of the bone marrow-derived stem cells prior to the induction of myocardial infarction in a murine model led to significant engraftment of bone marrow-derived cells into the injured myocardium *(35)*. Thus, myocardial injury is able to elicit the homing of bone marrow stem cells to the heart. Hematopoietic stem cells that are c-Kit$^+$ have also been shown to transdifferentiate into cardiomyocyte when directly transplanted into injured murine myocardial tissue *(77)*. The developing myocytes were small and resembled fetal and neonatal myocytes. They were positive for several myocyte-specific proteins, including cardiac myosin and connexin-43 and the transcription factors GATA-4, MEF2, and Csx/Nkx2.5 *(77)*. Jackson and coworkers demonstrated, using lethal irradiation and bone marrow reconstitution with labeled cells, that 0.02% of new cardiomyocyte and 3% of new endothelial cells after myocardial infarction are from the bone marrow *(43)*.

Evidence from humans also implicates the bone marrow as a potential source of cardiomyogenesis. Muller et al. *(78)*, Laflamme et al. *(79)*, and Quaini et al. *(80)* observed that male heart transplant recipients who had received a female heart had cardiomyocytes bearing the Y-chromosome, thus suggesting that cardiomyogenic precursors had been recruited from an extracardiac location. Conversely, cardiomyocytes bearing the Y-chromosome were discovered in female patients who had received bone marrow transplantation from male donors *(81)*, implicating the bone marrow as the extra-cardiac source of cardiomyogenic precursors.

Other models of tissue injury and repair have also highlighted the central role of bone marrow-derived cells. Sata et al. *(82)* demonstrated that the majority of smooth muscle cells involved in postangioplasty restenosis, graft vasculopathy, and hyperlipidemia-induced atherosclerosis were from the bone marrow. We also found, in a femoral angioplasty model in irradiated mice reconstituted with HSC from transgenic yellow fluorescent protein mice, that most smooth muscle cells within the intimal hyperplastic lesion had yellow fluorescence. This observation suggests that bone marrow-derived cells had migrated to the site of injury and had transdifferentiated into or fused with resident smooth muscle cells. Additionally, formation of intimal hyperplasia after vascular injury was absent in mouse models that bore a mutation in the signaling domain of c-Kit or that lacked the membrane isotype of its ligand, stem cell factor (manuscript in preparation).

Evidence outside the realm of cardiovascular medicine has also implicated bone marrow cells as important mediators of tissue regeneration. Models of bone marrow transplantation in animals with fumarylacetoacetate hydrolase deficiency have demonstrated significant engraftment of bone marrow-derived cells into liver parenchyma *(83,84)*. These cells produce albumin and phenotypically appear to be hepatocytes. Interestingly, evidence from the two separate labs also demonstrated that the new hepatocytes were the result of fusion between the bone marrow-derived cells and hepatocytes *(83,84)*. The new heterokaryons (products of cell fusion) expressed fumarylacetoacetate hydrolase. This latter observation suggests, as another editorial by Dr. H. Blau argues *(85)*, that fusion may actually be a physiologic event by which damaged cells receive fresh genetic material that may restore function. That is, fusion may be a mechanism by which epigenetic changes associated with a diseased phenotype are "reset", or new genetic functionality is added.

The mechanism of stem cell mobilization and homing to the injured organ is becoming increasingly elucidated, and some of these data are summarized below. The signals appear to consist of molecules involved in stem cell mobilization and release, migration, homing, and engraftment, the principle of which appears to be mediated through the c-Kit receptor.

An important signal appears to come from binding of the Kit receptor with its ligand, SCF. Lyman et al. *(86)* investigated the role of and the mechanism by which SCF mobilizes bone marrow-derived stem cells. Bone marrow suppression induced the expression of matrix metalloproteinase-9 (MMP-9) that caused the cleavage and release of SCF from the membrane of bone marrow cells, which in turn enhanced hematopoietic reconstitution by binding the kit receptor on the surface of the hematopoietic stem cells and promoted release and active proliferation of these cells. Furthermore, chemokine-induced mobilization of bone marrow repopulating cells by stromal-derived factor, VEGF, and G-CSF was impaired in MMP-9$^{-/-}$ animals.

SCF also appears to play a major role in peripheral mobilization of bone marrow cells. SCF administered to mice for 7 d resulted in the depletion of c-Kit$^+$ Sca$^+$ Thy^{lo} Lin$^-$ bone marrow stem cells in the bone marrow, but the multilineage, long-term reconstituting activity in the spleen and peripheral blood increased proportionally *(87)*. These observations suggest that systemic SCF administration caused redistribution of existing stem cells to peripheral sites, making them available for tissue repair. SCF may also be an important homing signal for the bone marrow-derived hematopoietic progenitor cells *(88)*. Indeed, administration of antibodies which block c-Kit resulted in reduced homing efficiency of progenitor cells *(89)*. Other investigators have shown than SCF also induces expression of very late antigen family of integrins, which mediate the adhesion of hematopoietic progenitor cell lines to fibronectin and vascular cell adhesion molecule-1 *(90–93)*. These proteins may play a critical role in the adherence and transmigration through the endothelial barrier of the HSC into injured tissue.

Recent findings suggest a role for SCF in myocardial injury as well, although this role needs to be fully elucidated. In a canine model of ischemia/reperfusion, Frangogiannis et al. *(94)* demonstrated upregulation of SCF mRNA 72 h postischemia. One possible mechanism is the aiding of mobilization and homing of c-Kit+ stem cells. The investigators identified a subset of tissue macrophages as the source for the SCF, thereby linking inflammation to stem cell mobilization. Considering the central role of antigen-presenting cell that tissue macrophages play in the immune system, one may hypothesize that these cells, recruited as part of the inflammatory response to any site of injury, can then initiate/propagate either an immune response or a repair response in a dichotomous fashion.

CARDIAC-DERIVED STEM CELLS

The hypothesis that the heart is also home to cardiac-specific stem cells that are capable of cardiomyogenesis is supported by recent evidence. Many terminally differentiated tissues have been shown to harbor cells with stem cell-like activity *(95)*. We have previously isolated myofibroblasts from the heart, which can be expanded ex vivo and will prevent functional deterioration when implanted into an infarcted region. Other investigators found a different cell population in the heart, SP cells, that may be cardiac-specific stem cells *(96)*. These cells were first identified, as detailed previously, in the bone marrow and were shown to have a high percentage of known HSC surface markers: c-Kit$^+$, Sca-1$^+$, CD43$^+$, and CD45$^+$. Hierlihy and colleagues *(96)* have been successful in isolating SP cells from single-cell preparations of murine heart. They showed that when the growth of the postnatal heart was attenuated in the dominant negative MEF2Cdn (cardiac-specific transcription factor) murine hearts, the SP cell population was depleted as the number of cardiomyocytes increased significantly. The authors were unable, however, to produce a direct link between SP cells and increased cardiomyogenesis.

Dr. M. D. Schneider's group from the Baylor College of Medicine recently provided the missing link connecting the myocardial SP cell population to myocardial regeneration *(97)*. A critical attribute of cells capable of self-renewal and extended proliferative capacity, as one would expect from stem cell or progenitor cells, is the capacity to prevent telomere shortening that leads to cell senescence. The Schneider group was able to identify a subset of the myocardial SP cell population as the cells that expressed 100% of the telomerase activity resident in the myocardium. Interestingly, the cell population was the Sca-1 positive subpopulation of myocardial SP cells. Characterization of these cells using a combination of gene-expression profiling, reverse-transcription polymerase chain reaction (RT-PCR), and protein expression analysis confirmed that these cells expressed a number, but not a complete set, of cardiac-specific transcription factors. The cells, however, did not express cardiac-specific structural proteins. These cells, when cultured in the presence of the demethylating agent 5-azacytidine, acquired the capability to differentiate to cardiomyocytes. When injected intravenously after an infarction, the cells homed to the infarct border zone and gave rise to new cardiomyocytes *(97)*.

The work of Dr. P. Anversa's group, from the New York Medical College, has recently proved the existence of cardiac-resident stem cells that appear to be less differentiated than the cells isolated by Schneider's group *(98)*. Examination of myocardial tissue from old rats revealed the presence of small c-Kit$^+$ cells that otherwise lacked markers of blood-derived cells. These round cells with little cytoplasm were isolated and grown in vitro at a single cell level. The resulting colonies formed spheroids that remained c-Kit$^+$ and undifferentiated, but also gave rise to satellite cells that became adherent to the culture dish. Immunohistochemistry demonstrated the production of smooth muscle actin, sarcomeric actin, and vWF—indicative of smooth muscle, cardiomyocyte, and endothelial differentiation, respectively—in a different subset of the satellite cells. These cells slowly lost their c-Kit expression and, as verified by the expression of cardiac-specific transcription factors and structural genes, readily formed cardiomyocytes. The transplantation of these cells into the infarct border zone, after myocardial infarction, ameliorated myocardial dysfunction induced by cell death, and over time allowed the synchronized beating of the transplanted area, as evidenced by echocardiography *(98)*.

The same group demonstrated that similar c-Kit$^+$ cells undergo rigorous cell proliferation in the left-ventricular biopsy samples of patients who had come to aortic valve replacement because of severe aortic stenosis *(99)*. Interestingly, in that study, the duration of symptomatic heart failure corresponded inversely to the number of dividing c-Kit$^+$ cells and directly to the degree of telomere shortening. These findings suggested, as would be expected from the limited capability of myocardial regeneration after injury, that the purported cardiac stem cells did not have unlimited proliferative capacity. These observations open the door, if the above findings are reproduced in magnitude by other groups, for strategies that use ex vivo expansion of these cells prior to implantation to prevent ongoing degeneration of myocardium.

However, we do not know the physiological role that these cardiac-derived stem cells play in response to myocardial infarction and progressive heart failure. Although the previously noted human studies, in addition to the data from rats, suggest an important role, the magnitude, time-line, and extent of the repair process caused by these cells remain unknown. The observation that these cells are not present uniformly in the myocardium (they are mainly concentrated in the atrial tissue, as well as in the left-ventricular apex) would also suggest some sort of mechanism for migration of these cells. These cells may either migrate through the interstitial space, or be mobilized into the blood stream with subsequent homing to the injured myocardium. If these cells are similar to hematopoietic stem cells, as suggested by phenotypic characterization and cell-surface protein expression, they may retain a similar capacity to be released from their immediate niche into the circulation. As suggested by chimeric bone marrow studies, these cells should also have the capacity to breach endothelial barriers and transmigrate back into myocardial tissue to undertake myocardial repair.

GENE-ENHANCED CELL TRANSPLANTATION TO REGENERATE THE HEART

Thus, the fields of cell transplantation and stem cell biology meet to provide promise for attempts at cardiac regeneration. The possibility that stem or progenitor cells are recruited to the area of cell transplantation where injury signals are once again generated by the transplanted cells may be the major mechanism by which cell transplantation of various cell types may impact cardiac function to a similar degree. Delineating the precise molecular mechanisms by which these cells are mobilized and recruited, and the subsequent signaling pathways that promote differentiation or transdifferentiation of the recruited cells to the cardiomyocyte lineage, are and will be areas of intense investigation. It is within this context that genetic modification of transplanted cells may hold significant potential (Table 2).

Gene-enhanced cell transplantation is still in its infancy, but already impressive results of its potential have arisen in the literature. Dr. V. J. Dzau's group from Harvard Medical School transfected rat MSCs with the *AKT1* gene, which is a serine-threonine kinase and is involved in survival signaling *(100)*. Transplantation of the transfected cell into the infarct zone within an hour of coronary ligation resulted in near normalization of both systolic and diastolic function in a dose-dependent manner at follow-up. Interestingly, the transplanted MSCs appeared to have transdifferentiated into cardiomyocyte-like cells. Furthermore, these cells appeared to express connexin 43 and N-cadherin at junctions with host cardiomyocytes. It is unclear from their data whether the cells had truly transdifferentiated, or had fused with native cardiomyocytes.

Recent evidence form the Cleveland Clinic has highlighted another utility of gene-enhanced cell transplantation. Askari and colleagues conducted a series of experiments that for the first time provided evidence for the recruitment of c-Kit[+] cells to the site of cell transplantation *(101)*. Chronic BrdU labeling after myocardial infarction resulted in the labeling of bone marrow cells and not cardiomyocytes. Eight weeks after myocardial infarction, and after BrdU administration was halted, transplantation of skeletal myoblasts resulted in an increase in the BrdU signal in the heart, suggesting that previously-labeled cells were recruited to the site of transplantation. Transfection of cardiac fibroblasts with stromal-derived factor-1 (SDF-1), a known stimulator of stem-cell homing which is expressed for up to 7 d after infarction *(101)*, and transplantation of these

Table 2
Protein- or Gene-Enhanced Cell Transplantation

Cells	Strategy	Results	Ref.
Fetal rat CM + bFGF microspheres	MI, rat	4 wk: improved function in combination therapy	107
Neonatal rat CM + HGF liposomes	MI, rat	4, 8 wk: increased angiogenesis and improved function in combination therapy	108
VEGF transfected rat adult CM	Cryo injury, rat	5 wk: increased angiogenesis but no improvement in function	17
VEGF transfected rat skeletal myoblasts	MI, rat	2 wk: reduced infarct size and improved function	102
CTLA4-Ig transfected rat fetal CM	Normal myocardium, mice	8 wk: reduced xenograft rejection	109
Akt transfected rat neonatal CM	Cryo injury, rat	4 d: increased survival of cells	110
Akt transfected rat MSC	MI, rat	2 ws: reduced infarct size and improved function	100
IGF transfected rat SMC	Cryo injury, rat	1 wk: increased survival of cells and increased angiogenesis	9
SDF-1 transfected Rat cariac fibroblasts and G-CSF admin	MI, rat	4 wk: increased homing of BM c-Kit$^+$ cells and improved function	101

CM, cardiomyocytes; bFGF, basic fibroblast growth factor; HGF, hepatocyte growth factor; VEGF, vascular endothelial growth factor; CTLA4-Ig, cytotoxic T lymphocyte late antigen-4 immunoglobulin; IGF, insulin-like growth factor; SMC, smooth muscle cells; SDF-1, stromal derived factor-1;

cells into the infarct region, resulted in a significant increase in the BrdU signal in the heart and improvement in cardiac function. Interestingly, a significant number of these cells were either CD34$^-$ or c-Kit$^+$, suggesting that they were endothelial progenitor cells or c-Kit$^+$ stem cells, although proof of this hypothesis was not provided.

CONCLUSION

Although cell transplantation was initially developed to directly replace lost cardiomyocytes after injury, the transplanted cardiomyocytes did not beat synchronously with the rest of the heart. We have discovered that the transplanted cells have a multitude of other effects that may account for the functional benefit seen with this therapeutic strategy. Angiogenesis and vasculogenesis occur to a significant degree in the recipient heart. We are also beginning to understand the extent of the influence of the transplanted cells on extracellular matrix remodeling. The role of cardiac-resident or bone marrow-derived stem cells in myocardial response to injury is becoming increasingly elucidated. The mobilization of the endogenous repair mechanisms that may involve stem cell recruitment may be a major mechanism by which cell transplantation arrests progressive heart failure. Once we understand the cross-talk signals that drive these mechanisms, we may be able to intervene and not only arrest progression of disease, but perhaps reverse it. A combination of cell- and gene-therapy may hold the future key to cardiac regeneration.

REFERENCES

1. Al Radi OO, Rao V, Li RK, Yau T, Weisel RD. Cardiac cell transplantation: closer to bedside. Ann Thorac Surg 2003;75:S674–S677.
2. Menasche P, Hagege AA, Vilquin JT, et al. Autologous skeletal myoblast transplantation for severe postinfarction left ventricular dysfunction. J Am Coll Cardiol 2003;41:1078–1083.
3. Assmus B, Schachinger V, Teupe C, et al. Transplantation of progenitor cells and regeneration enhancement in acute myocardial infarction (TOPCARE-AMI). Circulation 2002;106:3009–3017.
4. Stamm C, Westphal B, Kleine HD, et al. Autologous bone-marrow stem-cell transplantation for myocardial regeneration. Lancet 2003;361:45–46.
5. Strauer BE, Brehm M, Zeus T, et al. Repair of infarcted myocardium by autologous intracoronary mononuclear bone marrow cell transplantation in humans. Circulation 2002;106:1913–1918.
6. Tse HF, Kwong YL, Chan JK, Lo G, Ho CL, Lau CP. Angiogenesis in ischaemic myocardium by intramyocardial autologous bone marrow mononuclear cell implantation. Lancet 2003;361:47–49.
7. Koide M, Kawahara Y, Nakayama I, Tsuda T, Yokoyama M. Cyclic AMP-elevating agents induce an inducible type of nitric oxide synthase in cultured vascular smooth muscle cells. Synergism with the induction elicited by inflammatory cytokines. J Biol Chem 1993;268:24,959–24,966.
8. Ali S, Becker MW, Davis MG, Dorn GW. Dissociation of vasoconstrictor-stimulated basic fibroblast growth factor expression from hypertrophic growth in cultured vascular smooth muscle cells. Relevant roles of protein kinase C. Circ Res 1994;75:836–843.
9. Stavri GT, Zachary IC, Baskerville PA, Martin JF, Erusalimsky JD. Basic fibroblast growth factor upregulates the expression of vascular endothelial growth factor in vascular smooth muscle cells. Synergistic interaction with hypoxia. Circulation 1995;92:11–14.
10. Li RK, Jia ZQ, Weisel RD, Merante F, Mickle DA. Smooth muscle cell transplantation into myocardial scar tissue improves heart function. J Mol Cell Cardiol 1999;31:513–522.
11. Chiu RC, Zibaitis A, Kao RL. Cellular cardiomyoplasty: myocardial regeneration with satellite cell implantation. Ann Thorac Surg 1995;60:12–18.
12. Murry CE, Wiseman RW, Schwartz SM, Hauschka SD. Skeletal myoblast transplantation for repair of myocardial necrosis. J Clin Invest 1996;98:2512–2523.
13. Taylor DA, Atkins BZ, Hungspreugs P, et al. Regenerating functional myocardium: improved performance after skeletal myoblast transplantation. Nat Med 1998;4:929–933.

14. Scorsin M, Hagege A, Vilquin JT, et al. Comparison of the effects of fetal cardiomyocyte and skeletal myoblast transplantation on postinfarction left ventricular function. J Thorac Cardiovasc Surg 2000;119:1169–1175.

15. Menasche P. Skeletal muscle satellite cell transplantation. Cardiovasc Res 2003;58:351–357.

16. Suzuki K, Murtuza B, Smolenski RT, et al. Cell transplantation for the treatment of acute myocardial infarction using vascular endothelial growth factor-expressing skeletal myoblasts. Circulation 2001;104(12 Suppl 1):I207–I212.

17. Yau TM, Fung K, Weisel RD, Fujii T, Mickle DA, Li RK. Enhanced myocardial angiogenesis by gene transfer with transplanted cells. Circulation 2001;104(12 Suppl 1):I218–I222.

18. Kim EJ, Li RK, Weisel RD, et al. Angiogenesis by endothelial cell transplantation. J Thorac Cardiovasc Surg 2001;122:963–971.

19. Szmitko PE, Fedak PW, Weisel RD, Stewart DJ, Kutryk MJ, Verma S. Endothelial progenitor cells: new hope for a broken heart. Circulation 2003;107:3093–3100.

20. Choi K, Kennedy M, Kazarov A, Papadimitriou JC, Keller G. A common precursor for hematopoietic and endothelial cells. Development 1998;125:725–732.

21. Lin Y, Weisdorf DJ, Solovey A, Hebbel RP. Origins of circulating endothelial cells and endothelial outgrowth from blood. J Clin Invest 2000;105:71–77.

22. Murohara T, Ikeda H, Duan J, et al. Transplanted cord blood-derived endothelial precursor cells augment postnatal neovascularization. J Clin Invest 2000;105:1527–1536.

23. Eggermann J, Kliche S, Jarmy G, et al. Endothelial progenitor cell culture and differentiation in vitro: a methodological comparison using human umbilical cord blood. Cardiovasc Res 2003;58:478–486.

24. Gehling UM, Ergun S, Schumacher U, et al. In vitro differentiation of endothelial cells from AC133-positive progenitor cells. Blood 2000;95:3106–3112.

25. Hristov M, Erl W, Weber PC. Endothelial progenitor cells: isolation and characterization. Trends Cardiovasc Med 2003;13:201–206.

26. Peichev M, Naiyer AJ, Pereira D, et al. Expression of VEGFR-2 and AC133 by circulating human CD34(+) cells identifies a population of functional endothelial precursors. Blood 2000;95:952–958.

27. Iwaguro H, Yamaguchi J, Kalka C, Murasawa S, Masuda H, Hayashi S et al. Endothelial progenitor cell vascular endothelial growth factor gene transfer for vascular regeneration. Circulation 2002;105:732–738.

28. Kaushal S, Amiel GE, Guleserian KJ, et al. Functional small-diameter neovessels created using endothelial progenitor cells expanded ex vivo. Nat Med 2001;7:1035–1040.

29. Kawamoto A, Gwon HC, Iwaguro H, et al. Therapeutic potential of ex vivo expanded endothelial progenitor cells for myocardial ischemia. Circulation 2001;103:634–637.

30. Kocher AA, Schuster MD, Szabolcs MJ, et al. Neovascularization of ischemic myocardium by human bone-marrow-derived angioblasts prevents cardiomyocyte apoptosis, reduces remodeling and improves cardiac function. Nat Med 2001;7:430–436.

31. Kawamoto A, Tkebuchava T, Yamaguchi J, et al. Intramyocardial transplantation of autologous endothelial progenitor cells for therapeutic neovascularization of myocardial ischemia. Circulation 2003;107:461–468.

32. Fuchs S, Baffour R, Zhou YF, et al. Transendocardial delivery of autologous bone marrow enhances collateral perfusion and regional function in pigs with chronic experimental myocardial ischemia. J Am Coll Cardiol 2001;37:1726–1732.

33. Vicario J, Piva J, Pierini A, et al. Transcoronary sinus delivery of autologous bone marrow and angiogenesis in pig models with myocardial injury. Cardiovasc Radiat Med 2002;3:91–94.

34. Nishida M, Li TS, Hirata K, Yano M, Matsuzaki M, Hamano K. Improvement of cardiac function by bone marrow cell implantation in a rat hypoperfusion heart model. Ann Thorac Surg 2003;75:768–773.

35. Orlic D, Kajstura J, Chimenti S, et al. Mobilized bone marrow cells repair the infarcted heart, improving function and survival. Proc Natl Acad Sci USA 2001;98:10,344–10,349.

36. Hirschi KK, Goodell MA. Hematopoietic, vascular and cardiac fates of bone marrow-derived stem cells. Gene Ther 2002;9:648–652.

37. Kamihata H, Matsubara H, Nishiue T, et al. Implantation of bone marrow mononuclear cells into ischemic myocardium enhances collateral perfusion and regional function via side supply of angioblasts, angiogenic ligands, and cytokines. Circulation 2001;104:1046–1052.

38. Krause DS, Theise ND, Collector MI, et al. Multi-organ, multi-lineage engraftment by a single bone marrow-derived stem cell. Cell 2001;105:369–377.

39. Rafii S, Avecilla S, Shmelkov S, et al. Angiogenic factors reconstitute hematopoiesis by recruiting stem cells from bone marrow microenvironment. Ann NY Acad Sci 2003;996:49–60.

40. Mohle R, Bautz F, Rafii S, Moore MA, Brugger W, Kanz L. The chemokine receptor CXCR-4 is expressed on CD34+ hematopoietic progenitors and leukemic cells and mediates transendothelial migration induced by stromal cell-derived factor-1. Blood 1998;91:4523–4530.
41. Choi K, Kennedy M, Kazarov A, Papadimitriou JC, Keller G. A common precursor for hematopoietic and endothelial cells. Development 1998;125:725–732.
42. Orlic D, Kajstura J, Chimenti S, et al. Bone marrow cells regenerate infarcted myocardium. Nature 2001;410:701–705.
43. Jackson KA, Majka SM, Wang H, et al. Regeneration of ischemic cardiac muscle and vascular endothelium by adult stem cells. J Clin Invest 2001;107:1395–1402.
44. Tomita S, Li RK, Weisel RD, et al. Autologous transplantation of bone marrow cells improves damaged heart function. Circulation 1999;100(19 Suppl):II247–II256.
45. Tomita S, Mickle DA, Weisel RD, et al. Improved heart function with myogenesis and angiogenesis after autologous porcine bone marrow stromal cell transplantation. J Thorac Cardiovasc Surg 2002;123:1132–1140.
46. Wang JS, Shum-Tim D, Chedrawy E, Chiu RC. The coronary delivery of marrow stromal cells for myocardial regeneration: pathophysiologic and therapeutic implications. J Thorac Cardiovasc Surg 2001;122:699–705.
47. Conget PA, Minguell JJ. Phenotypical and functional properties of human bone marrow mesenchymal progenitor cells. J Cell Physiol 1999;181:67–73.
48. Prockop DJ. Marrow stromal cells as stem cells for nonhematopoietic tissues. Science 1997;276:71–74.
49. Pittenger MF, Mackay AM, Beck SC, Jaiswal RK, Douglas R, Mosca JD et al. Multilineage potential of adult human mesenchymal stem cells. Science 1999;284:143–147.
50. Gojo S, Gojo N, Takeda Y, et al. In vivo cardiovasculogenesis by direct injection of isolated adult mesenchymal stem cells. Exp Cell Res 2003;288:51–59.
51. Jiang Y, Jahagirdar BN, Reinhardt RL, et al. Pluripotency of mesenchymal stem cells derived from adult marrow. Nature 2002;418:41–49.
52. Ross RS, Borg TK. Integrins and the myocardium. Circ Res 2001;88:1112–1119.
53. Hornberger LK, Singhroy S, Cavalle-Garrido T, Tsang W, Keeley F, Rabinovitch M. Synthesis of extracellular matrix and adhesion through beta(1) integrins are critical for fetal ventricular myocyte proliferation. Circ Res 2000;87:508–515.
54. Lukashev ME, Werb Z. ECM signalling: orchestrating cell behaviour and misbehaviour. Trends Cell Biol 1998;8:437–441.
55. Lundgren E, Terracio L, Mardh S, Borg TK. Extracellular matrix components influence the survival of adult cardiac myocytes in vitro. Exp Cell Res 1985;158:371–381.
56. Kim HE, Dalal SS, Young E, Legato MJ, Weisfeldt ML, D'Armiento J. Disruption of the myocardial extracellular matrix leads to cardiac dysfunction. J Clin Invest 2000;106:857–866.
57. Spinale FG. Matrix metalloproteinases: regulation and dysregulation in the failing heart. Circ Res 2002;90:520–530.
58. Goodell MA, Brose K, Paradis G, Conner AS, Mulligan RC. Isolation and functional properties of murine hematopoietic stem cells that are replicating in vivo. J Exp Med 1996;183:1797–1806.
59. Spangrude GJ, Heimfeld S, Weissman IL. Purification and characterization of mouse hematopoietic stem cells. Science 1988;241:58–62.
60. Matsui Y, Zsebo KM, Hogan BL. Embryonic expression of a haematopoietic growth factor encoded by the Sl locus and the ligand for c-kit. Nature 1990;347:667–669.
61. Morrison SJ, Shah NM, Anderson DJ. Regulatory mechanisms in stem cell biology. Cell 1997;88:287–298.
62. Morrison SJ, White PM, Zock C, Anderson DJ. Prospective identification, isolation by flow cytometry, and in vivo self-renewal of multipotent mammalian neural crest stem cells. Cell 1999;96:737–749.
63. Goodell MA, Brose K, Paradis G, Conner AS, Mulligan RC. Isolation and functional properties of murine hematopoietic stem cells that are replicating in vivo. J Exp Med 1996;183:1797–1806.
64. Ferrari G, Cusella-De Angelis G, Coletta M, et al. Muscle regeneration by bone marrow-derived myogenic progenitors. Science 1998;279:1528–1530.
65. Petersen BE, Bowen WC, Patrene KD, Mars WM, Sullivan AK, Murase N et al. Bone marrow as a potential source of hepatic oval cells. Science 1999;284:1168–1170.
66. Eglitis MA, Mezey E. Hematopoietic cells differentiate into both microglia and macroglia in the brains of adult mice. Proc Natl Acad Sci USA 1997;94:4080–4085.
67. Mezey E, Chandross KJ, Harta G, Maki RA, McKercher SR. Turning blood into brain: cells bearing neuronal antigens generated in vivo from bone marrow. Science 2000;290:1779–1782.

68. Brazelton TR, Rossi FM, Keshet GI, Blau HM. From marrow to brain: expression of neuronal pheno-types in adult mice. Science 2000;290:1775–1779.

69. Gussoni E, Soneoka Y, Strickland CD, et al. Dystrophin expression in the mdx mouse restored by stem cell transplantation. Nature 1999;401:390–394.

70. Jackson KA, Mi T, Goodell MA. Hematopoietic potential of stem cells isolated from murine skeletal muscle. Proc Natl Acad Sci USA 1999;96:14,482–14,486.

71. McKinney-Freeman SL, Jackson KA, Camargo FD, Ferrari G, Mavilio F, Goodell MA. Muscle-derived hematopoietic stem cells are hematopoietic in origin. Proc Natl Acad Sci USA 2002;99:1341–1346.

72. Bjornson CR, Rietze RL, Reynolds BA, Magli MC, Vescovi AL. Turning brain into blood: a hemato-poietic fate adopted by adult neural stem cells in vivo. Science 1999;283:534–537.

73. Blau HM, Brazelton TR, Weimann JM. The evolving concept of a stem cell: entity or function? Cell 2001;105:829–841.

74. Anversa P, Nadal-Ginard B. Myocyte renewal and ventricular remodelling. Nature 2002;415:240–243.

75. Kajstura J, Leri A, Finato N, Di Loreto C, Beltrami CA, Anversa P. Myocyte proliferation in end-stage cardiac failure in humans. Proc Natl Acad Sci USA 1998;95:8801–8805.

76. Beltrami AP, Urbanek K, Kajstura J, et al. Evidence that human cardiac myocytes divide after myo-cardial infarction. N Engl J Med 2001;344:1750–1757.

77. Orlic D, Kajstura J, Chimenti S, Bodine DM, Leri A, Anversa P. Transplanted adult bone marrow cells repair myocardial infarcts in mice. Ann NY Acad Sci 2001;938:221–229.

78. Muller P, Pfeiffer P, Koglin J, et al. Cardiomyocytes of noncardiac origin in myocardial biopsies of human transplanted hearts. Circulation 2002;106:31–35.

79. Laflamme MA, Myerson D, Saffitz JE, Murry CE. Evidence for cardiomyocyte repopulation by extracardiac progenitors in transplanted human hearts. Circ Res 2002;90:634–640.

80. Quaini F, Urbanek K, Beltrami AP, et al. Chimerism of the transplanted heart. N Engl J Med 2002;346:5–15.

81. Deb A, Wang S, Skelding KA, Miller D, Simper D, Caplice NM. Bone marrow-derived cardiomyocytes are present in adult human heart: a study of gender-mismatched bone marrow transplantation patients. Circulation 2003;107:1247–1249.

82. Sata M, Saiura A, Kunisato A, et al. Hematopoietic stem cells differentiate into vascular cells that participate in the pathogenesis of atherosclerosis. Nat Med 2002;8:403–409.

83. Vassilopoulos G, Wang PR, Russell DW. Transplanted bone marrow regenerates liver by cell fusion. Nature 2003;422:901–904.

84. Wang X, Willenbring H, Akkari Y, et al. Cell fusion is the principal source of bone-marrow-derived hepatocytes. Nature 2003;422:897–901.

85. Blau HM. A twist of fate. Nature 2002;419:437.

86. Heissig B, Hattori K, Dias S, et al. Recruitment of stem and progenitor cells from the bone marrow niche requires MMP-9 mediated release of kit-ligand. Cell 2002;109:625–637.

87. Fleming WH, Alpern EJ, Uchida N, Ikuta K, Weissman IL. Steel factor influences the distribution and activity of murine hematopoietic stem cells in vivo. Proc Natl Acad Sci USA 1993;90:3760–3764.

88. Okumura N, Tsuji K, Ebihara Y, et al. Chemotactic and chemokinetic activities of stem cell factor on murine hematopoietic progenitor cells. Blood 1996;87:4100–4108.

89. Broudy VC, Lin NL, Priestley GV, Nocka K, Wolf NS. Interaction of stem cell factor and its receptor c-kit mediates lodgment and acute expansion of hematopoietic cells in the murine spleen. Blood 1996;88:75–81.

90. Papayannopoulou T, Craddock C, Nakamoto B, Priestley GV, Wolf NS. The VLA4/VCAM-1 adhe-sion pathway defines contrasting mechanisms of lodgement of transplanted murine hemopoietic pro-genitors between bone marrow and spleen. Proc Natl Acad Sci USA 1995;92:9647–9651.

91. Miyake K, Weissman IL, Greenberger JS, Kincade PW. Evidence for a role of the integrin VLA-4 in lympho-hemopoiesis. J Exp Med 1991;173:599–607.

92. Williams DA, Rios M, Stephens C, Patel VP. Fibronectin and VLA-4 in haematopoietic stem cell-microenvironment interactions. Nature 1991;352:438–441.

93. Hirsch E, Iglesias A, Potocnik AJ, Hartmann U, Fassler R. Impaired migration but not differentiation of haematopoietic stem cells in the absence of beta1 integrins. Nature 1996;380:171–175.

94. Frangogiannis NG, Perrard JL, Mendoza LH, Burns AR, Lindsey ML, Ballantyne CM et al. Stem cell factor induction is associated with mast cell accumulation after canine myocardial ischemia and reperfusion. Circulation 1998;98:687–698.

95. Korbling M, Estrov Z. Adult stem cells for tissue repair—a new therapeutic concept? N Engl J Med 2003;349:570–582.
96. Hierlihy AM, Seale P, Lobe CG, Rudnicki MA, Megeney LA. The post-natal heart contains a myocardial stem cell population. FEBS Lett 2002;530:239–243.
97 Oh H, Bradfute SB, Gallardo TD, Nakamura T, Gaussin V, Mishina Y et al. Cardiac progenitor cells from adult myocardium: homing, differentiation, and fusion after infarction. Proc Natl Acad Sci USA 2003;100:12,313–12,318.
98. Beltrami AP, Barlucchi L, Torella D, et al. Adult cardiac stem cells are multipotent and support myocardial regeneration. Cell 2003;114:763–776.
99. Urbanek K, Quaini F, Tasca G, et al. Intense myocyte formation from cardiac stem cells in human cardiac hypertrophy. Proc Natl Acad Sci USA 2003;100:10,440–10,445.
100. Mangi AA, Noiseux N, Kong D, et al. Mesenchymal stem cells modified with Akt prevent remodeling and restore performance of infarcted hearts. Nat Med 2003;9:1195–1201.
101. Askari AT, Unzek S, Popovic ZB, et al. Effect of stromal-cell-derived factor 1 on stem-cell homing and tissue regeneration in ischaemic cardiomyopathy. Lancet 2003;362:697–703.
102. Suzuki K, Murtuza B, Smolenski RT, et al. Cell transplantation for the treatment of acute myocardial infarction using vascular endothelial growth factor-expressing skeletal myoblasts. Circulation 2001;104(12 Suppl 1):I207–I212.
103. Tse HF, Kwong YL, Chan JK, Lo G, Ho CL, Lau CP. Angiogenesis in ischaemic myocardium by intramyocardial autologous bone marrow mononuclear cell implantation. Lancet 2003;361:47–49.
104. Perin EC, Dohmann HF, Borojevic R, et al. Transendocardial, autologous bone marrow cell transplantation for severe, chronic ischemic heart failure. Circulation 2003;107:2294–2302.
105. Tomita S, Li RK, Weisel RD, et al. Autologous transplantation of bone marrow cells improves damaged heart function. Circulation 1999;100(19 Suppl):II247–II256.
106. Tomita S, Mickle DA, Weisel RD, et al. Improved heart function with myogenesis and angiogenesis after autologous porcine bone marrow stromal cell transplantation. J Thorac Cardiovasc Surg 2002;123:1132–1140.
107. Sakakibara Y, Nishimura K, Tambara K, et al. Prevascularization with gelatin microspheres containing basic fibroblast growth factor enhances the benefits of cardiomyocyte transplantation. J Thorac Cardiovasc Surg 2002;124:50–56.
108. Miyagawa S, Sawa Y, Taketani S, et al. Myocardial regeneration therapy for heart failure: hepatocyte growth factor enhances the effect of cellular cardiomyoplasty. Circulation 2002;105:2556–2561.
109. Li TS, Hamano K, Kajiwara K, Nishida M, Zempo N, Esato K. Prolonged survival of xenograft fetal cardiomyocytes by adenovirus-mediated CTLA4-Ig expression. Transplantation 2001;72:1983–1985.
110. Zhang M, Methot D, Poppa V, Fujio Y, Walsh K, Murry CE. Cardiomyocyte grafting for cardiac repair: graft cell death and anti-death strategies. J Mol Cell Cardiol 2001;33:907–921.
111. Liu TB, Fedak PW, Weisel RD, et al. Enhanced IGF-1 expansion improves smooth muscle cell engraftment after cell transplantation. Am J Physiol Heart Circ Physiol Aug 26, 2004 [Epub ahead of print].

18 Embryonic Stem Cells and the Cardiovascular System

Neta Lavon and Nissim Benvenisty, MD, PhD

CONTENTS

SUMMARY

Human embryonic stem (ES) cells are pluripotent cells isolated from the inner cell mass of blastocyst-stage embryos. These cells are capable of self-renewal and can differentiate into many cell types. In vivo, human ES cells injected into immune-deficient mice yield teratomas with ectodermal, mesodermal, and endodermal cell derivatives. In vitro, spontaneous aggregation of human ES cells results in the formation of embryoid bodies (EBs) comprised of differentiated cells from the three embryonic germ layers. The addition of growth factors can induce the differentiation of human ES cells into specific populations of cells, among them the cells of the cardiovascular system, cardiomyocytes, and endothelial cells. Functional cardiomyocytes caused the EBs to exhibit rhythmic contractions. The cells of the cardiovascular system were distinguished by molecular markers and by their structural and functional characteristics. Human ES cells may serve as a source of cells for cellular transplantation in different pathologies, among them cardiovascular diseases, and as a model to study the embryonic development of human beings.

Key Words: Embryonic stem cells; differentiation; cardiomyocytes; endothelial; cardiovascular system.

From: *Contemporary Cardiology: Cardiovascular Genomics*
Edited by: M. K. Raizada, et al. © Humana Press Inc., Totowa, NJ

INTRODUCTION

Embryonic stem (ES) cells are line of cells derived from the inner cell mass (ICM) of blastocysts. ES cells were first isolated from mouse embryos *(1,2)*. The pluripotency of these cells is demonstrated by the use of three models: (1) embryoid body (EB)—a structure that is formed by the spontaneous aggregation of ES cells in suspension. The cells that comprise this EB propagate and differentiate, resulting in a cavitated structure that causes the EB to become cystic. It was shown that this cystic EB consists of cells from the three embryonic germ layers *(3)*. (2) Upon injection of the ES cells into immune-deficient mice, the cells form teratomas. These teratomas are differentiated tumors comprising many cell types *(3)*. (3) Chimeric mouse embryos may be achieved by injecting ES cells into blastocysts. The injected ES cells contribute to all embryonic tissues including the germ cells *(4)*. Various methods of genetically manipulating mouse ES cells were performed for the purpose of mutating an endogenous gene or introducing a transgene. This mouse ES cell system enabled the studying of interesting genes in vitro, but more importantly the creation of chimeras is an extremely useful tool for the analyzing of genes during the embryo development in vivo.

In this chapter, we will discuss the isolation of human ES cells, their spontaneous and directed differentiation, and the genetic manipulations induced in these cells. We will devote special attention to the differentiation of human ES cells into cells of the cardio-vascular system.

DERIVATION AND CHARACTERIZATION OF HUMAN EMBRYONIC STEM CELLS

Human ES cells were derived from spare cleavage-stage embryos of in vitro fertilized eggs, grown to the blastocyst stage *(5,6)*. Cells of the inner cells mass from these blastocysts were plated onto mitotically inactivated murine embryonic fibroblast feeder cells, and formed compact colonies of human ES cells. It was shown that these cells have a normal karyotype even when they are grown for an extended period of time in culture *(5,6)*. Human ES cells were found to have high activity levels of telomerase *(5)*, a protein responsible for maintaining the chromosome length and that is tightly correlated with immortality in human cell lines *(7)*. Undifferentiated human ES cells are characterized by specific cell surface markers and enzymatic activities. For example, the stage-specific embryonic antigens 3 and 4 and the markers TRA-1-60 and TRA-1-81 are expressed in human ES cells and are downregulated during their differentiation *(5)*. Pluripotency is defined as the ability of the cells to differentiate into cells comprising the three embryonic germ layers, namely, ectoderm, mesoderm, and endoderm. The pluripotency of human ES cells was proven both in vivo and in vitro. In vivo, injection of the human ES cells into immune-deficient mice generated teratomas harboring derivatives of all three embryonic germ layers *(5)*. In vitro aggregation of human ES cells brought about the formation of EBs *(8)*. The cells within the EBs acquired molecular markers specific for the three embryonic germ layers. The differentiating cells also acquired characteristic morphologies and further developed new functions. The functionality of cells, such as cardio-myocytes, is evident from the appearance of pulsing muscle cells *(8)*. Human ES cells were clonally derived either by dilution or by genetic selection in order to show the pluripotency of the single cells *(9,10)*. The different clonal cells also exhibited the creation of EBs that contained cells of the three embryonic germ layers.

DIFFERENTIATION OF HUMAN EMBRYONIC STEM CELLS

Growing the human ES cells in suspension caused the cells to aggregate and form EBs. This process was similar to that found in mouse ES cells *(8)*. Initially, the clusters of ES cells are composed of densely packed cells, creating simple EBs. After several days, the center of the bodies become cavitated and they begin to accumulate fluid and develop into cystic EBs. The cells within the EBs were shown to express α-fetoprotein, ζ-globin, or neurofilament 68 kd—molecular markers specific for the three embryonic germ layers *(8)*. In addition, rhythmic pulsation was observed, and cardiac muscle cells expressing α-cardiac actin were also demonstrated in these human EBs. Cells with various morphologies were revealed as a result of the dissociation of EBs and the plating of the differentiated cells as a monolayer *(11)*. The differentiation through EBs is spontaneous and seems stochastic. The effects of eight growth factors on human ES cells were assessed in order to direct the differentiation of the cells *(11)*. Analysis of cell morphology and the expression pattern of a large number of cell-specific markers confirmed the ability to induce specific differentiation by various growth factors. Thus, activin-A and transforming growth factor (TGF)-β mainly induce mesodermal cells; retinoic acid (RA), epidermal growth factor (EGF), bone morphogenetic protein 4, and basic fibroblast growth factor activate ectodermal and mesodermal markers; and nerve growth factor and hepatocyte growth factor allow differentiation into the three embryonic germ layers, including endoderm. Initial protocols were also established in order to induce the directed differentiation of human ES cells. For example, epidermal skin cells were enriched in the presence of EGF, myocardial cells were achieved by addition of TGF-β, and cartilage differentiation was evident when the cells were treated with bone morphogenetic protein 4 *(11)*. Further analysis showed that more molecular markers appeared upon differentiation of human ES cells, verifying the existence of many cell types such as hematopoietic cells *(12)* and cells with characteristics of insulin-secreting β-cells *(13)*. The differentiation of neuronal progenitor cells may be achieved even without the creation of EBs, because early stages of neuroectodermal differentiation were found in very dense cultures of human ES cells *(6)*. In serum-free media, the cells that were isolated from the culture created spherical structures that expressed early neuronal markers, and when plated and grown as a monolayer, these cells expressed more mature neuronal markers *(6)*. Neuronal differentiation may be induced by growth factors; thus, Schuldiner et al. *(11)* showed the ability of RA or nerve growth factor to induce neuronal differentiation under specific conditions. Moreover, RA supported the production of mature neurons that express dopamine or serotonin receptors, and the formation of complex plexuses of neuronal cells.

GENETIC MANIPULATION OF HUMAN EMBRYONIC STEM CELLS

Genetic manipulations of ES cells enable the introduction of foreign genes, such as marker or master genes, and the mutagenesis of endogenous genes. Marker genes are very useful for studying the expression profile of a gene during differentiation and for tracing and selecting a particular subset of the cells *(14,15)*. The overexpression of master genes in mice, such as certain transcription factors, can lead to differentiation into specific cell lineages *(16,17)*. The ability to mutate specific endogenous genes, either by homologous recombination or by gene trapping, changed the face of mammalian genetics *(18)*. Chimerism using ES cells allows germ line transmission of a transgene, thus enabling in vivo testing of the effect of the transgene or the mutation. The mutant knockout mice shed new light on gene function and enable the creation of many mouse models of human genetic diseases (19).

Eiges et al. (10) established a DNA transfection protocol for human ES cells that is different from the one used for murine ES cells. Human ES cells were also transduced by a lentiviral vector, resulting in the infection of almost 100% of the cells (20). The transfection of human ES cells with a reporter gene was the first attempt at utilizing genetic manipulation of cells in order to address a biological issue. Human ES cells were transfected with green fluorescent protein (GFP) while being controlled by Rex1, an ES cell-enriched gene. The transfected cells showed high levels of GFP expression, which were limited to the undifferentiated cells, and a fluorescence-activated cell sorter assisted in separating the differentiated cells from the fluorescent cells (10). This way, it was possible to sort out undifferentiated, potentially tumorigenic cells in order to prevent the risk of transformation of the cells during transplantation. In addition, the use of genetic manipulation in human ES cells should allow us to follow and select a desired subset of differentiated cells from a heterogeneous culture, thus purifying only a specific type of cells prior to transplantation. Protocols for homologous recombination in human ES cells, which were developed only lately, enable us to study gene function in humans more thoroughly (21). Figure 1 shows various ways of differentiating human ES cells and methods for selecting specific subsets of cells.

CARDIOMYOCYTES AND ENDOTHELIAL CELLS DERIVED FROM HUMAN ES CELLS

One of the most impressive evidences of differentiation of human ES cells is the creation of pulsing embryoid bodies that contain myocardial cells (8). The creation of spontaneously beating cardiomyocytes in mice was concomitant with rhythmic action potentials very similar to those described for embryonic cardiomyocytes and sinus-node cells (22). During formation of EBs, cardiomyocytes derived from mouse ES cells exhibit typical signal transduction pathways through adrenoceptors and cholinoceptors. Alterations in contractile sensitivity to Ca^{2+} during ES differentiation in culture provided functional evidence that cardiomyocytes derived from ES cells recapitulate embryonic cardiogenesis (23). Several distinct cell populations could be distinguished during cardiomyocyte differentiation through characteristic sets of ionic channels and typical action potentials, presumably representing cardiac tissues with properties of sinus node, atrium, or ventricle (24). Overall, the developmental program of mouse ES cells towards cardiomyocytes resembles that observed during cardiogenesis in vivo (25). Pure myocyte culture from differentiated mouse ES cells was established using the antibiotic selection of ES cells carrying sequences encoding for antibiotic resistance under the control of α-cardiac myosin heavy chain promoter. The selected cells were able to form stable intracardiac grafts in the hearts of adult dystrophic mice (14). The previously mentioned selection method was recently combined with a large-scale process, using stirred suspension cultures and deriving higher amounts of purified cardiomyocytes from mouse ES cells (26). Nkx2.5 is a transcription factor that plays a fundamental role in the transcriptional regulation of cardiac-specific genes. Lately, a Nkx2.5/GFP+ mouse ES cell line was established by knocking in an endothelial GFP reporter gene into the Nkx2.5 locus. These cells were proven to be precursor cells of sinoatrial node, atrial or ventricular cell types (27).

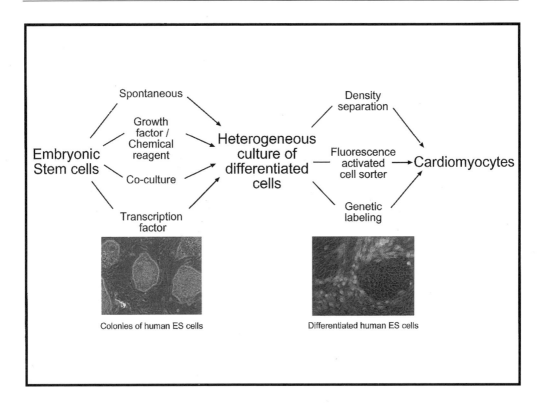

Fig. 1. Differentiation and selection of embryonic stem (ES) cells. Schematic representation of various ways to differentiate ES cells and methods for purifying specific subset of cells. Also shown are colonies of human ES cells on a feeder layer of mouse embryonic fibroblasts and heterogeneous population of nondifferentiated and differentiated green fluorescent protein (GFP)-positive human ES cells.

Cardiomyocyte loss in the adult mammalian heart may be irreversible, and frequently leads to diminished cardiac function. The ability to increase the number of functional cardiomyocytes in a diseased heart would have obvious therapeutic potential. Recent studies have suggested that cellular transplantation can be used to increase the number of myocytes in cardiac pathologies. Even though several different types of myocyte preparations were successfully engrafted in animals, it is difficult to obtain a sufficient number of donor cells in humans *(28)*. ES cells may serve as an alternative renewable source of donor myocytes. Rhythmic pulsation of myocytes was observed in cystic human EBs, and *in situ* hybridization with a marker of embryonic myocardial cells revealed that the central cavity of the pulsing EB was in fact surrounded by cardiomyocytes *(8)*. In addition, cells from the spontaneously contracting areas were positive to many cardiac-specific genes and transcription factors that are involved in cardiogenesis *(29,30)*. Morphologically, the cells presented varying degrees of myofibrillar organization, which were mainly consistent with early stage cardiomyocytes. Electrophysiological tests presented a relatively long action potential duration, characteristic of cardiomyocytes that are significantly different from noncardiac muscle, and the cells also presented normal chronotropic effects to drugs *(30)*. Furthermore, it may be possible to achieve induction of differentiation into cardiomyocytes by treating the ES cells with

Table 1
The Properties of Cardiomyocytes Derived From Human Embryonic Stem Cells

Methodology		Evidence for active cardiomyocytes
Molecular markers	RNA	α-cardiac actin (8,11); atrial myosin light chain, ventricular myosin light chain, α-myosin heavy chain, atrial natriuretic peptide, cardiac troponin T and I, GATA-4, Nkx2.5 (30); α-myosin heavy chain, atrial natriuretic factor, Nkx2.5 (32)
	Protein	α, β-myosin heavy chain, cardiac troponin I, desmin, atrial natriuretic peptide, α-actinin (30); α-actinin (29) α, β-myosin heavy chain, cardiac troponin I and T, sMHC, desmin, tropomyosin, α-actinin, GATA4, MEF2, N-cadherin, creatine kinase-MB, myoglobin, α1 and β1 adrenoreceptors (32)
Morphology and physiology	Cell morphology	Mononuclear and round or rod-shape (30)
	Electron microscopy	Immature phenotype of disorganized myofibrillar stacks in early stage EBs and more organized sarcomeric structure in older EBs, also Z bands and intercalated disks (30), poor sarcomeric banding pattern (29)
	Rhythmic contractions	30 pulses/min (8); 8.1% of 22-d-old EBs contained contracting areas, usually in the outgrowth of the EB with 94 ± 33 pulses/min (30); 60 pulses/min (29); up to 70% of the EBs contained contracting areas, rate of 40 ± 10 pulses/min (32)
	Electrophysiology	Relatively long action potential duration characteristic of cardiomyocytes (30)
	Pharmacological studies	Positive and negative chronotropic responses were observed (30), ion blocker decreased the contraction rate, adrenoreceptors agonists enhanced contraction rate (32)
Induction of differentiation	Growth factors	Induction of differentiation by TGF-β (11) 5-aza-dC, a demethylation reagent, enhanced cardiomyocytes differentiation (32)
	Coculture	Induction of differentiation by mouse visceral endoderm-like cell line End-2 (29,31)
Enrichment of cardio- myocytes	Percoll gradients	Fourfold enrichment from 17 to 70% cardiomyocytes using percoll gradient separation (32)

MEF, murine embryonic fibroblast; TGF, transforming growth factor; EB, ebryoid body.

TGF-β (11), or co-culturing the cells with END-2 cells (visceral endoderm-like cells similar to those normally adjacent to the region of heart development) (29,31). Treatment of the cells with 5-aza-2'-deoxycytidine, a demethylation reagent, could also enhance cardiomyocyte differentiation, which was shown to be enriched by Percoll density centrifugation to give a population containing 70% cardiomyocytes (32). The functional hetrogenenecity of cardiomyocytes derived from human ES cells was demonstrated by typical action potential of nodal-like, embryonic atrial-like, and ventricular-like cardiomyocytes in different outgrowths of beating EBs *(33)*. Table 1 presents the phenotypic and functional properties of cardiomyocytes derived from human ES cells.

Increasing the number of cardiomyocytes requires induction of new vascular structures. Tissue engineering approaches have already reported the production of vascular graft material from smooth muscle and endothelial cells *(34)*. Endothelial progenitors were also shown to have a therapeutic potential for myocardial ischemia *(35)*. Mouse ES cells may differentiate into endothelial *(36,37)* and smooth muscle cells *(38,39)*, and serve as a potential source of cells to form vascular structures. Yamashita et al. *(40)* established a system for induction and purification of vascular progenitors (flk1+ cells) from mouse ES cells. Flk1, one of the receptors for vascular endothelial growth factor, is a marker for lateral plate mesoderm *(41)*, and the earliest differentiation marker for endothelial and blood cells *(42,43)*. Indeed, the flk1+ cells gave rise to two major vascular cell types (endothelial cells and smooth muscle cells) in vitro *(36,44)* and in vivo *(40)*.

Endothelial cells were also derived from human ES cells. These cells were isolated from 13- to 15-d-old EBs by using platelet endothelial cell-adhesion molecule-1 (PECAM1) antibodies, and further characterized in vitro and in vivo *(45)*. PECAM1 is a marker for mouse embryonic endothelial cells *(46)* and is expressed in human EBs in correlation with vascular endothelial-cadherin *(45,47)*, suggesting that it could serve as a marker for human embryonic endothelial cells as well. The endothelial cells were found in groups within these EBs, organized in specific channel-like structures, and thus may show spontaneous differentiation to endothelial cells and blood vessel-like structures. In vivo, when PECAM1[+] cells were transplanted into immune-deficient mice, the cells appeared to form microvessels. Some of the human vessels had mouse blood cells in their lumen, suggesting that they had become functional *(45)*.

The accumulating data on the differentiation of human ES cells into the different populations of cells within the heart suggests that these cells may harbor a huge therapeutic potential. Thus, in the future, differentiated human ES cells may be used as an ultimate source of cells for transplantation cardiovascular medicine.

ACKNOWLEDGMENTS

We thank members of our laboratory for their critical reviewing of the manuscript. This research was partially supported by funds from the Herbert Cohn Chair (Hebrew University), by a grant from the Juvenile Diabetes Fund (USA), by a grant from the Israel Science Foundation (grant no. 672/02-1), and by funds from the United States–Israel Binational Science Foundation (grant no. 2001021).

REFERENCES

1. Evans MJ, Kaufman MH. Establishment in culture of pluripotential cells from mouse embryos. Nature 1981; 292:154–156.
2. Martin GR. Isolation of a pluripotent cell line from early mouse embryos cultured in medium conditioned by teratocarcinoma stem cells. Proc Natl Acad Sci USA 1981;78:7634–7638.
3. Wobus AM, Holzhausen H, Jakel P, Schoneich J. Characterization of a pluripotent stem cell line derived from a mouse embryo. Exp Cell Res 1984;152:212–219.
4. Bradley A, Evans M, Kaufman MH, Robertson E. Formation of germ-line chimaeras from embryo-derived teratocarcinoma cell lines. Nature 1984;309:255–256.

5. Thomson JA, Itskovitz-Eldor J, Shapiro SS, et al. Embryonic stem cell lines derived from human blastocysts. Science 1998;282:1145–1147.
6. Reubinoff BE, Pera MF, Fong CY, Trounson A, Bongso A. Embryonic stem cell lines from human blastocysts: somatic differentiation in vitro. Nat Biotechnol 2000;18:399–404.
7. Kim NW, Piatyszek MA, Prowse KR, et al. Specific association of human telomerase activity with immortal cells and cancer. Science 1994;266:2011–2015.
8. Itskovitz-Eldor J, Schuldiner M, Karsenti D, et al. Differentiation of human embryonic stem cells into embryoid bodies comprising the three embryonic germ layers. Mol Med 2000;6:88–95.
9. Amit M, Carpenter MK, Inokuma MS, et al. Clonally derived human embryonic stem cell lines maintain pluripotency and proliferative potential for prolonged periods of culture. Dev Biol 2000;227:271–278.
10. Eiges R, Schuldiner M, Drukker M, Yanuka O, Itskovitz-Eldor J, Benvenisty N. Establishment of human embryonic stem cell-transfected clones carrying a marker for undifferentiated cells. Curr Biol 2001;11:514–518.
11. Schuldiner M, Yanuka O, Itskovitz-Eldor J, Melton DA, Benvenisty N. Effects of eight growth factors on the differentiation of cells derived from human embryonic stem cells. Proc Natl Acad Sci USA 2000;97:11,307–11,312.
12. Kaufman DS, Hanson ET, Lewis RL, Auerbach R, Thomson JA. Hematopoietic colony-forming cells derived from human embryonic stem cells. Proc Natl Acad Sci USA 2001;98:10,716–10,721.
13. Assady S, Maor G, Amit M, Itskovitz-Eldor J, Skorecki KL, Tzukerman M. Insulin production by human embryonic stem cells. Diabetes 2001;50:1691–1697.
14. Klug MG, Soonpaa MH, Koh GY, Field LJ. Genetically selected cardiomyocytes from differentiating embronic stem cells form stable intracardiac grafts. J Clin Invest 1996;98:216–224.
15. Gossler A, Joyner AL, Rossant J, Skarnes WC. Mouse embryonic stem cells and reporter constructs to detect developmentally regulated genes. Science 1989;244:463–465.
16. Grepin C, Nemer G, Nemer M. Enhanced cardiogenesis in embryonic stem cells overexpressing the GATA-4 transcription factor. Development 1997;124:2387–2395.
17. Levinson-Dushnik M, Benvenisty N. Involvement of hepatocyte nuclear factor 3 in endoderm differentiation of embryonic stem cells. Mol Cell Biol 1997;17:3817–3822.
18. Capecchi MR. The new mouse genetics: altering the genome by gene targeting. Trends Genet 1989;5:70–76.
19. Smithies O. Animal models of human genetic diseases. Trends Genet 1993; 9:112-6.
20. Pfeifer A, Ikawa M, Dayn Y, Verma IM. Transgenesis by lentiviral vectors: lack of gene silencing in mammalian embryonic stem cells and preimplantation embryos. Proc Natl Acad Sci USA 2002;99:2140–2145.
21. Zwaka TP, Thomson JA. Homologous recombination in human embryonic stem cells. Nat Biotechnol 2003;21:319–321.
22. Wobus AM, Wallukat G, Hescheler J. Pluripotent mouse embryonic stem cells are able to differentiate into cardiomyocytes expressing chronotropic responses to adrenergic and cholinergic agents and Ca2+ channel blockers. Differentiation 1991;48:173–182.
23. Metzger JM, Lin WI, Samuelson LC. Transition in cardiac contractile sensitivity to calcium during the in vitro differentiation of mouse embryonic stem cells. J Cell Biol 1994;126:701–711.
24. Maltsev VA, Wobus AM, Rohwedel J, Bader M, Hescheler J. Cardiomyocytes differentiated in vitro from embryonic stem cells developmentally express cardiac-specific genes and ionic currents. Circ Res 1994;75:233–244.
25. Klug MG, Soonpaa MH, Field LJ. DNA synthesis and multinucleation in embryonic stem cell-derived cardiomyocytes. Am J Physiol 1995;269:H1913–H1921.
26. Zandstra PW, Bauwens C, Yin T, et al. Scalable production of embryonic stem cell-derived cardiomyocytes. Tissue Eng 2003;9:767–778.
27. Hidaka K, Lee JK, Kim HS, et al. Chamber-specific differentiation of Nkx2.5-positive cardiac precursor cells from murine embryonic stem cells. FASEB J 2003; 17:740–742.
28. Soonpaa MH, Daud AI, Koh GY, et al. Potential approaches for myocardial regeneration. Ann NY Acad Sci 1995;752:446–454.
29. Mummery C, Ward D, van den Brink CE, et al. Cardiomyocyte differentiation of mouse and human embryonic stem cells. J Anat 2002;200:233–242.
30. Kehat I, Kenyagin-Karsenti D, Snir M, et al. Human embryonic stem cells can differentiate into myocytes with structural and functional properties of cardiomyocytes. J Clin Invest 2001;108:407–414.
31. Mummery C, Ward-van Oostwaard D, Doevendans P, et al. Differentiation of human embryonic stem cells to cardiomyocytes: role of coculture with visceral endoderm-like cells. Circulation 2003;107:2733–2740.

32. Xu C, Police S, Rao N, Carpenter MK. Characterization and enrichment of cardiomyocytes derived from human embryonic stem cells. Circ Res 2002;91:501–508.
33. He JQ, Ma Y, Lee Y, Thomson JA, Kamp TJ. Human embryonic stem cells develop into multiple types of cardiac myocytes: action potential characterization. Circ Res 2003;93:32–39.
34. Niklason LE, Gao J, Abbott WM, et al. Functional arteries grown in vitro. Science 1999;284:489–493.
35. Kawamoto A, Gwon HC, Iwaguro H, et al. Therapeutic potential of ex vivo expanded endothelial progenitor cells for myocardial ischemia. Circulation 2001;103:634–67.
36. Hirashima M, Kataoka H, Nishikawa S, Matsuyoshi N. Maturation of embryonic stem cells into endothelial cells in an in vitro model of vasculogenesis. Blood 1999;93:1253–1263.
37. Vittet D, Prandini MH, Berthier R, et al. Embryonic stem cells differentiate in vitro to endothelial cells through successive maturation steps. Blood 1996;88:3424–3431.
38. Wobus AM, Guan K, Yang HT, Boheler KR. Embryonic stem cells as a model to study cardiac, skeletal muscle, and vascular smooth muscle cell differentiation. Methods Mol Biol 2002;185:127–156.
39. Drab M, Haller H, Bychkov R, et al. From totipotent embryonic stem cells to spontaneously contracting smooth muscle cells: a retinoic acid and db-cAMP in vitro differentiation model. FASEB J 1997;11:905–915.
40. Yamashita J, Itoh H, Hirashima M, et al. Flk1-positive cells derived from embryonic stem cells serve as vascular progenitors. Nature 2000;408:92–96.
41. Yamaguchi TP, Dumont DJ, Conlon RA, Breitman ML, Rossant J. flk-1, an flt-related receptor tyrosine kinase is an early marker for endothelial cell precursors. Development 1993;118:489–498.
42. Eichmann A, Corbel C, Nataf V, Vaigot P, Breant C, Le Douarin NM. Ligand-dependent development of the endothelial and hemopoietic lineages from embryonic mesodermal cells expressing vascular endothelial growth factor receptor 2. Proc Natl Acad Sci USA 1997;94:5141–5146.
43. Shalaby F, Rossant J, Yamaguchi TP, et al. Failure of blood-island formation and vasculogenesis in Flk-1-deficient mice. Nature 1995;376:62–66.
44. Nishikawa SI, Nishikawa S, Hirashima M, Matsuyoshi N, Kodama H. Progressive lineage analysis by cell sorting and culture identifies FLK1+VE-cadherin+ cells at a diverging point of endothelial and hemopoietic lineages. Development 1998;125:1747–1757.
45. Levenberg S, Golub JS, Amit M, Itskovitz-Eldor J, Langer R. Endothelial cells derived from human embryonic stem cells. Proc Natl Acad Sci USA 2002;99:4391–4396.
46. Vecchi A, Garlanda C, Lampugnani MG, et al. Monoclonal antibodies specific for endothelial cells of mouse blood vessels. Their application in the identification of adult and embryonic endothelium. Eur J Cell Biol 1994;63:247–254.
47. Lampugnani MG, Resnati M, Raiteri M, et al. A novel endothelial-specific membrane protein is a marker of cell-cell contacts. J Cell Biol 1992;118:1511–1522.

Index